Illustrated Nurses Dictionary

Illustrated Nurses Dictionary

G.N. Prabhakara

Principal
Professor of PSM
SDM College of Medical Sciences and Hospital
Manjushree Nagar, Sattur
Dharwad-580 009

PEEPEE

PUBLISHERS AND DISTRIBUTORS (P) Ltd.

Illustrated Nurses Dictionary

Published by:
Pawaninder P. Vij
Peepee Publishers and Distributors (P) Ltd.
Head Office: 160, Shakti Vihar, Pitam Pura, Delhi-110 034
***Corporate Office:* 7/31, Ansari Road, Darya Ganj**
Post Box-7243, New Delhi - 110002 (India)
Ph: 9811156083, 55195868
e-mail: peepee160@yahoo.co.in
peepee160@rediffmail.com
peepee160@gmail.com
www.peepeepub.com

Reprint:* *2008

ISBN 81-88867-60-8

Printed at:
Lordson, C-5/19, Rana Pratap Bagh, Delhi -110 007.

PREFACE

Medical Dictionary has always been first hand reference to Nurses and now an **"Illustrated Nurses Dictionary"** with routine Nursing Procedures shall form Prime reference to all Nursing Staff and Students in the country. Illustrations add to their good understanding and quick thinking which can lead good decision.

Initiation, motivation, guidance, proof reading and specific appropriations are from my wife Mrs. Malathi Prabhakara, Ex-Scientist CFTRI, CSIR, Mysore and my son Dr. Bharat M.P. PG-cum-Tutor in Radiodiagnosis and Imaging at SDM College of Medical Sciences and Hospital, Dharwad.

Nursing staff and students in my walks of life to whom I taught are responsible to bring out my experience.

My high appreciation and heartfelt thanks to Mr. Pawaninder P. Vij, M/s Peepee Publishers and Distributors (P) Ltd. New Delhi in giving a good commendable shape to my modest work.

G.N. Prabhakara

CONTENTS

A

A-scan It is the display of *Ultrasonograph*, which helps to measure the size and thickness of tissues and organs.

AV block It is the block in conduction from auricle to ventricle i.e., impulses do not reach ventricle from auricle. They are classified into *first degree, second degree and third degree* heart blocks.

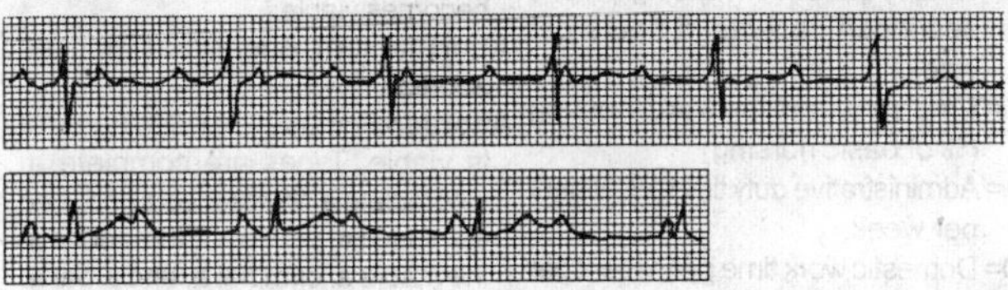

A V block

AA Alcoholics Anonymous, a group of alcoholics that helps other alcoholics.

AAMIH American Association for Maternal and Infant Health.

AAOHN American Association of Occupational Health Nurses.

Aasmus Greek word denoting Asthma.

Abacterial Clinical condition not caused by bacteria.

Abatement Severity of symptom or pain decreased.

Abbess Nursing among Christian duties by an elderly Christian woman in monasteries.

Abbott life care controller Used to control the delivery rate by monitoring and adjusting the drop rate in infusion set. It automatically stops the delivery of solution and sounds an alarm to alert the nurse.

Abbott life care pump These infusion pumps are indicated for clients who need accurate and carefully monitored flow rates, as well as those for whom positive pressure is required for the delivery of highly viscous solutions.

Abdomen It is the cavity between diaphragm and the pelvis. It is colloquially called *belly*.

Abducent To lead away from midline of our body. The muscle that rotates the eyeball outward is supplied by the cranial nerve which is called abducent nerve.

Abduction pillow It is an A-shaped pillow, of foam construction, foam straps that wrap around the clients upper thigh and ankle, used after hip repair or replacement.

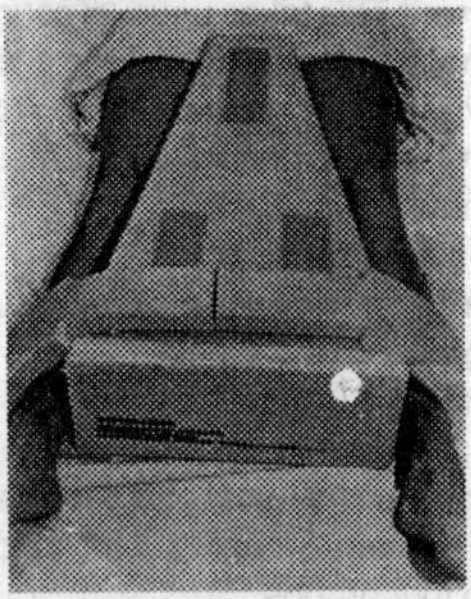

Abduction pillow

Abductor It is a muscle that draws a limb away from the body midline (helps in abduction).

Aberdeen estimation of manpower (Manpower requirement for Ward work)

W = N (B+T) + A + D + E gives nursing workload for one week in hours.

W=Weekly nursing workload mean hours.

N= No. of patients in ward, mean value.

B=Time required for nursing care of bedridden patients in hours per week.

T=Time required for ward nursing (% of basic nursing)

A= Administrative duty time per patient per week.

D= Domestic work time per patient per week.

E=Dependency factor for the ward.

ABER Annual Blood Examination Rate is an indicator used in malaria

$$ABER = \frac{\text{No. slides examined}}{\text{Population}} \times 100$$

Aberrant This takes unusual course.

Aberration Used in mental and optics; deviation from normal.

Ability Able to perform an act, mental or physical.

Abiosis Absence of life.

Ablatio placentae Premature separation of placenta.

Ablation Surgical or radiological destruction of cancerous tissue.

Abnormal Not usual or not regular.

ABO system Grouping human blood into four groups.

group	*red cell antigen*	*plasma antibody*
AB	A and B	—
A	A	anti β (beta)
B	B	anti α (alpha)
O	—	anti α and anti β (both alpha and beta)

Table: A B O system

Abort Foetus is expelled before it becomes viable.

Abortifacient Agent that induces abortion.

Abortion Foetus is expelled before it is viable. Types are complete **a.** incomplete **a.** threatened **a.** induced **a.** missed **a.** septic **a.** therapeutic **a.** inevitable **a.** criminal **a.** and tubal **a.**

Abortive polio Early form of polio with mild symptoms and no neurological involvement.

Abrasion A scraped or scratched skin wound.

Abruptio placenta Premature separation of placenta.

Abscess It is a collection of pus in a cavity.

Abscissa Horizontal of two coordinates in a graph.

Absenteeism Sick absence of workers in their scheduled work.

Absolute poverty It is the lack of basic necessities like food, shelter and access to clean water and health care.

Absolute scotoma Scotoma with light perception lost.

Absorbent Substance that absorbs or promote absorption.

Absorption Suction of fluid, mental concentration, uptake of radiation.

Abstinence Denial of indulgence of appetite from food, alcohol, drink, and sex.

Abuse It means maltreatment or misuse. Types are Child **a**. Drug **a.**

Acanthoma Skin cancer with no histological evidence. It is epidermoid which is keratinised, cornified squamous cells.

Acapnia Lowered content of CO_2 in the blood.

Acardia Congenital absence of heart in the newborn.

Acarus Genus of itch mite, *Acarus scabiei*.

Accessory Extra or supplementary, name of 11th cranial nerve.

Accident Sudden untoward event. Used in emergency medicine.

Accommodation Refers to adjustment of ciliary muscle of eye.

Accoucheur One who conducts delivery, obstetrician.

Accreditation Evaluation of an institution through regular appraisal.

Acetabulum Cup like socket in which head of femur bone fits and moves.

Acetate Acetic acid salt is called acetate.

Acetoacetic acid It is produced in fat metabolism, especially in starvation and diabetes giving rise to acetone bodies in urine.

Acetone Blood and urine contain traces of acetone. Chemically it is colourless inflammable liquid with characteristic odour. Increased in starvation and diabetes.

Acetylcholine Released by cholinergic nerve endings, e.g. parasympathetic nerves, lower motor neurones to skeletal muscles. Cholin-esterase destroys acetylcholine.

Acetyl coenzyme A It converts carbohydrate, fat and amino acid which are not needed for protein synthesis.

Acetylsalicylic acid Pharmacologically is an analgesic, antipyretic and anti-rheumatic. Commonly called *aspirin*.

Achalasia Muscle sphincter do not relax causing dilation of part above the sphincter. E.g., dilatation of oesophagus above the cardiac sphincter.

Ache A continuous pain which is dull in nature.

Achilles Achilles was a Greek hero who could be injured in the heel. Achilles tendon connects muscles of calf to the heel bone.

Achlorhydria Conditions like cancer stomach, pernicious anaemia and pellagra produce a condition where free chlorine is absent in stomach.

Acholuric Absence of bile in the urine

Achondroplasia arrested growth is seen where early union of epiphysis and diaphysis of long bones. The condition is inherited.

Achylia Enzymes and HCl are absent in gastric juice.

Acid A substance which will turn blue litmus red. It will form salt with an alkali.

Acid burn Corrosive acid burns are severe. Comes under special varieties of burns.

Acid-fast Bacteria causing tuberculosis and leprosy are acid-fast bacilli. Because they are not decolourised by mineral acids after staining

Acidity Refers to more acid secretion in stomach. Also when the state of being acid.

Acidosis pH of blood is disturbed. An increase of hydrogen ion concentration is observed. Incomplete fat metabolism causes acidosis as in diabetes.

Acid stomach Vague term to mention a symptom which could be due to any condition like ulcer, rebellious gallbladder, a stomach cancer, inflamed appendix, emotional disturbances or special form of anaemia.

Acme Peak stage of an infection.

Acne An inflammatory disease of the sebaceous gland, occurring mostly about the face, chest or back.

Acosmia Refers to ill health. Also an irregularity in disease process.

Acoustic Anything related to the sense of hearing.

Acquired Immunity developed, habit developed or illness developed in our environment.

Acrocephalia Head (skull) is pointed, is due to malformation.

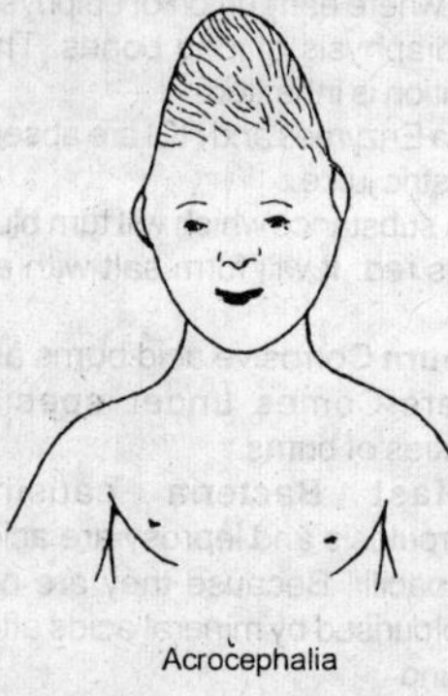

Acrocephalia

Acrodermatitis Dermatitis of upper and lower extremities.

Acrodynia It is called pink disease, is caused by mercury poisoning among children, manifested in pain and redness of fingers and toes.

Acromegaly Gigantism, over activity of anterior lobe of pituitary gland.

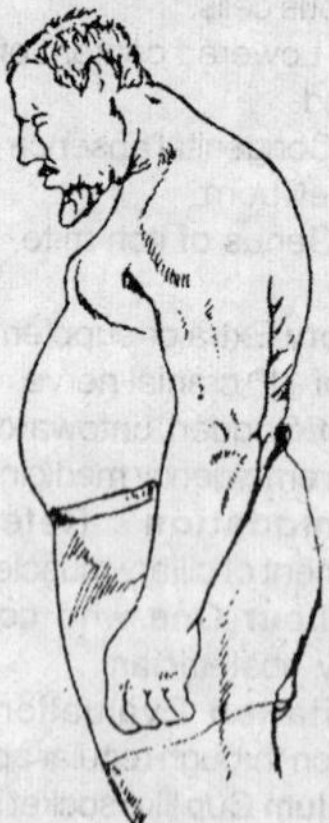

Gigantism

Acromion It is the point of the shoulder, formed by the projecting spine of the scapula.

Acrophobia Fear developed when a person claims the height.

ACTH Is a corticotrophin called *Adreno Cortico Trophic Hormone*.

Actinomyces A spore forming parasite which produces actinomycosis, from which streptomycin is produced.

Actinomycin An antibiotic used as bactericidal.

Actinomycosis Any infection with actinomyces which is chronic in nature colloquially it is called as lumpy jaw, wooden tongue.

Action Performance of a function by organ or part of body.

Activator It renders other substances active.

Active citizen The citizen with prescribed duties and responsibilities for his society.

Acts Enacted by the court of law like The Factory Act, The Food Act, The MTP Act etc., a performance involving motor activity in our body.

Acuity Clear, distinct and sharp like visual **a**. hearing **a**. etc.

Acupuncture In Chinese medicine, special needles are inserted to specific points for treatment of ailments, and relief of pain.

Acus A needle like process.

Acute Short and severe course of illness.

Acyclic Occurring independent of menses.

Adams apple Thyroid cartilage prominence in front of the neck.

Adaptation Adaptation of animal to environment, accommodation of individual to a given situation like colour **a**, light **a**.etc.

Addiction Habitual use of drug. It is psychological dependence.

Addison's disease Hypofunction of adrenal gland characterized by skin pigmentation, prostration, anaemia, low blood pressure, diarrhoea, digestive disturbances.

Adducent Turns inwards, performing adduction.

Adductor That which adducts, opposite of abductor.

Adenine It is 6 amino purine found in vegetable and animal tissue, also found in urine as decomposed product of nuclein.

Adenitis Inflammation of gland, like cervical **a**. salivary **a.**

Adenocarcinoma Glandular pithelial cancer.

Adenocele Cystic tumour of an adenoma.

Adenofibroma Benign tumour of connective tissue which shows glandular structure.

Adenoid Hypertrophy of pharyngeal tonsil present in children. Any structure which resembles a gland.

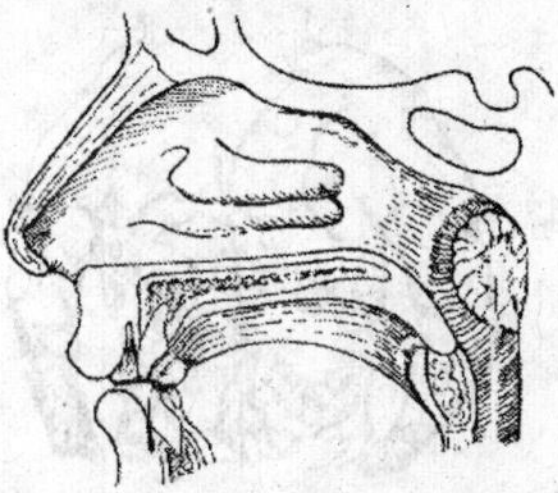

Adenoids

Adenoma Benign tumour of a glandular tissue.

Adenomyoma Common site is uterus and uterine ligaments. A tumour of endometrium and muscle tissue.

Adenosarcoma Malignant tumour of connective tissue and glandular tissue.

Adenosine Adenine d-ribose, a nucleotide is derived from nucleic acid.

Adenovirus Commonly cause ARI. Some strain cause eye infection and intestinal infection.

Adenosine diphosphate Hydrolysis of adenosine triphosphate gives rise to this product.

Adenosine triphosphatase It is the enzyme which liberates inorganic phosphate from ATP.

ADH *Anti Diuretic Hormone.*

Adhesion To remain in close approximation, common term used in GI tract.

Adipocele A hernia containing fatty tissue.

Adiposis dolorosa Clinical condition characterised by painful localised fatty swellings and by nerve lesions.

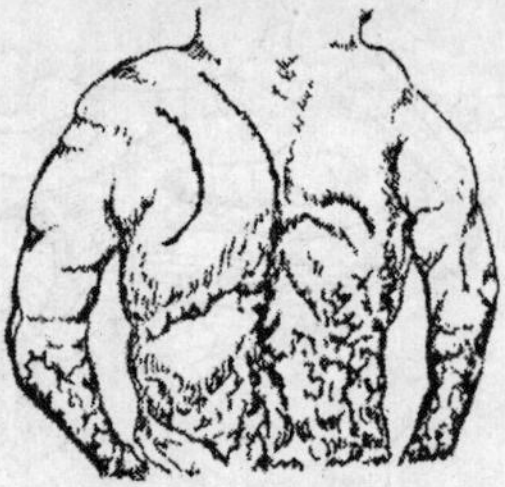

Adiposis dolorosa

Adiposity Excessive accumulation of fat in the body, obesity.

Adjuvant Which assists or which aids, which reduces solubility, which enhances antigenicity.

Admission of emergency case Nurse taking the message has to prepare special requirement, prepare bed, take care of the valuables.

Adnexa Appendage of an organ, like ovary fallopian tube of uterus.

Adolescence Period of life when physical growth and secondary sexual characteristics appear.

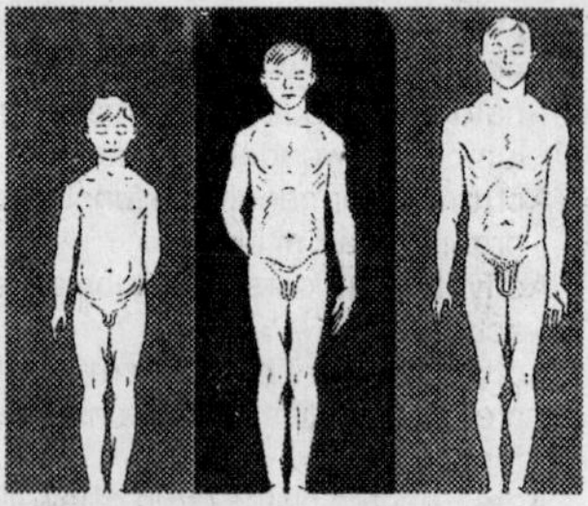

Secondary sexual characters in male

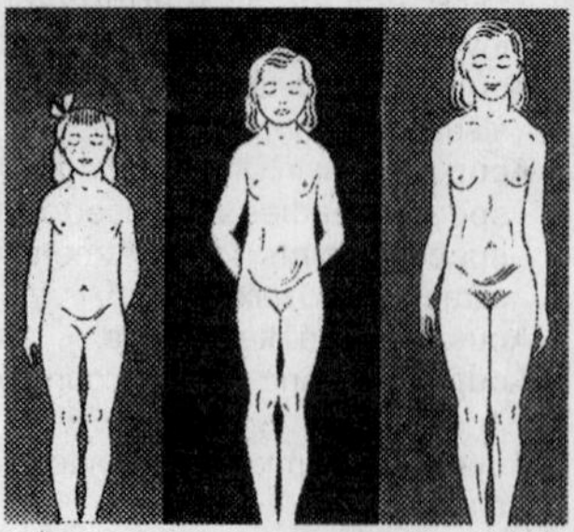

Secondary sexual characters in female

Adrenal Meaning nearer to kidney, refers to endocrine glands called adrenal glands.

Adrenaline A hormone secreted by adrenal glands, a powerful vasopressor drug, also called epinephrine.

Adrenergic Means activated by epinephrine, refers to the sympathetic nerve fibres.

Adrenocorticotrophin It is the extract from anterior pituitary gland (first extracted in the year 1933).

Androcentric Viewing the things from a male perspective.

Adsorbent A substance that absorbs fluid to itself.

Adsorption Power of a substance to attach another substance to their surface, has an application in chromatography.

Adult Human attaining full maturity

Adulteration Addition, substitution and misbranding of usable items, which cause harmful effect to the body.

Advanced life directive Procedure in terminal care, living will, euthanasia.

Advanced trauma life support A set of protocol used by nurse in an accident, trauma or injury.

Adventitia The outer coat of any tubular structure, usually referred to as tunica adventitia.

Adventitious breath sound Added or abnormal breath sounds.

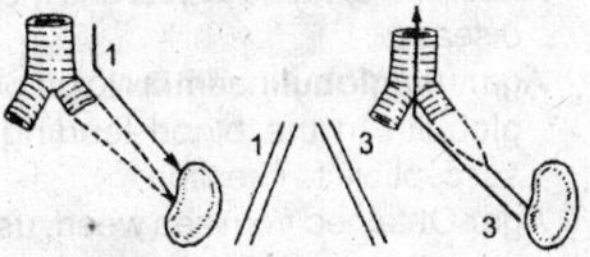

(a) 1 = tubular phase
3 = on expiration
Bronchial breath sound (no alveolar phase)

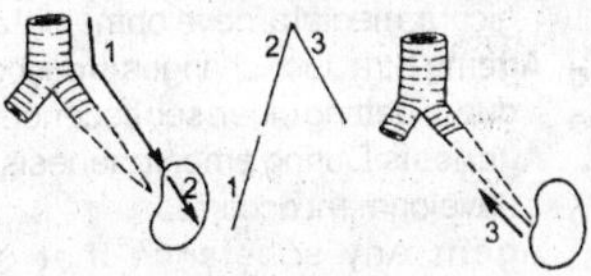

(b) 1 = tubular phase
2 = alveolar phase
3 = on expiration
Alveolar breath sound

Aedes Genus of mosquito which transmit dengue, yellow fever.

Aeration Refers to blood oxygenation.

Aerobe Organism which live in the presence of oxygen.

Aerobic exercise Done to increase the effectiveness of heart and lungs. Effective maintenance is seen without discomfort in this type of exercise.

Aeroplane splint Used in the treatment of fracture of upper end of humerus.

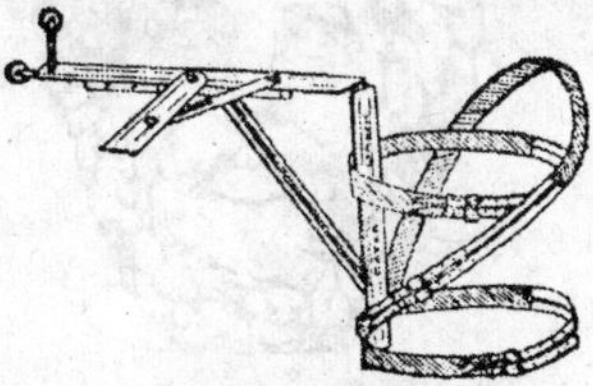

Aeroplane splint

Aerosol face mask Is a plastic face mask with two large exhalation ports which connect the patient to a neubuliser.

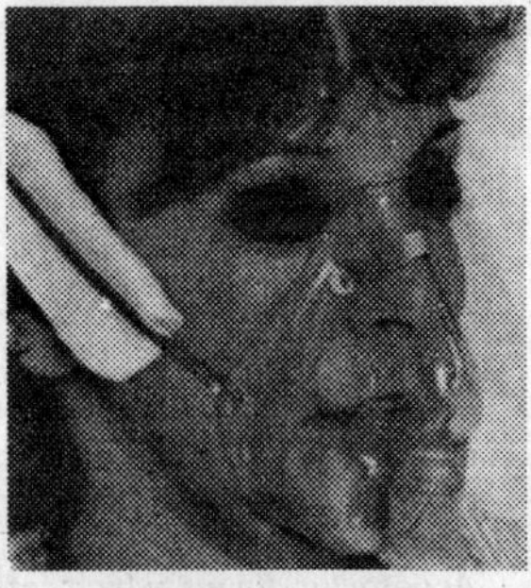

Aerosol face mask

Aerosol therapy Administering oxygen, aerosol either through low flow system or through high flow system through face mask.

Aerosol Droplets are used in administration of drugs by inhalation

Aesculapius Name of God of Healing in Roman Mythology.

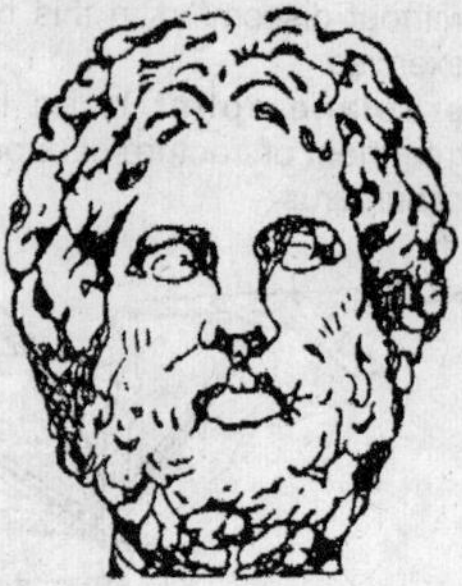

Aesculapius

Aetiology The cause of illness is described in this science.

Afebrile There is no raised body temperature.

Affect Pleasant or unpleasant is felt by a stimulus, an experience felt by an emotion.

Afferent Anything conveyed towards the centre, referable to nerve, vessel or lymphatic.

Affiliation University adopts and guides colleges with a view to issue of a maintenance order.

Affluent society High wages to many manual workers so that prosperity reached further down the class structure than ever before.

Aflatoxin It is fungal toxin by *Aspergillus flavus* which infests foodgrains particularly groundnut.

AFP surveillance In polio eradication, to strengthen the surveillance of *acute flaccid paralysis,* field surveillance and institutional surveillance are instituted.

African tick fever Tropical disease caused by *Borrelia duttonii*, a vector borne disease transmitted by ticks.

Afterbirth Description of afterbirth material which include placenta, umbilical cord and membrane.

Aftercare Follow-up done of the patient after his/her discharge from hospital.

Afterimage After the cessation of sensory stimulus there remains a visual impression that remains in the mind.

After pain Pain due to uterine contraction in third stage of labour.

Aftosa Other name for foot and mouth disease.

Agammaglobulinaemia No gamma globulin in the blood leading to susceptible to infection.

Agar Obtained from sea weed, used in culture medium, used as a common laxative.

Age It is the measure of time spent by human beings, animals and plant. Types are gestational **a.** chronological **a**. mental **a**. developmental **a.**

Ageing Structural changes in our body due to getting older, senescence.

Agenesis During embryogenesis no development occurred.

Agent Any substance that can produce physical, chemical, biological, social or mental hazard.

Agglutination A process where agglutinin when comes in contact with human serum, they get clumped.

Seen in Widal test and in blood grouping.

Agglutinin It is a substance that cause agglutination.

Agglutinogen Any substance when present in blood that produce antibody, which produces agglutinin.

Agitation Extreme restlessness.

Aglutition Difficulty in swallowing.

Agnosia Objects are not recognised due to non-interpretation of sensory stimulus, even when sensory organ is normal.

Agony Extreme physical and mental suffering.

Agranulocyte Monocytes and lymphocytes which do not have granules.

Agranulocytosis Marked increase of monocytes and lymphocytes as seen in irradiation or drug toxicity.

Agrarian society Major form of employment in a society is agriculture.

Ague Other name for malaria infection.

AHF Clotting factor VIII which is called *Anti Haemophilic Factor*.

AID Denote *artificial insemination* of woman by the semen of a *donor*.

AIDS End stage of HIV infection called *Acquired Immuno Deficiency Syndrome*.

AIH Denote *artificial insemination* of woman by the semen of her *husband*.

Ailment Describes the ailment of our body.

Ainhum A condition where construction and amputation of little toe among Negroes is seen.

Air embolism Sudden blocking of an artery or a vein by air, a risk in IV infusion.

Air hunger Fighting for the breath, a symptom in severe bleeding and in acute respiratory distress.

Air rings They are used in special bed making in nursing care, by inflating the air ring by a bicycle pump.

Airway It is the passage where air enters the lung and leaves the lung.

Akinesia Loss of muscular function as seen in anaesthesia, in spinal injury.

Akinetic A condition where loss of muscular movement is seen.

Alanine It is an amino acid.

Albinism A clinical condition where skin pigment is lost, sometimes changes in hair or in eyes are seen.

Albino Person affected with albinism.

Albumin Referred to animal protein and vegetable protein.. It is water soluble and coagulable by heat.

Alcohol It is the basis of wine and spirits, distilled from fermented saccharine. Is a common preservative and antiseptic.

Alcoholism Body changes due to excess intake of alcohol.

Aldehyde Meaning away from hydrogen, substance containing–CHO.

CH_3CHO = acetic aldehyde
$CH_2OH.CHOH.CHO$ = glycericaldehyde
$C_6H_4OH.CHO$ = salicylic aldehyde

Common aldehyde

Aldosterone Hormone of adrenal cortex, has Aldehyde group at C-18, control mineral balance particularly sodium and potassium.

Alternative medicine Holistic approach of medical treatment which consists of homeopathy, aromatherapy, hypnosis, acupuncture, etc.

Algae Chlorophyll containing water plants in sea or fresh water, both microscopic and macroscopic.

Algid Chilly or very cold.

Algor Gradual decrease of body temperature after death.

Alienation A symptom of schizophrenia,depersonalisation.

Alignment Arranged in a line, refers to anatomical position, alignment.

Alimentary Refers to the tract from mouth to anus, system of nutrition.

Alkali When it unites with acid it produces salt, substance which turns red litmus to blue.

Alkaline bath it is ordered in nursing care for the relief of irritation in skin conditions or to aid the removal of crusts, it uses 6 ounces of sodium bicarbonate in 30 gallons of water.

Alkaline When it has the reactions of an alkali.

Alkalinity When the quality of alkaline exists.

Alkaloid Morphine, cocaine, atropine, quinine, nicotine and caffeine are referred to as alkaloid because they are active nitrogenous compounds, are bitter and show physiological activity.

Alkalosis If blood reserve of alkali is increased.

Alkaptonuria Abnormal product of protein metabolism is seen in urine, when urine is exposed to air (oxygen) it becomes dark brown.

Alkylating agent An agent that damages DNA of the cell, a drug used in cancer treatment.

All or none phenomenon Individual cardiac muscle or skeletal muscle has this phenomenon which states that they react to the fullest or not at all.

Allantoin It is glyoxylic acid derivative present in allantoic fluid, foetal urine and in plants.

Allantois Membranous sac of foetus in early development.

Albuminuria Presence of albumin in the urine, seen during pregnancy, high fever and renal conditions.

Allele Pair of gene that occupies the homologous chromosome to produce altogether different effect in development.

Allelomorph One or more contrasting genes situated at the same locus in homologous chromosomes which determine alternative characters in inheritance.

Allergen Agent that produce allergy or alter immunity.

Allergy Hypersensitive state produced by the exposure of an allergen.

Allocate When assigned for a particular purpose.

Allocation Process of allocating.

Allograft tissues are taken from one person to another for grafting.

Allopathy To cure a disease by inducing different kind of action in the body.

Allopurinol Drug used in the treatment of gout.

Alopecia Baldness. Types are: alopecia areata, alopecia cicatricia, male pattern alopecia.

Alpha Denote first letter in Greek: alpha cells, alpha fetoprotein, alpha receptors seen with this prefix.

Aldosterone Secreted in adrenal cortex which helps in electrolyte balance.

Alter To castrate.

Alveolar Pertaining to the alveolus of lung.

Alveolitis Inflammation of alveoli.

Alzheimer's disease A condition with neuronal degeneration of brain which leads to dementia or forgetfulness in elderly people.

AMA American Medical Association.

Amantadine Drug used in viral infection and in Parkinson's disease.

Amaurosis Loss of vision due to no apparent cause or lesion in the eye.

Amaurotic Of the nature of amaurosis.

Ambivalence Simultaneous existence of two opposite attitudes like love and hate on an object.

Ambivert Who is not either an extrovert or an introvert.

Amblyopia Dimness of vision without detectable organic cause.

Ambu resuscitator Used in the management of routine tracheostomy care, is a manual resuscitator which will be attached to a source oxygen.

Ambulance loading Nursing principles are followed in the transport of patient either by manual or by stretcher method.

Ambulance unloading Nursing principles similar to Ambulance loading.

Ambulant One who is able to walk.

Ambulatory Patient who has the capacity to walk.

Amelia No limbs are developed in a child.

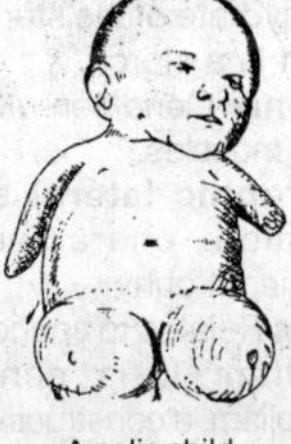

Amelia child

Amelioration Improvement in symptoms of a disease.

Amenorrhoea When there is no menstruation. Types are: primary **a**. secondary **a**.

Amentia Subnormal state of mind.

Ametropia Denotes defective vision, imperfection in refractive power of eye.

Amine Any organic compound containing nitrogen, according to number hydrogen atoms replaced they are termed *primary*, *secondary* or *tertiary* amines, e.g. are allylamine, phenylamine, propylamine.

Amino acid Chemical containing NH_2 and COOH group, types are essential and non-essential amino acids.

Arginine
Histidine
Isoleucine
Lysine
Leucine
Methionine
Phenylalanine
Threonine
Tryptophan
Valine

Table: Essential amino acids

Amino glycoside Bacterial antibiotics which interfere in function of bacterial ribosome. e.g. Gentamicin.

Aminophylline Alkaloid from camellia which is used as bronchodilator and as coronary vasodilator.

Aminosalicylic acid Its derivative is used in the treatment of tuberculosis (PAS).

Amitosis Not occurring by mitosis.

Amitriptyline An antidepressant drug.

Ammonia Colourless pungent gas used as cardiac stimulant (NH_3).

Ammonium Hypothetical radical NH_4, forms salts with metals.

Amnesia Loss of memory.

Amniocentesis Drawing amniotic fluid through abdominal wall.

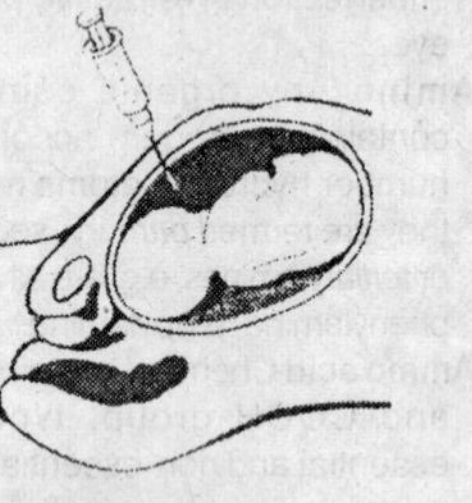

Amniocentesis

Amnion Thin, transparent, silvery and tough membrane lining the chorion laeve and placenta, that produce amniotic fluid.

Amnioscope Instrument to examine foetus and amniotic fluid through a tube.

Amniotic fluid Albuminous fluid contained in the amniotic sac.

Amniotic Pertaining to amnion.

Amoeba Protozoan parasite which cause amoebiasis.

Amoebiasis Infection caused by amoeba *E.histolytica*.

Amorphous Referred to powder particle, one which does not have shape.

Amoxicillin Penicillin analogue antibiotic.

Amphetamine Drug that stimulates the CNS.

Amphotericin Antifungal antibiotic.

Ampicillin Broad-spectrum penicillin antibiotic.

Ampoule Glass phial in which sterile drug or distilled water is sealed.

Ampulla Flask like dilatation of a canal, uterine tube.

Amputation stump dressing Many tailed bandage is used in special dressing in case of amputation stump.

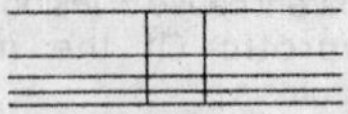

Many tailed

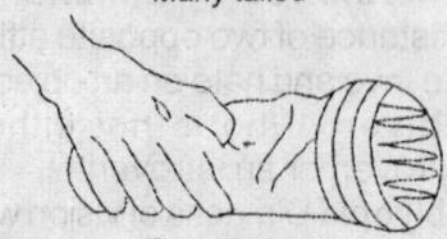

Recurrent

Many tailed bandage for amputation stump and recurrent bandage for amputation stump

Amputation Surgical removal of a limb or an organ.

Amyl nitrite Vasodilator and cardiac stimulant.

Amyl Derived from starch, univalent radical C_5H_{11}.

Amylase Present in saliva and pancreatic juice which digests starch, enzyme that reduces starch to maltose.

Amyloid Related to starch.

Amylose A polysaccharide, any carbohydrate of the starch group.

Amylum Is a starch.

Amyotonia Condition with loss of tone in muscles.

Amyotrophic lateral sclerosis Condition characterised by muscular atrophy.

Anabolic Related to anabolism.

Anabolism It is constructive metabolism, a constructive process in body.

Anacrotism An anomaly in pulse tracing, show additional wave or notch.

Anaemia Quality or quantity of RBC is deficient. Types are Microcytic **a**. Hypochromic **a**. Macrocytic **a**. Aplastic **a**. Haemolytic **a**. Pernicious **a**. Sickle cell **a**.

Anaerobe Microbe that can live without oxygen.

Anaesthesia Loss of sensation or feeling by drug or by pathological condition.

Anaesthetist Consultant who administers anaesthesia.

Anal Pertaining to anus.

Analeptic That stimulates CNS.

Analgesia Absence of sensibility to pain.

Analogous Resemblance present to some extent.

Analogue Same function through differ structurally.

Analysis Indepth study, break up to smaller component for the study.

Anaphase It is a stage in mitosis in which the halves of the divided chromosomes move apart towards the pole.

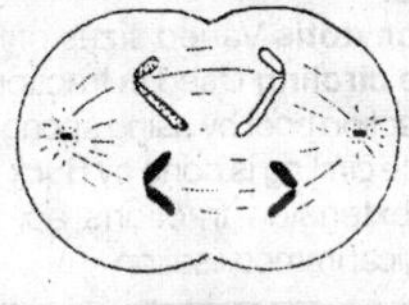

Anaphase

Anaphylactic reaction Exaggerated reaction of man or animal to a foreign protein or any allergen.

Anaplasia Loss of normal differentiation in tumour cells, undifferentiation.

Anastomose To communicate with one another, in arteries and vein.

Anastomosis Surgical formation or pathological formation of a passage.

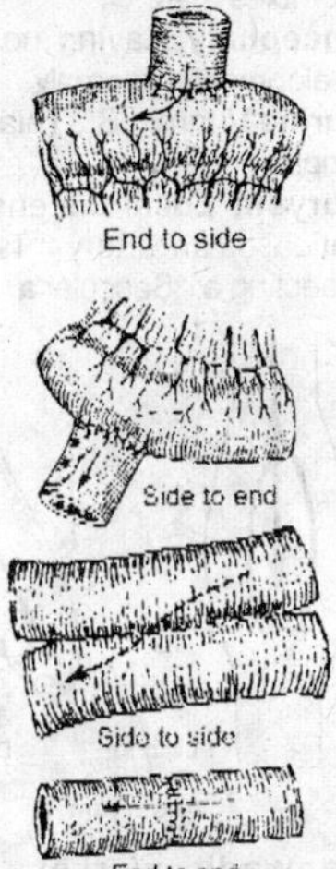

Common types of anastomosis

Anatomical Gift Act Any person above 18 years can donate his organ which is taken effect upon his death.

Anatomy Science that deals with the structure of our body.

Ancient society Greek and Roman society which was slave based production.

Ancylostoma Hookworm which comes under nematode, common cause of anaemia in tropical countries.

Androgen Hormone secreted by testes and adrenal cortex, responsible for secondary male sexual characters.

Androgenic Producing male characteristics.

Android Have male characters, resembles man.

Anencephaly Having no brain, a developmental anomaly.

Aneurine Vitamin B_1, Thiamine a B complex.

Aneurysm Local distension and dilation of an artery. Types are: Dissecting **a**. Saccular **a**. Fusiform **a.**

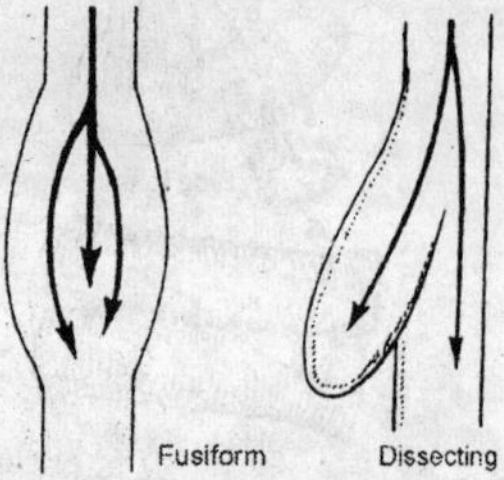

Aneurysm

Anganwadi worker Female voluntary worker work in Anganwadi the peripheral unit of ICDS activity under social welfare department.

Angioma Tumour where blood vessels or lymph vessels cells congregate.

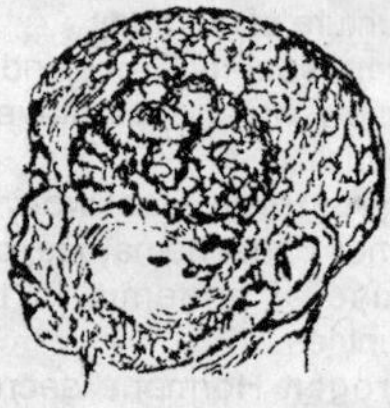

Cavernous angioma

Angina A suffocating pain, like Pectoral **a**. Parotid **a**. Abdominal **a**.

Angiocardiography By using opaque contrast and catheterisation radiological examination of heart and vessels is done.

Angiocath Inserting an over-the-needle catheter for administration of IV fluid and medications.

Angiography Radiological examination of vessels by using opaque contrast medium.

Angioneurotic Pertaining to angioneurosis, angioneurotic oedema.

Angioplasty To promote normal blood flow surgery of narrowed artery is done, balloon angioplasty.

Angiotensin Produced by the action of renin on plasma globulins, that which raises the B.P.

Anhidrosis Deficient sweat secretion.

Anhydrous Contain no water.

Aniline A coal tar derivative, dyes of aniline is occupational source of bone marrow depression.

Animal experiment Comes under research ethics where faithfully discrimination of doing right or wrong in professional activities is used.

Anisocytotis Varied sizes of RBC.

Ankle circling Used in traction care in traction boot by using sponge boot Ankle circling is done by Buck's boot for extension tractions as a pre-surgical immobilisation.

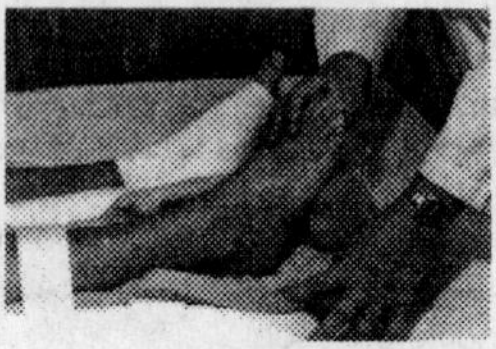

Buck's boot as traction boot

Ankle exercise Part of exercise in nursing care to assist patient in positioning and mobilisation.

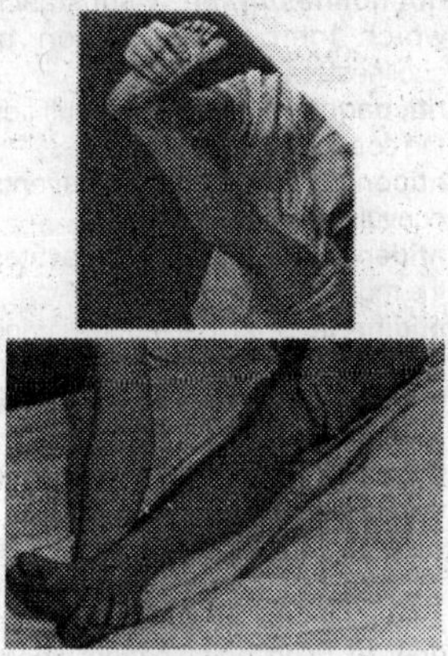

Ankle exercise

Ankle jerk A brisk tap to tendo Achilles produce plantar flexion of foot, done in neurological examination of the patient.

Ankle reflex To test S1 and S2 innervations. Percussion on Achilles tendon, Patient's ankle should plantar flex.

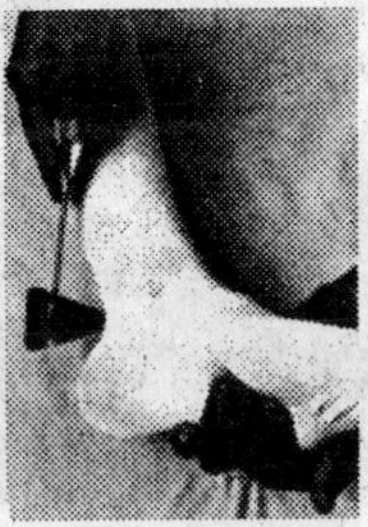

Ankle reflex testing

Ankle Part of the leg just above the foot including ankle joint.

Ankylosis Abnormal immobility of a joint.

Annelida Segmented worms like leeches.

Anodyne That which relieves pain, medicine that relieves pain, opium, morphine, hyoscine,etc.

Anomaly Too much deviation from the normal, commonly refers to developmental anomaly.

Anopheles A genus of mosquito, which transmits malaria.

A. anularis	*A. culicifacies*
A. fluviatelis	*A. minimus*
A. stephensi	*A. sundiacus*

Table: Common species of Anopheles mosquito.

Anophthalmia Congenital absence of eye.

Anorexia Loss of appetite, common clinical condition is anorexia nervosa.

Anosmia Sense of smell is lost.

Anovular Uterine bleeding without ovulation, contraceptive induced bleeding.

Anoxia Lack of oxygen to the tissue.

Antabuse Used in the treatment of alcoholism, disulfiram.

Antacid Drug used to neutralise gastric acidity.

Antagonist Drug inhibiting the action of another drug, enzyme inhibiting the action of another enzyme, muscle that has opposite action of another muscle.

Ante cubital fossa Space situated in front of the forearm, triangular in shape, bounded by brachioradialis laterally and pronator teres medially.

Anteflexion Abnormal forward curvature, normal forward flexion of uterus, displacement of a portion of an organ.

Antenatal Care provided during pregnancy to effect normal delivery.

Antepartum Shortly before birth like APH.

Anterior horn cell Nerve cells of anterior horn of spinal cord from which efferent fibres emerge.

Anterior Situated in the front.

Anteversion Forward tilting, usually refers to anteverted uterus.

Anthelmintic Chemotherapeutic agent used to kill helminths.

Anthracosis Inhalation of coal dust produces this type of pneumoconiosis.

Anthrax Disease caused by anthrax bacteria, is a zoonotic disease.

Anthropocentric Viewing the human race in contrast to other species.

Anthropology Science that studies origin, history, culture of human beings. Types arep hysical **a**. Cultural **a**. Social **a**. Medical **a.**

Anthropometry Study of measurement of human parts, height, weight, head circumference, chest circumference, mid upper arm circumference, etc.

Anti D gamma globulin Given to Rh negative mother within 72 hours of delivery to prevent haemolysis, used in Rh incompatibility.

Antibacterial Drug used to kill bacteria or to halt the growth of bacteria.

Antibiotic Substance produced from a bacteria or a fungi, is used to destroy another bacteria or fungi.

Antibodies They are immunoglobulin, types are IgA, IgG, IgM, IgD, and IgE.

Anticholinesterase A substance which inhibits the action of cholinesterase.

Anticoagulant That which nullifies the coagulation of the blood.

Anticonvulsant Drug that prevents convulsion.

Antidepressant Drug that elevates the mood.

Antidiuretic Drug that reduces urine output.

Antidote Drug used to counter the effect of a poison.

Antiembolic Hose or stockings used to prevent embolism.

Antiembolic cuffs To minimise venous stasis, applying intermittent pneumatic compression cuffs are applied, used for the patient who is bedridden for a long time.

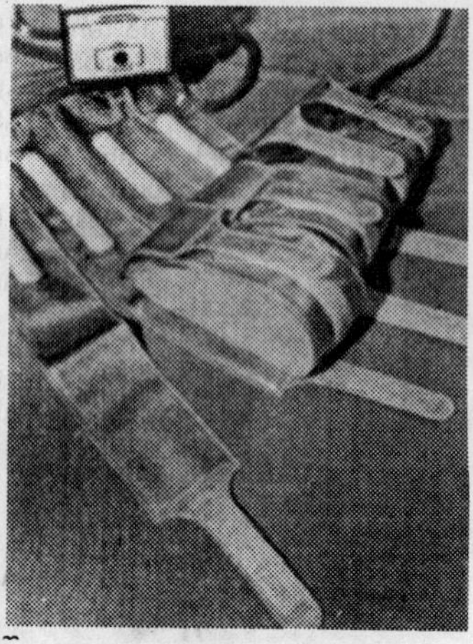

Antiembolic cuffs

Antiembolic stockings Applying elastic stockings to a patient with vascular disorders to prevent embolism.

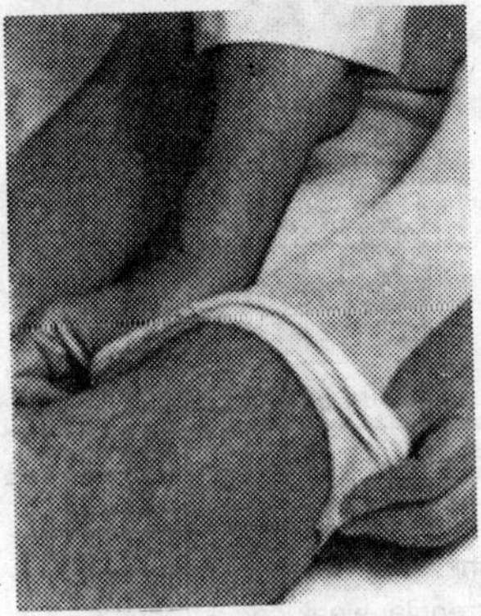

Antiembolic stockings

Antiemetic Drug used against nausea and vomiting.

Antigen A substance that produces antibody, which produce immune response.

Antihaemophilic Antihaemophilic globulin used in haemophilia, agent that counteracts the bleeding in haemophilia.

Antihistaminic Drug that block the tissue receptors for histamine, drugs used in allergic conditions.

Antihypertensive Agent that reduces the elevated blood pressure.

Anti-inflammatory Drug which counter acts inflammation.

Antimicrobial cleansing agents Soap and water, antiseptic solutions.

Antimycotic Drugs used against fungus.

Antiperspirant Preparations that reduce the amount of perspiration.

Antipruritic External application that relieves itching, drug which control itching.

Antipyretic Agent used to reduce body temperature as in fever.

Antisepsis Procedure to prevent infection by killing germs and by halting their growth.

Antiseptic Substance that kill or inhibit the growth of bacteria.

Antiserum Blood serum of man or animal which contains antibodies against toxin or infection.

Antisocial Individual who refuses to accept the normal obligations.

Antispasmodic Measures undertaken to relieve the spasm of muscles.

Antistin cream Is a soothing application in case of stings caused by bees, wasps, mosquitoes, or a biting insect.

Antitoxin A chemical substance in cells and blood serum produced as a defence reaction to a poisonous substances (toxin).

Antitussive Drug used to suppress cough.

Antrum It is a cavity in a bone like Maxillary **a.** Mastoid **a.**

Anuria Cessation of urine secretion, urine output is nil.

Anus The end portion of alimentary canal, outlet for stool.

Anxiety Chronic psychological disturbances, which lead to neurosis.

Aorta Main arterial trunk from which the systemic arterial system proceeds.

Aortic stenosis Narrowing of aortic valve leading to cardiac disturbances.

Aortocoronary bypass Surgical treatment of coronary obstruction by putting saphenous vein graft or by putting mammary artery graft

APA American Physiotherapy Association

Apex Top of an anatomical structure, apex of the heart, apex of the lung

Apgar score A system of newborn assessment

Apical pulse Palpating or auscultating the apical area to assess duration and strength of heart beat.

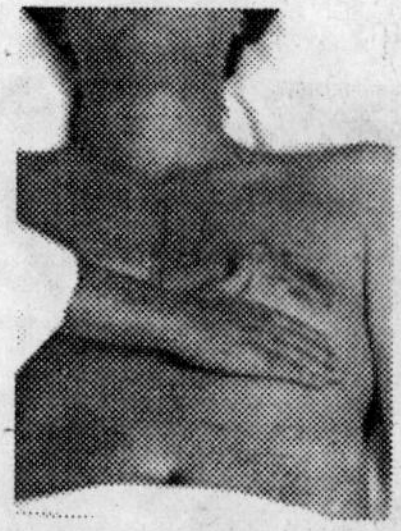

Palpating apical area

Sign	Score 0	Score 1	Score 2
Colour	blue, pale	body pink, limbs blue	completely pink
Respiratory effort	absent	slow, irregular weak cry	strong cry
Heart rate	absent	slow below 100	above 100
Muscle tone	limps	some flexionment	good move
Response to flicking foot	nil	grims the face	cries

Table: Apgar scoring

APH Ante Partum Haemorrhage.

Aphagia Loss of swallowing function.

Aphakia No lens in the eye, condition after cataract operation.

Aphasia Communication disorder due to brain damage, disturbed language no expression or no comprehension.

Aphonia Unable to produce sound, symptom of larynx diseases.

Aphrodisiac Drug used to excite sexual desire.

Aphthous Recurrent stomatitis.

Apical expansion exercises In case of lobectomy, mastectomy, gross pleural effusion, deep breathing exercises are applied for lung inflation.

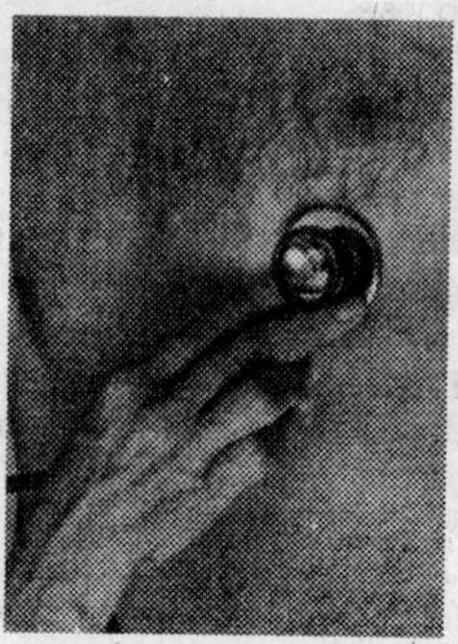

Auscultating apical area

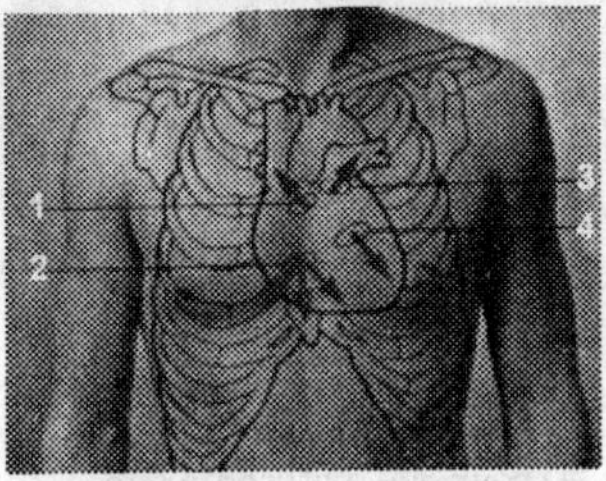

Areas of auscultation

1. Aortic
2. Tricuspid
3. Pulmonic
4. Mitral

Apical At the apex of the heart, pertaining to apex of a structure.

API A parasitological indicator in malaria.

$$\text{API} = \frac{\text{Confirmed cases during 1 yr}}{\text{Population under surveillance}} \times 1000$$

Aplasia Incomplete development, absence of growth.

Aplastia Having no tendency to develop into new tissue, refers to aplastic anaemia.

Apnoea Cessation of respiration, Cardiac **a**. Sleep **a**. Prematurity **a.**

Apocrine Modified sweat glands in hair follicles in axillary and pubic areas.

Apomorphine A derivative of morphine.

Aponeurosis Tendon like tissue that connects muscles to the parts that they move.

Apoplexy Stroke due to rupture of cerebral artery.

Apparatus suction Used in cavity drainage or to suction of emphymata.

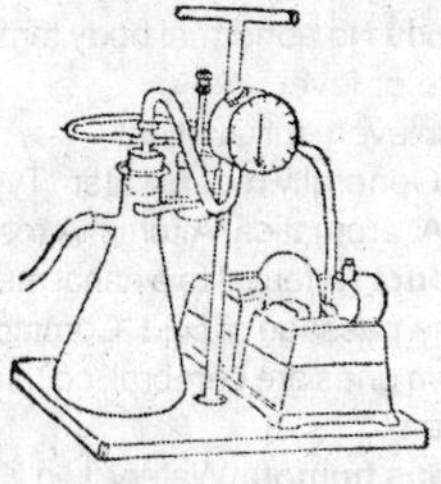

Suction apparatus

Appearance of patient Important physical sign of shock, coldness, paleness and beads of sweat are observed.

Appendicectomy Surgical removal of appendix in appendicitis.

Appendicitis Infection and inflammation of appendix, usually an acute condition, may be chronic in nature.

Appendicular skeleton Refers to the bones of arms, hands, legs, feet, shoulder and pelvis.

Appendix An additional or supplementary part.

Appetite It is the desire for the food, feels like eating.

Appliance A device meant for performing a function.

Applicator Device to apply medication.

Apraxia Mind blindness, unable to perform intricate skilled acts.

Apron Working white coat used by doctors, nurses and other para medical personnel.

APT Alum Precipitated Toxoid.

Aptitude Ability to acquire skill, both mental and physical ability skill acquiring.

Apyrexia No abnormal body temperature or fever.

AQ Achievement Quotient.

Aqua Generally mean water. Types are: A. aromatica, A.fortis, A.rosae.

Aqueduct Referred to a canal meant for the passage of fluid. Commonly known ones are cerebral, cochlear, sylvian.

Aqueous humour Watery fluid filling the eye between the lens and the cornea.

Aqueous Watery substance.

Arachis Plant from which ear wax and skin medications are produced.

Arachnodactyly A congenital condition where fingers and toes are thin and long when compared to normal individual.

Arachnoid Resemblance to a spider, membrane between pia and dura mater.

Arbovirus They are arthropod borne viral infections like yellow fever, encephalitis, sand fly fever, dengue fever, etc.

ARC American Red Cross.

Arcus A bow like or arch like.

Arcus senilis Opaque arch appearing round the cornea in elderly.

ARDS Acute Respiratory Distress Syndrome.

Areola Pigmented ring around nipple of female breast.

Arginine Is an essential amino acid.

Argyll Robertson pupil One of the sign in syphilis where light reflex is absent and accommodation reflex persists.

ARI Acute Respiratory Infection, common paediatric morbidity.

Arithmetic mean Average, measure of central tendency, sum up of all observation and dividing it by the number of observation.

Arm board It is used to prevent the needle or catheter from dislodging. A short cloth splint used to immobilise the extremity.

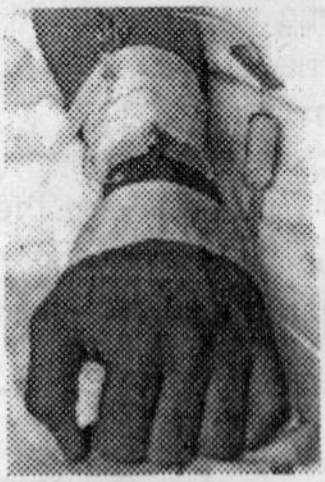

Arm board or splint

Arm exercises It is taught to patient under arm exercises to assist the patient with positioning and mobilisation.

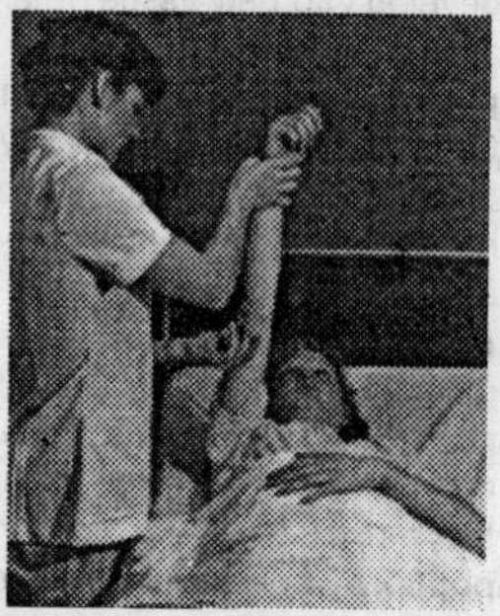

Arm exercise

Arm immobilizer Used in cases of shoulder dislocation, clavicular fracture, shoulder surgery. It is an elasticised fabric with a chest band and a humeral cuff to keep shoulder immobilised.

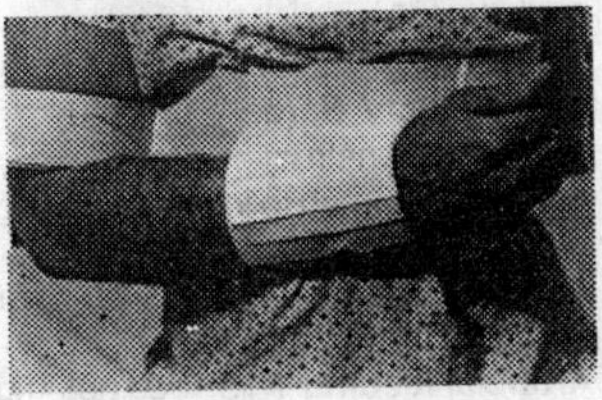

Arm immobiliser

Arm sling A versatile bandage with sturdy cloth used to support and immobilise hand, elbow and shoulder.

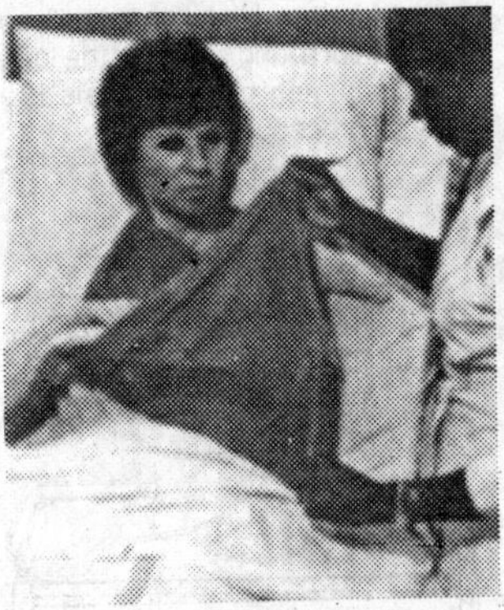

Arm sling

Aromatic Having spicy odour, spicy and stimulant quality of a medicinal plant.

Arousal It is an increased response to a stimulusa.

Arranged marriage Common in royal and aristocratic families where parents choose the marriage partner.

Arrector pili Muscle of the hair follicle which helps in hair erection, gooseflesh.

Arrhythmia Abnormal rhythm in heart function.

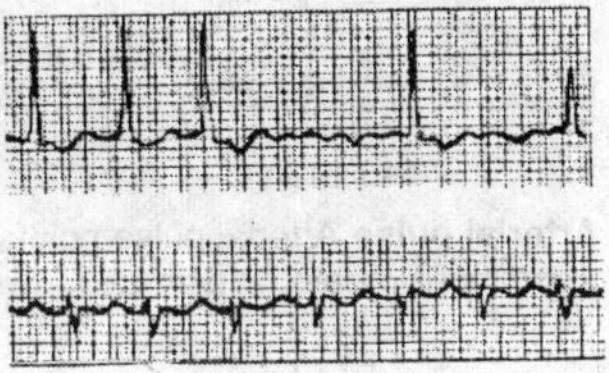

Arrhythmia

Arsenic An element which is poisonous, was used as medicinal preparation.

Art therapy When a patient cannot express feeling verbally, he is taught the art of using the art to express.

Artefact Artificial one, man made, not natural.

Arteries Largest class of vessels carrying blood away from the heart capillary, arteriole and artery are small, large and largest respectively.

Arteriography Radiograph of artery is taken after injecting radio-opaque contrast medium.

Arteriole A minute arterial branch.

Arterioplasty Arterial reconstruction by vascular surgery.

Arteriosclerosis Thickening and calcification of arterial wall.

Arteriovenous Connected with both artery and vein.

Arteritis Inflammation of an artery, common cause of partial occlusion of an artery.

Artery A vessel through which blood flows from heart to various parts of our body.

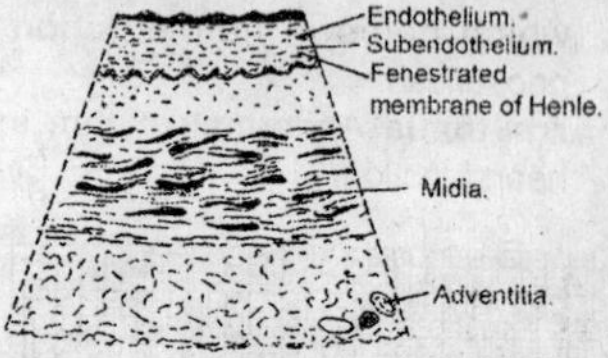

Cross-section of an artery

Arterial pulse Arterial pulse points commonly located in practice.

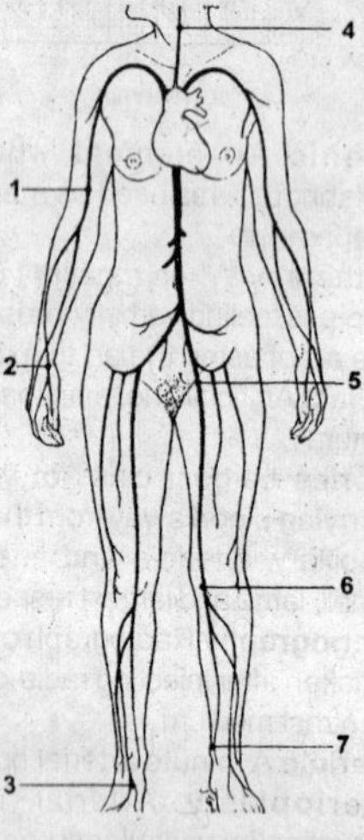

Anatomical landmark for palpating arterial pulses:

1. Brachial
2. Radial
3. Dorsalis pedis
4. Carotid
5. Femoral
6. Popliteal
7. Posterior tibial

Arthralgia Joint pain.

Arthritis Inflammation of joint.

Arthropathy Diseases of joint.

Arthroplasty Surgery undertaken for the reconstruction of joint.

Articular Related to joint, pertaining to joint.

Articulation Place of union of two or more bones, enunciation of words.

Artificial feeding This does not find its place in the context of exclusive breastfeeding, artificial feeding or bottle feeding are indicated only in breast disease, inverted nipple, etc.

Artificial pneumoperitoneum Introduction of air into the peritoneal cavity may be undertaken to produce collapse of a lung or part of the lung in the treatment of tuberculosis, is a special procedure.

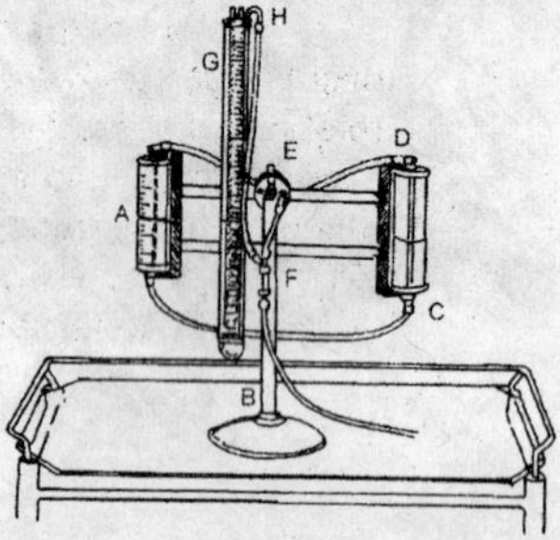

Stott's artificial pneumothorax apparatus:

A = glass cylinder
B = central column
C = rubber tubing
D = connection

E = slide valve
F = filter
G = monometer
H = 'u' tube

Artificial respiration Method to keep patient breathing when respiration has failed, means of resuscitation from asphyxia.

Artificial Not natural.

Arytenoids Shaped like a jug, arytenoids cartilage.

Asbestosis Pneumoconiosis caused by inhalation of asbestos fibres.

Ascariasis Roundworm infestation in intestine.

Ascites Free fluid collection in the peritoneal cavity.

Ascorbic acid Vitamin C.

Asexual Without sex, referred to asexual reproduction.

Asepsis Free from pathogens or micro-organisms.

Aseptic Made free from sepsis.

Aspartame Low calorie sweetener, it is aspartyl phenylalanine methylester.

Aspergillosis Fungal infection of lung caused by Aspergillus fungus.

Aspermia Absence of sperm in the semen.

Asphyxia Blood is without oxygen causing cyanosis.

Aspiration of chest Removing a collection of fluid from the pleural cavity.

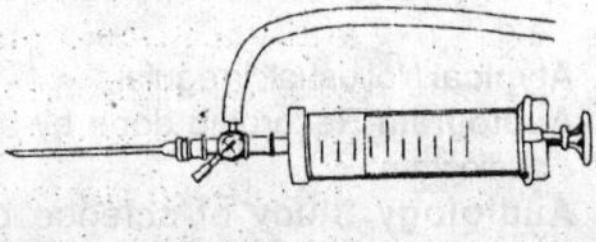

Martin's syringe for aspiration of chest

Aspiration Suction of fluid from a cavity.

Aspirin Acetyl salicylic acid, pain reliever, reduces temperature.

Aspirator Device to remove fluid by suction from a cavity.

Assay Assessment of safety, potency and clarity of a drug.

Assessment Judging a situation, critical analysis of a situation, skill assessment of nursing students.

Assimilation Absorption and utilisation of food by the tissue.

Asthenia Debility, loss of strength.

Asthma Dyspnoea with wheezing and difficulty in expiration difficulty in breathing as in allergy.

Astigmatism Rays of light is not sharply focused on the retina, diffused image is focussed, seen either vertical or horizontal at a point of time.

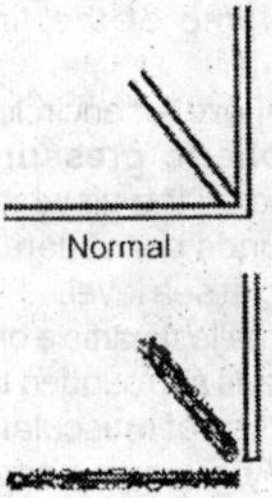

Normal and astigmatic error (line as seen)

Astringent Causing contraction and arresting discharges, agent with astringent action.

Astrocytoma Tumour of brain or spinal cord, brain cancer.

Asymmetry Unequal in size and shape of two halves of a structure.

Asymptomatic Without any symptoms.

Asystole No heart beat or cardiac arrest.

At risk Vulnerable to hazard, injury or disease.

Ataxia Irregular jerky movement because of poor muscular coordination.

Atelectasis Collapse of the lung due to injury or disease.

Atheroma Lipid with fibrous covering present within the artery.

Atherosclerosis Lesion of medium and large sized arteries with plaques of lipoid material and cholesterol in intima.

Athetosis Post-hemiplegic chorea in children which produce movements of hands and feet.

Athletes foot Tinea pedis a fungal infection in website of toes.

Atlas Name of the first cervical vertebra.

Atmosphere Air encircling the earth.

Atmospheric pressure Pressure exerted by the air which is usually 15 pounds per square inch or 760 mm Hg at sea level.

Atom Smallest particle of an element, a nucleus surrounded by electrons.

Atony Loss of muscular tone.

Atopy Allergic to some allergens which produce asthma, hay fever or eczema.

ATP Adenosine Tri Phosphate.

Atresia Birth defect where natural orifices are closed, common atresia are anal, vaginal and ear.

Atrial gallop It is represented as S_4 which has a higher pitch and if present it is elicited in the mitral area (apex) it sounds like 'dee-lub-dub' ($S_4 - S_1 - S_2$) that means atrial gallop follow-by heart sounds lub and dub indicate CCF.

Atrial Relating to the atrium, atrial flutter, atrial fibrillation, atrial septal defect, etc.

Atrioventricular Connected with both atrium and ventricle, AV node, AV block, AV valve, etc.

Atrium Auricle the upper chamber of the heart.

Atrophy Malnourishment, degeneration or lack of use leads to wasting of a tissue.

Atropine A drug derived from the deadly nightshade plant *atropa belladonna*. It has the following major functions in the human body: papillary dilation, muscular relaxation and reducing the gastric secretion.

ATS Anti Tetanus Serum a passive immunisation agent is given when a person is exposed to the risk of developing tetanus following injury or accident.

Attack Getting an episode of illness, usually refer to heart attack.

Attenuation Process of making a pathogen, non-pathogenic by repeated passage in culture either natural or artificial, vaccine is an attenuated preparation.

Attitude Positive or negative attitude in mental health, foetal position in the womb, position of human body in a given situation.

Attribute Characters that are not measurable, sex, death, survival, etc.

Atypical Not usual, irregular.

Audiogram Recording done by an audiogram.

Audiology Study of science of hearing, useful in evaluation of impaired hearing.

Audiologist Health professional or consultant in Audiology.

Audiometer An instrument to test the threshold of hearing in a patient suffering from hard of hearing.

Audit Review and evaluation of records done systematically.

Auditory assessment Assessing auditory function by Watch test or Weber and Rinne test.

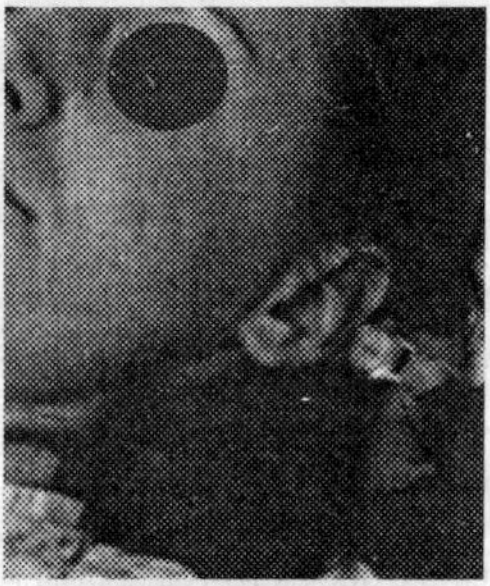

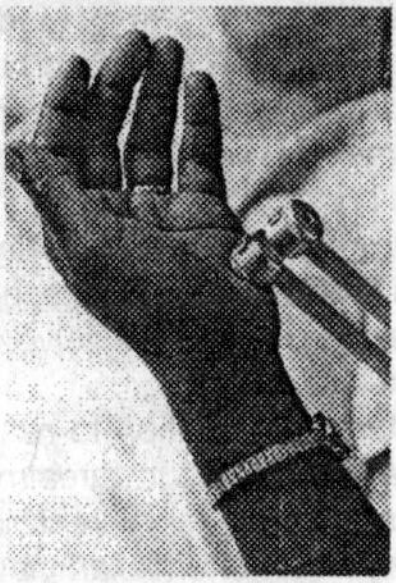

Watch test and Weber Rinne test

Aura Subjective manifestation experienced by a patient before getting fits, early premonition to epileptic fits.

Aural Pertaining to the ear.

Aureomycin Chlortetracycline effective in the treatment of some penicillin resistant infections.

Auricle Name for the external ear, old nomenclature for atrium.

Auricula Refers to auricle.

Auriscope Otoscope used in the examination of ear drum.

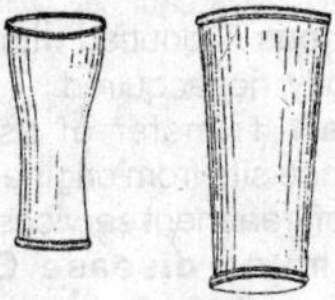

Foetoscope

Auscultation Listening to the sounds of internal organ by ear or stethoscope.

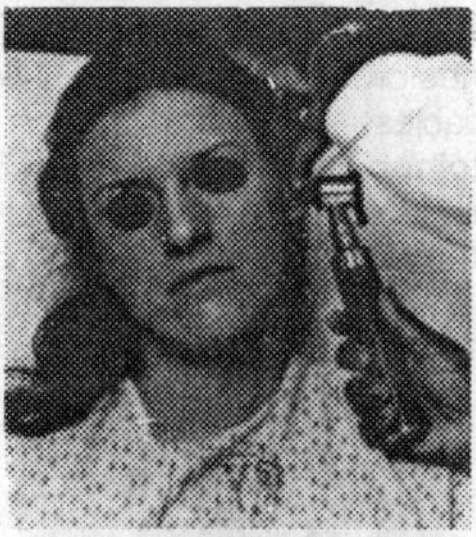

Otoscope

Australia antigen Present in serum of patient suffering from hepatitis B, hepatitis B surface antigen.

Autism It is subjective self centered trends of thought or behaviour.

Autoagglutination Agglutination occurring without the presence of an antigen, e.g. autohaemagglutination.

Autoantibody Antibody developed in an individual in response to his own tissue response, autoimmune.

Autoantigen Antigen present in one's own body that can produce antibody, autoimmune.

Autoclave It is a sterilising apparatus, common sterilising practice in a hospital.

Autogenous Produced within ones own body, not acquired.

Autograft Transfer of tissue to difference site from original site as a part of treatment services.

Autoimmune disease Clinical condition where ones own body develops antibody from its tissue culminating in self-destruction, Hashimoto's disease.

Autoimmunisation Formation of antibody against ones own tissue

Autoinfection Infection spread in ones own body e.g., thread worm, scabies.

Autoinoculation Self-introduction of micro-organisms in the body.

Autolet An automatic device called autolet used by diabetic patients who can self-monitor their blood glucose.

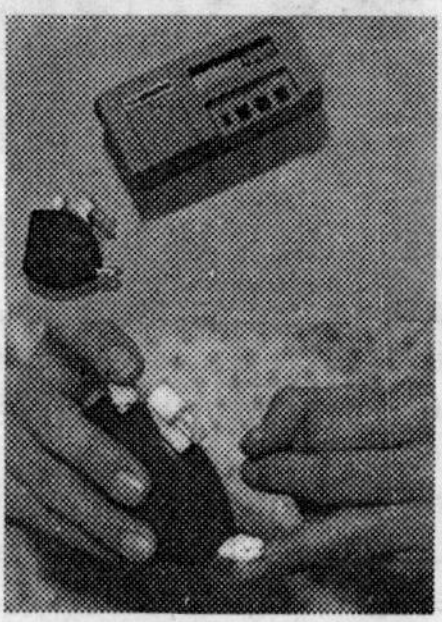

Autolet for diabetes

Autolysis Destruction of living tissues, common in pancreatic rupture.

Automatism Post-epileptic complication where patient performs an action of which he is entirely ignorant at that time.

Autonomic nervous system Nerves which control the smooth or involuntary muscle tissue of the internal organ.

Autonomic Self-governing control, autonomic nervous system activity sympathetic and parasympathetic actions work independently in our body.

Autonomous ethics Autonomic ethics deals with desirability of a thing particularly useful in health practice which is independent of others or under one's own law.

Autonomy of decision A patient taking a decision about his illness, for selecting a system of medicine, for selecting a doctor, for changing a doctor, for opting type of treatment is termed having *The autonomy of decision*.

Autonomy Full freedom, right of individuals to make choice, right to make decision for themselves, self-determination.

Autoplasty Adaptation to reality in mental health, autograft treatment in a person as a surgical treatment.

Autopsy Postmortem examination of dead to establish the cause of death, medico-legal procedure.

Autosomes Regular chromosomes excluding sex chromosome, 22 pairs autosomes in human body.

Auxiliary temperature Useful in caring of the newborn, recording auxiliary temperature will readily alert the nurse to rapid temperature changes that frequently occur in the newborn, useful than rectal temperature in the newborn care.

Avascular Not containing blood, no vessels present, necrotic tissue.

Avitaminosis Deficiency disease due to non-availability of vitamin.

Avulsion Tear occurred in a tissue or an organ, scalp aversion, phrenic nerve aversion, etc.

Axial skeleton Those bones including the spinal column and rib cage.

Axilla The armpit.

Axis Second vertebra in cervical region, line through the centre of a structure.

Axon A nerve fibre, nerve impulse pass through this cell fibre.

Ayurveda Native Indian treatment by plants and drugs, Indian system of medicine.

Azoospermia Absence of sperms in the semen, infertility.

Azotaemia Presence of urea and other nitrogenous waste material in the blood.

AZT Drug called Zidovudine, used in the treatment of HIV/AIDS.

Azygos Unilateral or unpaired, usually refers to azygos vein.

B

Babesiosis A protozoal infection which attack RBC.

Babinskis sign Great toe bends upwards when a stroke is made on the sole, Babinski positive indicate upper motor neurone lesion, physiological Babinski is present in babies.

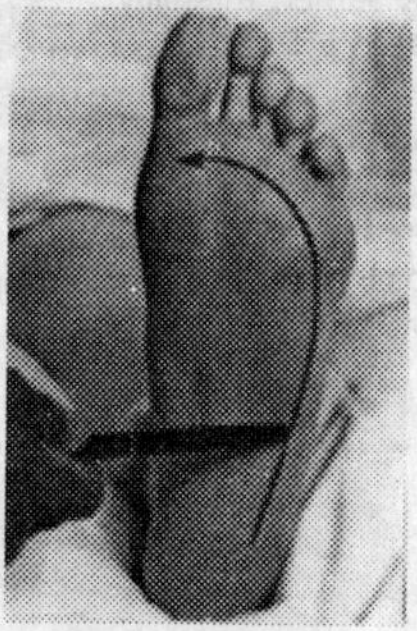

Babinski sign

Baby An infant. Types are: Battered **b**. Blue **b**.

Baby Friendly Hospital Initiative UNICEF's initiative which consists of following steps:

1. Breastfeeding policy available which is communicated to all staff.
2. All health care staff trained to implement the policy.
3. All pregnant women informed of the benefit and management of breastfeeding.
4. Mothers assisted to commence breastfeeding within half an hour of delivery.
5. Education of mothers for breast-feeding and maintenance of lactating even if they are separated from their babies.
6. Neonates to be given nothing other than breast milk unless medically necessary.
7. 24 hour rooming in.
8. On demand breastfeeding.
9. No teats or pacifiers to be given to breastfeeding babies.
10. Establishment of breastfeeding support groups.

Babylon Hammurabi able ruler of Babylon drew up a code of Law which was engraved on a pillar of hard stone and set up in the temple of Babylon, Oldest known medical ethics.

Bach remedies Flower remedy developed by Dr.Edward Bach who has used 38 types of flowers to treat emotional disturbances.

Bacillus Rod-shaped micro-organism which causes disease.

Bacilli
Coliform
Tetanus
Tuberculosis
Diphtheria

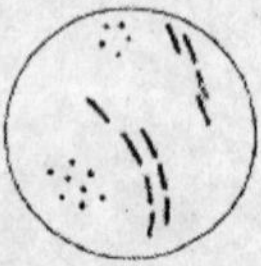

Bacteria

Back Posterior portion of the trunk from neck to pelvis.

Backache Common ailment called lumbago, pain in the back.

Bacteiostatic Chemotherapeutic agents and antibiotics which inhibits the growth of bacteria.

Bacteraemia Bacteria is present in the blood.

Bacterial As related to or with bacteria.

Bactericidal Chemotherapeutic agents and antibiotics which kills bacteria.

Bacteriology The study that deals with the scientific analysis and study of bacteria.

Bacteriophage They are used for phage typing, virus that infect bacteria.

Bacterium Organism that live on organic matter. Some are pathogenic and some are not. Types are *cocci, bacilli* and *spirilla*.

Bacteroid Structurally modified bacterium.

Bag technique Bag made of canvas, leather or light metal is used in home visiting. Specifications are made with bag and its content use by the public health nurse who visits families for primary health care.

Bag A sac or a pouch. Types are: Urine **b**. Ileostomy **b**. Colostomy **b**. Ice **b**.

Bagassosis Inhalation of sugar cane dust produces Bagassosis, Industry hazard in paper, card board and rayon factory.

Baker's cyst Synovial cyst in popliteal fossa common in bakers.

Balanced diet Diet containing required proximate principles, calories, vitamins, minerals and trace elements that can meet the requirement for healthy life.

Balanced diet for an adult.

Items(G.)	*Sedentary man*	*Sedentary woman*
Cereals	460	410
Pulses	40	40
Leafy veg	40	40
Other veg	60	40
Roots, tubers	50	50
Milk	150	100
Oil and fat	40	20
Sugar and jaggery	30	20

Balanitis Inflammation of glans penis secondary to phimosis.

Balantidiasis a protozoal infection causing dysentery, colitis.

Baldness Alopecia, no scalp hairs.

BAL British Anti Lewisite, Dimercaprol, antidote used in warfare.

Balloon technique The use of inflated balloons to apply medication or to change the temperature in hollow organs such as stomach or bladder.

Ballottement A test used in pregnancy, abdominal palpation of uterus, in P.V. examination a finger push upwards rebounds back.

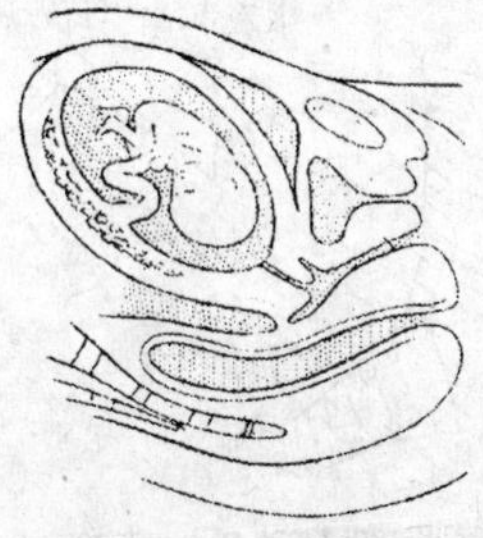

Ballottement

Balm Asmoothening agent used for external application.

Balneology Science that deals with different kinds of bathing.

Balneum vaporis Vapour bath, a bath therapy, a bath treatment:

Balsam Resins combined with oil from vegetable is extracted. Types are Canada **b**. Mecca **b.** Sulphur **b.**

Bandage Piece of gauze to wrap over any part of the body commonly Used in first aid treatment. Types are Abdominal **b.** Circular **b**. Elastic **b**. Plastic **b**. Pressure **b**. Spica **b**. Triangular **b**.

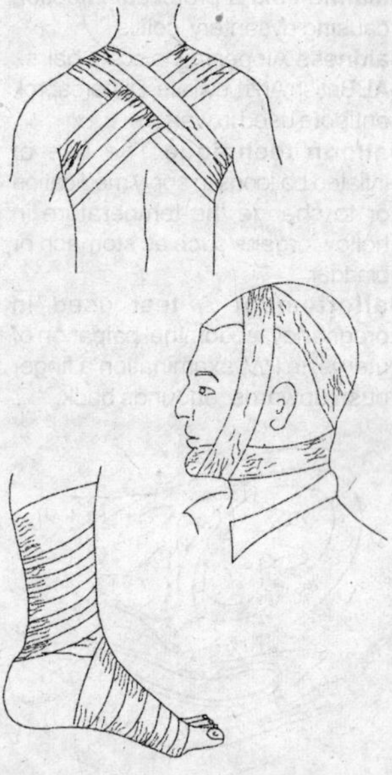

Different types of bandages

Banding Applying a band to stop the flow of blood in a vessel.

Bang's disease Brucella infection, a zoonotic disease, Malta fever, Produce abortion in animals and hence the name.

Bar diagram A diagram for data presentation, indicate the frequency of a character. Types are: *Simple, Multiple* and *Component* bar diagrams.

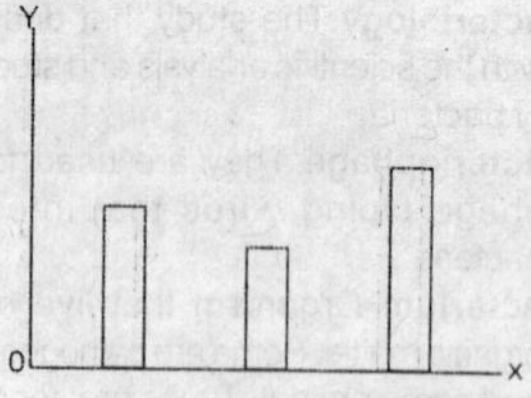

Bar diagram

Barber's itch Infection of the hair follicle by staphylococci bacteria.

Barbiturate A sedative and hypnotic drug, referred to phenobarbitone.

Barium Silvery metallic element used in radiology as contrast medium, barium enema, barium meal.

Barometer Instrument used to measure the atmosphere pressure.

Baroreceptor Receptors situated in carotid sinus and aortic arch, which control blood pressure, they are controlled by glasso-pharyngeal nerve and vagus nerve.

Barr body Present in female cell nuclear membrane, inactive X chromosome.

Barrel chest Normal elliptical shape is lost and has become rounded, Emphysematous chest.

Barrier Created obstruction. Types are Nursing **b**. Blood brain **b**.

Placental **b**. Protective **b**. Contraceptive **b.**

Bartholin duct Sublingual salivary gland duct.

Bartholin gland Glands in labia majora which open into vulva.

Bartonella Sand fly transmitted pathogens, Rickettsiales.

Bartter's syndrome Pathological changes in juxtaglomerular cells produce hyperaldosteronism.

Basal ganglia Nerve cell collection in base of the cerebrum, help in voluntary muscular movement.

Basement membrane Supporting cell layer at the base of epidermis and mucous membrane.

Basilar One situated in the base e.g., basilar artery.

Basiotribe Instrument used in crushing the head of dead foetus, used in stillbirth delivery.

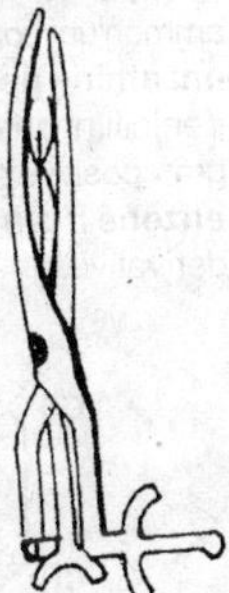

Basiotribe

Basophilia Abnormal increase of basophils as in severe anaemia, leukaemia, lead poisoning.

Bath Apparatus to immerse items, body wash for cleansing purpose, therapeutic bath with vapour, mud, aroma.

Bath by sponge Patient's body wiped with sponge.

Battered child syndrome Injuries inflicted on the body of children.

BBT Basal Body Temperature.

BCG BCG vaccine, named after Bacille Calmette Guerin.

Beanpole family It is the result of one child families in the society.

Bearing down Pain experienced during second stage of labour, child labour, pain of labour.

Beaver respirator Respirator used in bulbospinal polio paralysis, with tracheostomy beaver type of positive pressure respirator is used, used when controlled respiration is required over a long period, needs tube feeding.

Bicarbonate A parameter in acid and base balance, salt containing HCO_3.

Bed making A nursing skill to suit the bed to the sick, clean, smooth linens, covers of the right warmth for the season, protective rubber pads, making one half of the bed while the patient lies on the other, rolling the patient gently to the made-up side and finishing up the other.

Bed scale When patient is to be weighted in the bed like nephrotic syndrome immobile patient, bed scale is used.

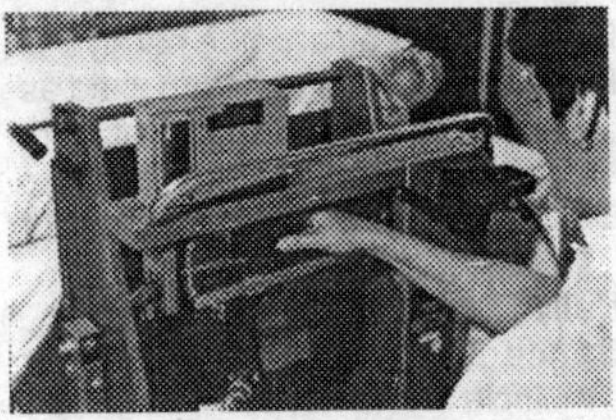

Bed scale

Bed wetting Unreadiness of the child to control bladder evacuation, no bladder control.

Bed A tissue is supported by supporting structure, a couch to sleep.

Bedboard Hard board as support below the mattress.

Bedding care Mattress and pillow protected by short mackintosh.

Bedpan A shallow vessel to bedridden patient for toilet in the bed.

Bedrest Restriction of patient movement by bedrest on therapeutic ground.

Bedsore Decubitus ulcer, semicomatous patient or comatous patients develop pressure sore.

Behaviour Reaction of human beings to external stimulus or an internal stimulus, event of an individual which are not intended or planned

Benign Not progressive, not cancerous.

Bejel A non-venereal disease caused by *Treponema pertenue*.

Belching Stomach gas is expelled through mouth.

Belief Whatever we feel true and hold true.

Beliefs Ideas developed by an individual over a period of time this is influenced by culture, literacy and religion.

Bell's palsy Facial nerve paralysis.

Belladonna A plant extract used as antispasmodic and pupil dilatation. Active ingredient is *atropine*

Bellini's tubule Connecting tubule of the kidney.

Belly The abdomen, bulging muscle.

Bence Zones protein Present in multiple myeloma, heated urine do not show this protein.

Benedict's test A qualitative test to find out the presence of a reducing agent like sugar present in urine 5 CC Benedict's reagent in a test tube + 8 drops urine observe for red, yellow or green precipitate.

Benedict's solution Solution containing:

- Sodium citrate.
- Sodium carbonate.
- Potassium sulfocyanate.
- Copper sulphate.

Used for urine test for sugar.

Beneficence One of the major principles of bioethics, "The principle of doing good which is called Beneficence in ethics".

Benign hypertrophy of the prostate Enlargement of prostate in elderly causing obstruction of urethra, a surgical condition in elderly males.

Benzalkonium chloride A surface disinfectant from quaternary ammonium compound.

Benzathine penicillin A long-acting penicillin antibiotic used against grampositive organisms.

Benzene It is a solvent from coal tar derivative.

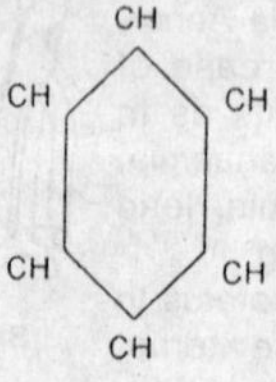

Benzene

Benzhexol Drug used in Parkinson's disease.

Benzocaine Local anaesthetic used as surface anaesthetic.

Benzoin A resin extract from plant, in ulcer treatment it is used as ulcer protectant.

Benzyl benzoate External applicator in the treatment of scabies, emulsion.

Benzylpenicillin Soluble penicillin used for quick absorption and for high blood level.

Bereavement Death or separation of loved ones.

Beri beri Thiamine deficiency state, may be dry or wet beri beri.

Berylliosis A pneumoconiosis by occupational inhalation of beryllium produces a chronic lung disorder.

Bestiality Sexual offence with lower animals.

Beta adrenergic receptor blockers These receptors are activators of adrenaline and noradrenaline, they are present in intestine, bronchi, heart and blood vessels.

Beta blockers Drug used in blocking the action of adrenaline on beta-adrenergic receptors in heart muscle.

Beta lactose An isomer of lactose which is more soluble and sweeter than lactose.

Betamethasone It is a synthetic glucocorticoid.

Betz cells Pyramidal cells with their axon in pyramidal tract in motor cortex.

Bezoar Mass of hair in the stomach, a surgical condition.

BHC Benzene Hexa Chloride a residual insecticide spray.

Bhore committee Survey report of health survey and development committee 1946 is a major document which has provided health planning in India.

Bias When difference occurs between observed value and true value it is said to be biased, research findings.

Biceps Powerful flexor muscle of the arm which has 2 heads.

Biconcave Both the surfaces of the lens are hollow.

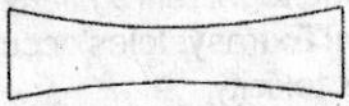

Biconcave lens

Biconvex Both the surfaces of the lens are bulged.

Biconvex lens

Bicornis Two horns are present in a uterus, incomplete union of Mullerian ducts leads to bicornis uterus.

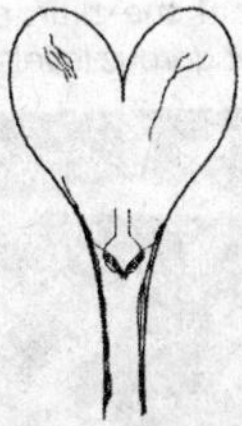

Bicornuate uterus

Bicornuate Similar meaning to bicornis.

Bicuspid Mitral valve, premolar teeth, one which has two projections.

Bicycle ergometer Fixed bicycle used for cardiac exercise at diagnosis and at post-operative follow-up.

Bifid When a part is divided into 2 parts, cleft lip, bifid tongue.

Bifocal Spectacle with two foci one for near vision and the other for distant vision.

Bifurcate To divide into 2 branches like artery, vein or nerve.

Bigeminal Occurrence twice, 2 pulse, 2 heart beat, 2 impulse occurring together regularly.

Bigemini Extrasystoles occurring in digitalis toxicity.

Biguanide Oral hypoglycaemic agent used in the treatment of diabetes.

Bilateral On both sides of a structure, similar on either side.

Bile Greenish yellow secretion of the liver which is collected in the gallbladder, related words are *bile duct, bile pigment, bile salt.*

Bilharzias Helminthic infestation by blood fluke, schistosomiasis.

Bili lites Infant's skin surface is exposed to the light for prescribed time called phototherapy. This is to help prevent the bilirubin from reaching dangerous levels.

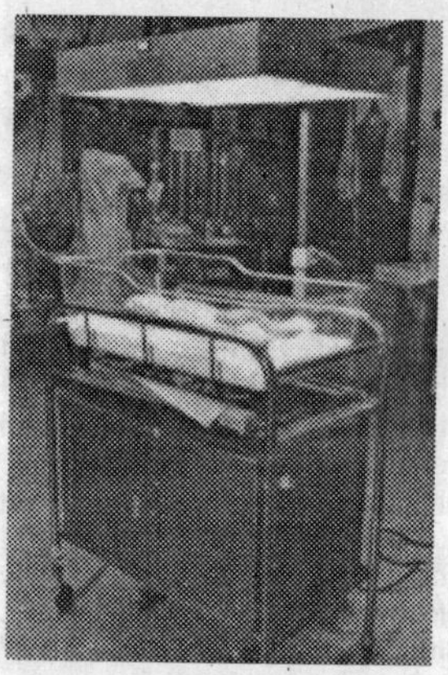

Bili lites phototherapy

Biliary Connected with bile, biliary fistula, biliary colic.

Biliousness An obsolete term formerly applied to all sorts of digestive disturbances.

Bilirubin Bile pigments produced by breakdown of haem. Types are direct and indirect bilirubin.

Biliverdin It is oxidised form of bilirubin.

Billings's method of contraception Ovulation time is found out by observing changes in cervical mucus, now rarely used method of contraception.

Bimanual Examination done by using both hands, gynaecological examination, examination by one hand on abdomen and the other in the vagina for internal genital organs.

Binary A structure made with 2 parts, binary scale, and binary fission.

Binet's test Method developed by Dr. Binet to assess mental age of a child.

Bing negative This suggests that it is normal ear, in which increase and decrease in loudness is perceived when a vibrating tuning fork is held on mastoid process and auditory meatus is closed and opened frequently.

Bing positive This suggests that there is hearing impairment which is sensineural in nature.

Binocular Pertaining to both the eyes, to visualise in both eyes, to see through both eye pieces provided in a microscope.

Binovular Outcome from two ova as in case of twins.

Bioethics Enunciated by Beauchamp and Childress. It deals with problems that have risen out of recent developments in science and technology.

Bioassay Biological assessment is made through animal experiments, testing the effect of a drug on an organ or in animal.

Biochemistry The study of chemistry of living beings, both of animals and human kingdom.

Biofeedback Medical evidence which can show that there is satisfactory performance of autonomic nervous system.

Biogenesis Genesis of life, life is possible only by living things and not by nonliving things in this universe.

Biohazard Hazards occurring due to auto-inoculation, during surgery, working with radioactive material by contamination by hospital waste material, hospitals cross infection, needle stick injury resulting in HIV infection, etc.

Biological transmission Disease transmission by arthropod vectors through propagative cyclo-propagative and cyclodevelopment methods as seen with plague, malaria and filaria respectively.

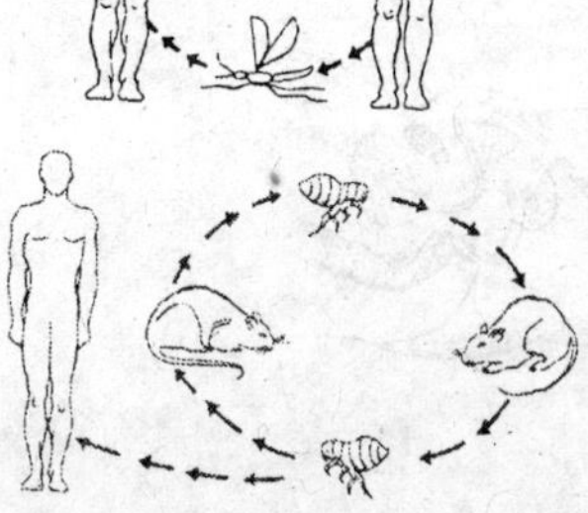

Biological transmission

Biology Study of evolution structure and function of living organisms.

Biomedicine Clinical medicine which is based on the proved principles of biochemistry and biophysiology.

Biometry Mathematical analysis of biological data, determination of expectation of life, application of statistics in biosciences.

Bionursing Biology knowledge is used in nursing practice.

Biopsy Removal of tissue from an organ for the purpose of pathological diagnosis.

Biostatistics Statistics that deals with the statistics of births, deaths, morbidity, fertility and demography of man, branch of biometry.

Biotherapy Treatment with serum and vaccine, treatment with live organism like lactobacillus, treatment with body secretions like bile.

Biotic Related to the living organism.

Biotin Part of vitamin B complex and is present in normal diet.

Biparietal Related to either parietal bones or parietal eminence.

Biparous Giving birth to two off-springs, producing two ova.

Bipedal By both legs, pertaining to both feet.

Birth and death registration A source of vital statistics, reliable source of statistics, it is compulsory to register these in India.

Birth control Pregnancy is avoided through contraceptives.

Birth defects Childhood medical problems, physical defects and organ defects occurring due to malformation.

Birth marks Colouration from the tiny vessels concentrated in a small area of skin, caused by patches of pigment in the skin, freckles, pigmented patches.

Birth A vital event that indicates the delivery of human baby either by natural or artificial confinement, prefixing birth many words are used in medical field like birth rate; birth control; birth mark, etc.

Birthing chair Special chair used in labour ward.

Birthing pool A pool of water is used for allowing a woman to deliver her baby.

Bis in die Twice a day.

Bisexual Person who has both male and female gonads.

Bisgard's treatment A treatment for varicose ulcers by using Bisgard's solution and gauze dressing in wet condition, worn from morning to evening, each fresh dressing is covered with elastic bandage.

Bitot's spot Shiny greyish spots on the cornea a sign of vitamin A deficiency.

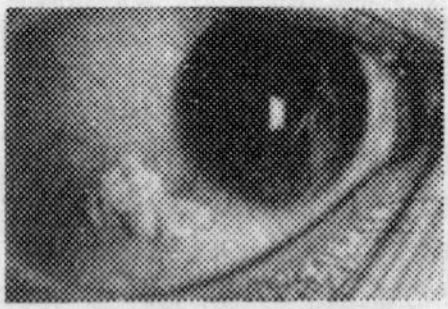

Bitot's spot

Black eye It is due to a blow on the eye resulting in bruising of the lid.

Black measles Severe haemorrhagic rashes in measles infection.

Blackhead A plug of dried sebum in excretory duct of the skin, comedo.

Blackout Diminished vision and momentary unconsciousness in aviators due to reduced circulation to brain and retina.

Blackwater fever Severe form of malaria caused by *Plasmodium falciparam* causing dark urine.

Bladder irrigation Done for cystitis, include catheterisation and irrigation of bladder.

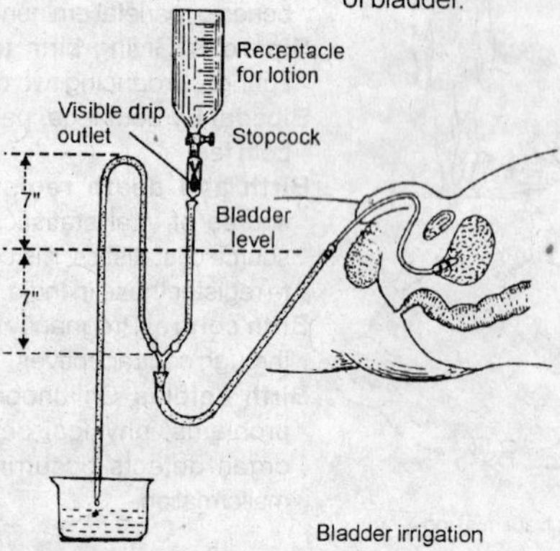

Bladder irrigation

Bladder Any membranous sac which holds gas or liquid, urinary bladder, gallbladder.

Blakemore tubes Triple lumen oesophageal nasogastric tube developed by Blakemore, used as a tamponade for the control of oesophageal bleeding.

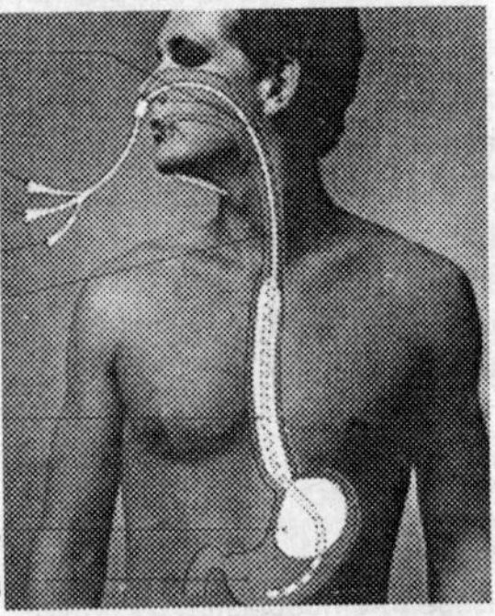

Oesophageal tube

1. Pharynx
2. Oesophageal balloon
3. Gastric aspirate
4. Gastric balloon
5. Oesophagus
6. Oesophageal balloon
7. Gastric balloon
8. Stomach

Bland diet Diet which do not contain spices or hard food stuffs, a therapeutic diet.

Blanket Along with position, warmth by blanket is the treatment for internal haemorrhage to avoid overheating the body.

Blastocyst A stage in the development of fertilised ovum, blastula.

Blastoma Cancerous tumour containing immature undifferentiated cells.

Blastula Blastocyst, a stage in the development of fertilised ovum.

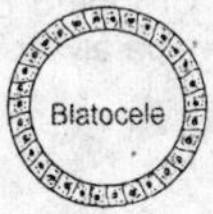

Blastula

BLB mask Oronasal apparatus used for oxygen therapy, Boothby Lovelace and Bulbulian apparatus.

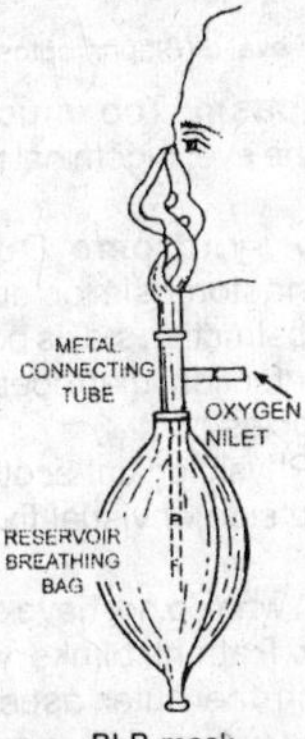

BLB mask

Bleaching powder Common disinfectant used in the disinfection of water, $CaOCl_2$, one ounce per 1000 gallons used.

Bleb Name given for a blister.

Bleeder Haemophilia patient, artery or vein which is difficult to ligate during operation.

Bleeding time Lab test done to find out the time taken for the bleeding to stop after a pin prick, 1 to 3 minutes.

Blepharitis Infection and inflammation of the eyelids.

Blepharophimosis Abnormal narrow eyelid aperture due to congenital condition or due to chronic inflammation.

Blepharoptosis Drooping of an eyelid due to nerve paralysis.

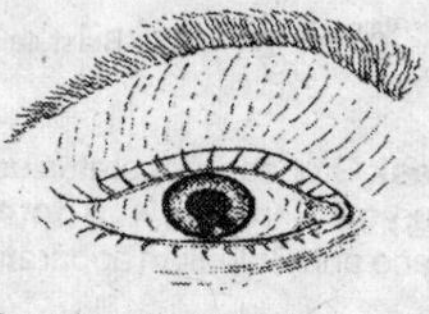

Drooping of eyelid (Blepharoptosis)

Blepharospasm Too much of winking of the eye, trigeminal nerve disease.

Blind loop syndrome Due to surgical anastomosis or due to intestinal obstruction stasis occurs leading to infection, diarrhoea and salt deficiencies.

Blind spot Physiological scotoma, scotoma outside of visual fixation point.

Blind Person who do not have sight.

Blink reflex Patient blinks when gently touch the outer aspect of each cornea with a wisp of cotton, absence indicates trigeminal nerve lesion.

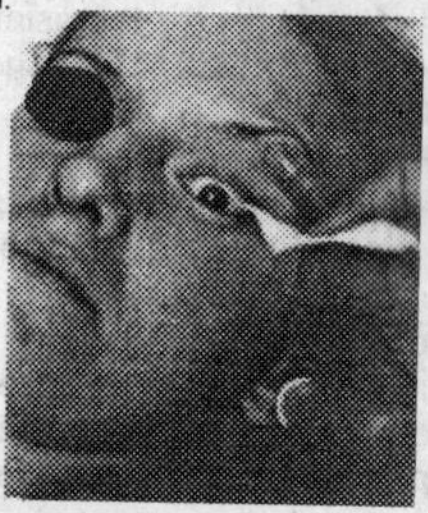

Blink reflex

Blister A bleb or a vesicle caused by a bruise.

Bloch' scale A series of solutions of tincture of benzoin in glycerinated water used to determine albumin precipitated in urine.

Block Obstruction, heart block, nerve block, regional block by anaesthesia.

Blood bank Blood collection, storage and distribution in a systematised way in the hospital.

Blood brain barrier A permeable membrane between blood and brain, barrier which separates blood and the brain.

Blood clotting It is natural defence mechanism of human body to prevent the bleeding, if it occurs inside the vessel then it could block the blood flow, it is influenced by plasma coagulation factors.

Coagulation factor	*Designated number*
Fibrinogen	I
Prothrombin	II
Tissue thromboplastin	III
Calcium	IV
Factor seven	VII
Antihaemophilic factor	VIII
Christmas factor	IX
Stuart factor	X
Plasma thromboplastin antecedent	XI
Hageman factor	XII
Fibrin stabilising factor	XIII

Table: Plasma coagulation factors

Calcium
Vitamin K → → Prothrombin
Thrombokinase
↓
Thrombin + Fibrinogen
↓
Fibrin + Blood cells
↓
Clot

Blood clotting process

Blood count Expression of blood cells per litre of blood, RBC count, WBC count, platelet count, etc.

Blood dyscrasia Abnormality of blood clotting mechanism of blood cells.

Blood fractions Separated blood portions of the blood used for purposes other than transfusion.

Blood group Human show 4 blood groups A, B, O, and AB, Rh sub-systems are known, helpful in blood transfusion.

Blood urea Nitrogenous waste material which ranges from 3 to 7 mmol per litre, increases in renal failure.

Blood platelets Small greyish discs in the blood which collect at the site of any wound and appear to assist in forming clots.

Blood pressure The pressure of blood against the inner walls of the blood vessels as it is being pumped through the circulating system.

Blood sugar Refers to the level of glucose in the blood, upper limit is 116 mg per dL in fasting and upper limit is 140 mg/dL post-prandial.

Blood transfusion Giving blood to patients in selected indications like surgery, injury, severe bleeding, severe anaemia, etc.

Blood typing The identification of blood with respect to the group in which it belongs.

Blood The fluid that circulates through heart, arterial and venous blood, oxalated blood is collected for lab examination.

Bloom's approach It is an approach in lesson plan popularly known as Bloom's evaluation approach, a methodology in teaching.

Blue baby Cyanosis of the newborn due to congenital malformation of the heart.

Blue cross The title and emblem of plans organised to insure the costs of hospital care.

Blue shield The title and emblem of medically organised plans to insure the costs of medical and surgical treatment.

Blush Redness of face due to emotional condition, heat flush.

BMI Weight/height^2 used as an index to assess obesity.

BMR Basal Metabolic Rate.

BTB Bobath technique of bath approach for physiotherapy to neurological conditions.

Boa's point Pain to touch on the left of 12th dorsal vertebra, diagnostic of gastric ulcer.

BOD Biological Oxidation Demand, sanitary indicators of sullage and sewage.

Body ketone Acetone, acetoacetic acid and beta-hydroxy butyric acid are called body ketone.

Body language Signs of communication, communication through gestures.

Body Mass of material, major part of an organ, thorax and abdomen.

Boil Skin infection caused by staphylococci, a furuncle, germ infection of skin.

Bolus A big tablet for swallowing, masticated food ready for swallowing.

Bone Connective tissue of skeleton, common words are bone marrow and bone graft.

Bordetella Name of the genus of bacteria which causes whooping cough.

Boric acid It is a mild antiseptic powder.

Both's respirator It is a negative positive pressure apparatus used as mechanical respirator, artificial aid for respiration over a long period.

Botulism Food poisoning due to clostridium botulinum, poisoning is due to a neurotoxin called *botulin*.

Bougie A flexible instrument used to dilate urethra or oesophagus.

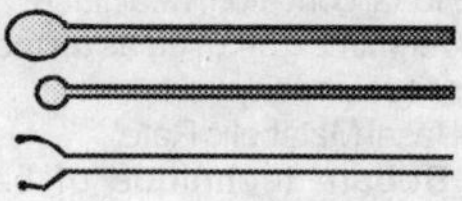

Bougie

Bout It refers to an attack of bleeding, convulsion, vomiting and diarrhoea.

Bovine Related to cows, bovine tuberculosis.

Bowel habit One of the principles of personal hygiene.

Bowel Refers to intestine.

Bowline traction knot This is the best knot that do not slip and hence is used in traction.

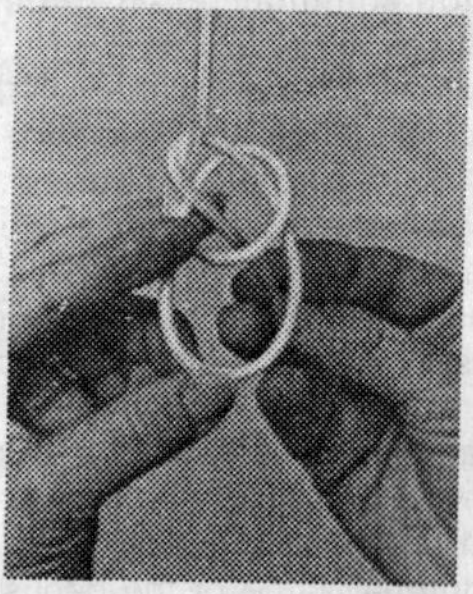

Bowline traction knot

Bowman's capsule Expanded end of kidney tubule which surrounds the glomerulus.

BP It is the pressure exerted on artery wall by the blood when it is flowing, systolic and diastolic BP, normally 120/80 mmHg.

BPL inactivated vaccine Cheap and cost benefit inactivated nervous vaccine used as vaccination of persons bitten by infected dog.

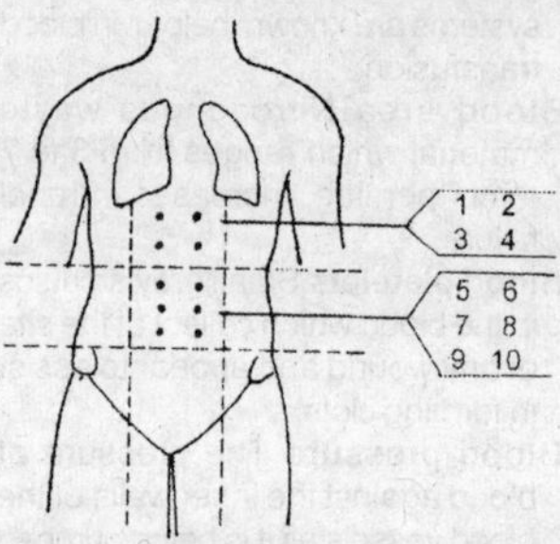

Site for BPL inactivated ARV vaccine

Branchial Related to brachia of developing embryo, branchial cyst, branchial sinus.

Brachioradialis reflex Evaluating deep tendon reflex, testing brachioradialis (supinator) reflex for C5 and C6 innervations.

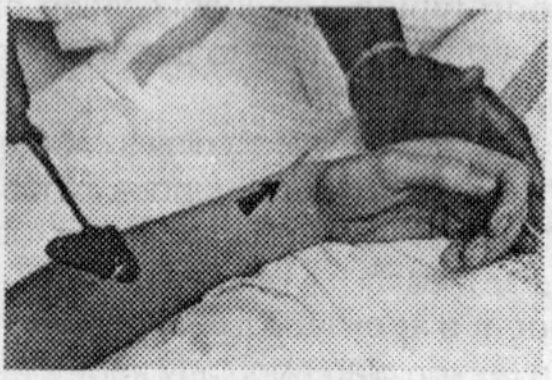

Testing brachioradialis reflex

Bracycardia Other name for bradycardia, low heart rate.

Bradycardia Low heart rate, low pulse rate.

Bradykinin Powerful vasodilator from degradation of protein by enzymes which causes smooth muscle contraction.

Bradypnoea Abnormal low respiratory rate, slow breathing.

Braille Louis Braille developed this method of printing useful for blind, raised dots feeling for reading.

Brain death Straight line in isoelectric EEG for 30 seconds defines definite death of human being.

Brain waves Tiny recordable electrical impulses reflecting activities in brain.

Brain Part of nervous system which is located in the skull.

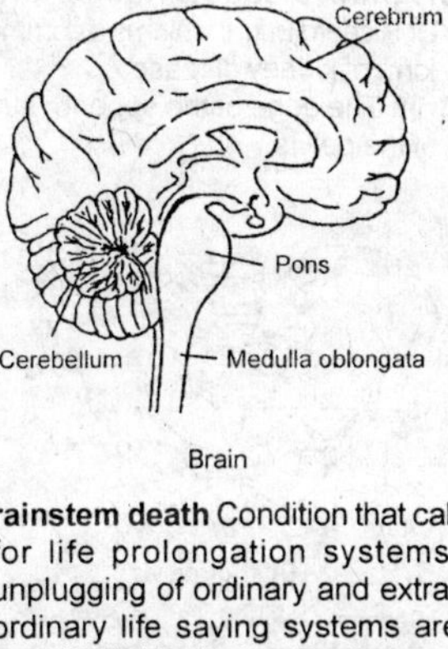

Brain

Brainstem death Condition that call for life prolongation systems, unplugging of ordinary and extraordinary life saving systems are permitted at Brainstem Death.

Bran bathe A bath for the relief of eczematous skin conditions, bran used is 2 lb in 30 gallons of water.

Bellows A modified bag used to produce positive pressure ventilation as an alternative to the first aiders own breath, porton bellows.

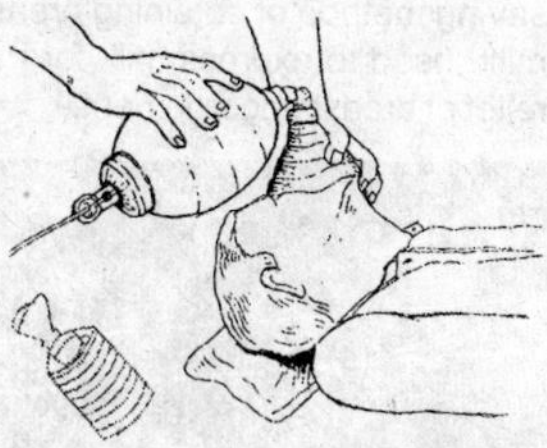

Bellow in Ambu resuscitator

Break bone fever Dengue fever caused by Arbovirus which belong to B group.

Breakpoint chlorination Best method of chlorination of water in large scale supply.

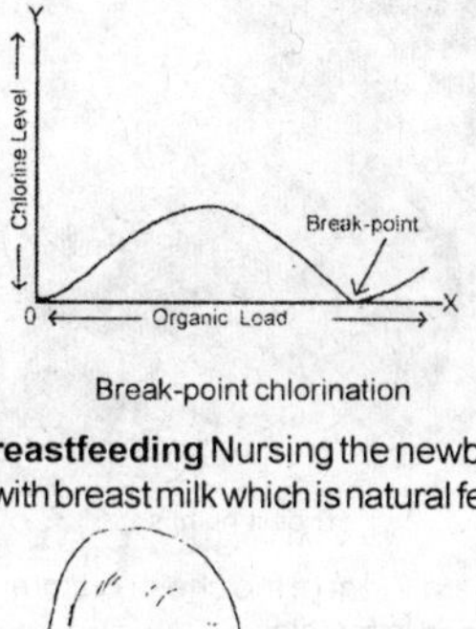

Break-point chlorination

Breastfeeding Nursing the newborn with breast milk which is natural feed.

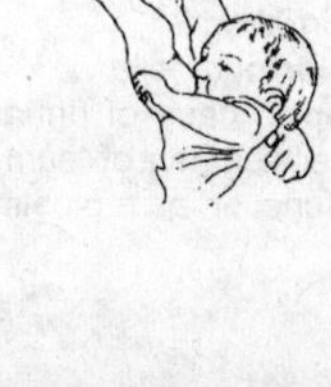

Breastfeeding

Breast pumps Efficient and time saving method of obtaining breast milk, used to express milk for the relief of breast engorgement.

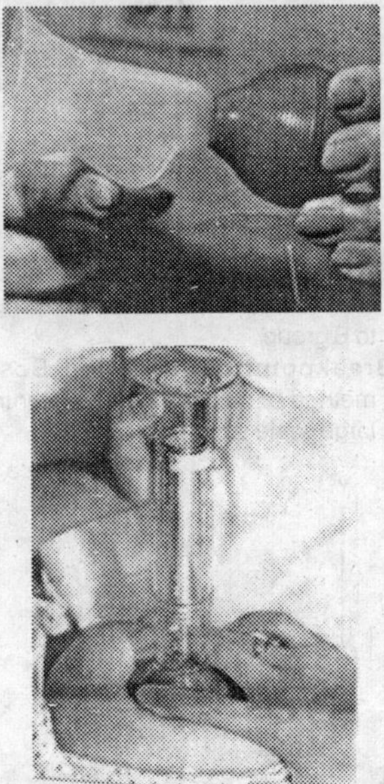

Breast pumps

Breast Front of the chest, mammary gland in females.

Breath Inspiration and expiration, normal breathing.

Breech Meaning buttocks, breech presentation in labour.

Bregma Anterior fontanelle.

Bricker's loop In case of urinary bladder cancer, segment of ileum is removed to function as a pipeline for the urine.

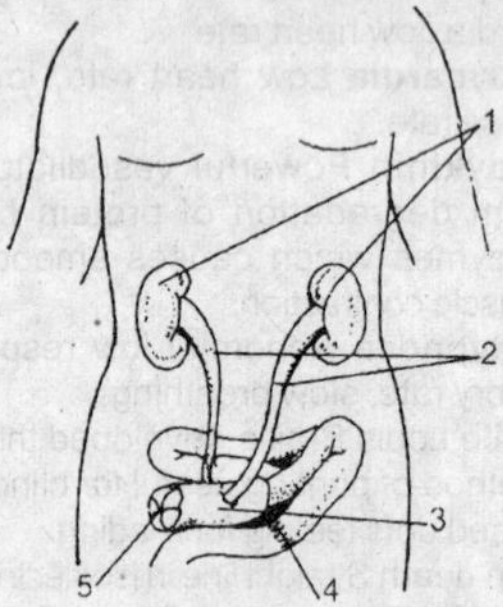

Bricker's loop

1. Kidneys
2. Ureters
3. Ileal conduit
4. Anastomosis of ileum
5. Stoma

Bridge Gap left after tooth extraction.

Bright's disease Named after Dr.Richard Bright which is a common form of kidney disease.

Brim The edge of the superior strait of the pelvis.

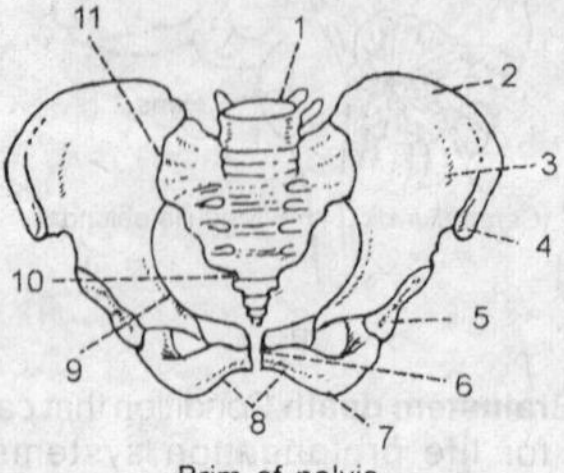

Brim of pelvis

1. Sacrum
2. Crest of Ilium
3. Iliac Fossa
4. Anterior Spine of Ilium
5. Acetabulum
6. Symphysis Pubis
7. Ischial Tuberosity
8. Sub-Pubic Angle
9. Brim of Pelvis
10. Sacro-Coccygeal Joint
11. Sacro-Iliac Joint

Broad ligament Peritoneal folds from uterus to sides of pelvis including vessels.

Broca's area Speech area, area in the left cerebral hemisphere, lesion of the area causes speech impairment.

Brodie's abscess Bone abscess which is chronic in nature named after Dr. Brodie.

Brompton cocktail Used in the relief of pain in terminal illness, morphine in chloroform water, morphine cocaine and diamorphine.

Bromsulphathalein Dye used in the laboratory while testing liver function

Bronchi Plural form of bronchus.

Bronchiectasis Destruction and dilatation of bronchioles, congenital or acquired.

Bronchitis Infection and inflammation of bronchi.

Bronchodilator Drug used for dilatation of bronchi.

Bronchography Radiological examination of bronchi by using radio-opaque medium.

Bronchopneumonia Descending infection from bronchi to bronchiole and to alveoli.

Bronchoscope Endoscope used by the surgeon to visualise bronchi during surgical intervention.

Bronchospasm In allergic conditions, sudden constriction of plain muscles of wall of bronchi causing difficulty in breathing.

Bronchus Larger passage of bronchi which allow air entry.

Broviac catheter Special catheter used to provide central venous line.

Brown fat Adipose tissue on the body of the newborn, help in hypothermia.

Broxton Hicks contraction Intermittent contraction of the uterus after the third month of pregnancy, a pregnancy sign.

Brucella A zoonotic disease which attack man, genus of bacteria.

Brucellosis Infection by Brucella, undulant fever, Malta fever, Mediterranean fever.

Brudzinski's sign A test for detection of meningeal irritation, flexion of one thigh cause the flexion of other thigh, flexion of neck cause bilateral flexion of hips and knees.

Bruise A contusion injury, superficial abrasion.

Bruit An abnormal murmur heard on auscultation.

Bryant's traction Employed for infants with fractured femurs, bilateral traction modified in congenital dislocation of hips.

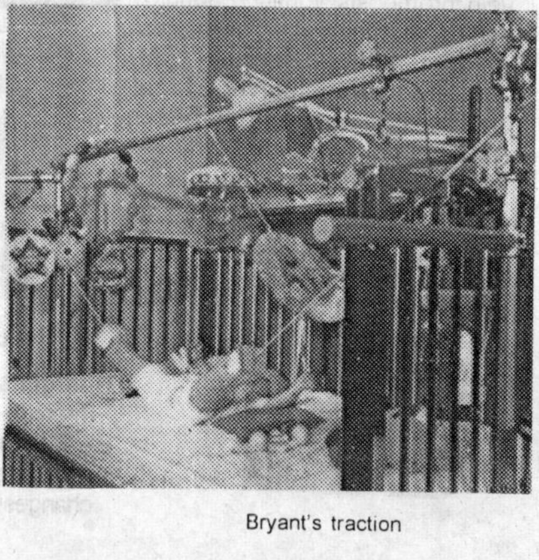

Bryant's traction

Bubo Inguinal lymphadenitis, axillary lymphadenitis, bubonic plague.

Bubonic Characterised by the appearance of bubo.

Buccal Related to mouth, related to cheek.

Buccinator It ridges mandible; alveolar process of maxilla and pterygo-mandibular ligament, help in compression of cheek, helps in retraction of mouth.

Buck's boot An extension traction by adhesive straps, indicated in patients who require presurgical immobilisation of fracture hip.

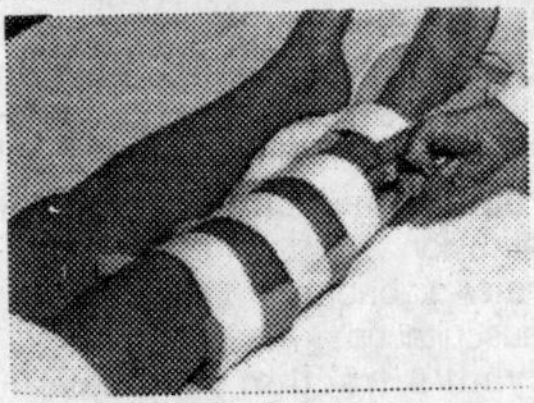

Buck's boot

Budd-Chiari syndrome Hepatic vein thrombosis, vomiting jaundice and hepatomegaly follows ascites.

Buerger Allen exercise It is indicated in occlusive arterial disorders like Buerger's disease or Raynaud's disease.

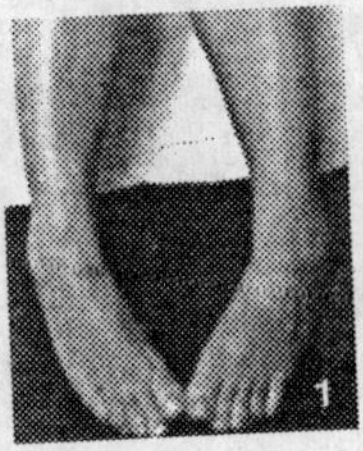

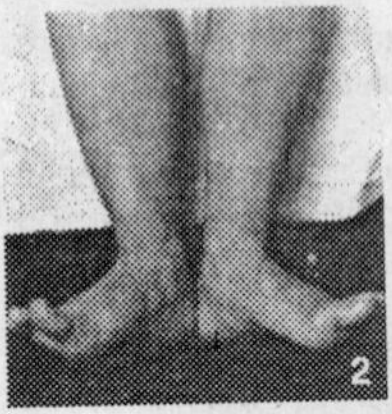

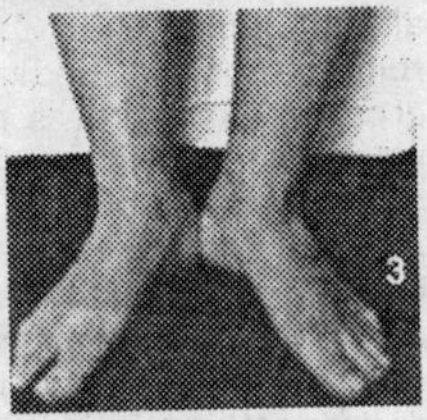

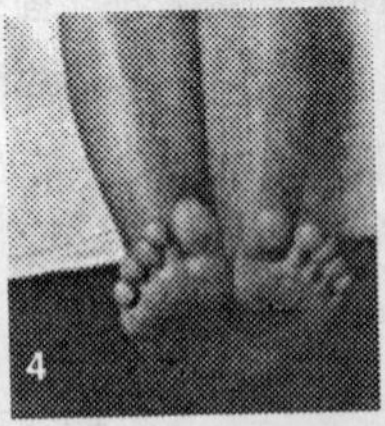

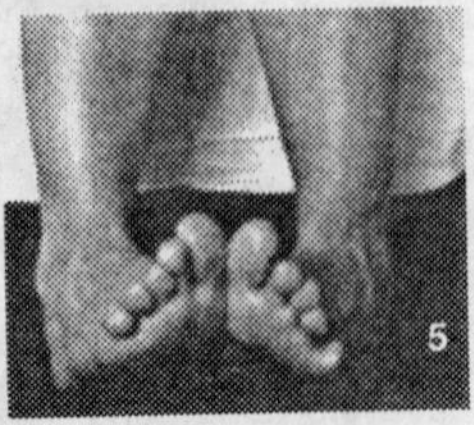

Buerger Allen exercise

Buerger's disease Other name for thrombo-angitis obliterans.

Buffer Physiological system which protects from unnatural body changes, shock preventing, $NaHCO_3$

as a buffer of blood, which do not allow concentration of chemicals.

Bulb Rounded organ, rounded mass, bulb of aorta, bulb of ovary.

Bulb syringe Normal item kept in newborn's crib for removing secretions in the nose and mouth.

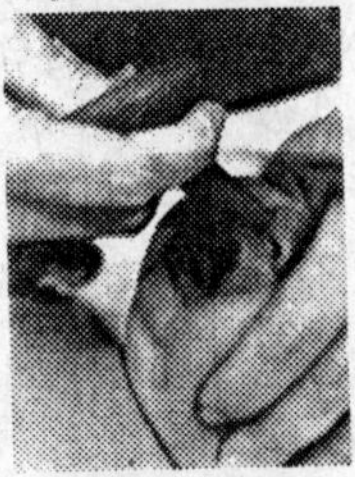

Bulb syringe

Bulbar Related to round organ, related to medulla oblongata.

Bulbourethral Related to round organ of urethra, bulb of urethra, bulb of penis.

Bulla A blister containing considerable quantity of fluid.

BUN Blood Urea Nitrogen.

Bundle A band composed of nerve fibres.

Bundle of His Contains 4* parts, it is muscular band with nerve fibres which connect the auricle to the ventricle, its degeneration produces heart block.

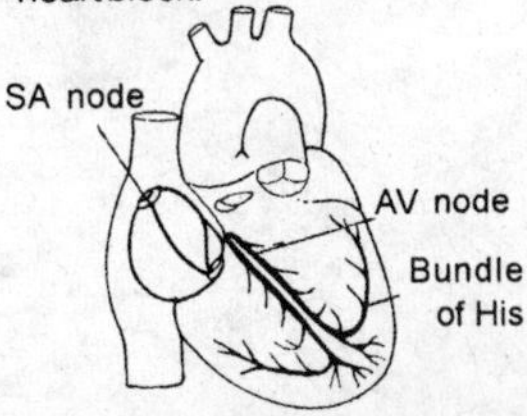

Bundle of His

- * The A V node (main bundle).
- * The right septal division.
- * The left septal division.
- * The terminal divisions.

Bundle Unidirectional nerve fibres.

Bunion Swelling of the bursa of metatarsophallangeal joint, swelling due to misfit shoes.

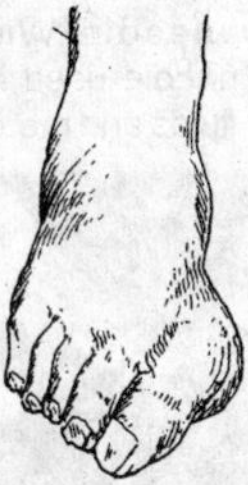

Bunion

Buphthalmos Manifestation of congenital glaucoma, enlarged eye ball.

Burr It is surgical drilling done on bone and teeth, burr hole.

Burkitt's lymphoma Lymphoblastic lymphoma of undifferentiated nature, lymphoma of non-lymphatic area, tumour associated with EB virus.

Burkitt's tumour African lymphoma a lymphosarcoma.

Burn Damage by sun burn, damage by radiation burn, injury by chemicals, electrocution, tissue injury by any type of burns.

Burning foot syndrome Vitamin B deficiency and chronic renal failure produces this symptom.

Burning tongue Painful burning sensation in the tongue.

Bursa Sac of synovial membrane, situated in joint for easy movement.

Bursitis Infection and inflammation of bursa, inflammation of bursa lined with smooth lubricating membrane (serous).

Burton's line Character of lead poisoning on the gum, blue line on the gum.

Butterfly needle Wing tipped butterfly needle used in administering I V fluids and medications.

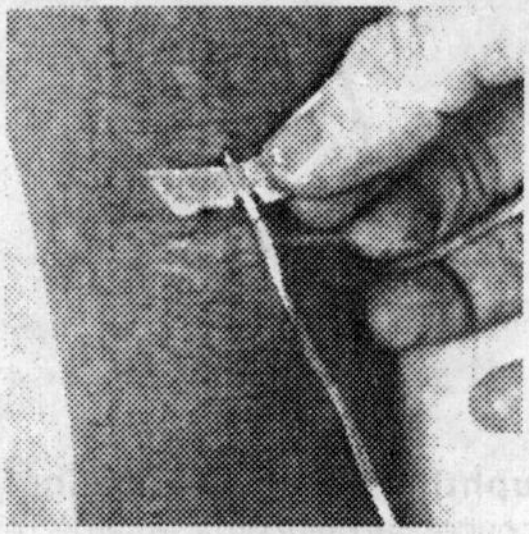

Butterfly needle

Butterfly rash Skin rash of cheeks which is like a butterfly.

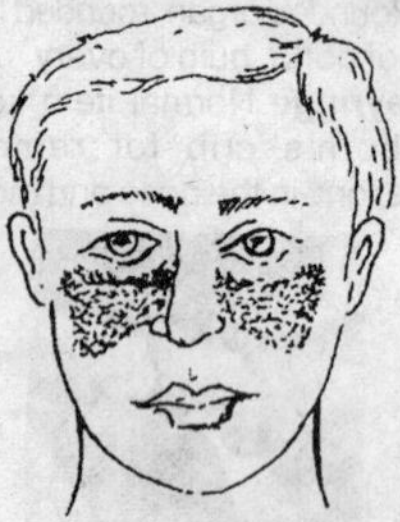

Butterfly rash

Buttock One of the gluteal prominence on the back of loin.

Bypass Flow of liquid is diverted, arterial graft, bypass surgery of heart, bypass surgery of lower limb.

Byssinosis Cotton dust inhalation in cotton industry causes this type of pneumoconiosis.

Bystanders Helpers are used in casualty management, used in first aid of natural calamities, bystanders are different types to help in first aid.

C

Carbohydrate Major proximate principle, and major source of calorie in the diet, synthesised by plants and stored in our body as glycogen.

Crohn's Disease A chronic condition of the terminal portion of the ileum in which granulation and oedema may give rise to obstruction.

Corticotrophin Adreno Cortico Trophic Hormone, ACTH.

CPM Critical Path Method under Management Technique in Nursing. It is the longest path which will delay the nursing activity.

Cacation Other name for defecation.

Cachet A coated cover which is used to administer bitter medicine.

Cachexia Severe debility, commonly late stage of illness, severe malnutrition, severe muscular wasting.

Cacosmia Odour which is not pleasant, sometimes it is by hallucinations.

Cactus Thorny plant from which vasomotor stimulants are prepared.

Cadaver Name for the dead body, human body kept for dissection.

Caduceus Wand of Hermes or Mercury the messenger of Gods which is used as Medical symbol, is an official symbol of the medical profession.

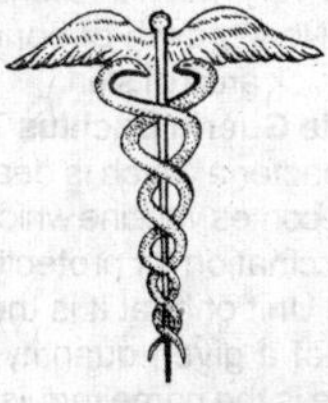

Caduceus

Caecum Colon begins as the caecum in the lower part of the right side of the abdomen to the caecum is attached the small cul-de-sac called appendix.

Caesarean section Delivery through abdominal wall incision and uterus wall incision, indicated in foetal distress and maternal distress, Julius Caesar was born this way and hence the name.

Caesium It is a chemical element, C-137 is radioactive Caesium, used in radiotherapy.

Caffeine Alkaloid of coffee which is nerve stimulant and diuretic, APC an analgesic contains aspirin, phenacetin and caffeine.

Caisson disease It is decompression sickness, found in people working in low altitude with high atmospheric pressure, in lower altitude with high atmospheric pressure gases are in liquid form; if air pressure is rapidly reduced it produces symptoms due to bubbling out of dissolved nitrogen, it is also called *divers' disease*.

Calamine It is an astringent and antipruritic used for external application, it contains zinc oxide and ferric oxide.

Calcaneus Heel bone which is joined with talus and cuboid bones.

Calciferol chemical name and dispensing name for vitamin D it is ergocalciferol or Vitamin D_2.

Calcification Callus formation, lime salt deposition in cartilage in the process of bone formation, it is a natural process.

Calcitonin It regulates blood calcium level and is secreted by C cells of thyroid gland.

Calcium oxalate Commonest form of urinary deposits:
A. Envelop form.
B. Dumb-bell form.
C. Biscuit form.

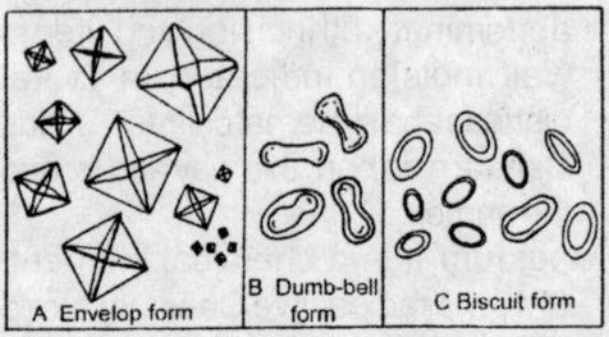

Calcium oxalate crystals

Calcium channel blockers They are pharmaceutical agents that act by slowing the influx of calcium ions into the muscle cells which causes arterial resistance reduced and also decreases myocardial oxygen demand.

Calcium Calcium which is constituent of bone and teeth is prime element in physiological function of the body. Muscular function and blood clotting is regulated by this element

---

Calcium carbonate is the chalk.
Calcium gluconate is antacid.
Calcium lactate is coagulant.

Calculus Stone in kidney, in urinary bladder, in gallbladder, on the surface of teeth.

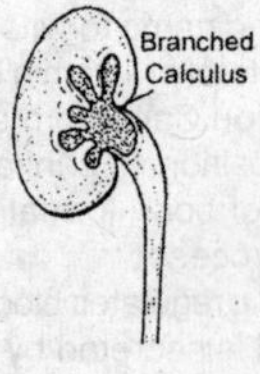

Stag horn calculus in the kidney

Calf It is formed mainly by gastrocnemius and soleus muscles on the back of leg.

Calibrator To measure the size of opening of an anatomical structure we use instrument which is called calibrator, often calibrator is used to dilate urethral stricture or any other body tubes.

Calliper Instrument with 2 prongs is used to put traction on an anatomical part, Callipers (pleural) is a compass for measurement of diameter of any item.

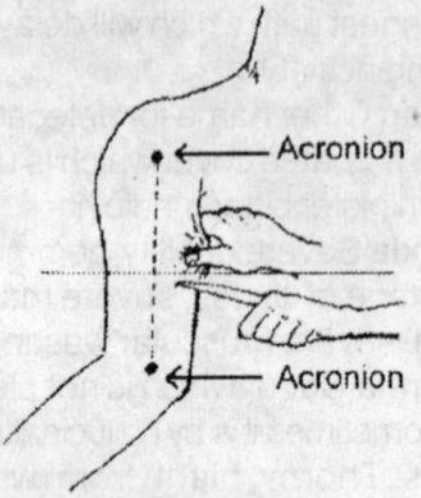

Skin fold calliper used for triceps skin fold thickness

Callosity Area of our body which is subject to friction develops callosity like palm, sole, plaque of thickened skin.

Callous Very much thickened item.

Callus New growth of bone tissue, hard thick area of skin.

Calmette Guerin Bacillus Tuberculosis bacteria which is deactivated and becomes vaccine which is used for vaccination for protection.

Calorie Unit of heat it is the energy value of a given quantity of food. Calorie is the prime requisite of the body for effective growth and development. Calorie available for proximate principles is:

Protein	4 calorie (17 Joule)*
Fat	9 calorie (37 Joule)*
Carbohydrate	4 calorie (17 Joule)*

*per gram of proximate principles.

Calorimeter Heat measurement instrument or an apparatus.

Camphor It is carminative in its property, prepared from camphor laurel.

Campylobacter Gram-negative motile spirally curved non-spore bearing bacteria which causes intestinal disturbances, common source is milk, meat and poultry.

Canal Tubular passages of the body like *alimentary canal, cervical canal, semicircular canal of Schlemm*, etc.

Canaliculous Represents small canal in the body.

Cancellous Spongy tissue of bone which looks like lattice work.

Cancer education An educational programme which provide study of cancer situation for a better development of responsible attitude towards cancer control.

Content of cancer education
Warning signs of cancer.
Risk factors.
National cancer situation.
Political commitment for cancer centres.
Educational goal of cancer centres.
Benefits of simple living.
Economics of smoking.
Economics of alcoholism.
Occupational aspects of cancer.
Carcinogens in atmosphere.
Cancer screening programmes.
Available treatment for cancer.

Cancer General term to denote cancer growth of any tissue, denotes wild and uncontrolled growth of cells, originally from Latin word meaning *crab*.

Cancroid One which resembles cancer.

Cancrum oris Mouth ulcer secondary due to debility, stomatitis which is gangrenous .

Candida Is a fungus which cause human infection, old name is Monilia, *Candida albicans* is common fungal infection seen in the community.

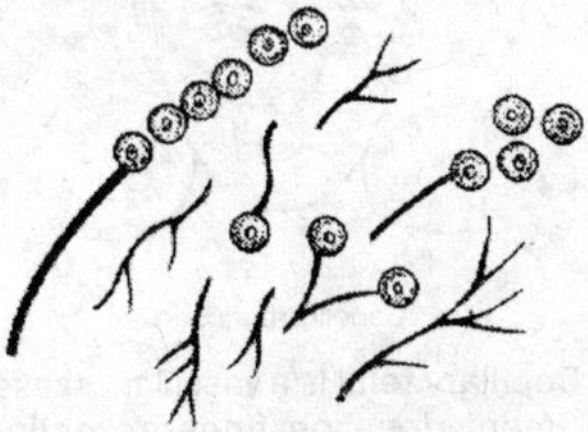

Candida

Candle Wax in cylindrical form with a wick for burning to furnish illumination.

Candy striper Girls who help in hospital work who wear pink and white striped uniforms.

Canine Refers to dog family which have eye tooth.

Canker sore Sore in the mouth for which cause is not known.

Cannabis Is a hallucinogen; it produces sense of well being followed by lethargy and ill effects, colloquially it is named as marijuana, hashish, ganja, bhang.

Cannula It is meant for either to introduce or to remove fluid into an organ or to the body.

Canoeing Canoeing, rowing and sailing provide vigorous exercise, outdoor exercise.

Canthus Angle at either end of the slit like eyelids.

CAPD Continuous Ambulatory Peritoneal Dialysis.

Capeline bandage Used for fixing a dressing to the head with the help of two roller bandages.

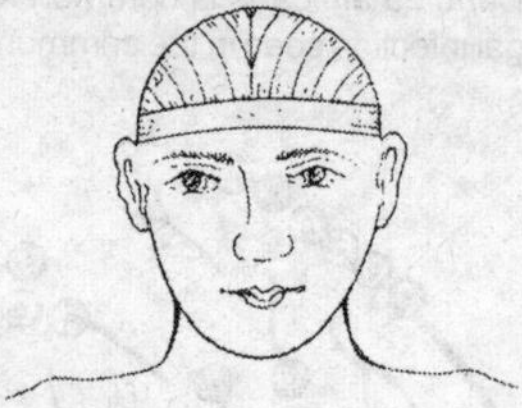

Capeline bandage

Capillary refill Is a vascular assessment done on fingers, testing adequate circulation.

Capillary tube Used in the collection of blood sample with a pin prick of finger.

Capillary It refers to minute vessel which connect venule and an arteriole.

Capital It is a social force in terms of money, machinery and plant to produce goods.

Capitulum Eminence on a bone by which it articulates with another bone.

Caplan's syndrome Progressive massive lung fibrosis in pneumoconiosis along with rheumatoid arthritis.

Capsid Virus particle is protected by a protein covering which protects it from destructive enzymes.

Capsular It is related to articular capsule.

Capsule A membranous sac which enclose an organ, a tissue or a cell gelatine enclosure for drug delivery.

Caput Refers to head or main portion.

Carbachol Acetylcholine like substance which contracts plain muscle and relaxes voluntary sphincter.

Carbamazepine Drug used in epilepsy, in acute pain, in neuralgia.

Carbamino haemoglobin It is a compound containing carbon di oxide and haemoglobin.

Carbohydrase Group of enzymes which catalyze the hydrolysis of higher carbohydrates to lower forms.

Carbol fuchsine Staining used in histology which is made up of the following:

- Fuchsine.
- Alcohol.
- Phenol.

Carbon dioxide Gas resulting from the oxidation of the carbon formed in tissues and excreted from lungs, *carbon dioxide snow* is used in skin disorders.

Carbonet dressing It is an open mesh gauze dressing impregnated with water soluble non-adherent polyethylene glycol, a surgical dressing.

Carboxy haemoglobin Present in condition where carbon monoxide positioning occurs.

Carbuncle Acute staphylococcal infection of subcutaneous tissues multiple boils which tend to undermine the skin.

Carcinogen An agent that produces cancer.

Carcinoid syndrome Bowel tumours spreading to other organs and producing various clinical manifestations like skin changes, diarrhoea, asthmatic condition, fall in BP, ascites, etc.

Carcinoma Malignant cancer growth of epithelial tissue, cancer arising from skin cells or lining cells of inner organs like:

- Adenocarcinoma.
- Basal cell carcinoma.
- Epithelioma.
- Squamous cell carcinoma.

Carcinomatosis Secondaries in many organs, metastasis, cancer spread.

Carcinosis Widespread dissimination of cancer throughout the body, Other name for carcinomatosis.

Cardia Cardiac orifice of the stomach.

Cardiac catheterisation Is an invasive procedure performed to assess cardiac anatomy and function in patients with CCF, congenital heart disease, assessment of cardiac surgery.

Cardiac cirrhosis Liver disorder secondary to heart disease.

Cardiac cycle It is the time taken and duration of period from one heart beat to another heart beat, the phases are:

- Atrial contraction about 0.1 seconds.
- Ventricular contraction about 0.3 seconds.
- Ventricular relaxation about 0.5 seconds.

Cardiac failure Heart fails to function normally or fails to pump sufficient blood to meet the requirement of the body.

Cardiac massage This technique was first described in 1960 in America by Kouwenhoven after experience with animals and later with man, it is a life saving technique.

Cardiac output Quantity of blood ejected from the ventricle every minute, it is calculated by:

(Heart rate) × (stroke volume)

72 × 70 = **5.0 litres per minute**

Cardiac index Cardiac output expressed per square meter body surface area:

C.I = cardiac output / body surface area

= 5 / 1.7

= **3.3 Ltr/M^2**

Cardiac plexus Branches of vagus nerve and sympathetic nerve which encircles the base of the heart.

Cardiac reserve Capacity of the heart to meet the requirement of the body by raising the level of critical level of function.

Cardiac sphincter Muscle surrounding the entrance to the stomach which permits food to enter and retains it after it has been admitted.

Cardinal Meaning fundamental, main, chief such as:

- Cardinal signs.
- Cardinal ligoments

Cardiogenic Started or originated from the heart.

Cardiograph Recording of heart's contraction and relaxation in the graph:

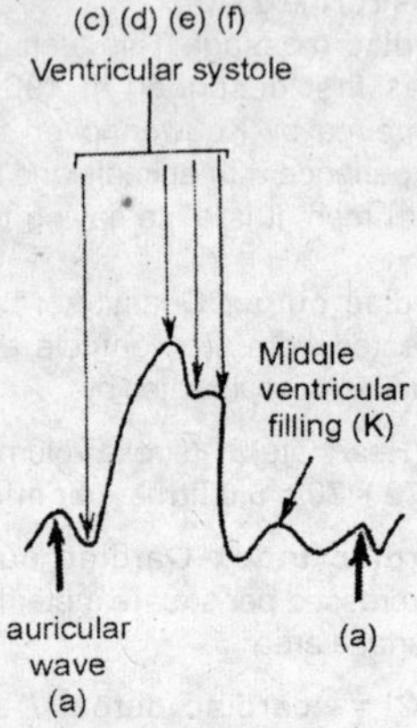

Cardiogram

Cardiologist Consultant in cardiac illness diagnosis and its treatment.

Cardiology It is the study of structure and function of the heart.

Cardiomyopathy Heart muscle disorder which is chronic in nature.

Cardio-omentopexy Surgical suturing of a portion of the omentum to the heart:

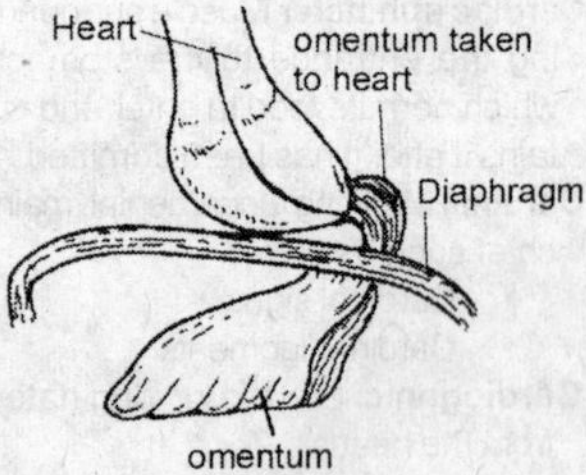

Cardio-omentopexy

Cardiopulmonary resuscitation It is called CPR, cardiac massage and artificial respiration are common tool of CPR, it is a medical emergency care.

Cardiotoxic Substance which is toxic to the heart.

Cardiovascular Related to heart and blood vessels.

Carditis Inflammation of the heart.

Care in the community Is a *deinstitutionalisation* policy for the care of sick and injured in their family and in their community.

CARE A major relief organisation called Co operative for Assistance and Relief Everywhere (from USA).

Carer Refers to elderly person who takes care of the members of the family, non-professional who takes care of patients in their homes.

Caries It signifies decay of bones, decay of teeth.

Carminative Used in the relief of flatulence and associated colic drug that helps in expelling gas from gastrointestinal tract.

Carnivorous Animals that eat flesh.

Carotid body Sensitive structure at the bifurcation of carotid bifurcation, which controls pressure and hypoxia condition of the blood.

Carotene It is provitamin A, present in carrots and tomatoes pigment in plant and animal tissue which gets converted into vitamin A in the liver.

Carotenoid Marked by yellow colour similar to the one that is produced by carotene.

Carotid sinus At the bifurcation of common carotid artery an area richly supplied with nerve endings which controls concentration of oxygen and blood pressure.

Carotid Main artery on either side of the neck called carotid arteries, originally meaning principal item.

Carpaine An alkaloid used like digitalis which is extracted from papaw, $C_{14}H_{25}NO_2$.

Carpal tunnel syndrome Pressure on the medial nerve in carpal tunnel giving rise to a clinical condition with pain, tenderness and muscle weakness of thumb muscles.

Carpal tunnel A tunnel where flexor tendons and median nerve pass through. The canal is below the flexor retinaculum of the wrist.

Carpal Related to the wrist:

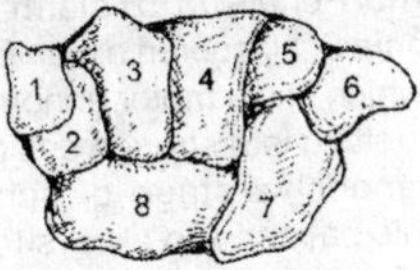

Carpal bones

1. Pisiform 2. Triquetral
3. Hamate 4. Capitate
5. Trapezoid 6. Trapezium
7. Scaphoid 8. Lunate.

Carpus Consists of eight small bones forming the wrist.

Carrier Person who harbours the pathogens and do not manifests the illness, carrier stage is known in infectious diseases and in hereditary abnormalities.

Carrot Is an umbelliferous plant, used as vegetable, its seed is diuretic.

Cartilage Specialised connective tissue in adults in the form of hyaline cartilage, elastic cartilage and fibro-cartilage colloquially called gristle, less hard and more elastic than bone, commonly seen in joints.

Carbolic acid Other name for phenol.

Case control It is a type of research study where a study group and a control group are selected.

Case study In depth study of a group or an event case study in case of nursing profession can include the following:

- Sickroom.
- Bed making.
- Patient toilet.
- Observation of the sick.
- Injections.
- Surgical techniques.
- Diet.
- Medicine.
- Special conditions and bandaging.
- Case study refers to in depth study of any such component.

Case Designated patient with a disease in hospital management.

Caseation When tissue becomes cheesy mass due to degeneration after the disease.

Casein Milk protein.

Casoni's test A skin test with hydatid fluid, if positive indicates the infection of *Echinococcus granulosus* infection

Cast Shed shapes or mould of a hollow organ:

A. Waxy casts C. Granular casts
B. Epithelial casts D. Hyaline casts.

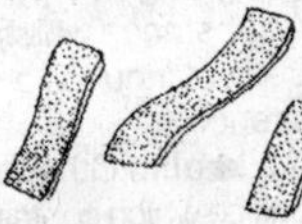

A. Waxy casts

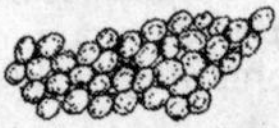

B. Epithelial casts

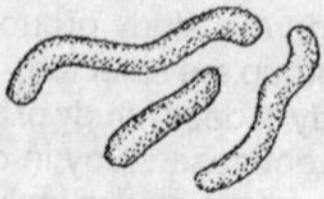

C. Granular casts

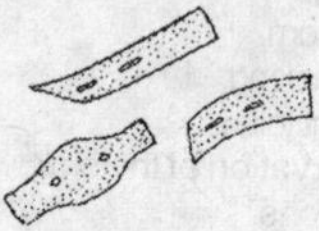

D. Hyaline casts

Casts

Caste Is a system where social stratification is done in India.

Castor oil Vegetable oil which when taken internally is a purgative and is a smoothening agent when applied externally.

Castration Removal of male or female organs viz., testes and ovaries.

Casts Is used for immobilisation and as comfort device, used in the treatment of fractures.

Casuality It denotes accident or trauma or injury or death, area of emergency treatment.

CAT Computerised Axial Tomography.

Catabolism Breakdown of body substances giving energy.

Catalyst A substance which is inactive by itself but induces a reaction by its presence.

Cataplasma kaolini Other name for Kaolin Poultice which contains china clay, glycerine, menthol and methyl salicylate, it is analgesic and heat retaining poultice, requirements are:

- Tin containing cataplasma kaolini.
- Saucepan containing boiling water.
- Lint or old linen.
- Palette knife.
- Jug containing boiling water.
- Poultice board.
- Warmed plates, trays dishes to carry the poultice to bed side.

Cataplexy Loss of muscle power which occurs all of a sudden.

Cataract A preventable blindness coagulation of lens or clouding of lens of the eye.

Catarrh Chronic inflammation of mucosa with discharge inflammation of mucous membrane of nose and throat.

Catarrhal Pertaining to catarrh.

Catatonia Schizophrenia manifestation which show motor abnormalities, getting into strange positions unresponsive stage of schizophrenic patient who always tends to resume a fixed posture.

Catchment area Refers to water table in the ground, refers to percolation area which can contaminate drinking water of a well.

Catecholamine They stimulate sympathetic nerves, adrenaline and noradrenaline.

Catgut Used for ligation and sutures which are prepared from sheep intestine.

Cathartic Drug that stimulates the action of the bowel.

Catheter strap By using two pieces of tape one 10 × 10 and the other 10 × 25 cm, similar to Montgomery strap, used to anchor patient with Foley catheter, helpful in eliminating the need for repeated removal and reapplication of tape when frequent repositioning of the Foley is necessary.

Catheterization Employment or passing a catheter.

Catheter Flexible rubber tube used to drain bladder or any body cavity.

Cat scratch fever Fever by cat scratch though to be viral in origin, benign subacute regional lymphadenitis.

Cauda An appendage which looks like a tail, terminal portion of spinal cord.

Caudal Related to cauda or tail like appendage.

Caul Unruptured amnion which envelop foetal head.

Causalgia Post-nerve injury burning pain.

Cause That which brings out a condition in clinical practice.

Caustic Acid or alkali which can burn tissue.

Cauterization Using cautery tissue destruction is undertaken.

Cautery Application of heat, electric current or carbon dioxide for destroying tissue it is a means of destroying tissues, by means of heat, current or carbon dioxide.

Cava Pleural form of cavum, vena cava.

Cavern A pathological cavity in the organ or body, lung abscess.

Cavernous The one which has hollows, cavernous sinus, cavernous breathing.

Cavities of trunk There are three cavities of the trunk

- The thoracic cavity.
- The abdominal cavity.
- The pelvic cavity.

Cavity Potential space in the body, pleural cavity, abdominal cavity, cavity caused by caries.

CBI Continuous Bladder Irrigation.

CCU Coronary Care Unit.

CD_4 cell count It is a diagnostic tool in case of HIV/AIDS.

CDD Control of Diarrhoeal Diseases

CDP Community Development Programme.

Cefataxime Third generation antibiotic used in infections.

Celiac disease Gluten induced malabsorption syndrome of the intestine.

Celiac plexus Plexus near celiac artery origin which are sympathetic nerves.

Celiaca refered to the belly or abdomen.

Celioma Tumour of the abdomen.

Cell membrane Cell covering which covers the cell which is made of carbohydrate fat and protein.

Cell Basic unit of living organisms.

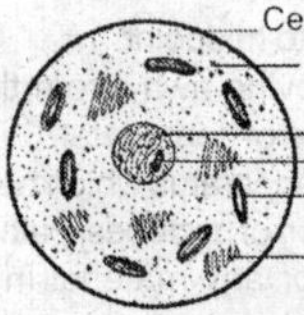

Cell and its parts

Cellular immunity T cell mediated cellular immunity, it is the basis of organ transplantation.

Cellulitis Diffuse inflammation of connective tissue.

Cellulose Type of carbohydrate which becomes covering of vegetable cells, bulk and roughage food.

Ceisius scale Temperature scale which fixes melting point of ice and boiling points of water as under:

Ice 0^0 C ..... melting point

Water 100^0 C ..... boiling point.

Celsius Degree centigrade a scale for measurement of heat.

Cementum Bone like structure which covers the root of tooth.

Censor Critical examination of medical, nursing professional acts.

Census Enumeration of population at a given point of time once in 10 years in our country, recent census was held in 2001a major source of vital events which is done once in 10 years.

In India

First census 1881.

Latest 13th census 2001.

Centigrade Unit for the measurement of temperature, a scale.

Centile Connected with percentile.

Centimetre One hundredth of a meter or 10 mm.

Central Refers to midpoint.

Centrifugal Moving away from the centre, reverse of centripetal.

Centrifuge An apparatus which help in sedimentation of microbes, pathogens, solids or any material in a liquid when rotated at a given speed.

Centriole They are substances to which spindle fibers get attached during mitosis, they are minute organelle with its hollow cylindrical body one end closed and the other end opened.

Centripetal Moving from periphery to centre, opposite of centrifugal.

Centromere In mitosis or meiosis chromosomes gets allied with spindle fibres.

Cephalexin An antibiotic.

Cephalgia Experiencing aches in the head, headache.

Cephalhaematoma By the pressure during labour bleeding occurred beneath the pericranium is common among newborn babies , which gets absorbed during a course of time.

Cephalic Refered to the head end of the body or towards the head.

Cephalin Monoamino monophosphatide existing in brain, nerve and egg, has haemostatic property.

Cephalothoracopagus Union from crown of the head to the middle abdominal region in case of birth defect, double monster united as described.

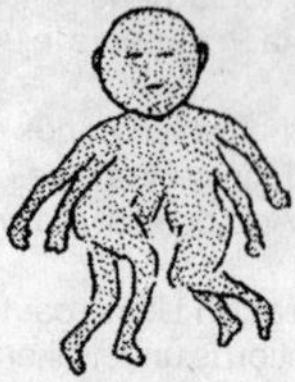

Cephalothoracopagus

Cercaria Intermediate stage in the life cycle of trematode or flukes which are free swimming forms.

Cereals Edible grain, rice, ragi, jowar, food grains.

Cerebellum Portion of the brain below cerebrum and above medulla oblongata.It is responsible for posture and voluntary fine movements.

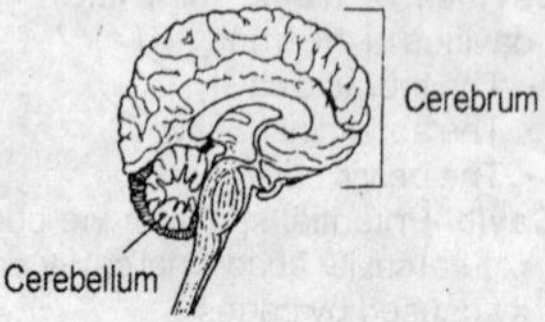

Cerebrum and cerebellum

Cerebellar ataxia Failure of muscle coordination in cerebellar pathology or pathology due to cerebellum.

Cerebral palsy Condition caused by injury to the brain of newborn at birth where coordination of movement is affected and child is flaccid or athetoid.

Cerebral Related to cerebrum like cerebral hernia, cerebral haemorrhage, cerebral irritation, cerebral palsy etc., pertaining to brain or forebrain which controls the body.

Cerebrospinal fluid Fluid from choroids plexus which circulates in subarachnoid space.

Cerebrospinal related to spinal and brain

Cerebrovascular Related to vein and artery of brain like cerebrovascular accident, cerebrovascular disease.

Cerebrum Large portion of brain which has two hemispheres, which again are divided by fissure.

Cerumen Ear wax soft brown wax like secretion of external auditory meatus.

Cervical cap Method of family planning by vaginal method which is not widely available in India.

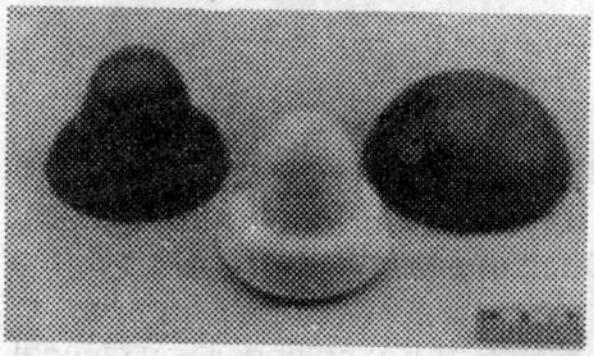

Cervical cap

Cervical collars Soft cervical collar is used intermittently on a short-term basis for the relief of muscle spasms or for cervical immobilisation after an injury to cervical region. Hard cervical collar is used frequently for long-term use in cervical fractures or fusions.

Cervical plexus First 4 cervical nerves join by their anterior rami to form plexus, they are communicated with sympathetic ganglia.

Cervical spondylosis Osteoarthritic changes in the cervical vertebra which leads to osteophytic growths, they may cause nerve root compression.

Cervical traction Is applied for patients with cervical spine disorders , neck muscle spasm, neck pain.

Cervical uterine radiation implants Providing care for patients with cervical uterine radiation implants, treatment of endometrial cancer by implants with radioactive isotopes.

Cervical Related to neck or uterine cervix like cervical vertebra, cervical canal, cervical spondylosis, cervical smear, etc.

Cervicitis Infection and inflammation of cervix.

Cervix Constructed portion i.e., neck of uterus, it is 2 inches long and projects into vagina, its physiological dilatation is useful in childbirth.

Cestoda They are tapeworm group in helminths under parasites tapeworms which show scolex and proglottids, a group under helminths

Cetyl Univalent alcohol radical.

$C_{16}H_{33}$.

CFT Complement Fixation Test.

Chafe Irritation of skin of moist area

of the body, skin changes in skinfold areas, friction caused skin irritation.

Chaga's disease Other name for African Trypanosomiasis.

Chain Bacteriae attaching end to end, atoms linked together in a compound.

Chalazion Swollen sebaceous gland in eyelid, meibomian cyst or tarsal cyst swelling of meibomian gland of eyelid which secrete hard substance, look like hard tumour.

Challenge An immunological term where specific antigen administration can produce immunity in the body.

Chamber It refers to closed compartment, e.g., anterior chamber and posterior chamber of the eye.

Chancre Syphilis manifestation at the site of initial inoculation of infection, hard syphilitic primary ulcer.

Chancroid VD Ulcer due to *Haemophilus ducreyi* soft sore or genital ulceration caused by *Haemophilus ducreyi* a gram-negative bacteria.

Chandler index It is an index for the community diagnosis and community treatment of hookworm infection:

Chandler index	*Inference*
300 and above	major public health problem
250 to 299	minor public health problem
200 to 249	potential danger with community
Below 200	not significant

Character Traits and other qualities of man specific to him or her, it also can denote normal or abnormal character of man or woman.

Charcot Leyden crystal They are needle like crystals which are hexagonal double pointed and colourless, they are found in the following conditions:
- Intestinal amoebiasis.
- Sputum of chronic asthma patients (bronchial asthma).

Charcot's joint Originally identified when syphilis caused chronic progressive and degenerative joint disease, of late it can also occur in leprosy and diabetes which is due to underlying neurological disorder degenerated and denerved joint which has hypermobility in conditions like:
- Tabes dorsalis.
- Spinal cord injury.
- Syringomyelia.

Charcot's triad Sign of disseminated sclerosis (multiple sclerosis), they are :
- Nystagmus.
- Intension tremor.
- Scanning speech.

Charging fee Care given to the sick is charged and this charge is called fee. Code of conduct are laid down for charging the fee in medical and nursing practice.

Charle's law It postulate that gas expands in direct proportion to absolute temperature provided pressure remain constant.

Charms Worn round the neck to ward off illness, a medical folklore.

Charting Maintenance of patient's record of health and disease or of prognostic condition, it is a clinical record of patient under care tabulated record of pulse, temperature, BP, body look, skin change and other relavent observable changes of a patient in the hospital in morning rounds by the nurse.

CHD Coronary Heart Disease.

Cheek Fleshy wall on either side of the oral cavity.

Cheilitis Infection and inflammation of lips.

Cheilosis Due to vitamin riboflavin deficiency and general debility we notice maceration at the angles of the mouth.

Chelating agent Chemical agent that can act as antidote in poisoning, they combine with poisonous material in the body and hasten their excretion from the body, e.g., dimercaprol, D - penicillamine, EDTA, etc.

Chemical burns Burns by acids, alkalis, iodine and phosphorus mustard and lewisite.

Chemical warfare Toxic chemicals are used as weapons in war ,nerve gas use in warfare..

Chemise A dressing prepared by a muslin cloth used in rectal surgery.

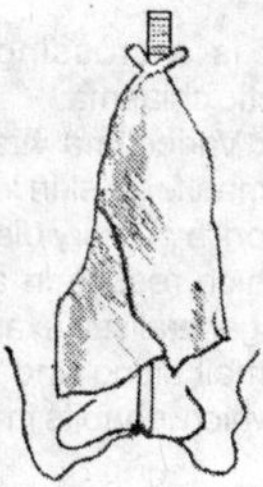

Chemise

Chemistry Science that deals with elements, compound and their reactions and formation of new compound.

Chemocephalia Flat head.

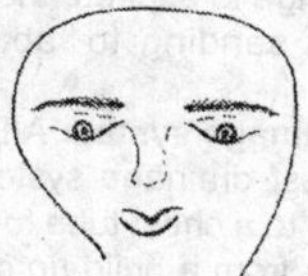

Flat head

Chemoreceptor Sensory nerve endings that gets activated by stimuli to produce required physiological action, e.g., of chemoreceptor are (specialised sensory nerve ending which converts chemical stimuli into an electrical stimuli producing specific chemical sensation):

- Olfactory cells.
- Carotid body.
- Aortic body.
- Taste buds.

Chemosis Oedema of conjunctiva.

Chemotaxis Cellular reaction to chemical stimuli, reaction with acid, alkali or other chemical substances.

Chemotherapeutic index An index used in relation to chemotherapy prognosis.

Chemotherapy Chemical agents given as treatment agent in case of illness treatment of disease by drugs and chemicals.

Cheopis index One of the useful rat flea index in public health practice:

Cheopis index

$$= \frac{\text{No. of X.cheopis counted on rats}}{\text{No. of rats examined}}$$

Cherry red spot Fundoscopic findings of retina in Taysach's disease, red spot in retina.

Chest drainage specimen By inserting 20 gauge needle attached to a syringe to aspirate the specimen for sending to laboratory testing.

Chest drainage system A Disposable chest drainage system that attaches to a chest tube to relieve pressure from a build-up of air or fluid in the pleural space as in thoracic trauma, pleural tears, spontaneous pneumothorax, haemothorax etc. It contains:

- Suction control chamber.
- Water seal chamber.
- Collection chamber.

Chest tube Tube which is used in chest drainage system to relieve pressure in the chest and which is connected to a drainage system.

Chest Anatomical name is thorax; types are: barrel chest, flail chest, pigeon chest and normal chest.

Chest bandage First aid measure in chest injury.

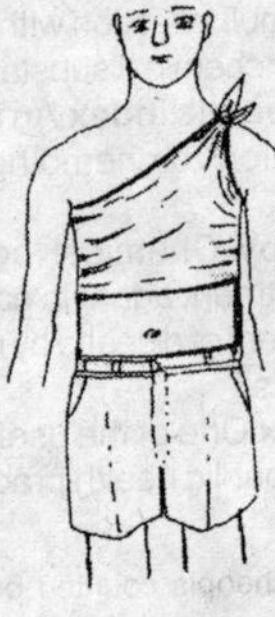

Chest bandage

Chest circumference One of the anthropometric measurement in nutritional assessment, its crossing over with head circumference is an indicator.

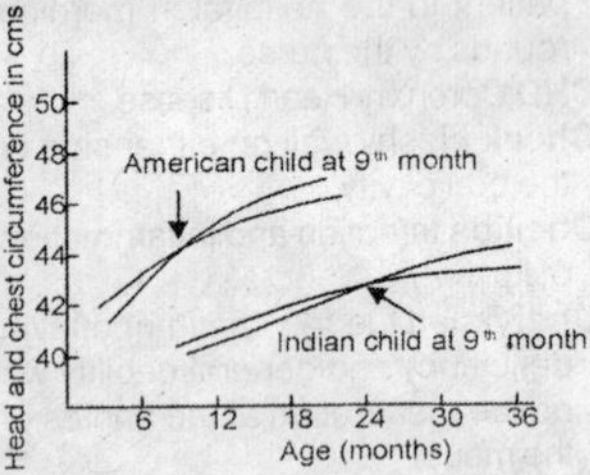

Crossing over of head and chest circumference

Cheyne Stokes respiration Colloquially it is called tidal respiration, it is irregular rhythmic breathing with temporary apnoea, causes are:

- Narcotic poisoning.
- Arteriosclerosis.
- Uraemia.
- Cerebral tumours.

Chi Square test A Significant test to test the goodness of fit or association of attributes, a non-parametric test.

Chiasma It is a crossing point, refers to optic chiasma.

Chickenpox Varicella a viral infection which manifests skin lesions a viral infection, a primary disease of children which results in a highly contagious generalised exanthema.

Chiggers Small biting and burrowing insect which inhabits in vegetations.

Chilblain Vasoconstriction of exposed parts like hands, feet causes local changes like swelling and inflammation, itching and burning.

Child guidance clinic It is run in team spirit by child psychologists, psychiatrists, psychosocial workers, paediatrics speech therapists, neurologists and occupational therapists for:

- Child counselling.
- Play therapy.
- Parental counselling.

Child psychology Understanding of mind and behaviour of a child for normal growth and developing and skills.

Child Refers to the period covering neonate, infant, childhood, and part of adolescent period between the age of 0 to 14 years, paediatric age group.

Chinese medicine Traditional system of medicine from China which has the principle of Yin and Yang , herbal medicine, animal medicine and acupuncture.

Chiropody Care and maintenance of feet and its disorders.

Chiropractice Traditional healers who practice the treatment of illness.

Chiropractor Traditional healer who has unscientific theory and unproved assumptions for illness.

Chlamydia Group of bacteria which cause diseases in man:

Chlamydia Trachomatis	LGV Trachoma Conjunctivitis Non-gonococcal urethritis
Chlamydia psittaci	Parrot fever (psittacosis)

group of pathogen which cause LGV, trachoma, ornithosis and genital infections.

Chlopheniramine Is an antihistaminic drug.

Chloral hydrate Used as a hypnotic agent.

Chlorhexidine Common antiseptic solution used in:

- Surgical scrub.
- Preoperative skin preparation.
- Wound dressings.

Chlorination Process of using chlorine in water purification as a supplement to sand filtration, types are:

- Prechlorination.
- Postchlorination.
- Combined chlorination.
- Super chlorination.
- Break point chlorination.

Chlorine Gas in its natural form, available in different compound, used in disinfectants and sterilisation in the form of hypochlorite.

Chloroform Volatile liquid used in G.A. liquid anaesthetic agent used in anaesthesia for surgery.

Chloroma Skull bone tumour which is greenish in colour and is associated with myeloid leukaemia.

Chloroquin Drug used in the treatment of malaria and arthriti common antimalaria drug used in NMEP, it is also a therapeutic agent in amoebic hepatitis, rheumatoid arthritis and lupus erythematosus.

Chlorosis Green sickness in girl who suffers from anaemia due to defective blood formation.

Chlorothiazide Oral diuretic agent used in hypertension.

Chlorpromazine Therapeutic agent in vomiting, anxiety and agitation, enhances the action of other analgesics and anaesthetics.

Chlorpromazine Drug that produces tranquillity.

Chlorpropamide Oral hypoglycaemic agent used in diabetes.

Chondroma Hyperplastic growth of cartilage tissue.

Chokes Burning sensation beginning in substernal region.

Choking Obstruction in respiratory passage, neck constriction which obstruct breathing and circulation.

Cholangiography X-ray of biliary tract in radiological examination.

Cholangitis Infection and inflammation of bile duct.

Cholecystectomy Surgical excision of gallbladder.

Cholecystitis Gall induced inflammation of gallbladder.

Cholecystogram Examination of gallbladder and bile ducts by I V biligrafin.

Cholecystokinin Hormone released in duodenum when fat content is passed through duodenum, cholecystokinin causes contraction of the gallbladder, duodenum secretes this hormone which stimulates gallbladder contraction and secretion of the pancreas.

Cholelithiasis Gallstones present in gallbladder or in the bile ducts.

Cholera Acute intestinal infection caused by *Vibrio cholerae* bacteria, it is notifiable disease, it is quarantinable disease.

Cholestasis Because of obstruction of bile duct bile cannot flow and stasis occurs.

Cholesteatoma Tumour containing cholesterol, common sites are:

- CNS.
- Skull bone.
- Middle ear.
- Meninges.

Cholesterol It is precursor of steroid hormones and bile acids, Source:

- RBC.
- Nervous tissue.
- Animal fat.
- Bile juice.

Other area where cholesterol present:

- Gallstones.
- Atheroma of arteries.
- Various cysts.
- Carcinomatous tissue.

Choline An amine which help in fat metabolism, commonly found in urine, CSF and blood.

Cholinergic Related to nerve which release acetylcholine.

Cholinesterase This is an enzyme which destroys acetylcholine.

Chondrin It is the basic substance of cartilage which can be obtained by boiling cartilage.

Chondroma Benign tumour of cartilage.

Chondromalacia Softening of cartilage which is an abnormal condition.

Chondrosarcoma Malignant tumour of cartilage.

Chorda Denoting cord.

Chordae tendinea These connect A V valves to papillary muscles.

Chorda That which is cord like, a tendon.

Chordee Downward curvature of penis by hypospadias.

Chorea Spasmodic involuntary rapid movements of face, hip and shoulder which is due to pathology of basal ganglion, two clinical entities of chorea are seen in practice:

- Huntington's chorea – in middle age and is hereditary.
- Sydenham's chorea – in children and is St.Vitus dance.

extra-pyramidal damage produce this movement disorder. Movement which quasipurposive, involuntary, non-repetitive limb movement.

Choriocarcinoma Malignant neoplasm from trophoblast of hydatidiform mole rare cancer found in women after pregnancy.

Chorion Outer membrane covering the foetus an extra-embryonic membrane that covers outer wall of blastocyst from which chorionic villi is developed.

Choroiditis Inflammation of choroid.

Choroid Dark brown vascular layer in the eyeball which is in between sclera and retina.

Christmas disease Hereditary bleeding disease similar to haemophilia.

Christmas seal Employees of affiliated local organisation working under National Conference of Tuberculosis, Workers rely on the Christmas seal for financial support.

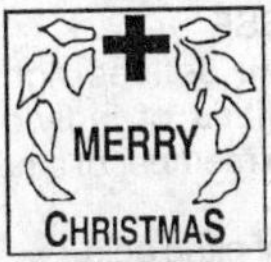

Christmas seal

Chromatin DNA present in cell nucleus, chromatin positive and negative are used in case of females and males respectively.

Chromatography It is a method of chemical analysis, substance in solution is separated when they are percolating to get absorbed to paper by capillary traction, definite pattern is produced and gives recognition of the substance laboratory procedure to separate more than two chemical compounds in solution by passing across the surface of an absorbent paper.

Chromosome They are present in the nucleus of a cell, DNA of chromosome transmits genetic information and is associated with RNA man contains 22 pairs of autosomes and two sex chromosomes (XX and XY) the structure that store genetic information, there are 22 pairs of autosomes and one pair of sex chromosomes in man.

Chronic obstructive lung disease Chronic bronchitis and chronic asthma which cause poor FEV_1 they are called COLD by abbreviation.

Chronic Disease which lasts longer and suffering is for many years.

Chronological Described in a natural sequence.

Chronology Historical highlights in ascending order of an event or of facts.

Chyle Lymph drain to left subclavian vein via thoracic duct which is rich in fat and protein.

Chyme Food with gastric juice is semi-digested which is seen in intestine after passing from stomach.

Chymotrypsin Enzyme secreted by pancreas, chymotrypsin is activated by trypsin and help in protein metabolism

Cicatrix Keloid, it is the scar of healed wound.

Cilia Other name of eyelashes, filaments of ciliated membrane they are projecting items of epithelial cells of bronchi to propel mucus and foreign particle.

Ciliary ganglion This is present in orbital fossa from which ciliary nerves emerge, which supply ciliary muscles, sphincters of iris and smooth muscles of blood vessels.

Ciliary muscle They are smooth muscles of ciliary body which help in accommodation.

Ciliary process Anatomical process with 70 or more folds meridionally arranged to secrete nourishing fluid to cornea, lens and vitreous homour.

Cinchona Cinchona bark containing quinine and cinchonine which are anti-malarial drugs.

Cinnamon Dried inner bark of *cinnamomum*, carminative and astringent.

Ciprofloxacin Broad-spectrum antibiotic.

Circle Body which is round or which is circular like circle of Willis.

Circle bed An electrically operated bed which provides a vertical alteration of patient's position from either supine or prone via a supporting mattress and an anterior frame that attach to a circular outer frame.

Circle of Willis Branches of internal carotid artery and basilar artery join at the base of the brain, (anastomosis of branches of internal carotid artery and basilar artery).

Circulation Any circular motion of fluid in canals or tubes , circulation of the heart, common types of circulation in clinical practice are:

- Coronary circulation.
- Pulmonary circulation.
- Portal circulation.
- Systemic circulation.
- Lymph circulation.
- Extracorporeal circulation.
- Collateral circulation.

Circulatory failure Cardiac pump action is not sufficient to meet oxygen demand.

Circumcision Surgical excision of foreskin of penis done on religious ground or as part of treatment of phimosis. Female circumcision is found in tribes which include excision of labia majora, labia minora and clitoris, surgical removal of prepuce for religious purpose or for therapeutic purpose.

Circumduction Joint movement at the apex of a cone where circular movement is performed.

Circumflex Winding is done around any substance or item.

Cirrhosis Degenerative changes of liver due to infection or alcohol. Common clinical types of cirrhosis are:

- Alcoholic cirrhosis.
- Pulmonary cirrhosis.
- Cardiac cirrhosis.
- Posthepatic cirrhosis.

Cisternal puncture insertion of hollow needle into cisterna magna to take out CSF.

Citizenship It defines rights and responsibilities of individual by becoming a member of a nation or state.

Citrate Salt of citric acid.

Citric acid cycle Popularly known as Kreb's cycle, metabolism of pyruvic acid in presence of oxygen to release carbon dioxide and water plus energy.

Citric acid Antiscurvy substance present in citrus fruits (lemon, orange).

City A large urban area with exciting and vibrant places.

Civil defence Defence by civil administration in case of disasters .

Civilisation A complex cultural and social entity which cover a society.

Clamp Surgical instrument to compress tissue in surgery.

Class culture Is shared meanings and patterns of behaviour associated with a particular social class.

Classical sociologist Early sociologists who developed distinctive way to look at society.

Claudication Severe pain at walking which produce lameness, suggest artery block painful condition on walking in calf muscle due to poor blood circulation.

Clavicle splint Has padded straps that encircle anterior axillae to provide compression at the clavicular area, is applied in clavicle fracture.

Clavicle Collar bone which form part of the shoulder girdle.

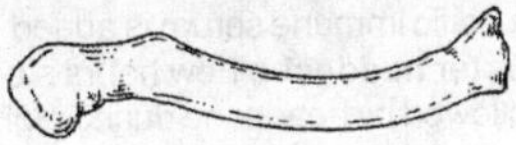

Clavicle

Clavus Horny tubercle of the skin.

Clawfoot Planter arch is abnormally raised, pes cavus high longitudinal arch of foot with dorsal contracture of toes.

Clawhand Hyperflexon of proximal phalanges and extreme flexion of middle and distal phalanges.

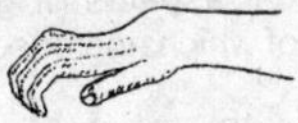

Claw hand

Clean catch method Urine specimen is collection in antiseptic precaution or without contamination.

Cleavage Complex molecule is converted into simple molecule.

Cleft palate Longitudinal fissure of embryonic age remained after birth in the case of palate.

Cleft Connote longitudinal opening, common clinical usage are:

- Cleft palate.
- Cleft lip.

Clenching Forcible contraction of jaw muscles by keeping teeth intact position.

Cleptomania It is an impulsive act of stealing by a person who has no motive of stealing or even do not know the value of stolen item.

Clergy Person who is sympathetic and helpful in dealing with emotional problems like grief.

Climax Highest peak of disease, highest peak of sex act (orgasm).

Clinic Place of clinical practice by a doctor or nurse, place for the treatment of illness, bedside teaching to medical and health science students in a teaching hospital.

Clinical sociology An intervention to solve social problems in clinical practice.

Clinical Bedside clinical examination for diagnosis and treatment.

Clip Device to hold blood flow in artery or vein, device to hold the lips of a wound.

Clitoris crises Involuntary orgasm in females, common symptom in tabes dorsalis.

Clitoris Erectile tissue situated at the anterior junction of the labia minora in female.

Clitorism Opposite to priapism of males, it is repeated painful erection of clitoris in females.

Cloaca Common opening for intestine and urogenital system.

Clone III meningitis Type which caused epidemic of meningococcal meningitis which is known as *Mecca epidemic of 1987*.

Clone Cells that are genetically identical to each other and have descended by asexual reproduction from parent cell.

Clonic Characters of clonus is present, second stage of fits.

Cloning Development of a replica (without a natural biological process) when vector with marker is inserted into host cell by micro-injection.

Clonus Muscle getting rigid and relaxed spasmodically, clonus is seen in upper motor lesion where alternate contraction and relaxation of muscle occurs

Closed glove technique It is the skill of putting on sterile attire, when the nurse is required to assist surgical procedures in O T.

Closed chain Method of linking together of atoms of a compound

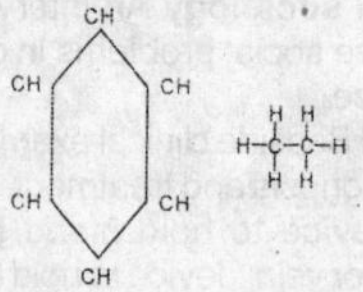

Closed chain and open chain

Closed society Where little social mobility is seen.

Clostridium Anaerobic spore forming bacteria found in intestine and soil.

Clot Blood when exposed becomes semisolid mass by coagulation.

Clove hitch Commonly made from broad flannel bandage to use in the treatment of fractures by splints.

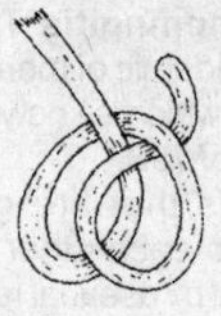

Clove hitch

Club foot Weight bearing arch of foot is abnormal, talipes.

Clubbing Thickening and broadening of tip of fingers secondary to poor circulation by heart diseases, lung diseases and tuberculosis tip of finger and toe gets bulbous enlargement with more of longitudinal curvature, clubbing is common findings in:

- Cyanotic heart disease.
- Congenital heart disease.
- Suppurative lung disorders.
- Infective endocarditis.

Clumping Due to agglutination reaction cells, RBCs join together grouping of bacteria occurs when specific immune serum is added.

Cluster headache Few hours sleep followed by headache during nights continuing for many months, watering in the eye is also present.

Clutton's joint Manifestation of congenital syphilis where hydroarthrosis of knee joint is seen, this is also associated with interstitial keratitis.

CNS Central Nervous System which contains brain and spinal cord.

Coaching Competent instructors in the technical aspects of game, ignorance of which, increases the injuries.

Coagulation Process of blood coagulation refers to blood clotting, refers to protein coagulation.

Coarctation Constriction of vessel as in coarctation of aorta stricture or constriction of vessels as seen in coarctation of aorta.

Coat and poles stretcher An improvised stretcher with the help of overcoats, sleeves and Poles for the transport of the sick and injured.

Coxa Refers to hip or hip joint.

Cobalt 60 Used in cobalt therapy for malignant lesions.

Cobalt Metal, in traces required for affording pigments in the body. Isotope is used as radiation therapy for cancers.

Cocaine extract from cocoa leaves, drug from cocoa leaves used in local anaesthesia,it is a nerve stimulant in small dose, in large dose it is toxic causing depression, respiratory depression and cardiac arrhythmia.

Coccus Spheroid-shaped bacteria like streptococci and staphylococci.

Coccygeal body Arteriovenous anastomosis at the level of coccyx.

Coccyx terminal bone of spinal cord which is formed by four rudimentary vertebra.

Cochlea Canal of internal ear which is spiral in shape.

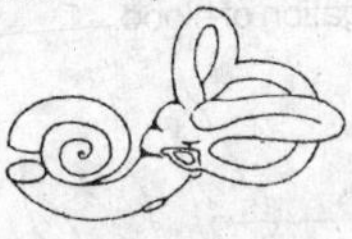

Inner ear which shows cochlea an organ of hearing.

Cocktail Beverage containing many ingredients.

Cock-up splint It is a malleable metal splint used to maintain the wrist and hand in the position of extension.

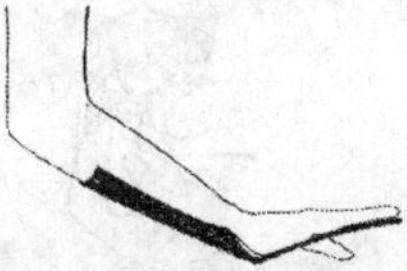

Cock up splint

Cod liver oil Purified form of codfish liver oil which is the source of vitamin A and D.

Codeine Opium alkaloid which is analgesic and antitussive.

Code It refers to code of conduct in medical and nursing practice, well known codes are Nuremberg Code, International Code of Medical Ethics and Medical Council of India and Nursing Council of India Code.

Coefficient Ratio between two different quantities like calorie coefficient.

Coenzyme An activator for protein enzyme for enzyme action

Cognition It is nervous function of conscious mind which give knowledge.

Cogwheel Tremor and rigidity seen together as clinical manifestations, In Parkinson's disease because of extrapyramidal pathology the symptom is described.

Cohabitation Couple live together who are not legally married.

Coherent Characterised by adhesiveness of matter.

Cohort Group of individual who have common characteristics for the selection for a study, types of cohort are:

- Birth cohort.
- Marriage cohort.
- Female cohort.

Cohort study A prospective study where a Cohort is selected which is a group of people experiencing common characteristics e.g., those who are born on 3rd Feb 2005 is a birth cohort.

Coitus Sexual intercourse in natural course by married couple or between male and female.

Colchicine Alkaloid used in the treatment of gout, $C_{22}H_{25}O_6N$.

Cold chain A system of storage and transport of vaccines at low temperature from the site of manufacture to the site of vaccination.

Cold compress Alternative treatment in case of injuries to the joints by application of cold compresses to relieve pain and to reduce swelling.

Cold cream They are cleansing agents which are water-in-oil type of emulsion which acts in two different ways.

i. mineral oil portion dissolves set bum and loosens the particles of grime.
ii. suspending effect of the formula facilitates the removal of dirt with a soft towel or tissue.

Cold pack It is a common nurse care which is provided by cloth dipped in cold water or ice to reduce fever, to reduce pain or to reduce the swelling in bruise.

Cold Means low temperature, also means viral cold involving URT.

Coldlite instrument Instruments used for diagnostic purpose are made of plastic parts which require special care in sterilisation, e.g. are Rectal speculum, Vaginal speculum, Auriscope.

Colic Abdominal pain and spasm which is severe form of abdominal distress due to spasm or obstruction of intestine, gallbladder or ureter.

Coliform It is a group of organisms, main type is *E.coli* which cause GE.

Colitis Infection and inflammation of colon due to various reasons, inflammatory changes in large bowel, emotional and bacterial causes are known.

Collagen disease They are types of rheumatic diseases , collagen is applied to the term connective tissue of the body, e.g.:

- Bursitis.
- Fibrositis.
- Tenosinovitis.
- Lumbago.

Collagen Fibrous structure in tendon, bone, cartilage and other connective tissue, structural tissue of human body other than bone, cartilage, membrane or tendon, a type of fibrous tissue.

Collar bone Other name for clavicle which is the set of shoulder girdle.

Collateral Meaning accessory to some thing like collateral circulation.

Collection of blood sample Capillary blood collection for routine lab investigation of blood.

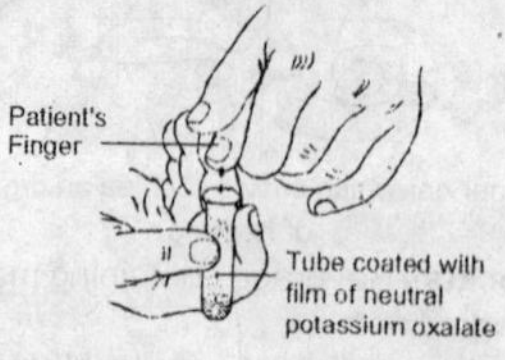

A. Blood collection from finger

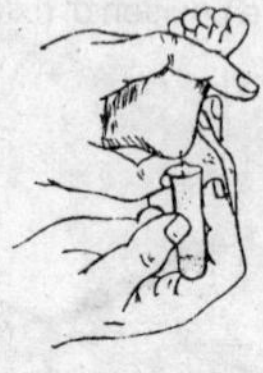

B: Blood collection from heel of infant

Collective behaviour The action of mob or a crowd in a society.

Colles' fracture Fracture of lower end of radius at the wrist when a person falls on outstretched hand, we see *dinner fork* deformity:

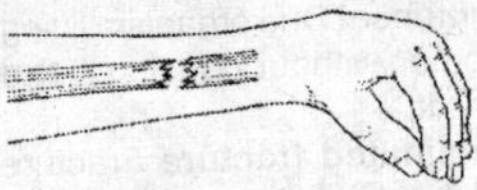

Colles' fracture

Colloid Gelatinous substance by colloid degeneration, any substance which is glue like in appearance, colloid is not influenced by gravity and hence do not settle in a liquid, colloid cannot permeate through semipermeable membrane like dialysis a special type of chemical solution, an oatmeal bath.

Coloboma Congenital fissure affecting retina and choroid coat:

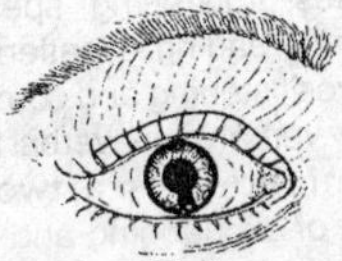

Coloboma of iris

Colon It refers to the portion from *caecum to rectum* called large intestine:

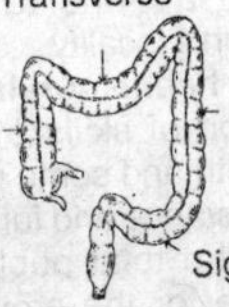

Parts of colon

Colonic irrigation High enemas promoted by cults and quacks, it has limited use, dangerous unless administered under medical supervision.

Colonic lavage Indicated for sigmoidoscopy or barium enema requirements:

- A rubber catheter size l4 or rectal tube.
- A length of rubber tubing.
- A tubing clip.
- A glass connection to fit the rubber tubing and the catheter.
- Lubricant and swabs.
- A larghe jug containing the wash out fluid, usually water or normal saline about 6 pints.
- An irrigating can, a large funnel a pint measure.
- A pail to receive returned fluid or a bed pan.
- Receiver for soiled swabs and catheter.
- The water or lotion is prepared at 105°F and used at 100°F.

Colony When bacterial growth is allowed under favourable conditions, growth of bacteria are seen as colonies.

Colostrum Initial secretion of breast following delivery which contains high protein and low lactose and contain immunity producing substances.

Colostomy Done on ascending colon, transverse colon or sigmoid colon, indicated in trauma, obstructed colon, rectovaginal fistula, and inoperable tumours.

Colour It is the tint of any object.

Colour blind Usually hereditary disease which may be for 2 colours or for 3 colours, also called achromatopsia.

Colour index It gives the amount of haemoglobin present in RBC.

Colpitis Infection and inflammation of vagina.

Colpopexy Surgical suturing of prolapsed vagina to the abdominal wall.

Colporrhaphy Surgical repair of vagina, if it is for retrocele it is posterior colporrhaphy, if it is for cystocele it is anterior colporrhaphy.

Colposcope Instrument used to examine vagina and cervix through magnified lens, helpful for detecting malignant conditions.

Column Round pillor, vertical items.

Coma Deep unconsciousness where patient cannot be aroused with no spontaneous eye movement and no response for painful stimuli, deep and continuous unconsciousness formerly common in diabetes.

Combined pill Oral contraceptive tablets which contain two hormones similar to the natural hormones in a woman's body.

Comfort zone Criteria for thermal comfort which is measured by Corrected Effective Temperature and Predicted Four Hour Sweat Rate as under.

	CET	P_4SR
Comfortable	77 to 80°F	—
Comfort zone	—	1 to 3 litres
Hot, uncomfortable	81 to 82°F	—
Just tolerable	—	3 to 4.5 litres
Intolerable	86°F	4.5 + litres

Comfort Relief from pain, depression, anxiety, discomfort and uneasiness, physically comfort from reasonable temperature and humidity of working place physical and thermal comfort under environmental health.

Commensal One organism living on another without causing harm or benefit.

Comminuted fracture Fracture in which a bone is broken and there are more than two fragments.

Commissure When corresponding parts unite like angle of eyelid or angle of lip, etc.

Common cold A virus infection of the upper respiratory tract.

Communicable disease Infectious diseases that is transmitted from one person to another directly or indirectly, which usually have vector for the transmission.

Communication skill Involve processes of listening, speaking, writing and reading in patient-care in involves listening and communicating by verbal or nonverbal forms.

Communication Is a two way process of exchanging and shaping ideas, feelings and message and is for:

- Acquiring knowledge.
- Learning skills.
- Develop good attitude.

Community action Community organised actions to achieve objectives in a locality.

Community health nursing It is the combination of skills of nursing, public health and some phases of social assistance and functions as a part of the total public health programme for the promotion of health, improvement of social conditions, prevention of illness disability and rehabilitation.

Community People living in one area, who have common interest and belong to same organisation, group of individuals and families living together in a defined geographic area, usually comprising a village, a town or a city.

Compartment syndrome When blood or drainage collect under the tissue of the injured extremity, resulting in swelling and diminished blood flow which is a medical emergency.

Compatibility Suitable for one to one in a society, suitability is mutual, mixing together easily in case of blood grouping and cross-matching.

Compatible The one that mixes easily, blood is compatible means it can be transfused since it matches by blood grouping and cross-matching.

Compatible blood Blood from individuals of the same blood group or type, that can be given safely in blood transfusion.

Compensation for workmen Indemnities paid by employers through insurance or otherwise to workers injured on the job.

Compensatory education Education which has as its main aim the overcoming of perceived deficiencies in a child's education.

Competence Performing professional act in an agreeable manner, role of health professional is met with by professional skill in duties and responsibilities.

Complement A lytic substance which is present in serum, when it combines with antigen antibody complex it produces lysis, there are 4 complements viz., C'_1, C'_2, C'_3, and C'_4 serum contain substance called complement which combines with antigen and antibody reaction to overcome bacteria, they are enzymatic proteins in human serum, when they are activated they stimulate immunological status, it is explained that bacterial opsonisation and leukocyte chemotaxis as mechanism of process in immunological events.

Complement fixation In antigen antibody reaction complement is fixed for the completion of reaction, e.g., Wasserman reaction done in syphilis.

Compliance Measures required for occurrence of physiological process, force is required for lung expansion; here force is a compliance for lung expansion.

Complication Problems encountered during the course of a disease, sequence of events sometimes fatal or serious following the primary condition.

Component It refers to a constituent element or part of a referred item.

Compound family Is a reconstituted family and is a feature of high divorce society which include step families.

Comprehension What we grasp by our mental acumen to understand a situation.

Compression Pressure by one on the other, state of being pressed, in embriogenesis compression means omission of some development.

Compulsion The necessity for repeated actions such as washing the hands repeatedly, checking up again and again on whether all the lights are turned out, checking again and again whether properly locked.

Computer An electronic device with multiple uses like information storing, information retrieval, DTP, net working, e-mail services, etc.

Comte A French sociologist who developed the idea of positivism.

Concave Both side of lens hollowed out, opposite of convex.

Conceive To have a stretch of imagination, to have an image, to form an idea, to become pregnant.

Concentration Strength of a chemical solution in chemistry, mind fixation on one thought by allowing other thought excluded.

Concept Getting an idea of a situation in mind.

Conception Becoming pregnant with the implantation of fertilised ovum, obtaining or arriving at a concept.

Concha Inner aspect of nasal cavity which is divided into upper, middle and lower by their anatomical position and which is turbinate

Concussion Violent jerk to brain by sudden jolt, brain injury produced by the shock of explosion or violent blow without external injury.

Condensation Act of becoming thick, like water condenses to ice.

Condenser Device in microscope which condenses the light on object.

Condom catheters Indwelling catheter used in male patients for external collection urine drain, Texas catheters.

Condom Barrier sheath used for contraception in male and female, male condom is under national FP programme a sheath or covering made of thin latex rubber for men as a barrier method of family planning, Nirodh under national F P programme.

Conductive hearing loss Type of auditory dysfunction, there is physical obstruction of the sound such as fusion of stapes or a foreign body in external ear, tested with the help of tuning fork.

Condyle Round eminence at the end of a bone or at the site of articulation with another bone, smooth surfaces of a bone which articulate with other bone, lower extremity of femur has two condyles which articulate with the tibia to form the knee joint.

Condyloma Wart like elevated lesion of the skin, types clinically identified are :

- Condyloma acuminata.
- Condyloma lata.
- Growth in the skin around anus and external genitalia.

Cones Special cells in retina of eye which are able to distinguish colours.

Confabulation Memory loss of a patient who fills that loss of memory with inappropriate thoughts.

Confidentiality A patient has every right to privacy over the issue of truth. This aspect of professional secrecy is called confidentiality.

Congenital dislocation of hip It is one of the immediate care of the newborn, to assess for congenital dislocation, perform the Ortolani click test by positioning your middle fingers over the greater trochanters and your thumbs along the medial thighs. Then flex the hips and knees.

Congenital Clinical condition or lesion present since birth, names are in use in clinical practice are:

- Congenital heart defect.
- Congenital dislocation of the hip.
- Congenital infection.

Congestion Abnormal accumulation of fluid in organ, congestion of lung excess of fluid accumulation in a tissue or organ, usually post-inflammatory in nature; congested lung, congested heart, etc.

Congress Refers to an assembly, needed for health legislation.

Coniology The scientific study of dust which cause pollution effects.

Conjugation The act of joining together, chemical conjugation and biological conjugation are known in many fields.

Conjunctiva Mucous membrane covering the front of eyeball and lining of eyelids,the membrane which covers the eyeball and lines the eyelids.

Conjunctivitis Infection and inflammation of conjunctiva, clinical types are:

- Purulent conjunctivitis.
- Phlyctenular conjunctivitis.
- Catarrhal conjunctivitis.
- Granular conjunctivitis.

Connective tissue Areolar tissue, bone and cartilage are examples which are developed from mesenchyme , matrix containing cells and fibres they are building tissue of the body holding other tissues together or in proper relation to each other.

Consanguinity Near relative relationship, blood relationship, marriages within the family circle.

Consciousness Person who is in proper orientation of time, place and person, person who is having a state of awareness, person who is having normal motor and sensory responses.

Consent Voluntary agreement with action proposed by another, presently it is suggested to go for informed consent, this gives the patient freeness to and capacity to make decision for his treatment. *Informed consent* is quite agreeable ethical issue in professional activities.

Conservative Aiming at preserving as much as possible.

Conservative treatment Non-radical method of treatment to restore health.

Consolidation Substance becoming solid, lung consolidation in infection by becoming solid and by the presence of exudate.

Constipation Incomplete movement of bowel, motion not fully passed and feeling to pass motion frequently, inability to perform normal bowel elimination functions.

Constitution Functional habit of human body, routine adjustment of body.

Consultation Qualified professional giving opinion on diagnosis and treatment.

Consumer Patient is the consumer in health care services.

Consummation The first act of sexual intercourse after marriage.

Consumption Being utilised, act of consumed, washed away from the body in the form of excretion.

Contact lens Fexible non-reactive device kept on the cornea which facilitate and correct the refractive error.

Contact receptors Nerves which transmit stimuli only on contact e.g., touch.

Contact When an individual is in association with or in contact with another person who is infectious.

Contagion Infectious disease when spread from one person to another by direct contact.

Contagious disease That which spreads by contact like scabies, skin infection.

Contagious Refers to disease which easily gets transmitted from one person to another either by direct or indirect contact.

Containment To help to retain an infection not to spread to other places by available control measures in public health practice.

Continence Ability to control the act of urination or sex act.

Continent ileostomy Draining the internal pouch (kock pouch), faecal content drainer with the help of the patient.

Continent One who is capable of controlling certain physiological processes like defecation, urination or sexual indulgence.

Continuing education Facility made available to professionals to update their knowledge by attending arranged formal programmes.

Continuum A social phenomenon showing variation between two opposite characteristics e.g., hermaphrodite in between male and female.

Contraculture An alternative vision by a subculture in a society.

Contraception Measures undertaken to prevent the occurrence of pregnancy by available methods and measures of family planning.

Contraction This refers to muscular action or muscle contraction which usually of shorter duration and repetitive in nature, when applied to uterus this is called labour pain.

Contract Arrangement between doctor and patient, between nurse and patient for treatment and care with dignity.

Contracture It is the process of fibrosis because of permanent contraction of any tissue, especially of skin and muscle, two common clinical conditions worth mention are:

- Volkmann's ischaemiac contracture.
- Dupuytren's contracture.

Contraindication Clinical condition which makes the mode of treatment not practicable circumstances which suggest avoidance of certain medical or surgical or OBG procedures.

Contralateral Any thing or any change that occurs on the opposite side in reference to anatomical position, opposite side of the body.

Contrast bath Use of alternating hot and cold water usually as a spray.

Contrast medium Chemical substance used in radiological diagnosis to make any organ to make visible.

Contrecoup injury Left side brain injury leading to damage on right side, backside injury of skull leading to damage in front of the brain, injury on one side and damage is on the other side of the brain.

Control Refers to disease control, restrain from the act, a group with similar characteristics as study group for a case control study.

Controlled trial To have unbiased study, in a research trial one group is not given actual medicine or investigations to see whether the difference occurred in study group and control group is by chance.

Contusion Other name for bruise, superficial injury.

Convalescence Recovery period after illness, after injury or after operation.

Conversion Emotion becoming manifestations, foetal parts getting changing, tuberculin conversion.

Conversion hysteria Psychoneurotic condition where patient has found his fears unbearable and has converted them into a physical disability.

Convex Refers to lens whose curvatures are blown outwards, opposite of concave.

Convolution Refers to folds in the brain or in the renal tubules, twist or coil of any organ, especially one of the prominent convex parts of the brain.

Convulsion It is a state of involuntary contraction of voluntary muscles due to organic causes or sometimes by unknown causes, common clinical types are major convulsion and minor convulsion unconsciousness accompanied by muscular twitching.

Cookery In nursing care it refers to sick-room cookery, simple digestible foods are needed for invalids which must be fresh and of best quality. They include the following:

- Barley water.
- Imperial drinks.
- Diluted milk for infants.
- Butter flour mixture.
- Thickened milk feed.
- Lactic acid milk.
- Milk vegetable soup.
- Baked custard.
- Egg jelly.
- Orange jelly.
- Bread and butter pudding.
- Scrambled egg.
- Junket.
- Sauce.
- High protein drinks.

Cooley's anaemia It is an inherited disorder of haemoglobin synthesis called thalassemia major.

Coombs' test This is an immunological test to detect antibody on RBC to diagnose haemolytic anaemia or to check for incompatibility, laboratory test to detect autoimmune haemolytic anaemia.

COPD Chronic Obstructive Pulmonary Disease.

Copper T An intrauterine device used as conventional contraceptive device.

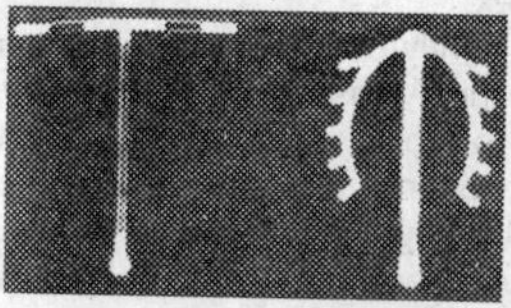

Copper T

COPRA The **CO**nsumer **PR**otection Act of 1986.

Copula Refers to a connecting part.

Copulation Other name for coitus or sexual intercourse, term applied to lower animals.

Coracoid Any structure which resemble a crow's beak.

Coramine Proprietary name of Nikethamide.

Corneal Referable to cornea like corneal graft or corneal ulcer.

Cornu It means a horn e.g., cornu of the uterus.

Coronal Related to head like coronal suture.

Cornification It is the process of convertion of squamous epithelian cells into hard horny substance, common examples are:
- Feather.
- Hair.
- Nail.
- Horn.

Core function of family The sexual, the reproductive, the socialisation and the economic.

Corpse It refers to dead body or a cadaver.

Corn Induration and thickening of skin, pressure points.

Cornea Transparent front portion of the eye, the clear window at the front of the eye.

Corneal reflex It is testing for blink reflex:
a. lightly brush fingertips across the eyelashes.
b. touching outer cornea with cotton.

It is absent in 5th cranial nerve involvement, diminished with contact lens put up.

Cornification Because of deposit of keratin, skin becoming horny or the process of cornification.

Cornu Any horn like projection.

Corona The head, the skull, the crown, the main portion of any organism.

Corona radiata Both ascending and descending fibres of internal capsule are called corona radiate, the fibres above the corpus collosum which connects from all direction to reach cerebral cortex is specifically called corona radiata.

Corona Structure which resembles a crown.

Coronal Related to skull or head.

Coronary angiography Injection of iohexol or urograffin which are contract medium to radiological diagnosis of coronary artery pathology.

Coronary thrombosis Clot formation and blocking of coronary artery which cause angina pectoris and M I.

Coronary Crown like and encircling feature, refers to the following:
- Coronary artery.
- Coronary bypass surgery.
- Coronary care unit.
- Coronary circulation.

Meaning crown like, describes arteries which supply blood to the heart muscle, connected with heart attacks.

Coronoid fossa It is a oval depression on anterior surface of distal end of humerus which articulates with coronoid process of ulna.

Corpse Cadaver, a dead body.

Corpulent Overweight or obese person.

Corpulmonale Due to pulmonary pathology right sided heart failure.

Corpuscle Small body or little units like RBC, WBC. Small cell, small protoplasmic body, RBC, WBC.
Common corpuscles are:
- Red blood corpuscle.
- White blood corpuscle.
- Malphigian corpuscle.
- Meissner's corpuscle.
- Pacinian corpuscle.

Corpus Main part of an organ such as:
- Corpus cavernosum.
- Corpus callosum.
- Corpus luteum.
- Corpus stratum.

Correlation Correlation is a technique to study relationships:

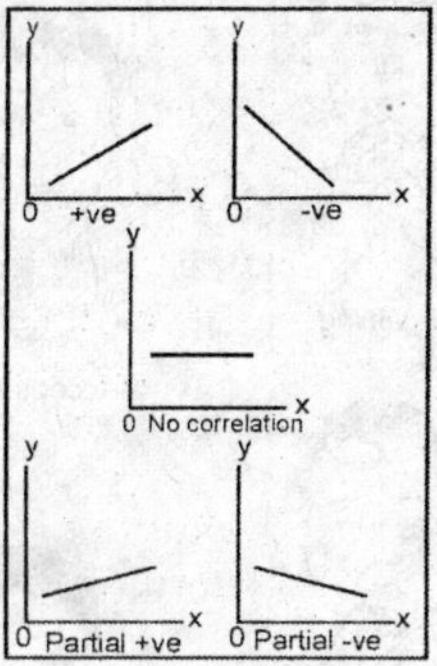

Correlation

Cortex Outer layer of the plant, outer layer of an organ, common reference is made for the following:

- Renal cortex.
- Cerebral cortex.
- Adrenal cortex.

The outer layer of cells of an organ such as the adrenal gland or kidney.

Corticosteroid Hormones from adrenal cortex, synthetic corticosteroid, they help in metabolism as under:

- Salt and water regulation by mineralocorticoids.
- Proximate principle regulation by glucocorticoids.

Cortisone Hormone of the adrenal cortex useful in certain forms of rheumatic illness and many other diseases.

Corynebacterium Slender, rod-shaped, gram-positive, non-motile bacteria which cause diphtheria infection in human beings.

Coryza Acute URI infection which is manifested with sneezing, discharge from nose, is equivalent to common cold.

Coxalgia Refers to the pain in hip joint.

Cosmetic surgery Plastic surgery and reconstruction surgery done to improve the appearance commonly done in birth defects and burns.

Cosmetics Beautifying substances or preparations, tending to preserve normalcy or originality.

Cost accounting How money is spent in each act of nursing when recorded becomes cost accounting, It helps in cost control.

Cost benefit The economic benefit of nursing service is compared with the cost of that nursing service.

Cost-effective Providing a value for money spent in medical practice, like OPV in prevention of polio lameness in community.

Cot death Sudden Infant Death Syndrome.

Cotrel dynamic traction It is prescribed for patients as preoperative management in scoliosis to enhance soft tissue stretching prior to spinal fusion.

Cottonpox Benign type of smallpox or alastrim

Couching Crude method in which displalcement of lens is done to improve vision in case of mature cataract.

Cough Voluntary explosive expulsion of air from lungs which help in the expulsion of foreign body or the mucous.

Counselling Listening and offering guidance and advice to a person in the case of illness, disease, operation or incurable disease, guidance and counselling of patients by nurse, doctor or health personnel, face to face communication by which one can help the person to make decision and to act on them.

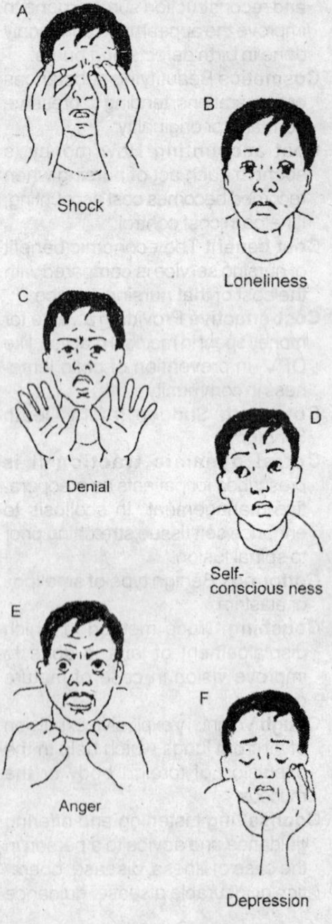

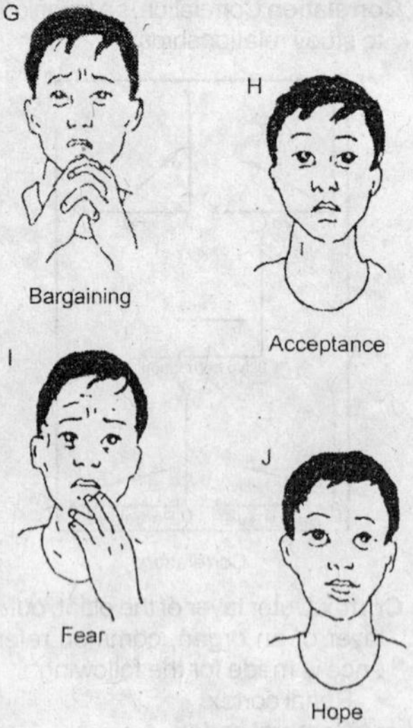

Counselling stages as a result of positive counselling (A to J)

Counter culture Ideas, beliefs and practices of a sub-culture.

Counterirritant A substance or a drug which when applied on the skin produces skin changes and removes pain by counter irritation.

Couple protection rate Is an indicator of the prevalence of contraceptives practice in the community. By 60% of CPR we can achieve NRR of 1.0.

Coupling Very common in digitalis overdose where we get extra-ventricular heart beat after a normal heart beat, term used in cardiology.

Courts Legal dais for dealing with criminality and offences through medical evidences.

Courtship Dating, sign of adolescence, developing interest in opposite sex.

Cow sociology Sociology of service of capitalist enterprises.

Cowper's gland Mucous gland below the bulb of male urethra just as Bartholin gland in females.

Coxiella A genus which cause Q fever, specific reference to *C.burnetti*.

Coxsackie Coxsackie's virus causing various types of infection, a group of virus which produces illness like meningitis, pleurodynia, acute myocarditis and acute pericarditis picorna virus group causing many pathological conditions like:

- Myocarditis.
- Epidemic conjunctivitis.
- Aseptic meningitis.
- Pleurodynia.
- Herpangina.

Crab louse Other name for pubic louse, except for physical nuisance, they do not transmit any disease, Phthirus pubis is its entomological name.

Cradle hold Commonly used position for breastfeeding in which mother is sitting upright, with the infant's head held in the crook of her arm and its buttocks cradled in her hand.

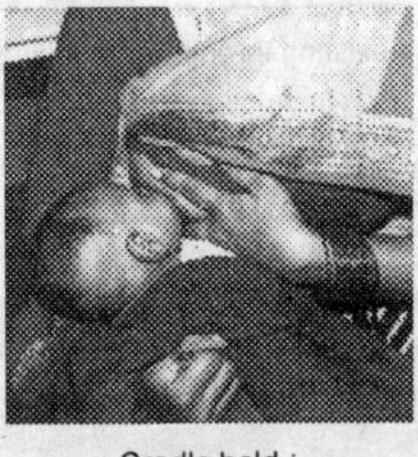

Cradle hold

Cradle splint Called Braun's cradle splint used in a plaster splint for the treatment of fractures of the lower limb.

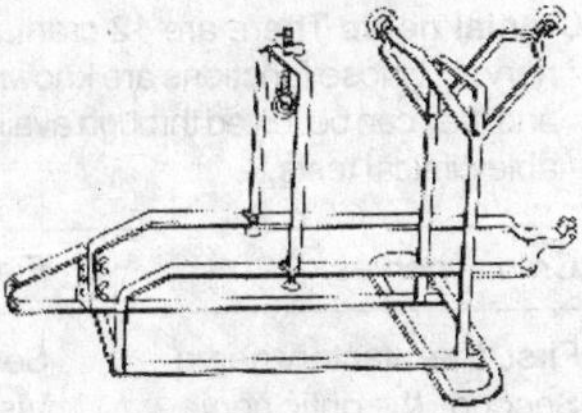

Cradle splint

Cradle Infant's bed with protective sides which is on rockers, to support on the arm, metallic frame on the bed of the patient to protect his injured parts.

Cradle carry A mode of transport of sick or injured by one man, rehearsed in first aid.

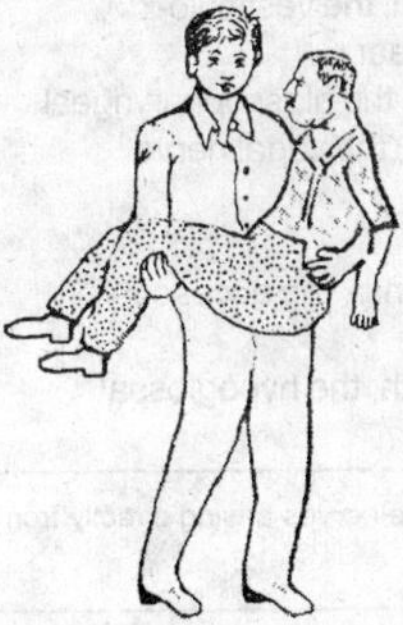

Cradle carry

Cramp Painful spasmodic muscular spasm, intense heat can cause muscle cramps.

Cranial Which are related to skull or head or crown like, cranial nerves.

Cranial drainage Observation of drainage from eyes, ears, nose for CSF is necessary indicated in craniocerebral injury or recovery from craniotomy.

Cranial nerve There are 12 cranial nerves whose functions are known and they can be tested through available clinical tests,

Cranioclast surgical instrument for crushing of foetal head in case of Intrauterine death.

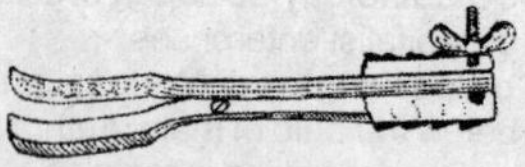

Cranioclast

Cranial nerves	*Function*	*Tests*
First, the olfactory nerve	Sense of smell	Smelling
Second , the optic nerve	Vision	Snellen's test
Third, the oculomotor nerve	Eye movement	Weakness of orbicular occuli
Fourth, the trochlear nerve	Eye movement	Intorsion
Fifth, the trigeminal nerve	Face sensation Mastication	Sensation Clenching
Sixth, the abducent nerve	Outward eye move	Movement
Seventh, the facial nerve	Facial expression Ant.2/3rd tongue Taste sensation	Eyebrow Raise
Eighth, the vestibulo-cochlear	Hearing, Equilibrium	Rinne, Webers caloric test
Ninth, the glossopharyngeal	Post. 1/3rd tongue	Taste sensation
Tenth, the vagal nerve	Sensory and motor to Viscera and resp. passage	heart, abdominal
Eleventh, the accessory nerve	Movement of larynx and pharynx	
Twelfth, the hypoglossal nerve	Protrusion and movements of tongue	

These nerves arising directly from the brain and existing through an opening in the skull.

Craniocleido dysostosis Defective ossification of bones of head, face and clavicle which is a birth defect or a congenital malformation.

Cranium Skull that contains the brain, the cavity that contains the brain, the skull.

Creatine It is the nitrogenous material present in the muscle, creatine is present in the urine in cases of fever and starvation.

Creatinine It is the product of protein metabolism which is normally present in the urine.

Crede maneuver It is manual pressure applied to the bladder employed to facilitate the removal of urine for patients whose bladder is flaccid.

Crede's method It is method of manual expulsion of placenta by putting downward pressure on uterus through anterior abdominal wall which allow a sort of squeezing of uterus.

Cremaster A type of fascia enveloping testicles and spermatic cord which also helps to suspend the testicles.

Crepitation Grating sound in fractured bone pieces, grating sounds fine or course crepitation is heard in lung disorders.

Crepitus Grating sound or sensation that can be heard or felt during joint movement.

Crescent Sickle-shaped structure e.g., menisci of knee joint, myopic condition due to atrophy of choroid.

Cresol Disinfectant containing 5% phenol which is a coal tar derivative.

Cretin Hypothyroidism, in children the condition is called cretinism.

Cretinism Hypothyroidism condition leading to lack of thyroid secretion , characterised by arrested physical growth and dull dry skin.

Cri du chat syndrome It is a chromosomal disorder characterised by:
- Microcephaly.
- Mental retardation.
- Dwarfism.
- Laryngeal defect with cat's cry.

Cribiform Organ or tissue which is sieve like in its appearance.
Examples are:
- Cribiform plate of ethmoid bone.
- Cribiform fascia of fossa ovalis.

Cricoid Signet ring like structure e.g., cricoid cartilage.

Crisis situation A brief psychological method of treatment for the person who is in an emotional crisis, it is a sudden event in one's life which disturbs the mental equilibrium.

Crisis Peak of disease which terminates either in death or survival, sudden paroxysmal intensification of symptoms of an illness, *Life crisis* when a family member dies, *adrenal crisis* due to adrenal failure, during adolescent period *identity crisis* refers to critical period of an illness like:
- Pneumonia crisis.
- Addisonian crisis.
- Sickle cell crisis.
- Thyroid crisis.
- Renal crisis.
- Bleeding crisis.
- Asthmatic crisis.
- Epileptic crisis.

Crista Ridge like structure, ampulla of semicircular canal, crista supraventricularis of heart.

Criteria Decision is made on specified criteria or standards for case diagnosis, case management and case prognosis.

Crohn's disease Other name for regional enteritis which involve all the coats of intestine.

Cross class family Husband and wife in different social class by their occupation.

Cross cultural comparisons Examination of two societies for similarities and differences.

Cross eye Squint or strabismus.

Cross-matching For the purpose of blood transfusion testing is done along with blood grouping for cross-match to identify compatibility.

Croup A closing of the voice box due to infection or spasm.

Croupette It is indicated for infant who needs high humidity, oxygen and temperature controlled environment by pneumatically powered system.

Crown Portion of teeth seen above the gum.

Crowning It is in the first stage of labour when the caput or head of newborn is seen protruding from vulva.

Crucial ligaments Ligaments inside the joint capsule in the form of a cross, run between the femur and the tibia in the knee joint.

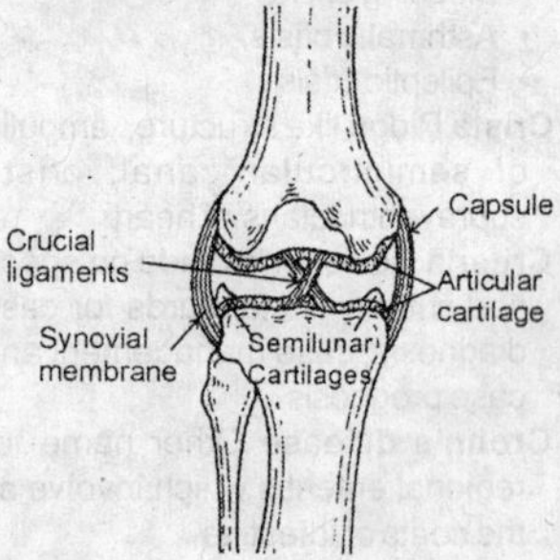

Crucial ligaments in knee joint

Crura Leg like resembling divergents, examples:
- Crura cerbri.
- Crura spinosa.
- Crura of diaphragm.

Crus Any organ which look like a leg, portion of body from knee to foot.

Crutches Walking aid for patients who have affected limbs. Assisting patients with crutches by the nurse: Nurse to stand on affected side and grasp the security belt in the midspine area at the small of the back, free hand is positioned at shoulder area so that the nurse can pull the patient toward her in the event that there is a fall forward, she should not obstruct the movement of arm, she should instruct the patient to look up and outward the destination rather than at feet.

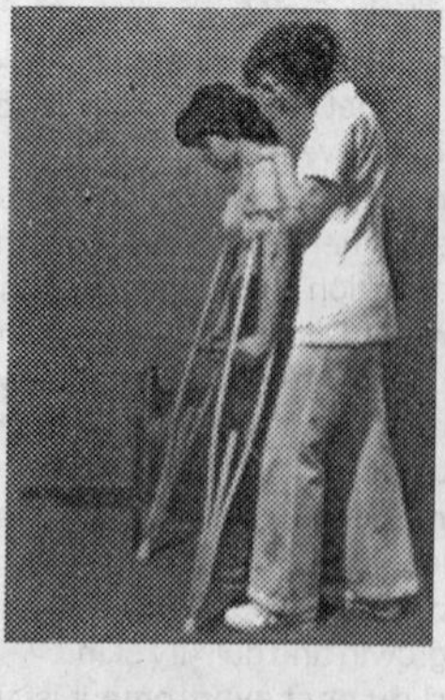

Crutches in use

Cryoglobulin It is an abnormal globulin found in the following conditions:
- Multiple myeloma.

- Leukaemia.
- Mycoplasma pneumonia.

Cryosurgery Use of extreme cold situation to destroy tissue employed in neuro-surgery.

Cryotherapy Cold usage for the purpose of treatment of illness.

Crypt Means hidden, minute tube like depression opening on the surface of anatomical part.

Cryptococcosis Common fungal infection by *Cryptococcus neoformans* which attack brain tissue in patients who are immunocompromised by certain diseases like AIDS.

Crypts of Lieberkuhn Mucous membrane glands which secretes intestinal juice.

Crystal Particles with definite angles and pattern like Charcot Leyden crystals, calcium phosphate crystals.

Crystalline That which resembles a crystal in nature or in clearness.

Crystalluria Urine containing crystals indicate specified pathology including sulpha drug administration.

CSF Cerebro Spinal Fluid.

CSSM Child Survival and Safe Motherhood, recently it is renamed as R.C.H.

Ctenocephalus Genus of fleas.

Cubital fossa Hollow anterior portion of elbow which has definite boundry; Pronater teres medially and Brachioradialis laterally.

Cubitus refers to elbow or forearm, when deformity is there usage of cubitus valgus and cubitus varus are used:

- Medial or lateral deviation of forearm which is abnormal.
- Lateral deviation of forearm is called *cubitus valgus*.
- Medial deviation of forearm is called *cubitus varus*.

Cul-de-sac A blind cavity or a blind sac.

Culdocentesis Perforating and draining fluid from rectouterine pouch for the purpose of diagnosis, perforation is through posterior upper vaginal wall.

Culdoscope It is a type of endoscopic examination for the purpose of diagnosis.

Culdoscopy Endoscopic examination of pelvic cavity through posterior vaginal fornix.

Culex One of the type of mosquito which transmits filaria and dengue .

Cult Group of people who follow their own ideal principles which have come from their ancestors.

Cultural taboos Aspects of social life which are considered forbidden by the norms of society.

Culture clash Is a cause of under achievement of working class and ethnic minority.

Culture medium Substance or preparation used for the cultivation of living cells.

Culture shock Disruption because of an alien culture.

Culture Growing pathogens in a favourable condition:

- Culture and sensitivity test.
- All acquired aspects of life in a society.
- Denotes the characteristics of a race, of a religion or of a social group.
- Way of life of a society.

Cuneiform Wedge-shaped anatomical structure; there is one cuneiform bone in wrist, there are three cuneiform bones in the foot.

Curare Historically known as arrow poison, now it is used in anaesthesia. Is a muscle relaxant used in surgery, originally it is extracted from a south American Plant used to poison arrows by tribes.

Curative Refers to medical treatment to cure an illness.

Curette Surgical instrument used to scrape unhealthy tissue during surgery which is shaped like a spoon.

Curie It is the unit of radiation expressed as disintegration per second. It is calculated at $10^{10} \times 3.7$ disintegration per second.

Curling ulcer Duodenal ulcer which occurs secondary to severe burns of the body.

Curriculum It refers to the course of study in educational system through Board or through University.

Curvature Bend of a line which is quoted as *curve of the line* which may be normal or abnormal, every organ has some curvature or the other like spinal curvature, lesser curvature and greater curvature of the stomach, etc.

Cushing's disease Clinical condition characterised by increased *corticosteroid-associated* clinical features secondary to **Pituitary** cause.

Cushing's syndrome Clinical condition characterised by increased corticosteroid associated clinical features, the cause lying within the **adrenal gland** like adrenal adenoma, bilateral adrenal hyperplasia and rarely adrenal carcinoma, *exogenous intake of Corticosteroids is the commonest cause.*

Cusps Component parts of heart valves.

Custom Is an established pattern and a traditional pattern of human behaviour.

Cutaneous ureterostomy Method of urinary diversion in intractable incontinence and malignancy; The ureters are resected from the bladder and one or both ureters are brought directly through the abdominal wall.

Cutaneous Related with the skin or its appendages.

Cuticle Outer layer of the skin , also referred to as epidermis.

Cutis It refers to true skin or derma.

CV A measure of variability by using a coefficient obtained from the. Mean and Standard Deviation:

$$C.V. = \frac{S.D.}{Mean} \times 100$$

CVP central venous catheter Semi-permanent indwelling central lines that are inserted into the right atrium via cephalic, subclavian or jugular veins, indicated in chemotherapy, transfusions and central venous pressure monitoring.

CVP It is the highest level of distension and pulsation in the internal jugular vein in centimetres, using the sternal angle (the point at which the clavicles meet) as reference point.

More than 3 cm indicate elevated CVP:

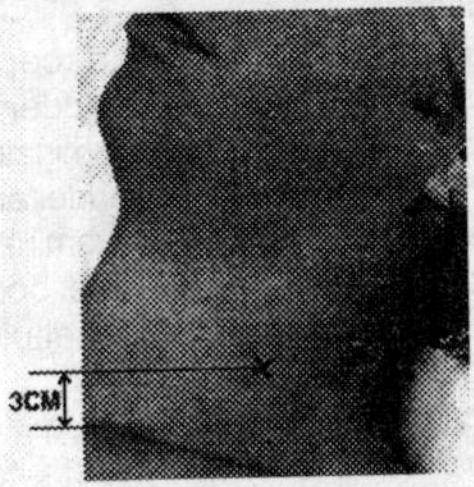

CVP

Cyanocobalamine Anti-anaemia factor vitamin B_{12} found in animal foods, this with intrinsic factor is essential for erythropoisis.

Cyanosis Bluish discolouration of skin and mucous membrane due to poor oxygenation of blood as in blue babies or circulatory failure.

Cycle Events occurring in a serial manner as seen in menstrual cycle or cardiac cycle.

Cyclopia Developmental anomaly where there is one orbital fossa, nose is absent and is seen as an appendage above the orbit.

Cycloplegia Dilatation of pupil due to paralysis of ciliary muscles.

Cyclops Tiny vector of the size of a pin head which transmits Guinea Worm infection.

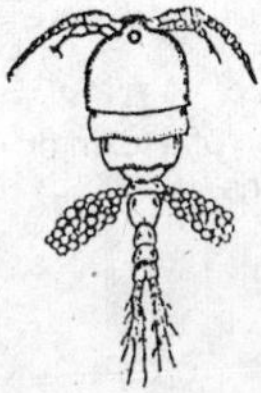

Cyclop

Cyesis Refers to pregnancy state, the false pregnancy is called pseudocyesis.

Cyst A cavity containing liquid or semi-solid material and is lined by epithelium, common cysts of clinical importance are:

- Thyroglossal cyst.
- Ovarian cyst.
- Dermoid cyst.
- Branchial cyst.
- Hydatid cyst.
- Meibomian cyst.
- Multilocular cyst.
- Sebaceous cyst.
- Sublingual cyst.

Cysts of intestinal protozoa They are findings of stool examination of patients who suffer from intestinal parasitism:

A. Uninucleate and quadrinucleate *E.histolytica*.

B. Uninucleate and *octonucleate* *E.coli*.

C. *Giardia intestinalis*.

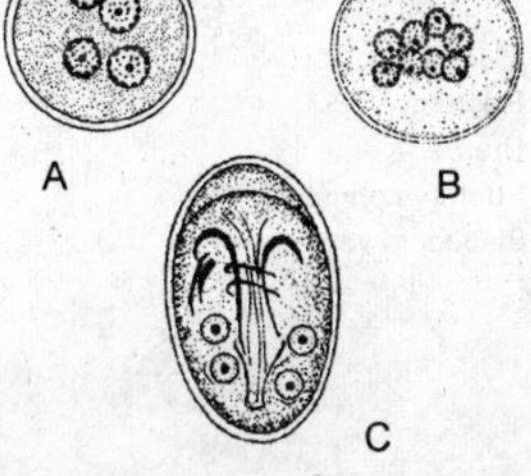

Cysts of intestinal protozoa of man

Cysteine Amino acid which contain sulphur which is produced by dietary protein.

Cystic fibrosis Also called mucoviscidosis or cystic fibrosis of the pancreas, hereditary disorder associated with accumulation of thick mucous and abnormal secretion of sweat and saliva.

Cysticercosis Pork tapeworm infection by *Taenia solium*.

Cysticercus Larval form of tapeworm.

Cystine Amino acid closely related to cysteine, when it is excreted in urine it is called cystinuria.

Cystitis Infection and inflammation of urinary bladder.

Cystocele Hernial protrusion of urinary bladder through vaginal wall:

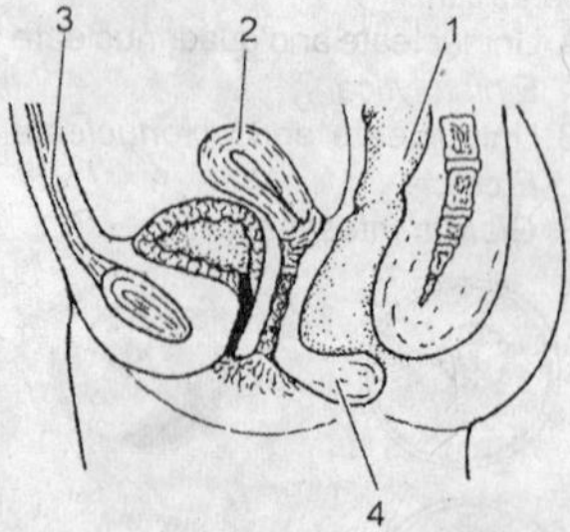

Cystocele

1. Rectum.
2. Uterus.
3. Pubi symphysis.
4. Bladder in vagina.

Cystolithiasis Clinical condition where stones are seen in urinary bladder.

Cystoscope When endoscopic examination of urinary bladder is undertaken an electrically illuminated instrument by which the bladder and the kidney can be visually examined.

Cytochrome Pigment in the body which is responsible for cellular respiration.

Cytogenetics Scientific study of living cells during mitosis for chromosomal examination to detect chromosomal abnormalities.

Cytology Microscopic study of structure and function of cells of living organisms, when done for detection of early cancer it is called exfoliative cytology.

Cytomegalovirus Virus belonging to herpes simplex group.

Cytopathogenic Producing pathological changes in cells, degenerative changes are seen in cells.

Cytoplasm Protoplasm of the cell which is seen around the nucleus.

Cytosine Pyrimidine base found in DNA.

Cytosis Describes the conditions of nucleus of WBC, common words that are expressed to describe the conditions are:

- Isocytosis.
- Anisocytosis.
- Hypercytosis.
- Hypocytosis.
- Normocytosis.

Cytotoxic Toxic action of a toxin on cells of special organs.

D

D & C OBG Procedure done for diagnosis and therapy, dilatation and curettage.

D N B Diplomate of National Board an examination taken by medical graduates after MBBS, which is conducted by Indian Academy of Medical Sciences, New Delhi, it is also an abbreviation for Di Nitro Benzene.

Dacryorrhoea It is a condition with profuse flow of tears.

Dactyl Refers to digit, which can be either a finger or a toe, refers to a finger or a toe, it also refers to the fruit of the date.

Dairy products It includes whole milk, skimmed milk, evaporated milk, buttermilk, butter, cheese, ice cream etc.

Dale reaction It is a test for sensitisation in guinea pig, uterine horn is removed and is immersed in a fluid containing an antigen will cause contraction of uterus.

Dalton's law It states that the weight of the absorbed gas rises and falls in proportion to the pressure though the volume of a gas absorbed by a liquid remains constant.

Dames de charite During 17th century in France a voluntary visiting service by influential ladies formed "Dames de charite" who nursed the sick at home, at hospital, at home for aged, at home for insane and in the battle field.

Damp A dangerous gas containing nitrogen, carbon dioxide and carbon mono-oxide present in the Mines.

Dander Skin particle of animals which cause allergy by inhalation.

Dandruff Cast-off cells from outer layer of skin of scalp.

Dane particle It is the particle of hepatitis B virus which has the sphere of 42 nm.

Dangerous Drug Act Drugs prescribed should be basic, indispensable and necessary to the sick and suffering, as per the Act "Dangerous Drug Act" 1965 it is an offence to obtain dangerous drugs for any purpose other than authorised.

Dangling of extremities On the day of the surgery patient is required to sit on the side bed and dangle their legs before getting out of bed, it is to protect the patient's back, minimise the strain to an abdominal or perineal incision and exercise the upper extremities as well.

Danida An assistance by Government of Denmark for the prevention of blindness, for the veterinary health (dairy development) and for higher studies in MSc ophthalmology for developing countries, an International Voluntary Organisation.

Dapsone It is sulphone drug which is used in the treatment of leprosy.

Daraprim Antimalarial drug pyrimethamine.

Dark circles of eye This does not have relation to diseases, it is dependent on anatomical factors and family traits, the skin of eyelids is thin and contains little fatty tissue, the blood which passes through the large veins close to the surface shows through to the surface of the skin. This produces a bluish-black tint in the skin, this is accentuated when fatigued, when anaemic, when pregnant and in later years of life.

Dark room This space is for processing X-ray films in radiology or in photography.

Darling's disease Histoplasmosis is known as Darling's disease.

Dartos The subcutaneous muscle of scrotum.

Data Facts collected in health practice which can be of two types:

- Continuous data..height and weight.
- Discrete data......hair colour.

Database Collected data is stored , reviewed and updated for the use of medical audit, data base is used in health planning, it is useful for evaluation of treatment given.

Dating Developing interest in other sex, sign of adolescence and adulthood, boys and girls meet in meeting places where they feel interested under desirable circumstances.

Dentifrices During 1960 dentifrice formulas were developed which apparently helped preventing dental decay. Tooth brush and tooth paste are common examples of dentifrices, devices to clean teeth.

Datura Datura plant is the source of anticholinergic drugs like scopolamine and hyosciamine.

Dawn phenomenon In diabetic patients growth hormone is released in the morning which influences hyperglycaemia in the morning which is called *Dawn phenomenon.*

Day care Care given to 0 to 4 aged children which is the substitution for family life.

Day light factor It is the ratio between instantaneous illumination indoors and simultaneous illumination outdoors, the formula is:

$$\text{Day Light Factor} = \frac{\text{Indoor illumination}}{\text{Outdoor illumination}} \times 100$$

recommended day light factors are:

8% for living room

10% for kitchen

Day nursery Day time care giving institutions for 0 to 5 year age children which also has non-formal education for kids.

Day patient care Specialised health care for patient during the day, admission and discharge will be on the same day since investigations, treatment or minor OPD surgery are undertaken.

DB Measurement unit for noise

Whispering	10 dB
Talking	60 dB
Speech	80 dB
Radio music	85 dB
Shouting	80 dB
Crying	80 dB
Road roller	120 dB
Planes take off	150 dB

DDT emulsion Under nursing care of the hair, when head is found to be infested with lice or nits they are treated with older methods like:

- Lethane oil application.
- DDT emulsion applicate.
- DDT application when done, the hair is washed 48 hours after the application.

DDT Dichloro Diphenyl trichloroethane, a Residual insecticide.

Deadly nightshade Produces food poisoning, children are occasionally affected through eating poisonous berries e.g., those of the deadly night-shade, or toadstool taken by mistake for mushrooms, in these cases symptoms of poisoning occur soon after the food has been eaten, staining of mouth and clothing round the neck may supply evidence that poisonous berries have been eaten.

Deafness conductive Hearing loss due to inability of ear to transmit sounds to the nerve endings of inner ear, conduction deafness.

Deafness nerve Inability of the hearing nerve to transmit sound stimuli to the brain, nerve deafness.

Deafness Person who is not in a position to hear, which may be of 2 types:

- Conduction deafness.
- Nerve deafness.

It is a state in which loss of hearing is there.

Deamination Breaking down of amino acids to form urea and this takes place in the liver, the process is called hydrolysis.

Death awareness Death awareness cannot be perceived in PVS stage (persistent Vegetative State) and in a state of irreversible unconsciousness. It is experienced by patients in advanced and terminal stages of illness, it is precipitated by illiteracy (fear of other world) and by literates (who know the true story of their organs and tissues) It is related to the Right of Information, Culture and Tradition influence death awareness.

Death of the family Family weaning by divorce, cohabitation and lone parent.

Death rate No. of deaths per unit of population in reference, rate is expressed per thousand.

Death In cellular component or in an organism if all physical, chemical and biological processes is stopped, common concepts are:

- Brain death.
- Clinical death.
- Cot death.
- Natural death.
- Unnatural death.

Debility Lack of physical tone and extreme weakness in the body.

Debridement Surgical intervention for quick and good healing of a wound, removal of traumatic wound tissue to all normal healing.

Decalcification Calcium salt is taken off from the bone in disorders of calcium metabolism.

Decapsulation Surgical removal of fibrous capsule.

Decay Decomposition of dead organic matter, gradual decomposition of dead organic matter, old ageing signs.

Decerebrate posturing This can occur with upper brainstem injury where we see extension of the extremities after a stimulus.

Decerebrate When there is no cerebral function due to brain damage, person show neurological disorders and no cerebral functions.

Decibel Is an expression of intensity of sound which is used in evaluation of state of deafness in a patient.

Deciduas Refers to temporary milk set in children.

Deciduous teeth Milk set of teeth in babies which are 20 in number as under:

Right upper 2,1, 2. ++ Left upper 2, 1, 2.

Right lower 2,1, 2. ++ Left lower 2, 1, 2.

Decision making Information of patient is used to arrive at treatment modalities.

Declaration of Geneva World Health Assembly in 1948 has adopted the declaration which declares that each member of medical profession pledge his life to the service of humanity.

Declaration of Hawaii This is declaration at Hawaii given by World Psychiatric Association.

Decline Progressive decrease of any item.

Decoction Medication prepared from chemicals or plant extracts in the, form of a liquid.

Decompensation Usually refers to heart which has failed to compensate to overcome increased work load.

Decompression Status when raised intracranial pressure is reduced by removal of flap of skull, gradual exposure to normal atmosphere from high altitude pressure.

Decongestant Drug which reduces swelling or congestion, usually refers to nasal decongestants, drug which helps in reducing swelling of tissues in inflammation.

Decontamination Making free atmosphere for persons or patients from pathogens, from radioactive substances, from nerve gas.

Decorticate posturing It is upper extremity flexion with lower extremity extension and it can occur with an injury to the cortex.

Decortications Surgical removal of outer layer of an organ as in decortications for chronic emphyema.

Decubitus Because of lying down posture changes that occur is explained.

Decubitus ulcer Bedsore in a chronic ill patient which is a pressure sore.

Deep tendon reflex They are present in all normal adults. Absence or heightened reflexes denote pathology associated with an interruption of an impulse at the associated anatomic site in the spinal cord

DTR scale	*Description*
0	non-reflexive
1	hypo-reflexive*
2	normal
3	brisk**
4	hyper-reflexive

*normally seen in old people

**not always associated with pathology

common deep tendon reflexes:

a biceps reflex.

b brachioradialis or supinator reflex.

c triceps reflex.

d patellar reflex.

e ankle reflex.

Deep veins These accompany the arteries of general circulation and are therefore called companion veins along with superficial veins they form the veins of the general circulation.

Deerfly fever Other name for tularaemia.

Defecation Elimination of waste material in the form of stool which is a process of body excretion.

Defence Body reaction to protect from injury, is a defence mechanism, refers to protective behaviour.

Defervescent Reduction in the severity of illness or of a fever in disease process.

Defibrillation Action taken to restore atrial fibrillation or ventricular fibrillation.

Deficiency disease Refers to dietary deficiency which cause clinical manifestations.

Deficit Not up to the mark when compared to normal , a deficiency.

Defluoridation Removal of excess content of fluorine from drinking water to prevent fluorosis, Nalgonda technique of Defluoridation.

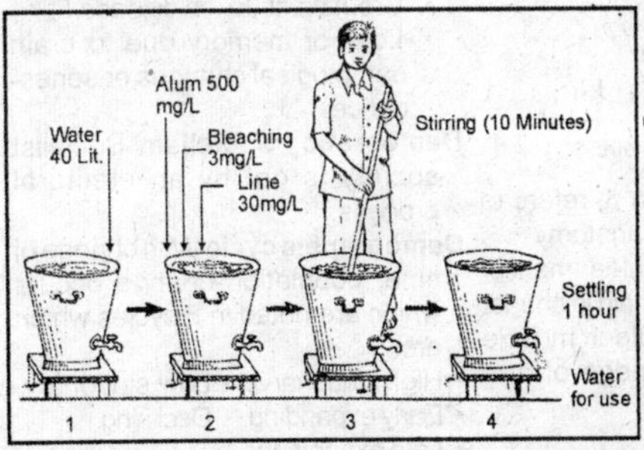

Defluoridation (Nalgonda technique)

Deflorescence After the active stage when skin rashes start disappearing as in the case of chickenpox, measles.

Deglutition Physiological function of swallowing.

Dehydration State of loss of fluid from the body, common causes are vomiting diarrhoea, sweating, shock and acidosis are its sequelae.

Dehydro cholesterol It is precursor of vitamin D

DeLee mucous Trap appliance used in providing neonatal care, A DeLee mucous trap is used when congestion is deeper in the nose and mouth and the secretion may potentially block the airway.

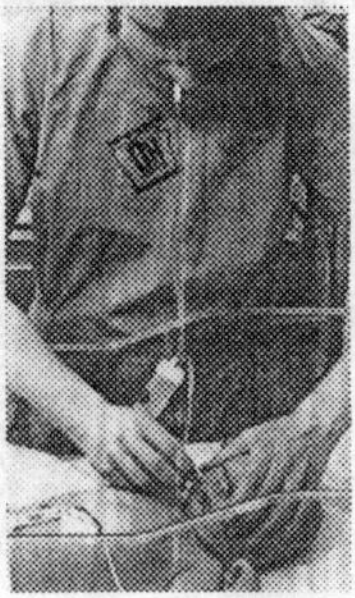

DeLee mucous trap

Deleterious Harmful to the body, substance which is harmful to the, body.

Delinquency Juvenile criminal activity, juvenile delinquency, antisocial, actions, Illegal antisocial and criminal conduct of a minor child.

Deliriant poison Belladonna or atropine which give dryness of the mouth, incoherent speech, unsteadiness and delirium is less common poison seen in clinical practice or emergency medicine

Delirium incoherent talk and delusion as seen in high fever or neurological disorders

Delivery word used for childbirth, it can be normal, assisted and abnormal.

Delouse Measure taken to take away of body louse or head louse

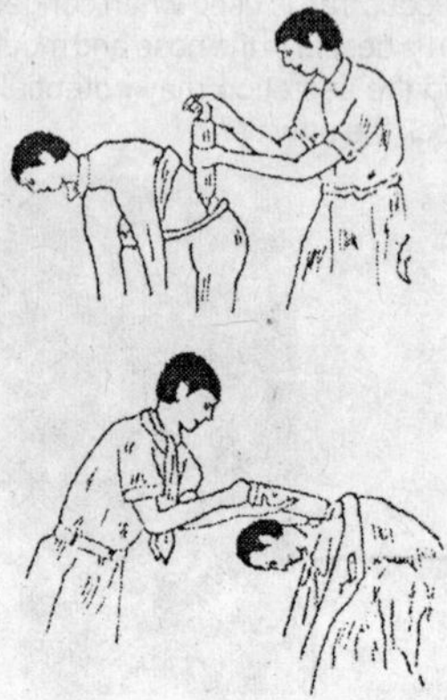

Delousing method

Delta Greek letter Δ or δ, refers to any triangular area in anatomy.

Deltoid ligament Lateral ligament of knee joint which is deltoid in shape.

Deltoid muscle Shoulder muscle attached to deltoid ridge of arm bone.

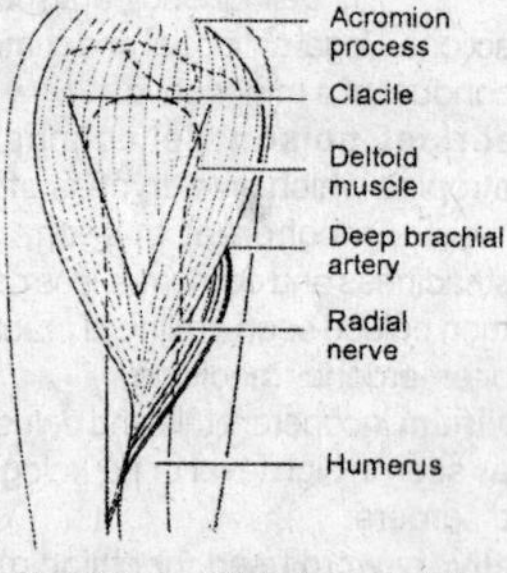

Showing site of injection used in I M injection to deltoid muscle

Deltoid Meaning triangular, refers to deltoid muscle which has origin from scapula and insertion to humerus.

Delusion False belief which cannot be corrected even by reasoning, it is a belief which occurs in non-existent situation.

Dementia Irreversible changes in mental acumen which give rise to loss of memory, loss of judgement, loss of emotional control, common clinical conditions are:

- Senile dementia.
- Presenile dementia.
- Atherosclerotic dementia.
- Alzheimer's disease.
- Creutzfeldt-Jakob disease.
- Loss of memory due to brain pathological changes or senescence.

Democratic Socialism Socialist society is got by an electoral process.

Demographic cycle With change of time, population change occurs which are noted in 5 cycles which are:

- High stationary. • Low stationary.
- Early expanding. • Declining.
- Late expanding.

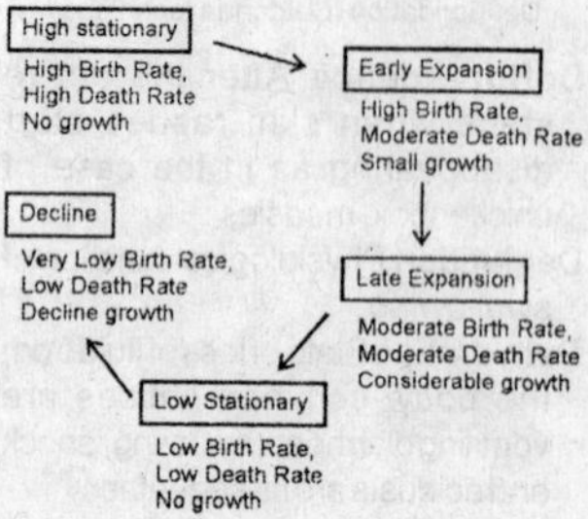

Demographic cycle

Demography Study of people with respect to age, sex, race, occupation or any specific conditions in their society.

Demyelination Destruction of myelin sheath of nerve fibres as seen in disseminated sclerosis.

Dendrite Protoplasmic filaments of nerve cell which is responsible for the transmission of impulses from neurone to neurone, fine interlacing branches of nerve cell, they pick up impulses and carry them into the cell.

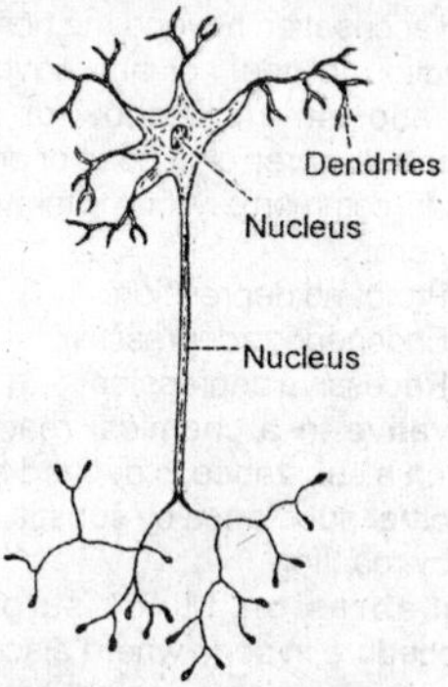

Nervecell showing dendrites

Dendrites Nerve fibres which extend from nerve cells called neuron, nerve fibres other than axon.

Dengue A viral disease that is seen in tropical countries which is transmitted by mosquito, colloquially known as *break bone fever*.

Denis Browne splint This splint is used in child below one year of age which has talipes deformity and is worn at nighttimes or during naps.

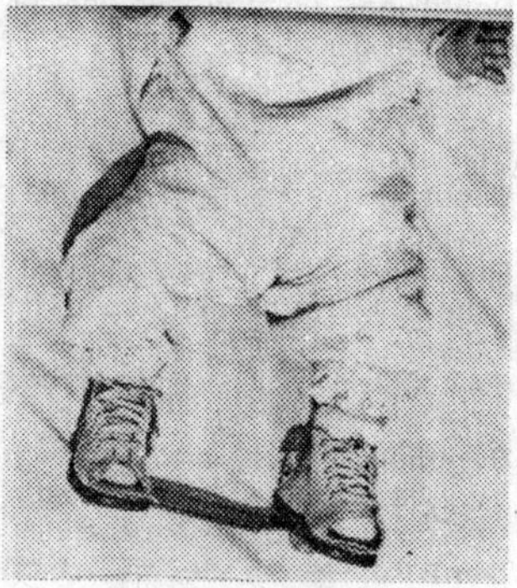

Denis Browne Splint

Density Describes urbanism.

Dental formula Formula to count dentition of animals and man.

Dental fluorosis It is manifested by white and yellow patches on teeth, corrosion in teeth and mottling of teeth.

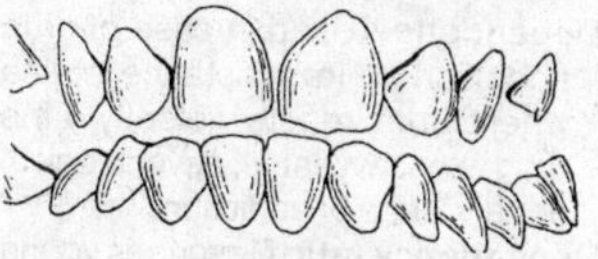

Dental fluorosis

Dental plaque Gummy hard mass which cause dissolution of enamel.

Dental pulp Central space within tooth which is richly innervated and vascularised.

Dental sealant Plastic film applied to cover pits where food debris gets lodged to prevent infection.

Dental Related to teeth such as dental hygiene, dental nurse and dental student.

Dentifrice Dental preparation for cleansing purpose.

Dentine Bulk of the teeth dentine is part existed between pulp and enamel.

Dentist Professional who is qualified to practice dentistry.

Dentistry Branch of dental science that covers the diagnosis and treatment of diseases of teeth, mouth and associated tissues and bones.

Dentition Teething process which can be primary in case of milk set or secondary in case of permanent set.

Denture Dental device which replaces the lost teeth, which may be fixed or movable, removable prosthesis of set of teeth.

Deodorant Cosmetic preparation which removes body odour due to sweat, substance which takes away offensive odour.

Deoxy corticosterone Renal hormone with mineral corticoid activity.

Dependence Used in case of drug addiction or in substance abuse where body reacts violently if the drug is not available, psychological dependence or addiction.

Dependency ratio Describes young and old dependents on head of family.

Depilatory Medical preparation which can help in removal of hair which are not wanted in the given area of the body, agent that can remove hair.

Depolymerisation Chemical reaction where the breakdown of polymers into monomers occurs.

Deposit It refers to sediment in a liquid, or organic matter collected in tissue, or hard material collected on the teeth.

Depressant Drug which is used to reduce body activity, a situation which brings down the body activity; such as anaesthetics, tranquilisers, sedatives and alcohol.

Depressed fracture Fracture in which one of the fragments is depressed below its normal level, example is when the vault of the skull has been fractured and a piece of the bone is pressed inwards, It is classified under complicated fracture.

Depression State of sadness and self accusation beyond the normal reaction to grief or any adverse situation in life, hollow or any depressed area on a bone or on an organ, common psychiatric terminology are:

- Profound depression.
- Endogenous depression.
- Recessive depression.

Derivative In a chemical reaction when a substance is derived from another substance by substitution or by reaction.

Dermabrasion Minor surgical procedure in acne where a scar is removed or improvement done in case of scar, removal of outer skin layer by friction.
Scraping or smoothening of skin to improve acne scars.

Dermacentor Means prick to the skin, it refers to a genus of tick.

Dermatitis Infection and inflammation of skin tissue, depending upon the cause of dermatitis we have the following types:

- Contact dermatitis.
- X-ray dermatitis.
- Varicose dermatitis.

- Traumatic dermatitis.
- Allergic dermatitis.
- Occupational dermatitis.
- Exfoliative dermatitis.

Dermatographia Skin reacts by producing wheals when a scratch is made by finger or by an instrument.

Dermatology Speciality in medical profession which deals with the diagnosis and treatment of ailments of skin, STD, RTI, and HIV/AIDS.

Dermatome chart Evaluation of sensory function is done by testing dermatome zones from Dermatome Chart.

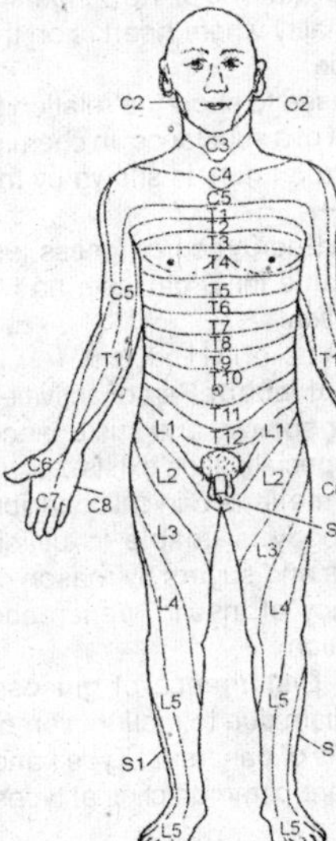

A. Front

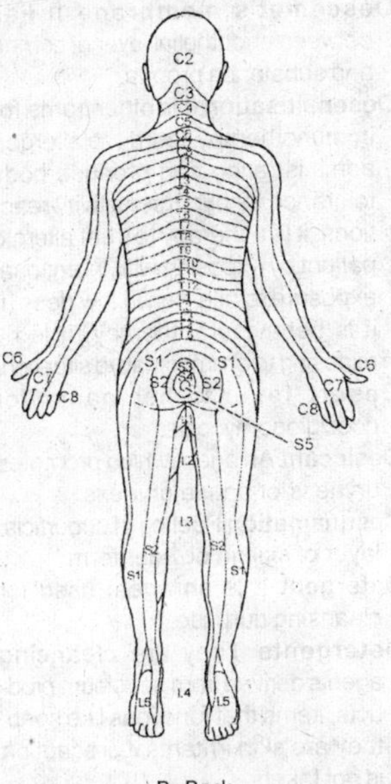

B. Back

Dermatome Chart

Dermatome an instrument used to cut or incise the skin, a sensory field of the skin which is supplied with afferent nerve fibres from posterior spinal root.

Dermatomycosis Fungal infection of skin.

Dermatosis Skin infection which do not produce inflammation.

Dermis Layer below the dermis which is called true skin, also called as corium or subsurface skin.

Dermoid Related to the skin and skin appendages, this resembles the skin.

Descemet's membrane It lies between endothelial layer of cornea and substantia propria.

Desensitisation It is other name for immunotherapy, low dose allergen administration can produce body tolerance for hypersensitivity reactions, it is a therapy to treat allergic patient by exposing with intentional exposure to allergen in low dose, if it is behavioural therapy it is by exposing to an imaginative situation.

Desert fever Other name for coccidiodomycosis.

Desiccant An agent which promotes dryness or cause dryness.

Desquamation Peeling of superficial layer of skin in powder form.

Detergent It is an agent used for cleansing purpose.

Detergents They are cleansing agents derived from petroleum products, items that functions like soap, they are skin irritants if precaution is not taken.

Detonation Explosive getting exploded producing bursting noise

Detoxication reduction in the toxic property of a poison.

Detoxification Other name for detoxication, chemical process of neutralising a toxic substance there by it is no longer a toxic substance.

Detrusor Muscle of urinary bladder which function for pushing the content of bladder downwards.

Dettol An antiseptic which is employed in the form of lotion, which are made by dissolving the remedy in water, thus making a solution of suitable strength, this is available for general and specific uses.

Development Refers to the skills of a child in the milestone along with physical growth process where society move to industrial state.

Deviance Deviation from normal behaviour which is accepted in a society, it speaks of standard of morality.

Dexterity It refers to motor skill.

Dextran Contain large glucose molecule given I V as plasma volume expander, increases the osmotic pressure of blood.

Dextrin It is a soluble carbohydrate, it is a product of breakdown of Starch and Glycogen.

Dextrocardia One of the congenital abnormality where heart is on the right side.

Dextro Used to show the relation to the right of a substance, in chemistry dextrorotatory is shown by the symbol +.

Dextrose Energy source for tissues, other name for D glucose, an I V preparation.

Dharma A belief in Hinduism.

Division of labour Part of activities done for survival and sustenance where specialisation exists.

Diabetes mellitus Clinical condition where body is unable to utilise starches and sugars by reason of deficiency of insulin, pancreatic dysfunction.

Diabetes Disturbance of glucose metabolism due to malfunction of beta cells of pancreas, Type I and Type II are common clinical types known.

Diabetogenic Attributed to an agent which induces diabetes such as drugs or physiological condition of pregnancy.

Diagnosis identification of illness in a patient, identification of abnormality in a patient by attending doctor, a necessity for illness treatment, common terms used are:

- Clinical diagnosis.
- Laboratory diagnosis.
- Provisional diagnosis.
- Final diagnosis.
- Nursing diagnosis.
- Differential diagnosis.

Diagram multiple bar It is a method of data representation in biostatistics.

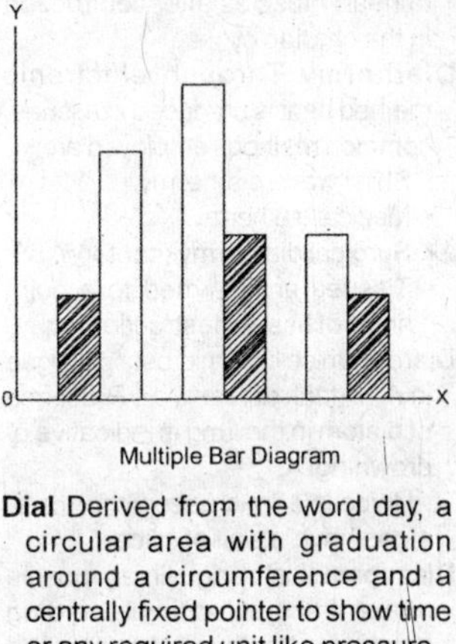

Multiple Bar Diagram

Dial Derived from the word day, a circular area with graduation around a circumference and a centrally fixed pointer to show time or any required unit like pressure.

Dialysate During dialysis the substance which passes through membrane is called dialysate.

Dialyser It implies to the membrane used in dialysis, it refers to artificial kidney (machine) used for dialysis.

DialysisProcess of removal of waste product by using semi-permeable membrane which do not allow colloids (nitrogenous waste material), other name for haemodialysis.

Diameter It is the line that passes through the central point of the circle which touches circle, common diameters frequently measured are:

- Pelvic diameter.
- Cranial diameter of foetus.

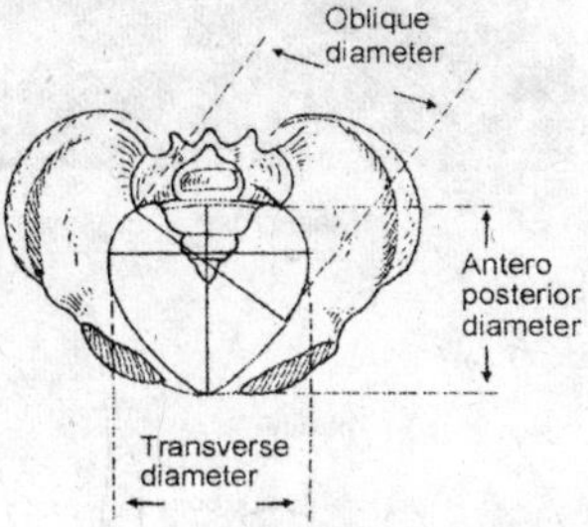

Diameter of pelvic inlet

Diaphoresis Profuse perspiration of a person.

Diaphragmatic breathing exercise It is a deep breathing exercise,if patient is taught diaphragmatic breathing he will breathe more efficiently and obtain better lung function by correctly using his abdominal muscles and diaphragm.

Diaphragmatic hernia Protrusion of abdominal organs into thoracic cavity through diaphragm.

Diaphragm It is colloquially called muscle of breathing, chest cavity and abdominal cavity are separated by diaphragm.

Diaphragm They are soft rubber cups that cover the cervix. It should be used with spermicidal jelly or cream. Checking proper placement of a diaphragm is very important.

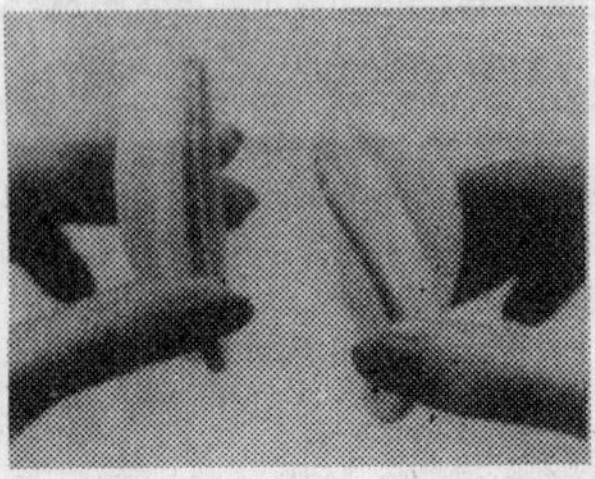

Diaphragm

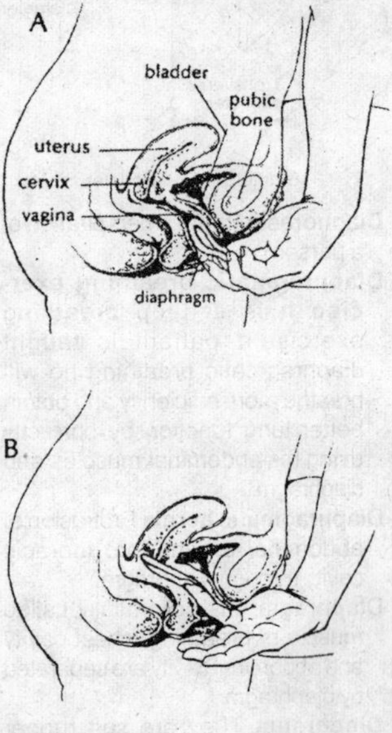

Checking proper placement of diaphragm or cervical cap

Diaphysis It refers to the shaft of a long bone.

Diarrhoea Frequent evacuation of loose stool which bring about body changes due to dehydration, loose watery stool which is passed frequently which can cause body dehydration and salt loss.

Diastase Pancreatic enzyme which is secreted into intestine, this has the ability to convert starch into sugar, common source is during the germination of seeds.

Diastole It is the state of relaxation of heart muscles after contraction in the cardiac cycle.

Diathermy Through electronic method heat is produced in tissues, common methods employed are:

- Short wave diathermy.
- Medical diathermy.
- Surgical diathermy (cautery).
- Tissues are warmed to a point short of tissue destruction.

Diatom Unicellular microscopic algae in river, tank or reservoir, Presence of diatom in the lung is indicative of drowning.

Unicellular microscopic forms of algae have a wall of silica.

Diazepam It is tranquilliser, muscle relaxant and anti-convulsive drug used in the treatment of anxiety and epilepsy.

Dichlorphenamide Drug used in glaucoma to reduce intraocular pressure.

Dichromatic Colour blindness where patient can see two primary colours.

Dick test Skin test done to find out susceptible to scarlet fever.

Dicrotic notch Notch which is found in descending limb of pulse wave.

Dicrotic It denotes double beats, refers to dicrotic pulse.

Dicyclomine An anticholinergic drug used in peptic ulcer and intestine spasm.

Didactic Theory class where one man goes on talking and which do not have interaction, Lecturer is the word used for this teaching technology.

Diet survey By enquiry and data collection on personal visit, information on food consumption is done in the following ways:

- Weighment of raw food.
- Weighment of cooked food.
- Oral questionnaire.
- Stock inventory.

Minimum of 7 days or 3 days data gives average value for

i. Per capita consumption of calories.
ii. Per capita consumption of nutrient.

Diet Food and drink taken or consumed by an individual in every day life, different types of diet used in practice are:

- Balanced diet.
- High calorie diet.
- Low calorie diet.
- Low fat diet.
- Low residue diet.
- Liquid diet.
- Hospital diet.
- High fibre diet.
- Elimination diet.
- Bland diet.
- Therapeutic diet.
- Therapeutic adaptation of normal diet.

Dietetics Dietary science which lays down the principles of nutrition for proper feeding of an individual in health and disease.

Diethycarbamazine It is an anti-filarial drug.

Diethylpropion It is an anti-obese drug.

Dieticians Nutritional expert who can help balanced diet, therapeutic diet and therapeutic adaptation of normal diet in hospitals, nursing homes and home care services, one who is specialist in dietetics.

Differential When we make out the differences we use this terminology, refers to differential diagnosis, differential count.

Diffuse Not localised, scattered all around, usually refers to infiltration.

Diffusion Spontaneous mixing of chemical molecules which gets distributed equally in the solution or in the gaseous material.

Digestion Conversion of eaten food into absorbable form for its utilisation by the body for energy, for body building or for protection of the body.

Digestive juices Secretions of the digestive tract which act chemically to help convert food to digestible forms which the body can use.

Digit It refers to a finger or a toe.

Digital radiography X-ray which is read by computerised imaging.

Digitalis Drug used in case of heart failure to strengthen the heartbeat and to slow down the conducting power of the AV bundle, specifically indicated in atrial fibrillation colloquially called fox-glove, basic drug used in heart diseases.

Digitalis effect ECG showing adequate digitalisation among heart patients.

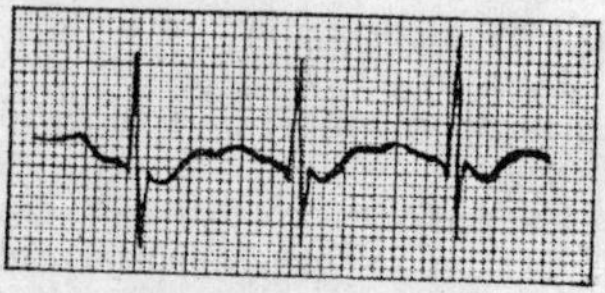

Digitalis effect showing

depressedST segment (scooped) thus dragging T wave downwards giving an appearance of V (Tick mark).

Digitalis toxicity Manifestations of digitalis overdose is identified early by the following ECG changes;-

- **Decreased rhythmic heart rate (sinus bradycardia*)**
- irregular heart rate and rhythm (supraventricular and ventricular arrhythmias)
- premature beats (uni or multifocal)
- very severe conditions – type I and II heart blocks or BBB (Bundle Branch Block)

*Clinically important in early identification

Clinically identified early by:

- gross irregularities in pulse rate and rhythm
- C N S signs

Digitalisation Administration of digitalis and attaining the optimal therapeutic blood concentration.

Digoxin Refers to digitalis drug.

Dilantin An antiepileptic drug, its toxicity can cause Nystagmus.

Dilatation Stretching or dilating a tubular structure or an orifice beyond its dimension.

Dilator An instrument used to dilate or stretch a tubular structure or an orifice.

Diluent An agent that reduces the concentration of a liquid or which can make an agent less harmfull.

Dimercaprol Known as BAL (British Anti Lewisite) which is used in the treatment of mercury poisoning or metal poisoning.

Dimethylphthalate Common mosquito repellent for external application to repel the mosquitoes.

Dimple sign Dermatofibroma becomes indented when pressure is exerted on lateral sides (produce dimple) as against melanoma which do not, it is a diagnostic sign for dermatofibroma.

Diopter Optical instrument for measuring angles, it also denotes the refractive power of a lens.

Dioptre Unit of measurement of lens in refractive error correction,
1 dioptre = parallel light after entering lens gets focussed at a distance of 1 metre.

Diphtheria Acute communicable disease caused by *Corynebacterium diphtheriae*, a bacteria, which has almost vanished due to potent vaccine.

Diphyllobothrium Genus belonging to large tapeworms leaf like organism with pits, refers to genus of tapeworms.

Diplegia Paralysis occurring in both sides of the body.

Diplococcus Genus diplococci which are spherical coffee bean-shaped found in pairs.

Diplococcus Spherical bacteria arranged in pairs, common examples are:

- Pneumococcus which is lanceolate in its form.
- Gonococcus which is coffee bean- shaped.

Diploid Refers to pair of chromosomes which are specific in number for given animals, human beings have 46 chromosomes.

Diplopia Double vision due to weakness of external ocular muscles.

Diprosopus Birth defect showing a monster with a single trunk and normal limbs but varying degrees of duplication of the face.

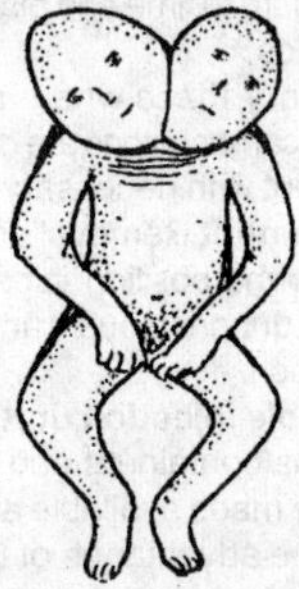

Diprosopus

Directorate of health and FP State level officer who directs and coordinates the health and family welfare activities in a state.

Directorate of Indian systems of medicine State level officer who directs and coordinates systems of Ayurveda, unani, tibb, homeopathy etc., which are other systems of medicine in a state.

Directorate of Medical Education State level officer who directs and coordinates systems of medical education in colleges which teach and train health science students which are affiliated to state university of health sciences and is directed by their respective National Councils like Medical Council, Dental Council, Nursing Council.

Dirt eating It is called pica a bad habit among children who eat dirt, Historically the word has come from Latin which refers to a bird that eats everything unfit for food– a magpie, Since mouth is main organ of tactile sensing child gets to dirt eating.

Disability Impairment leading to restriction for normal physiological function of an organ, part or body which can be physical disability or mental disability in its nature.

Disaccharide Two molecule containing saccharides like maltose, lactose.

Disaster Sudden natural calamity like storm, fire, earthquake or explosion which can produce high causalities.

Disc Circular structure which is flat in nature like optic disc or intervertebral disc.

Discharge of patient It refers to permission to treated patient to go home after complete treatment in a hospital be it a medical therapy or surgical therapy.

Discharge Substance which is excreted or evacuated from tissues, organ, particular reference to wound discharge, an excretory substance, matter set free by force.

Discus Refers to disk, intervertebral disk.

Disease Body show pathological changes from physiological changes culminating in structural and functional changes.

Disincentives Similar to incentives, disincentives are also measures to make couple to practice family planning as a strategy, e.g., are:
- Improvident maternity.
- No housing loan.
- No subsidised medical treatment.
- No free education.

Depending upon 2 child norm or 3 child norms, disincentives are made to force on these couple who have more than 2 or 3 children.

Disinfection To take away infection by means of available measures like physical disinfectants, chemical disinfectants, common types of disinfection are:
- Prophylactic disinfection.
- Concurrent disinfection.
- Terminal disinfection.

Disinfect Process of destroying or bringing to lowest count to make harmless or to stop the multiplication of micro-organisms.

Disinfectant Chemical agent that is used to disinfect an article, an item, a surface, an area or a place where pathogens cannot survive.

Dislocation Displacement of a bone on to other bone which is also called subluxation or luxation.

Following an injury if bone of a joint is wrenched out from its place it is called dislocation, this is always associated with tearing of joint capsule.

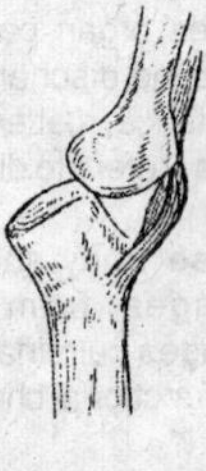

A

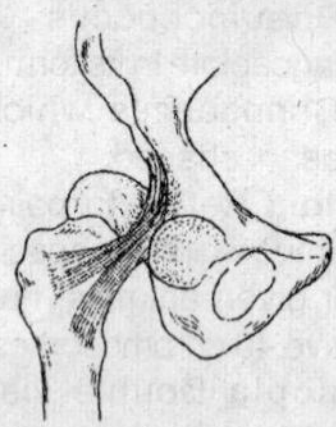

B

A: Posterior dislocation of knee

B: Posterior dislocation of hip joint

Disorientation Mental confusion for place, time and person, person who cannot identifies or has confusion with regard to time and place where he stands.

Dispensary Place where medicine or medicamentations are dispensed to patient with necessary advice.

Displacement Removal or taken to an abnormal position, in psychology it is an unconscious transference of emotion.

Disposable injection unit This unit contains containers and injectors that are made available and which have the advantages of providing sealed sterile equipment ready for immediate use, it reduces the risk of sensitisation dermatitis for doctors and nurses who have to give large number of these injections, They are called *single dose injection units, which prevents disease transmission.*

Disposable transfusion set This is helpful in preventing disease transmission and cross-infection among patients who receive blood transfusion. Usual indications are haemorrhage, burns and shock, transfusion service includes:

- Whole blood.
- Dried plasma and serum.
- Packed red cells.

Disposable polythene "giving" set includes.

- Needle with Luer fitting.
- Luer fitting mount.
- 2" of rubber tubing for drugs to be added.
- Clip for regulating rate of flow through polythene tubing.
- Filter and drip.
- Needle to pierce bung of sterile infusion container.
- Air inlet filter to be hooked above fluid level in the container.

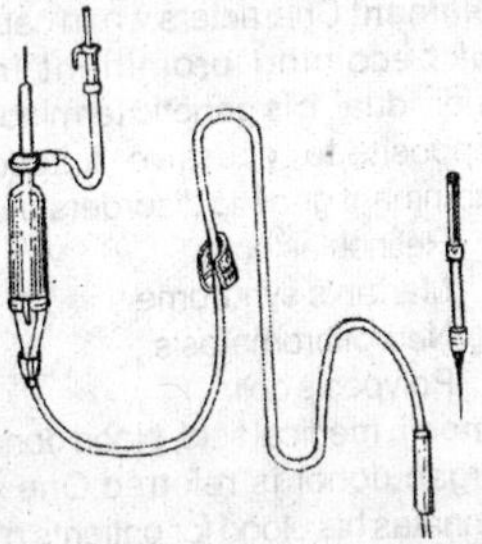
Disposable polythene I V set

Disposition Development of tendency to succumb to certain type of infection by man, predisposed to infection.

Dissect To cut open and see the structure in case of anatomy in cadaver, to cut open and observe and repair surgically in case of surgery on living body.

Disseminated Refers to widely distributed in human body in different organs, usually refers to malignancy or fibrotic conditions.

Dissociation Separation, molecular splitting in chemistry, emotions are separated from mind in psychiatry.

Distal When an organ is situated away from central portion of the body, not proximal.

Distance receptors Stimuli from a long distance is received or transmitted as in the case of eye vision, ear hearing, etc.

Distension Abnormal expansion or enlargement of an organ, abdominal distension, bladder distension, refers to intestinal distension due to fermentation and gas ccumilation. In nursing practice there are nursing relief measures in case of abdominal distension which are:

- Ox bile enema.
- Turpentine enema.

other nursing measure is passing a flatus tube for the relief of distension.

Distillation It is a process of condensing vapour, process of vaporisation.

Distribution It describes how a thing is spread out, population distribution, agent distribution, statistical distribution in case of characteristics.

Disulfiram Other name for antabuse which is used in alcohol addicts, that is used in de-addiction of alcoholics.

Diuresis Refers to increased urinary excretion in person or patient.

Diuretics They are medications which increase the amount of urine secretion from the kidneys.

Diurnal Period of activity in day time, diurnal variation is variation from change in man when he is not active in day and not resting in night.

Diverticulitis Blind pouches formed in intestine are diverticula and their infection and inflammation refers to diverticulitis.

Diverticulosis Presence of diverticula without inflammation or infection in intestine.

Diverticulum Single pouch in intestine, oesophagus, bladder etc., congenital abnormality like Meckel's diverticula.

Diving Under sports and physical fitness swimming is an excellent all-round exercise for body conditioning. Swimming pool sanitation is advocated from health point of view.

Divorce The legal termination of a marriage.

Dizygotic Derived from two separate fertilised ova, refers to twins.

Dizziness It is a feeling of haziness associated with anxiety commonly due to biliousness the digestive disturbances dizziness occurs, pathological causes of dizziness are:

- Significant changes in blood.
- pressure.
- Disease in the middle ear.
- Failure of fusion of visual images.
- Brain changes due to hardening of arteries.
- Brain tumours.

DNA **D**eoxyribo **N**ucleic **A**cid.

Doctors Qualified medical professionals who involve in diagnosis, treatment and follow-up of cases in illness.

Dog bite This is made equivalent to hydrophobia or rabies because the saliva of rabid dog can transmit rabies which can be fatal in most of the cases, all dog bite carry medical treatment including ARV injection.

Dolor Word refers to pain, following medical terminologies are worth observing:

- Dolores vagi = wandering pain
- Dolores coxae = sciatica
- Dolores capitis = headache.

Domiciliary Any service given at home or at family level, common terms used:

- Domiciliary treatment.
- Domiciliary midwifery.
- Domiciliary services.

Dominance One who controls others, Right sidedness or left sidedness, Genetic quality where allele expresses the characters.

Dominant Characters when capable of becoming prominent in an individual, it is genetic terminology, opposite to recessive, autosomal dominant genetic disorders are:

- Retinoblastoma.
- Marfan's syndrome.
- Neurofibromatosis.
- Polyposis coli.

Donor In medical field, blood donor or organ donor is referred,One who donates his blood for patients blood transfusion in the case of critical conditions.

Donovan body *Chlamydia trachomatis* which causes granuloma inguinale.

Dopa It is the precursor of dopamine, it is intermediate product in biosynthesis of adrenaline or noradrenalin, as drug it is used in Parkinson's disease.

Dopamine It is known to function in the transmission of nerve impulse, present in brain, present in adrenal medulla, it is used in cardiogenic shock, related to noradrenalin.

Dope Term in use for narcotic habit forming drugs.

Doping When sports person uses androgens or anabolic steroids to improve their performance.

Doppler effect it is radiological diagnostic term where wave frequency versus wave movement, relationship seen by radiologist for grouping into normal or abnormal.

Doppler US flow meter Doppler ultrasound flow meter is used in detection of intermitent claudication, deep vein thrombosis, a device that is used in recording pulsatic changes in blood flow in a vessel.

Dorsal column Dorsal column tract transmits the perceptions of light touch and vibrations, it is tested with a cotton wisp against patient's skin.

Dorsal gluteal injection site It is the diagonal line that extends from the posterior superior iliac spine toward the greater trochanter of the femur, and the horizontal line extending from the posterior superior iliac spine to the lateral hip two fingers' breadth below the iliac crest, from the boundary for the area that is safe for IM injections.

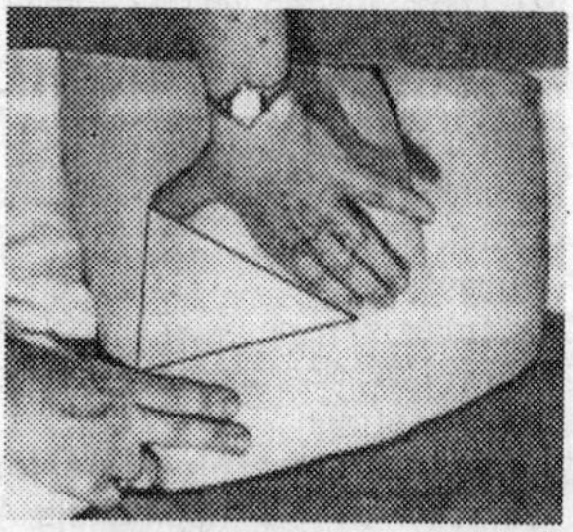

Area safe for gluteal injection

Dorsal position for examination This is common position for gynaecological examinations, Following specific nursing requirements are prescribed:

" The bed should be screened and nearby windows closed. The patient should lie on her back and knees slightly flexed and one pillow is kept under the head and shoulders,

Bedclothe is turned down to the thighs, patient is covered a sheet, nightgown is folded up to the breasts, a small shawl is covered to the chest, at examination, the urse should see that the area from breast to the pubes is bare,

Nurse stands at left hand side of bed at head end.

All gynaecological examination should be made "rectal examination set" ready.

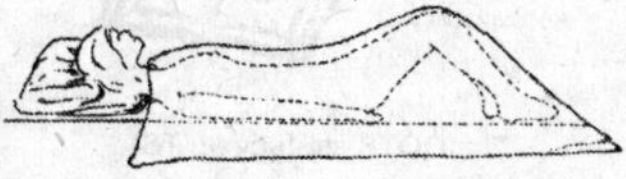

Dorsal position for gynaecological exam

Dorsal Posterior part or back part of organ or body.

Dorsiflexion In case of fingers bending backwards, in case of toes bending upwards.

Dorsum Means back or posterior.

Dose It is a portion or a quantity that is to be administered at one time for a patient who is on medication.

Dosimeter Device to measure exposure to radiation of person working in radiology department or in a place where radioactivity is present.

Dosimetry Accurate and systematic determination of drug dose in medical therapeutics.

Dossier Patient's case history are kept in the record form, it is a portfolio of patient in the hospital.

DOTS Is a strategy to ensure that by providing most effective drug and confirming that the drug is taken, the strategy are:

- political commitment.
- diagnosis by microscope.
- adequate supply of right drugs.
- directly observed treatment.
- accountability.

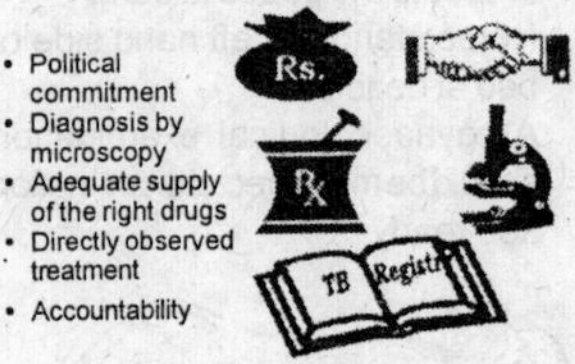

The DOTS strategy (in TB)

Double bagging contaminated supplies Contaminated hospital waste need to be enclosed in an impermeable bag before they are removed from patient who is in isolation, double bagging avoids spill of contaminants to outside of inner bag.

Double blind method Term used in clinical trial or drug trial where patient and researcher both do not know about real drug or otherwise, clinical trial for a new drug is conducted by double blind method in research.

Douche To flush out a cavity permitted fluids are used as flushing agent, vaginal irrigations are done for preoperative cleansing with providone iodine solution for smoothening inflamed vaginal mucosa and for applying medications to the vaginal mucosa.

Douching vaginal This is done for cleansing purposes in cases of vaginal discharge, before gynaecological surgery on female genital tract, cleansing measure for patients wearing vaginal pessaries.

Douglas's pouch This is the other name for rectouterine pouch.

Dover's powder It is the combination of two powders in medication which are Opium powder and Ipecac powder.

Down's syndrome Known as Mongolism or trisomy 21 syndrome, physical malformation , mental handicap, or both are seen in a child which has the defect in chromosome 21.

Downward social mobility Poor health and tough business allow a super ordinate to move downward.

DPT Triple antigen which contains active immunising agents which can prevent the occurrence of following three diseases:

- Diphtheria.
- Whooping cough.
- Tetanus.

Dracontiasis Guinea worm infection in man, one of the longest nematode infection of man.

Dracunculus Genus name for Guinea worm D.medinensis A filarial nematode parasite which looks like a little dragon.

Drag carry This is valuable to carry unconscious patient from a burning room or from a confined space which do not permit the first aide to stand upright.

Drain Refers to draining purulent material from a wound abscess or a cyst.

Drainage system portable Is used in case of postsurgical indwelling drain that connects to a portable vacuum container, portable wound drainage system.

Dramamine Long acting Dramamine which contain cyclizine is commonly used in the treatment of Travel Sickness: some drowsiness is expected.

Dressing for I V Antibiotic ointment is applied to the taped insertion site, area is covered with sterile gauze pad, this is covered with a 7.5 × 10 cm strip of tape.

Dressing Material applied to cover the wound.

Dressings They are requirements after surgery or injury, sterilised dressings.

Drift Movement which is due to external force, refers to antigenic drift.

Drinker's respirator This is negative-positive pressure respirator used in first aid, this mechanism apparatus is used where negative pressure applied to the chest wall causes inspiration and expiration is produced by a slight degree of positive pressure.

Drip IV Infusion of fluid in case of dehydration or sickness.

Drop Minute drop of a liquid, one drop is smallest quantity of liquid that can be taken at a time through an appliance, common drops of use are:

- Eye drops.
- Ear drops.
- Nasal drops.

It also means the permanent flexion of fingers or toes in some of t h e clinical conditions.

Droplet infection Suspended particles in the air is inhaled and infection is thus obtained, infection due to inhalation of pathogens.

Drops They are topical medications for eye (eye drops), for ear (ear drops) nose (nasal drops).

Dropsy Meaning oedema or excess fluid. It is a clinical condition where too much fluid is retained in the body causing water logging of the tissues.

Drowning Person when immersed in water gets suffocated due to inhalation of water into his lungs which may be suicide or homicide in nature.

Drug Medicamentations in sickness substances derived from chemicals, plant, or animals which are used in the treatment of diseases, substances that are used for the promotion of better health. Terminology in common use are:

- Drug interaction.
- Drug tolerance.
- Drug addiction.
- Drug abuse.
- Drug idiosyncrasy.

DT This is one of the available vaccine containing Diphtheria, Tetanus for adult above 12 years, double antigen for active immunisation.

Dubin Johnson syndrome Inherited defect of bile metabolism, conjugated hyperbilirubinaemia.

Duchenne dystrophy It is a childhood disorder characterised by progressive muscular dystrophy.

Duct Channel for the passage of secretion or fluid of an organ or gland.

Ductus venosus Venous duct through which umbilical vein drains to inferior vena cava, part of foetal circulation.

Ductus It means a duct, used term in ductus arteriosus

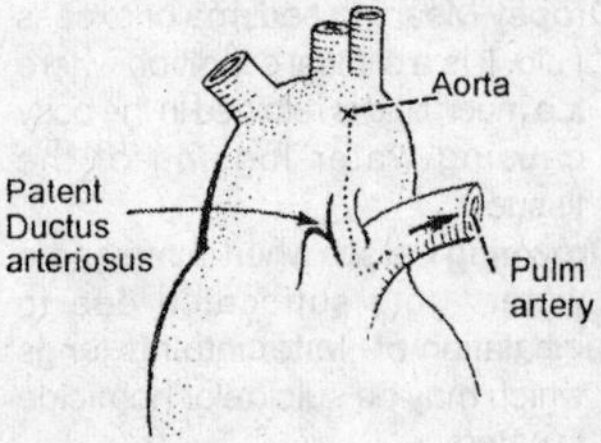

P D A (Patent Ductus Arteriosus)

Dumb-bell It refers to a mass consisting of two spherical portions connected by a narrow connector, if an organ in anatomy is shaped like dumb-bell it is referred to as dumb-bell shaped.

Dumping Colloquial term meaning quick evacuation of contents.

Duodenal Pertaining to duodenum, portion of small intestine.

Duodenum First 25 cm of small intestine from pyloric opening to jejunum, Portion of small intestine which lies immediately adjacent to the stomach.

Dupuytren's contraction Because of contracture of palmar fascia, fixed bending of one or more fingers.

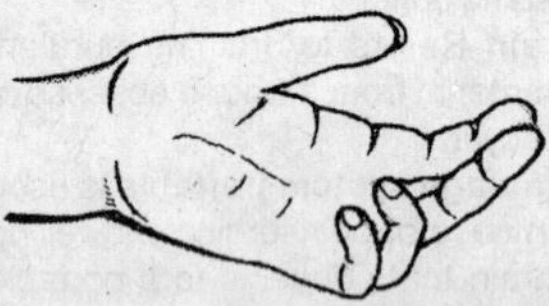

Dupuytren's contraction

Dura mater Outer covering of the brain which is strong fibrous in nature which even extends to spinal cord. The brain and cord are covered by three membranes called meninges; the outer coat is tough fibrous sheath which lines the cranium and is called the dura mater.

Durkheim French Sociologist who developed functionalism.

Dwarf Short stature of man or woman.

Dwarfism Short stature because of arrest of growth and development, Common causes are:

- Cretinism.
- Hypopituitarism.
- Renal rickets.

Dyad Refers to double chromosome in genetic process, when a chemical combines with 2 hydrogen it is referred to as dyad.

Dyne It is the unit of force, it is defined as the force which when acting continuously upon a mass of 1 gram, will impart to it an acceleration of 1 cm per second.

Dysarthrosis Deformed and dislocated joint.

Dysbasia A neurological pathology which give rise to difficulty in walking.

Dyschondroplasia When cartilage is deposited in the shaft of a bone it become short-ended and gets deformed.

Dyscrasia When there is imbalance in the components of a system, usually refers to blood dyscrasia.

Dysdiadochokinesis It is a cerebellar pathology manifestation where ability to perform rapid alternate movements are lost.

Dysentery Usually refers to inflammatory disease of colon frequently passed loose motion which is blood tinged, commonly either bacillary dysentery or amoebic dysentery.

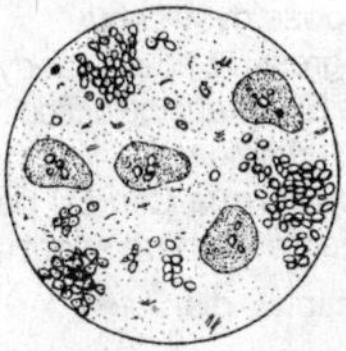

A : Stool in acute amoebic sentery

Scanty cellular exudates, clumped RBC, pyknotic bodies and trophozoites of *E.histolytica* with injected RBC.

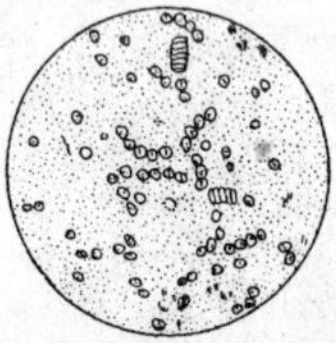

B: Stool in acute bacillary dysentery

Abundant cellular exudates containing pus cells, macrophages with phagocytosed RBC, ghost cells and discrete RBC with occasional rouleaux formation.

Dysfunction When there is impairment of function of an organ or tissue.

Dysgamma globulinaemia A clinical condition where person succumbs to infection due to deficiency of one or more immunoglobulin.

Dysgenesis Development is found defective.

Dysgerminoma Tumour of germinal cells of ovary or testicle which are yet getting differentiated, it is usually a cancerous growth.

Dyshidrosis Itching vesicular rash appear when there is disturbance in sweat secretion occurs, deranged sweat mechanism.

Dyskinesia When there is impairment of voluntary movement.

Dyslexia Reflex learning is lost where we see difficulty in reading, difficulty in learning, difficulty in writing and difficulty in spelling appreciation.

Dysmenorrhoea Clinical condition depicting painful menses, two common types are:

- Primary dysmenorrhoea.
- Secondary dysmenorrhoea.
- They are also called spasmodic and congestive dysmenorrhoea respectively.

Dysostosis When bone development is abnormal or defective.

Clinical condition of defective ossification which occur in foetal cartilage.

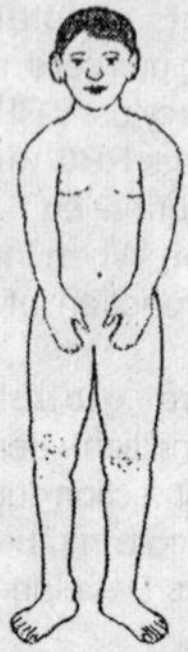

Cleidocranial dysostosis

Dyspareunia Experiencing painful intercourse by a woman.

Dyspepsia Manifested with nausea, vomiting and flatulence which is organic in nature, nervous dyspepsia is due to anxiety.

Dysphagia Experiencing difficulty in swallowing.

Dysphasia Experiencing difficulty in speaking.

Dysplasia Tissue development is found abnormal.

Dyspnoea Experiencing difficulty in breathing.

Dyspraxia Experiencing difficulty in performing coordinated movements.

Dysrhythmia Refers to abnormal pattern of pulse, of heart rate, of brain waves, where regularity of normal pattern are lost.

Dystaxia Experiencing difficulty in controlling voluntary movements.

Dystonia Lack of muscular tone.

Dystrophia Refers to dystrophy, refers to dystrophia myotonica.

Dystrophy Partial atrophy due to faulty nutrition of tissue or organ this refers to faulty development.

Dystrophy Refers to faulty nutrition as in case of:

- Elastic dystrophy.
- Adipose dystrophy.
- Progressive muscular dystrophy.

Dysuria Experiencing difficulty or pain during urination.

Dyszoospermia Clinical pathology or a disorder where spermatozoon formation is disrupted.

E

Eale's disease Thrombophlebitis of retinal vein causing retinal haemorrhage and vitreous haemorrhage.

Ear cartilage Ear cartilage is helpful in immediate care of the newborn, development of ear cartilage helps to gauge the gestational age of the newborn If ear stays in the position in which it is pressed or if it returns to its original position slowly it usually means that the gestational age is less than 38 weeks.

Ear plug In noise pollution area this device is used to plug the external ear to prevent sound access.

Ear wax The wax present in ear canal leading to the middle ear, the wax keeps the middle ear healthy by its protective action.

Ear Organ of hearing and organ of equilibrium which is made up of three parts.

a. External ear (outside to ear drum).
b. Middle ear (bones and upto pharyngotympanic tube).
c. Internal ear (bony and membranous labyrinth).

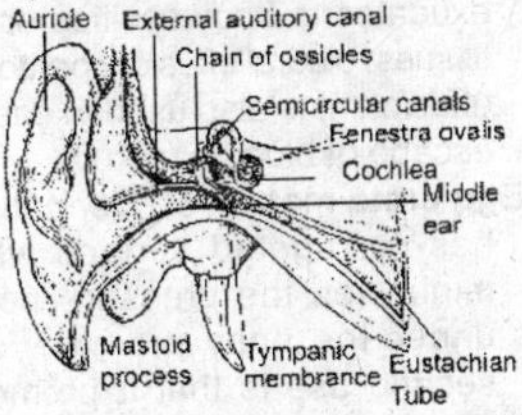

Structure of ear

Ebola virus Which cause viral haemorrhagic fever and rashes, prevalent in Central Africa, it is considered to be a zoonotic disease.

Ecchymosis A skin discolouration caused by effusion of blood below the skin due to a bruise.

ECG Abbreviation for Electro Cardio Gram.

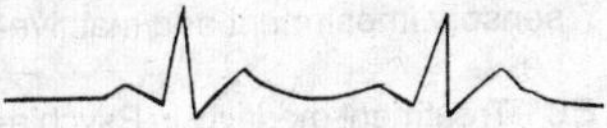

E.C.G.

Echinococcus One of the group of tapeworm called echinococcus, larval forms are present in hydatid cysts which involve organs like liver, lung, and brain.

Echo virus A virus related to influenza which causes obscure types of infection.

Echo Meaning sound, repetition of a sound or of a movement. Types of echo heard are:

- Amphoric echo ... oral voice echo.
- Metallic echo ... in pathological heart.

Echopraxia Involuntary movement of part or organ of the body.

Echovirus Group of enterovirus, ECHO is derived from Entero Cytopathogenic Human Orphan, cause diarrhoea and meningitis.

Eclampsia Toxaemia of pregnancy, apart from oedema, hypertension, albuminuria, patient will have convulsion, disease peculiar to pregnancy.

Eclecticism Therapeutic regimen is determined based on signs and symptoms rather than coming to a final diagnosis, old system of medicine in practice in general practice.

Ecology Study of the relation of environment and illness with respect to man.

Economy Money management in health and disease.

Ecstasy Exaltation feeling with sensory impairment and inactiveness.

ECT Treatment modality in Psychiatry, Electro Convulsive Therapy.

Ecthyma A pustular eruption seen in syphilis or tropical dermatitis.

Ectoderm Germinal layer from which skin and nervous system is derive.

Ectoparasite Parasite that harbours on the body of host like body louse.

Ectopia Any organ when situated in abnormal position like ectopia cardis, ectopia vesicae.

Ectopic Not in its normal position, common example is ectopic pregnancy.

Ectrimma It is an ulcer which is caused by friction in certain parts of the body.

Ectropion Evertion of eyelid secondary to paralysis or skin contraction.

Eczema Superficial inflammation of epidermis which is staged by redness papule, vesicle, crusting and scaling, allergic dermatitis is called atopic dermatitis,chronic skin lesion due to allergic origin.

Edentulous Loss of teeth.

Edema Tissue swelling due to retained fluid, can be inflammatory oedema or dropsy.

EDTA **E**thylene **D**iamine **T**etra **A**cetic acid, a chelating agent.

Educational objectives This refers to knowledge, skills and attitude which are otherwise called cognitive domain, psychomotor domain and affective domain.

Intellectual skill (Cognitive)	Practical skill (Psychomotor)	Communication skill (Affective)
Describe	Demonstrate	Participate group discussion
Explain	Inject	Appreciate art
Identity	Insert	Help patient
Infer	Palpate	Accept culture
Distinguish	Manipulate	Show concern

Educational objectives

EEG Abbreviation for Electro Encephalogram, recording of brain waves through an electronic device.

Efferent That which moves towards periphery from a centre, opposite of afferent, usage is efferent nerve.

Effluent This comes under waste management where sewage or industrial waste is treated as per the specification and the fluid supernatant is discharged for farming.

Effusion Escape of inflammatory exudates to body cavities or into tissues, pleural effusion, peritoneal effusion, it is also used in case of escape of blood or serum.

Egg crate mattress This mattress has corrugated surface which minimises the pressure points under the bony prominences, second use is that it promotes better air circulation to help prevent skin breakdown.

Eggs of helminths On stool examination by microscopic view, eggs of helminths can be diagnosed since they are specific to given helminth

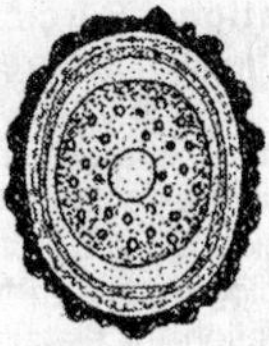

Egg of Round worm (Fertilised)

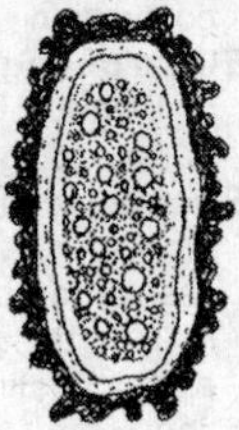

Egg of Round worm (Unfertilised)

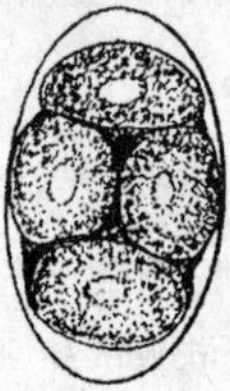

Egg of Hook worm

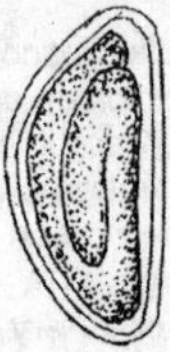

Egg of *E. vermicularis*

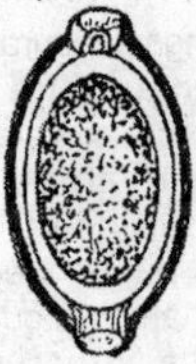

Egg of *T. trichura*

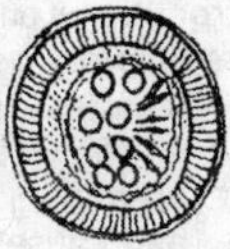

Egg of *T. saginata*

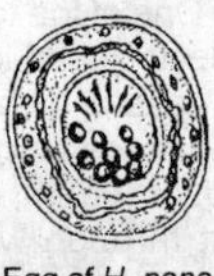

Egg of *H. nana*

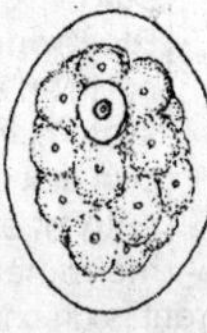

Egg of *F. buski*

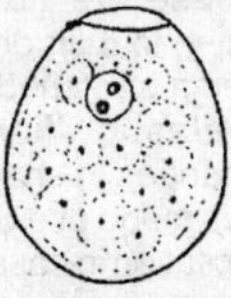

Egg of *D. latum*

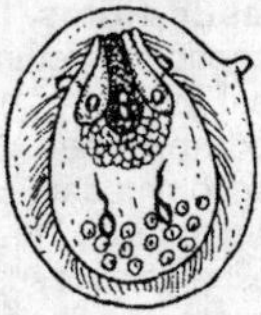

Egg of S. haematobium

Common eggs of helminths

Egg hygiene Cleanliness maintained for keeping egg clean by avoiding soil contamination, faecal matter contamination to prevent certain diseases.

Ego Part of our mind which identify as SELF, term used in psychoanalysis.

Egoism It is a cult of the individual.

Egyptian code The Egyptian code of medical ethics meted out punishments for malpractices which is more severe than those of the Babylonian code. This is described in Hermetic books of the God Thoth; which describes the punishment if physician departed in the least from the accredited methods of treatment and the case ended fatally, the Code specified that the life of physician is to be forfeited.

Eisenmenger's complex A congenital defect in the heart which has VSD and resistant of pulmonary vasculature.

Ejaculation Reflex action by sex stimulation which cause ejection of semen.

Elastic bandage They are applied to provide immobilisation and support and to minimise swelling. They are wrapped from limb part to central part of body, they are applied firmly but never tightly.

Elastic fibres These are fibres capable of returning to their original form after being stretched or compressed, elastic fibres accommodate changes in shape.

Elastic force This is made use of in exhaled air resuscitation in case of asphyxia, when there is failure of respiration and muscles of respiration are not functioning; the volume of air remaining in the lungs is maintained by a balance between the elasticity of lungs which tend to collapse and drive air out and the elasticity of the ribs or chest cage which keep the lungs expanded and tend to drawn air in the elastic force in the case of lung chest elasticity

Elastic Substance which is capable of stretching such as elastic bandage, elastic tissue, elastic stocking.

Elation Feeling of well being with a state of excitement, euphoria or mania.

Elbow The joint between arm and forearm.

Electric shock Shock produced by the conduction of electricity in the

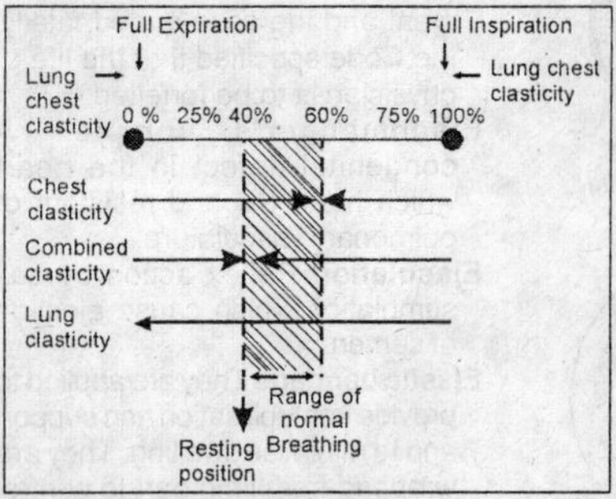

body which is called electrocution. First aid in nursing practice guides the nurse to save the life of a person who has touched the electric connection.

Electrocoagulation Surgical diathermy, high frequency current is used to coagulate the tissues.

Electroejaculation This is an electrical stimulation for ejaculation in case of paraplegics. Electric probe is used by keeping in rectum for electrical stimulation for ejaculation.

Electrokymograph Instrument used to demonstrate cardiac silhouette, parts of this instruments are:

- A fluoroscope
- A pick up unit
- A recording instrument
- Kymograph principally records the motion through density of organs.

Electrocautery An instrument which contains needle or loop which can be electrically heated to destroy tissues.

Electrocution It brings out paralysis of respiratory nerve centre and muscles, it produces electric shock which stops the breathing and heart beat and causes burns, electrocution can also occur by lightening, death occurring by electric shock or electric burn.

Electrode One of the terminal in an electric conducting system, in case of a battery or a cell electrode points to entry or exit of current, is an instrument through which current is discharged to a patient, in other words electrode is a medium between an electric conductor and patient (object).

Electrolysis Removal of unwanted hair by use of a negative galvanic current.

Electrolyte When chemical compound is dissolved in a liquid it liberates ions which are electrically charged and thus conduct electricity, electrolyte balance denotes the maintenance of balance between different elements in the tissues or organs.

E C G Electro Cardio Graphy, it is the tracing of heart contraction and relaxation in the cardiac cycle.

Electrocardiograph Electronic instrument for recording the action of heart.

Electron microscopy Instrument which is capable of enlarging extremely minute objects such as virus and thus helps in the scientific study of microbes.

Electron Electrons are negatively charged particles, they move around the nucleus of an atom, from this we have electron microscope.

Electrophoresis It is a biochemical process where current is passed through blood or serum to separate electrically charged particles, thus separated particles separate to bands for our identification of protein.

Element It is primary component of a compound, simplest chemical substance which cannot be further broken down.

Elementary Item which cannot be divisible into still finer particle, as simple as possible.

Elephantiasis Swelling in scrotum, leg, penis, breast, hand etc., due to lymphatic stasis secondary to filarial infection, hypertrophy of skin and subcutaneous tissue occurs.

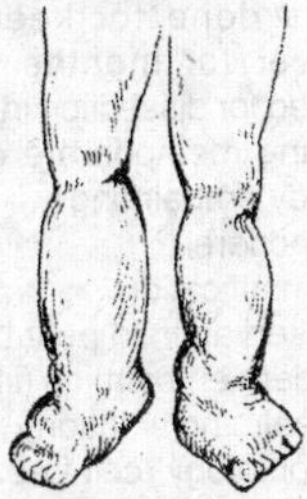

Elephantiasis of legs

Eligible couple They are women in the age group of 15 to 45 years of age from which following items are excluded;

Primary sterility
Secondary sterility
Early menopause.

Elimination Denotes the expulsion or extrusion of a substance from the body.

ELISA Enzyme Linked Immunosorbent Assay, a blood test in HIV or other specified viral infection which is not confirmatory test.

Elixir Sweetened liquid used as sweetening agent in case of drugs they are hydro-alcoholic liquid which gives flavour apart from its containing medications for oral use, common elixirs in use are:

- Amino acetic acid elixir.
- Five bromide or three bromide elixir.
- Diphenyl hydramine hydrochloride elixir.

Elliptical One which has the shape of ellipse, closed conic section shaped, a flattened circle.

Emaciation Very thin body, too much of wasting of body tissues.

Embalming Human body preservation is done for keeping the cadaver for months which is required for dissection in anatomy, following methods are employed for body embalming:

- Adipocere.
- Mummification.
- Preservation in peat bogs.
- Modern embalming (injection of embalming solution).
- Cryobiology (cell freezing).

Embolectomy Surgical removal of an embolus, surgical treatment in case of thromboembolism.

Embolism A loose blood clot which is in the circulation, which when blocks a vessel it may cause partial or complete block, is an emergency.

Embryo It is very early stage of development of organism, in case of man embryo period is from conception to end of second months

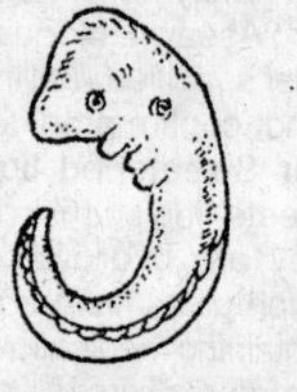

Human embryo

Embryology Scientific study of fertilised egg till its birth, in case of human foetus it is called human embryology.

Emergency It is a crisis due to natural calamity, acute illness, poisoning, accidents or trauma which require immediate intervention.

Emesis An act of vomiting.

Emetic A substance that induces vomiting.

EMF Electro motiveforce measured in volts which is the differential in potential that cause the flow of electricity.

Eminence It is usually a rounded projection, always referred to a bony projection.

Emission Ejection which is not voluntary such as like semen spill, dispersion of light.

Emollient Substance which is used to soften skin, pharmacy preparation which is used in softening the skin.

Emotion It is a state of feeling that produces emotional touch ending with cry, laugh, shout or getting depressed.

Emotional climate It is visible and occurs in extreme love or in extreme hatredness, growing adolescent experience most, next stage which experience is old age.

Emotions Feelings like love hate, etc.

Empathy Involving in others' feeling, show concern.

Emphysema Presence of air in a cavity or in a tissue which is abnormal or pathological, common terminology are:

- surgical emphysema
- pulmonary emphysema
- inflation of lung or stretching of lung which cause difficulty in breathing.

Empirical Experience based action or decision and not on scientific basis.

Emporiatrics This is the science which deals with health of travellers, common illness which a person comes across during travel are:

Malaria	STD
Giardiasis	HIV/AIDS
Dengue	Amoebiasis
Influenza	Typhoid
SARS	Hepatitis

Empowerment Permitting a patient to act or to control self-care and help nurses and doctors in the health care services including medical treatment.

Empty nest family Children moved out of adult partners.

Empyema Pus collection in the pleural cavity.

Emulsification It is a biological process by which the secreted bile acid lowers surface tension of fat; this brings out larger fat globules into smaller globules.

Emulsion A liquid mixture containing oil and water, oil gets suspended in water with the help of emulsi-fying agent.

Enamel Hard covering of the teeth, crown of the teeth is covered by enamel which is hard, dense and pure white glistening in nature.

Encapsulated That which is enclosed in a capsule.

Encephalitis Infection and inflammation of the brain, this can be septic, tubercular or parasitic in nature, infection and inflammation of brain covering, common causes are viral infection of the brain.

Encephalopathy When brain do not function because of brain damage, common types are:
- Wernick's encephalopathy.
- Dialysis encephalopathy.
- Hepatic encephalopathy.
- Hypertensive encephalopathy.

Encephalocele Protrusion of brain through skull opening, hernia of the brain.

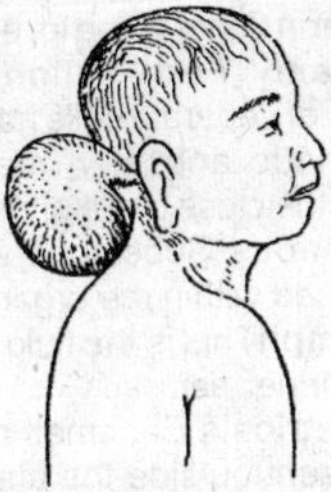

Encephalocele

Endarteritis Inflammation of inner coat of artery sometimes which blocks the arterial supply.

Endemic ascitis It is due to a food toxin, Millet (Panicum miliare = Gondhli) is contaminated with crotalaria seeds (Jhunjhunia) which contains hepatotoxin called pyrrolizidine alkaloid, ascitis and jaundice are common.

Endemic Refers to a disease which always lurking in a place and frequently cases do occur not equalling to public health problem.

Endocarditis Inflammation of the endocardium due to infection by bacteria, fungus or rickettsia infection and inflammation of inner lining membrane of the heart.

Endocrine Glands which do not have ducts and secretes the

hormone directly into the blood, examples of endocrine glands are:
- Pituitary.
- Suprarenal.
- Thyroid.
- Parathyroid.

Endocrinology Study of endocrine glands, their function, pathology and management in case of malfunction.

Endoderm Other name for entoderm

Endogamy Fertilisation by the union. of separate cells having the chromatic ancestry, marriages within the close circle of the family.

Endogenous Substance which is produced within the organism.

Endolymph This is the fluid present in the inner ear.

Endometriosis Endometrial tissue is present outside the uterus like intestine, urinary bladder or ovary etc, which causes pain and bleeding.

Endometrium Inner layer of mucous membrane lining the uterus.

Endoscope Medical instrument used for visual inspection of hollow organ or hollow cavity.

Endothelium Lining of the inner layer of circulating system which are made of simple squamous cells.

Endotracheal It refers to within the trachea, refers to endotracheal tube which is inserted for anaesthesia or for ventilation.

Enema Enema is an injection of fluid into the rectum and this is ordered for the following reasons:
- To empty the bowel of faeces.
- To relieve distension due to flatus.
- To introduce drugs or fluids.
- For diagnostic purpose.

In practical nursing common enema used are:
- Barium sulphate enema.
- Cortisone enema.
- Magnesium sulphate enema.
- Retention enema.
- Enema to relieve distension.
- Sodium polystyrene sulphonate enema.

Major group of enema are:
- Retention enema.
- Non-retention enema.

Energy consumption Human body system has the capacity of working by available energy. This sort of energy consumption is calculated by considering
(i) Age of the person.
(ii) Height of the person.
(iii) Weight of the person by using Harris Benedict formula.

Energy deficit When routine and normal demands of living are not met with.

Enophthalmos Abnormal sunken eyeball.

Entamoeba Some of the parasite belonging to this genus are pathogenic to man, common pathogenic protozoan parasite is *Entamoeba histolytica* causes intestinal amoebiasis, this can also cause of some of the cases amoebic hepatitis.

Enteric When it is related to the intestine, like enteric infection, enteric coated,

Enteritis Infection and inflammation of small intestine.

Enterobius Genus belonging to nematode worm, threadworm is the common example which is known as *Enterobius vermicularis*.

Enterocolitis Infection and inflammation of both small intestine and large intestine.

Enterogastritis Infection and inflammation of stomach and small intestine.

Enterotoxin Toxins produced by bacteria which infect intestine, that which produces food poisoning, that which produces gastroenteritis.

Enterovirus They are picorna viruses which infect intestine and produce nervous tissue pathology, common viruses are polio virus, coxsackie virus, echo virus andrhinovirus.

Entoderm Innermost germinal layer of the embryo, from entoderm future intestine, lungs and glands will develop.

Entomology It is the study of biology and control of insects of public health importance and about insect-borne diseases like plague, malaria, yellow fever, typhus, etc.

Entoplasm Other name for endoplasm, by staining a cell we observe the endo-plasm as blue staining and non-chromatinic.

Entropion Pathological condition where there is inversion of the eyelids is present which cause rubbing against eyeball.

Enucleation Surgical removal of eye-ball from the orbit for therapeutic purpose, removal of any organ en mass from its place or from its supporting tissue.

Enuresis Bed wetting during night either by organic cause or by psychologic cause.

Environment Surroundings which surround us influencing our health and illness, types of environment are:

- Physical environment.
- Chemical environment.
- Biological environment.
- Social environment.
- Spiritual environment.

Enzootic This refers to diseases occurring endemically among animals.

Enzymes They are substances produced by the living cells whose presence aids another process within the body, enzymes speeds other biological process to get completed, digestives juices.

Eosin Common dye used in staining biological specimen which is red in colour, it is derived from bromine and fluorescein.

Eosinophilia During blood examination, excessive eosino-phils are found in the blood smear, it is diagnostic of allergic manifestations.

Ephedrine Drug used in asthma and chronic bronchitis as antispasmodic drug and as bronchodilator

Epicanthus Vertical skin fold on either side of the nose, it is characteristics of some races, otherwise it is not normal in other races

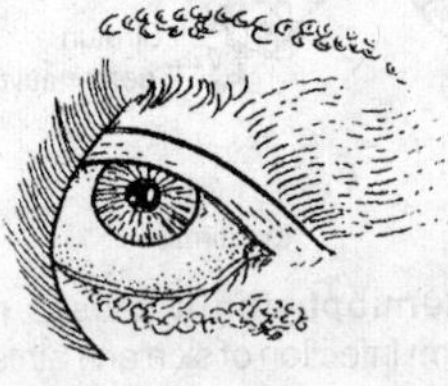

Epicanthus

Epicondyle Long bone protuberance on the condyle of that bone.

Epidemic dropsy It is due to food toxin by the contamination of mustard oil with orgemone oil, the toxin attributed is *sanguinarine*.

Epidemic Disease occurring in a community more than our expectation, common epidemics known are:
- Cholera.
- Gastroenteritis.
- Infective hepatitis.
- Epidemic conjunctivitis.

Epidemiology Study of the determinants and distribution of disease, this considers agent, host and environment (Epide-miological triad).

Epidermis Outer, non-vascular, non-sensitive layer of horny cells that protects the dermis or true skin

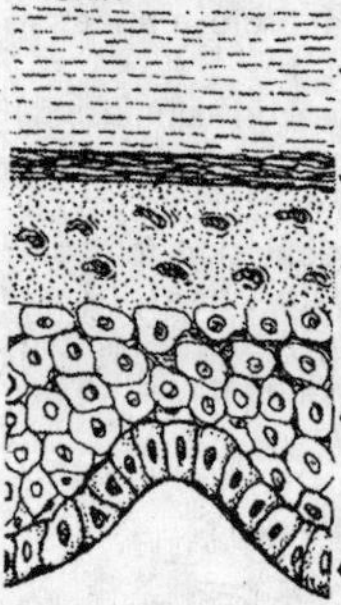

Epidermis

Epidermophyton It causes ringworm infection of skin and athlete's foot, it is a genus of fungi, skin manifestation is also associated with nail manifestations, hairs are usually not infected.

Epidiascope Is an audiovisual aid, opaque direct projector, used to project a diagram, a picture, data from a book or from journal

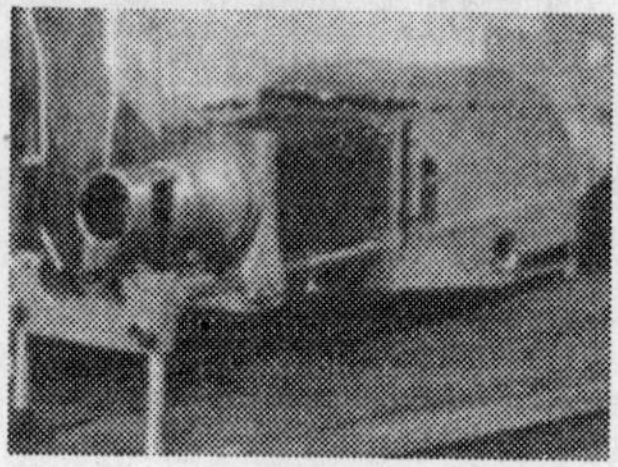

Epidiascope

Epididymis Convoluted tubule containing ducts of testes which end in spermatic duct anatomically situated along posterior border of testes which help in storing, transporting and maturation of spermatozoa, it is an elongated cord like structure.

Epididymo-orchitis Infection and inflammation of testes and epididymis.

Epidural Refers to epidural anaesthesia, meaning outside the dura mater,
Anaesthetic approaches are:
- Lumbar.
- Caudal.

Indications are during childbirth and in chronic pain.

Epigastrium Region of abdomen which is above the stomach

Epignathus It is soft palate tumour or hard palate tumour in the region of Rathke's pouch, after filling the buccal cavity it protrudes outside mouth.

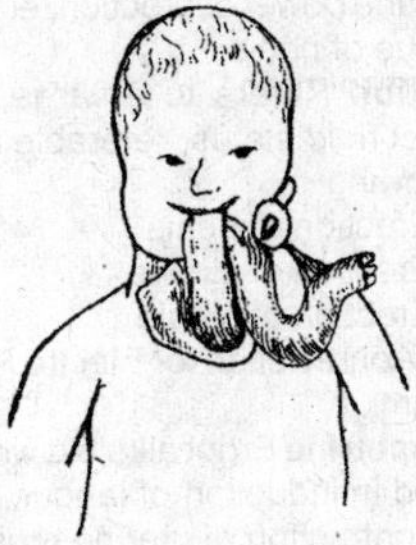

Epignathus

Epiglottis Is an anatomical structure made of cartilage which helps to prevent swallowing food into trachea, flap like anatomical structure that lies over the opening to the larynx, main function of this organ is to keep food and other foreign matter out of the air passage.

Epilation The process of removal of hair from the body.

Epilepsy A neurological disorder which is primarily disease of brain which can cause two types of fits *viz.*,

grand mal- convulsions followed by unconsciousness

petit mal - short partial blackouts and no loss of conciousness

Epileptiform That which resembles a fit.

Epinephrine Commonly called adrenalin which is produced by inner portion of the adrenal gland.

Epineurium Nerve sheath surrounding the nerve.

Epiphora Too much of shedding of tears, usual causes are obstruction in lacrimal duct and ectropion.

Epiphysis In early part it is end of a long bone which is united to the shaft through a cartilage, in early life it develops individually but unites with shaft of the bone at a later life, useful in age determination.

Episcleritis Inflammation of outer coat viz., episclera of the eyeball.

Episiotomy Surgical incision done during second stage of labour to facilitate childbirth in primigravida, this helps to avoid damage to perineal muscles during childbirth.

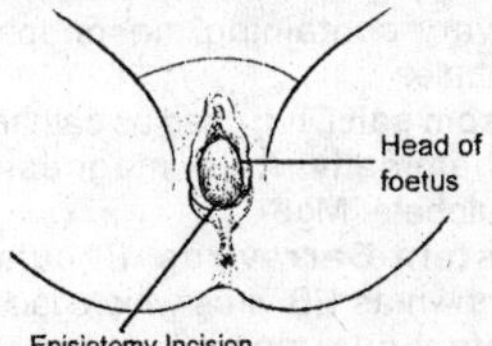

Episiotomy

Epispadias Condition where abnormal opening of urethra on the dorsal penis

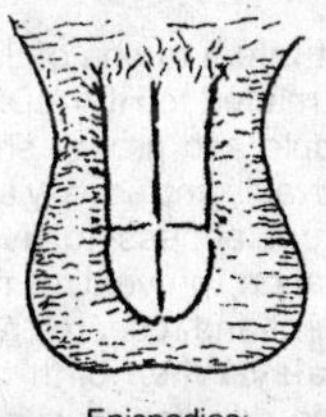

Epispadias

Epistaxis Clinical condition or traumatic condition where bleeding in the nose is seen.

Epithalamus It is part of diencephalons, this includes the following:
- Pineal body.
- Stria medullaris.
- Habenular trigone (habenula).

Epithelioma Tumour of the epithelium.

Epithelium Cells of the outer layer of the skin, sometimes cells of lining membrane.

Epituberculosis Pre-tuberculosis manifestation which show pulmonary congestion, in paediatric age this is manifested in the form of homogenous opacity which is from lung lobe to hilus.

Epoophoron A vestigial structure of the ovary which is situated on the ovary containing mesonephric tubules.

Epsom salt Drug used as cathartic, chemically it is magnesium sulphate, $MgSO_4$.

Epstein-Barr virus Popularly known as EB virus which causes infectious mono-nucleosis, it belongs to herpes virus, it is found to cause Burkett's tumour and nasopharyngeal cancer.

Epulis It is a tumour of lower jaw which is fibrous sarcomatous in nature.

Equity It refers to one of the major ethics related to HIV/AIDS,
All people and groups should be treated fairly and equally and have an equal access to available, information, prevention methods treatment and research results.

Erb's palsy When birth injury or assisted delivery causes injury it causes pressure on cervical nerve (roots of lower cervical nerves) or brachial plexus; it produces paralysis of the arm in the newborn.

Erectile Refers to muscles which has the power of erection, erectile-tissue of penis.

Erection Refers to enlarged and erect rigid status, referable to the following:
- Erection of penis.
- Erection of clitoris.
- Erection of nipple.

ERG Abbreviation for Electro Retino Gram.

Ergometrine Ergot alkaloid which is used in induction of labour, helps in contraction of uterine muscle.

Ergonomics It is the science of fitting a person to a job or fitting a job to a person for better efficiency, recent area of interest in occupational health, application of ergonomics influences the production of an industry.

Ergosterol It is present as sterol in plants and animals, becomes vitamin D_2 by U V irradiation.

Ergot A therapeutic agent produced from fungus and is used in inducing labour and in checking haemorrhage.

Ergotamine Ergot alkaloid used in the treatment of migraine.

Ergotism Clinically gangrene of limbs due to ergot poisoning.

Ergotoxine It is an alkaloid from ergot, formula is $C_{35}H_{39}N_5O_5$

Erosion Changes produced by ulceration in the tissue, common usage is cervical erosion.

Erotic That which produce sexual love or lust.

Erotism It is the act of sexual desire.

Erratic Not predictable, not in order, not to the acceptable norm, the one which is fluctuating in nature.

Eruption Tooth eruption, skin eruption, coming out by breaking tissue.

Erysipelas Skin infection causing redness due to group A haemolytic streptococci.

Erythema Abnormal condition of skin with fearful redness of the skin due to local congestion, common causes of erythema are:

- Sunburn.
- Inflammation.

Erythematous Clinically seen with erythema.

Erythroblast They are nucleated precursors from which RBC develops.

Erythroblastosis Blood examination show erythroblasts, if it is in foetus it is called erythroblastosis foetalis which is due to Rh incompatibility.

Erythrocyte It is a mature RBC responsible for transport of oxygen with the help of haemoglobin.

Erythrocytosis Abnormal raise of RBC in the blood which is also called erythrocythaemia.

Erythromycin Broad-spectrum antibiotic used against gram positive and gram-negative organisms.

Erythropoiesis Word is used for the production of RBC.

Erythropoietin It is a kidney hormone useful in stimulating bone marrow for RBC production,

Eschar When living tissues are destroyed we see slough which is called eschar, causes could be:

- Burns.
- Severe infection.
- Gangrene.

Escherichia Genus belonging to enterobacteriaceae, *E.coli* is common pathogen in clinical practice.

ESIS Abbreviation for Employees State Insurance Scheme for the welfare of industrial workers, comes under occupational health.

Esmarch's tourniquet A rubber bandage used to make a limb avascular during surgery.

Esophageal speech In case of cancer of larynx, removal of larynx produces speech less owing to loss of vocal cord, in such situations person learns to talk with the help of stomach and oesophagus which is in the place of windpipe.

Esophagus Anatomical structure stretching from pharynx up to stomach, it is a musculo membranous canal which measures about 9 inches.

ESR Abbreviation for Erythrocyte Sedimentation Rate.

Essence Refers to volatile oil in alcohol used for fragrance, also refers to an item which is an indispensable part.

Essential newborn care Under RCH this component is intended to reduce perinatal and neonatal mortality in the community, this includes:

- Resuscitation of newborn with birth asphyxia.
- Prevention of hypothermia.
- Prevention of infection.
- Exclusive breastfeeding.
- Referral of sick newborn.
- Care of low birth weight babies.

Essential obstetric care This refers to basic maternity service to all pregnant women in the country to ensure:
- Registration of pregnancy at 16 week.
- 3 antenatal check ups by ANM (MPW).
- Safe delivery either at home or at health centre.
- 3 postnatal check ups.

Essential Very much required or indispensable, like
- Essential amino acid.
- Essential fatty acid.
- Essential nutrients.
- Essential oils.
- Essential obstetrics.
- Essential paediatrics.
- Essential tool.

Ester Ester is the outcome by the elimination of water when acid and alcohol reacts.

Esterase It is an enzyme which is used in hydrolysis of esters, helpful in breaking ester into acid and alcohol.

EST Abbreviation for Electro Shock Therapy.

Estimates They are observed values of a sample or of a population, types are:
- Point estimates.
- Range estimates.

Estrogen They are female hormones responsible for female sexual characteristics.

Ethanol Other name for alcohol.

Ether An anaesthetic agent which is highly inflammable, a liquid anaesthetic which evaporates readily and is inhaled during anaesthesia.

Ethical issue Components of medical professional ethics which is in vogue e.g., ethical issues in genetic engineering include the following:
- Patenting of the biological system by big industries.
- Use of Human Genome Project for genetic discrimination.
- Genome based information used for LIC.
- Misuse of technology in general.

Ethics It is the regulation for moral obligation in nursing profession, this code of ethics controls the nurse's behaviour with patients and in management procedure, specific area of ethics for nurses is called *nursing ethics*.

Ethmoid It is a bone of the base of the skull which contains ethmoid sinuses, ethmoid sinus is situated between the eyes.

Ethnic This is a group with a social structure and functions forming a cultural group, a social group with common characteristics.

Ethnology Study of human race, human evolution and human relationships including his origin

Ethos Particular social and cultural characteristics and norms of a group.

Ethyl chloride It is a liquid anaesthetics, this evaporates rapidly, it produces cooling effect, used as local anaesthetic.

Ethyloestrenol It is an anabolic steroid used in the treatment of weight loss, debility, osteoporosis

Etiology Deals with the causation of illness and it's perpetuating factors, pathogenesis of a disease is studied.

Etiquette professional Rules of behaviour laid down in nursing profession,code of manners in nursing profession,ceremonial observed in profe-ssional duties of a nurse.

Eucalyptus oil Oil from eucalyptus tree which is antiseptic and a mild stimulant used in nasal catarrh.

Eugenics In the prevention of genetic disorders, measures taken to improve physical and mental environment, helpful to get good future generation.

Eunuch Male whose testes are removed, castrated.

Euphoria A good perceivable feeling of well being, usually by a drug.

Eustachian tube Partially collapsible canal which admits air from the throat into the middle ear, this helps to equalise the pressures on the eardrum.

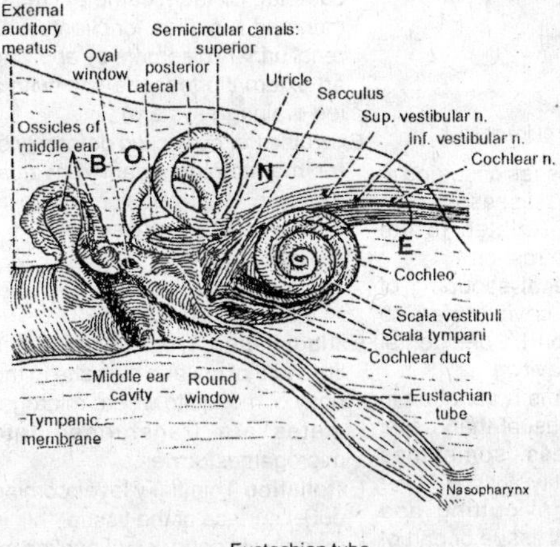

Eustachian tube

Euthanasia Euthanasia is the Act of deliberately ending the life of a patient which can be active or passive, " it is unethical procedure of taking life of a patient, with or without consent of the patient in irreversible/terminal illness"

Euthyroid Thyroid which is normally functioning, normal thyroid gland.

Evacuation Making discharge from natural orifices, bowel movement, removal of any material from the body organ.

Evaluation Critical appraisal of a clinical condition, assessment of a clinical condition, in nursing practice evaluation of patient is the later procedure.

Evidence based medicine Decision on diagnosis and treatment or management is done based on descriptive study and appraisal of research findings upto date, it is also called McMaster university approach since it was developed there, McMaster criteria for evidence based medicine are:

- available evidence of patient and population is taken
- patient's problem is taken than patient's protocol
- epidemiology, statistics, pathophysiology and clinical experience is best taken
- patients outcome is regarded as prime factor.

Evisceration It means removal of entire internal organ from its place, commonly used in case of evisceration of the eye.

Evolution Changes in the characteristics of an organism over a few generation is called evolution, this can refer to physical, mental and cultural aspect of the given organism.

Ewing's tumour It is sarcoma of the long bone.

Exacerbation This refers to the increased severity of clinical signs and symptoms in a patient who is suffering from an illness, acuteness of a clinical condition.

Examination of lower eyelid it is done to find out redness, congestion, watering, foreign body or any ulcer.

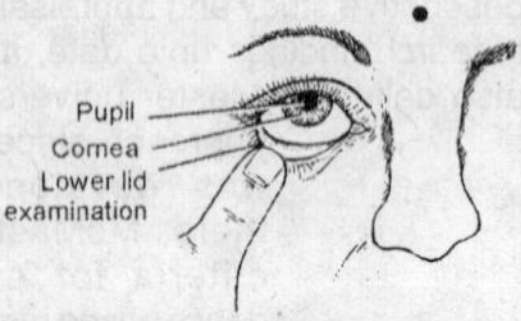

Examination of lower lid

Exanthem Skin rashes occurring in case of infectious diseases.

Exanthematous Related to the disease with skin rashes

Excavation Surgical scooping of material from a cavity, refers to dental excavation before dental filling of caries cavity.

Exception If there is a variation in clinical case, unusual than usual in case of illness, sometimes refers to rare entity.

Excision Surgical cutting and removal of part of tissue or part of organ tumour excision.

Excitation Stimulated, overwhelmed, it is an act of stimulating.

Excitement It is a response to a stimulus which is emotional and physiological in nature.

Exclusion Taken out or rejected, surgical separation of an organ from the main organ in human body.

Exclusive breastfeeding Only breastfeeding till 4 months and no other feed at that time constitute *Exclusive Breastfeeding.*

Excrement Metabolic secretions of the body like faeces, urine and sweat.

Excreta Discharge of excretory system like stool, urine and sweat.

Excretion Waste material which is thrown out of the body or expelled from the body.

Exdwelling catheter Other name for male urinary collection catheter, condom catheter, Texas catheter; it is used for clients with renal urinary disorders by applying an external urinary device (with a leg drainage system).

Exercise For correcting deformity or for maintaining health physical exercise or physical exertion is done, types of exercises are:

- Active exercise.
- Passive exercise.
- Isometric exercise.

Exflagellation This is seen in the life cycle of malaria parasite in the body of mosquito where microgametes are transformed into microgamestocytes.

Exfoliation Thin flaky layer coming out of surface of the tissúe, this is referable to dead tissue peeling off

Exhalation The act of expiration or giving out of breath, giving off of a vapour.

Exhibitionism To show off, one who is showing off for attention, under unacceptable circumstances a person exposes genitals in the public.

Exocrine Glands that have ducts to secrete their secretion like salivary gland.

Exogenous The origin is from outside, opposite of endogenous.

Exomphalos It is referred to congenital umbilical hernia, herniation of abdominal viscera into the umbilical cord.

Exophthalmometer Ophthalmic instrument which can measure the protrusion of eyeball.

Exophthalmos Abnormal protrusion of the eyeball seen in cases of thyrotoxicosis and injury.

Exostosis Bony growth from the surface of the bone.

Exotic That which is not native, that which is foreign.

Exotoxin Bacterial poison which is released to tissues around it.

Exotropia Outward turned eyes of a person, strabismus which is divergent.

Expanded role This word is used in nursing profession when the nurse takes the role play in her duties outside the duties and responsi-bilities of her working institution.

Expected outcome In nursing practice planning is done to have an expected result in case of case management.

Expectorant Drug which produce expulsion of phlegm or sputum in a patient who is having lung inflammation due to infection.

Expectoration Phlegm or sputum coughed out of lung passages.

Experimental design It is part of nursing research, used to fulfil the requirement of procedure and good design in research or experiment.

Characteristics of experimental design are:

- Random allocation of patients.
- No arbitrary correction.
- No bias in result noting down.
- Use of control with similar characteristics.

Common experimental designs are:

- One way approach.
- Two way approach.
- Latin square approach.
- Factorials design.
- Split plot design.
- Use of analysis of co-variance.

Experimentalism It is a philosophy of Nursing Education, it teaches that every thing is changing continually including man, mortality, democracy and education, according to this philosophy the experience is the only reality.

Experiment To demonstrate truth or fact, a procedure is followed in science.

Expiration Moving the inspired air out of the lung by the way of breathing.

Exploration Surgical opening of any tissue, part, organ for coming to final diagnosis, opening of abdomen to find out cause of acute abdomen.

Expression Facial expression during emotion in man, breast milk removal by manual pressure, prominent character seen in future generation in case genetic characters.

Extension traction It is indicated for patients who require presurgical immobilisation of a fractured hip or for patients with fractured femur, pelvic injury sciatica, muscle spasms degenerative arthritis of knee or knee injury which require immobility; extension traction is also known as buck's boot with the help of adhesive straps or a sponge rubber boot.

Extension Name given to the movement which cause straightening, like:
- Extension of the arm.
- Extension of the leg.
- Extension of the back.

Extensor It refers to a muscle which helps in the straightening of limb, muscle which extends the limb.

External respiration Regular breathing of man, this is visible form of expiration and inspiration.

External skeleton Bony framework which is carried by the organism on outside of its body, crayfish has an external skeleton.

External urinary device When prolonged use of indwelling catheter is needed external urinary collection device is used, male urinary collection system also called Texas catheter or condom catheter.

Extracapsular this refers to a type of cataract operation, it also refers to fracture of long bone which is outside the capsule.

Extracellular It refers to extra-cellular fluid, which means outside the cell.

Extramedullary situated outside medulla oblongata.

Extrasensory Thoughts coming out about future happening without any available means of communication, occurring beyond usual ordinary senses, extrasensory perception called ESP.

Extrasystole Contraction not occurring in cardiac cycle but occurring before regular contraction, premature contraction of the atrium or of the ventricle

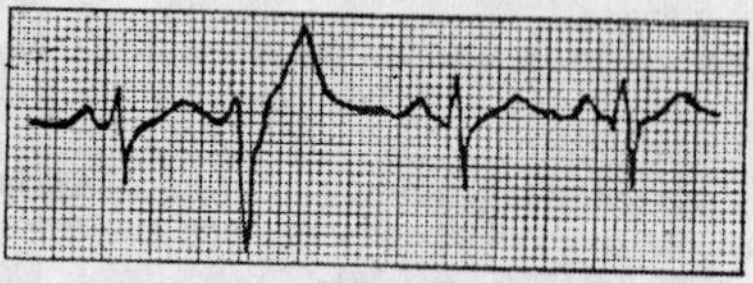

Extrasystole or premature VPB Ventricular premature beat

Extrauterine Refers to events occurring outside the uterus such as ectopic pregnancy.

Extra It is a prefix meaning additional such as extramural, extracellular, extracalorie, etc.

Extract Any substance when steeped in water or alcohol and then evoporation of fluid is done; it gives a concentrate which is called extract, e.g., belladonna extract, opium extract, etc.

Extraction When a concentrate is taken out from plant by extract, when breech is pulled out in breech extraction, when a thing is removed by applying vacuum called vacuum extraction.

Extrapyramidal When a thing is outside the pyramidal tract, nerves outside the pyramidal tract is called extrapyramidal system.

Extravasations Escape of fluid to its abnormal position, blood leak as in case of bruise or contusion.

Extremity Distal part of feet or the hand.

Extrinsic The origin is from outside, common usages are extrinsic muscle, extrinsic factors in disease causation.

Extroversion When an organ is turned inside out, extroversion of uterus.

Extrovert Is a type of personality where person mixes well in society, socialable and outgoing, opposite of introvert.

Extubation Tube is removed which is inserted for intubation.

Exudate Substance which is thrown out, substance which is deposited.

Exudation Discharge of serous fluid around tissue, discharge around RBC, WBC or any cell, discharge due to cell wall permeability.

Eye bandage It is used to retain a dressing on the eye.

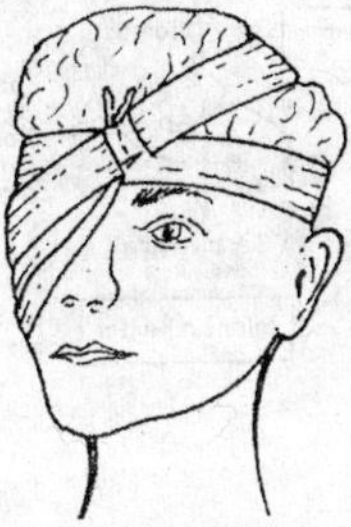

Eye Bandage

Eye bank Since 1944 we have eye banks which help in availability of qualified hospitals and surgeons a supply of fresh or preserved cornea for the corneal graft operation, they are for sight restoration.

Eye It is the organ of sight, special sense organ of human body or any living organism.

Eyedrops Medicamentation to the eye in case of infection or inflammation put through dropper.

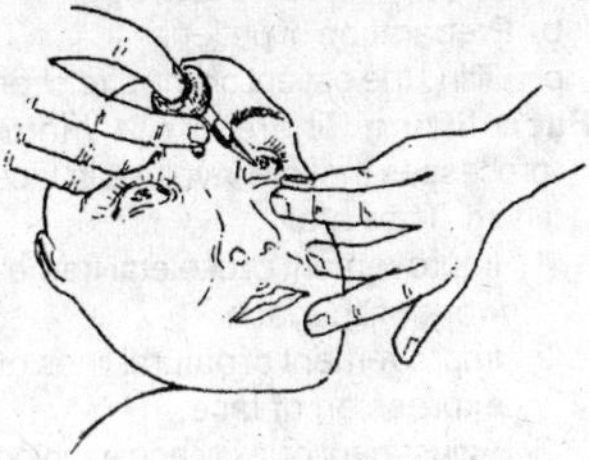

Application of eyedrops

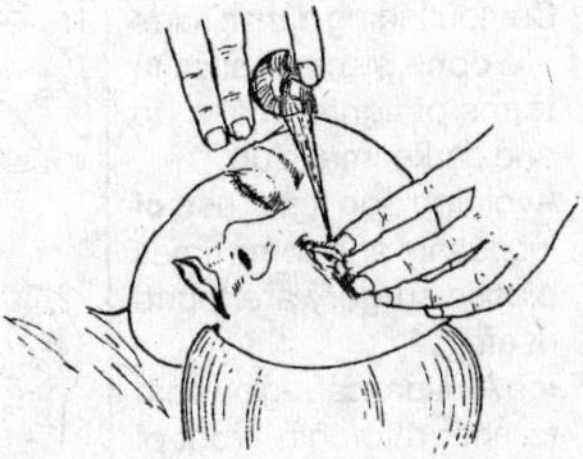

Irrigation of eye

Eyelid lids which cover eye is made up of connective tissue and muscle, lower and upper eyelid which protects the eye, the special sense organ.

Eye tooth This is the name given to upper canine tooth.

F

Face downward transport It is first aid in spinal injuries followed in coal mines,

First aid training gives the first aider three steps in this transport

a. Preparation of stretcher
b. Preparation of patient
c. Lifting the patient on the stretcher.

Face lifting There are 4 major processes that are involved in face lifting. They are:

1. Improvement of skeletal framework of the face.
2. Improvement of natural lines of expression of face.
3. Adjustment of laxity and sagging of folds and pouches.
4. Adjustment of skin colour of the face.

Camouflaging dark circles are done by cosmetics in terms of lighter make up and darker make up

Avoiding sun light, use of lubricants and some times plastic surgery are found useful.

Face Anatomical region from forehead to chin, front of the head.

Facemask In managing respiratory therapy simple facemask (low flow system) is used for short term therapy when moderate concentrations of oxygen are desired but it must be used cautiously on patient who might potentially vomit and aspirate. In case of patients requiring reliable, precise and controlled concentrations of oxygen (particularly patients with COPD) need Venturi (air entrainment) mask for highflow system.

Facet a Flat area on the surface of a bone, small abraded spot on teeth.

Facial nerve It is VII cranial nerve, it supplies facial muscles and platysma, it supplies submandibular gland and sublingual gland, taste sense from anterior 2/3rd of tongue is supplied by this cranial nerve.

Facial Related with or pertaining to face like face presentation.

Facilitation A quick fording for an action is called facilitation.

Factor To get the result, *factor* becomes very important element.

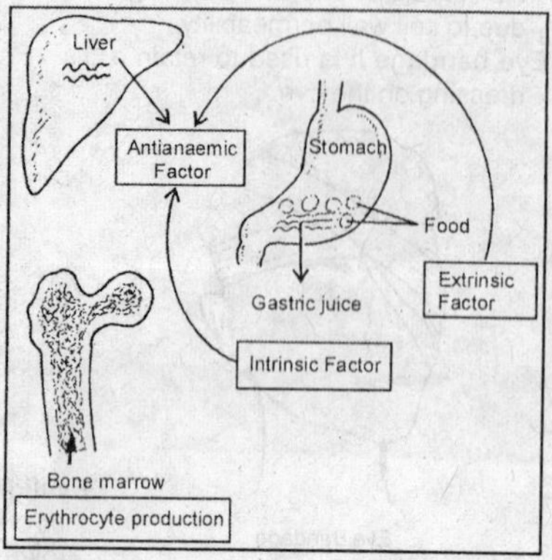

Factors in erythropoiesis

Facultative A biological condition where bacteria can survive with oxygen or without oxygen, natural ability to live in available circumstances.

Faculty Refers to teaching staff, it denotes mental status of a person.

Faeces Waste material excreted from bowel after metabolism which may contain undigested particles, water and pathogens, stool.

Faecalith Very hardened stool.

Fahrenheit scale This is the scale used to measure heat like
Human body temperature 98.4°F
Boiling water 212.0°F.

Fahrenheit German physicist who lived during 1686-1736 (G.D. Fahrenheit).

Failure Refers to an organ when it fails to perform its function, common usage are:
- Cardiac failure.
- Renal failure.
- Respiratory failure.

Fainting Other name is syncope which is a state of temporary unconscious ness due to diminished blood supply to the brain which may be due to
i. Exhaustion and fatigue.
ii. Emotion and fear.
iii. Accidents.
iv. High heat.
v. Long standing.

Faith Normal reaction in times of illness to seek out those persons who are trained in treating illness, the substance of things hoped for, the evidence of things not seen, faith healing by spiritual power.

Falciform ligament Refers to the ligament of the liver, it separates right and left lobes of liver, anatomically it is the reflection of peritoneum which attach liver to diaphragm.

Falciform Any thing which is sickle-shaped.

Fallopian tube It is called oviduct which carry ova from ovaries to uterus, uterine tube.

Fallot's tetralogy It is a congenital heart disease with the defects of
a) Pulmonary stenosis.
b) VSD.
c) Overriding of the aorta.
d) Hypertrophy of the right ventricle.

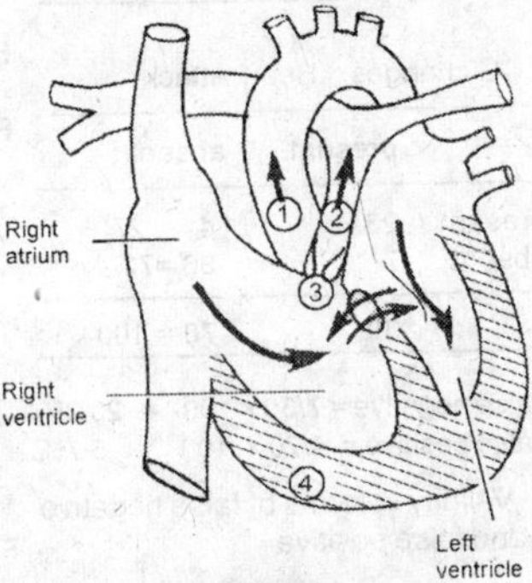

Fallot's tetralogy

1. Dextro- position of arota.
2. Pulmonary stenosis.
3. Ventricular septal defect.
4. Hypertrophy of right ventricle.

Fallout Result of nuclear war injuries, radioactive fallouts.

Falls Second highest cause of injuries result from falls which disable the industrial workers, as a result of stumbling, slipping or loss of balance.

False negative It is used in screening test, screening test is negative even when there is *disease* in the patient.

False positive It is used in screening

False positive It is used in screening test, screening test is positive even when there is *no disease* in the patient.

Test	Disease	
	present	absent
positive	a	b = (a+b)
negative	c	d = (c+d)
	a + c	b+d = (a+b+c+d)

ECG changes	Heart Attack	
	present	absent
present	23	4 = 27
absent	7	66 =73
	30	70 = 100

False negative = 7/30 × 100 = 23.3%
False positive = 4/70 × 100 = 5.7%

Validity in terms of false negative and false positive.

False ribs 8th rib to 12th rib which do not attach with sternum.

False teeth When a lost tooth is replaced by either fixed or removable appliance.

Falx Any anatomical structure which is shaped like sickle e.g.,
- Falx cerebri.
- Falx inguinalis.
- Falx cerebelli.

Familial Illness, disease, characteristics etc are occurring in a given family which is more than our expectation.

Family doctor Physician who looks after the health of a family, who examines illness in family background and who treats illness in family background.

Family planning It is now called Family Welfare Planning which covers the following.
- Family planning methods.
- Family planning measures.
- Artificial reproductive technologies.

It is a national health programme in India.

Family People related to by blood and marriage live under one shelter.

Family size Number of children born to a couple.

Family structure The composition of a group of people living together as family

Family types are:
- Single family.
- Joint family.
- Three generation family.
- Blended family.
- Extended family.
- Extended nuclear family.
- Single parent family.

Fantasy Imaginary visions which depicts unconscious conflicts.

Fantus test This is urine examination to find out level of NaCl which is normal constituent of urine. It can be reduced in certain diseases and in excessive loss of salt from the body, normal excretion of NaCl is 6.0 grams per day

Lab requirements for this titration are;

Test tube = 10 drops urine
+
drop Pot. chromate solution
+
silver nitrate (2.9%) 1 drop at a time
↓
Shaken well to observe the end point which is CHANGE

OF COLOUR FROM YELLOW TO BROWN

Inference – No. of drops = Grams of NaCl per litre

(e.g., 5 drops = 5 grams per litre)

FAO Food and Agriculture Organisation which is an International Organisation.

Farm life It is the rural home which has the family hazards due to chemicals, insecticide, animal disease and farm accidents.

Farmer's lung It is occupational hazard among farmers and agriculturists, also called hey fever.

Fascia Connective tissue sheath which encloses a muscle or an organ.

Fasciola A genus of flukes, Fasciola hepatica.

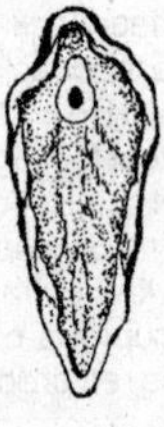

Fasciola hepatica

Fasting When a person do not accept food or drinks for reasons known or unknown.

Fat embolism This is common complications of severe trauma with multiple fractures, hip fracture and femur fracture should be followed for minimum 3 days to exclude fat embolism, early signs of fat embolism are:

- Raised temperature.
- Increased pulse rate.
- Precordial chest pain.
- Dyspnoea.
- Cough.
- Agitation.
- Disorientation.

Late signs of fat embolism are:

- Petechiae at buccal membranes.
- Petechiae at chest.
- Petechiae at hard palate.

Nursing care includes:

- Oxygen administration.
- Administration of diuretics.
- Administration of anti-inflammatory agents.

Fat emulsion Fat emulsions are indicated to patients who are deficient in essential fatty acids due to disorders such as severe burns, late stage of kidney disease, ulcerative colitis and cancers.

Fat soluble This word is used for vitamin A, vitamin D, vitamin E and K since they are fat soluble.

Fatal That which causes death and that which is deadly fatal haemorrhage, fatal accident, etc.

Fat An oily substance found in meat, fish, cheese, milk, some vegetables, energy yielding and gives essential nutrients, one of the proximate principle which yield 9 calories per gram.

Fat soluble Capable of being dissolved in the body fat.

Fatherhood Anticipated and required care for the child given by the father, involve some share in all of the tasks of baby care and child health.

Fatigue It is a state which vary from disinclination to exhaustion, mental fatigue, muscle fatigue.

Fatty acid Present in fat which is one of the proximate principles of the diet. They may be saturated or unsaturated in nature

Types are:
- Simple fatty acids.
- Compound fatty acids.
- Derived fatty acids.

Saturated fatty acids are:
- Lauric acid.
- Palmitic acid.
- Stearic acid.

Unsaturated fatty acids are:
- Oleic acid.
- Linoleic acid.

Fatty change When accumulation of fat occurs in a cell which is demonstrable.

Fatty That which contain fat, in case of degeneration by fatty infiltration term used is fatty degeneration.

Fauces An opening that lead mouth to pharynx, the boundaries are:
(a) Soft palate.
(b) Base of the tongue.
(c) Palatine arches.

Favism It is clinically seen as acute haemolytic anaemia due to ingestion of fava beans, this is related with the deficiency of glucose 6-phosphate dehydrogenase in red cells.

Favus Fungal infection of scalp by *Trichophyton schoenleinii*, ringworm infection of the scalp.

Fear It is a reflex response to external danger, manifested with apprehension.

Febrile convulsion When fever developed precipitates it causes fits, usually seen among children.

Febrile Related with fever like febrile convulsion.

Faeces Waste product of digestion which excreted as stool from bowel.

Fecundation Making pregnant, making fertile, impregnation, fertilisation.

Fecundity It is the physiological ability of a woman to produce children.

Fee splitting Dubious arrangements in medical profession like charging more fee, more of referral for commission, recommendation for over-investigation of patient constitute fee splitting, when a case is referred or transferred, the commission obtained by the transfere constitute fee splitting.

Feeble mindedness Lowered mental capacity or mental deficiency.

Feedback It is one of the monitoring process, it is seen in national health programmes, seen in physiological process, seen in enzyme reaction, Types are:
- Positive feedback.
- Negative feedback.

Fehling solution It is used in qualitative test for sugar, it contains two types of solution called Fehling A and Fehling B , when urine sugar is tested with Fehling by boiling it produces cuprous oxide which is observed as red precipitate.

Fehling A	*Fehling A*
Copper sulphate 34.66 grams Potassium iodide 173 grams Water 500 ml sodium hydroxide 50 grams Water 500 ml	

Female genital mutilation It exists as tradition and culture in some of the African countries, it includes excision of labia majora, labia minora, clitoris and partial closure of introitus.

Female reproductive system Understanding of female reproductive system is important for performing routine gynaecologic examinations,

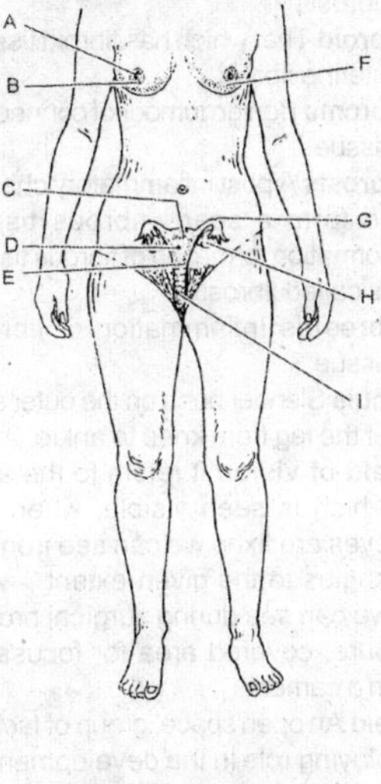

The female reproductive system

A Nipple
B Areola
C Uterine fundus
D Uterus
E Cervix
F Breast
G Fallopiantube
H Ovary
I Vagina

Femur Anatomically it is thigh bone.

Feminisation Physiological development of female sexual characteristics in girls.

Feminism When a man develops secondary sexual characteristics like loss of hair, breast development, feminine voice, etc.

Femoral Anything that is related with femur.

Fenestra An opening which looks like a window e.g., Fenestra ovalis.

Fenestration It is the surgical intervention by opening the obstructed window between inner and middle ear (Fenestra=window).

Fenugreek Plant which is hay like whose seeds are used for condiments, as known foodpad fenugreek is used as tea.

Fermentation Refers to enzymic decomposition, fermentation is seen in alcohol production, bread production, vinegar production, common types in medical practice are:

- Intestinal fermentation.
- Alcoholic fermentation.
- Lactic acid fermentation.

Fern Plants which do not yield flowers,fern extract is edicinally useful being antihelminthic.

Ferrous That which contains iron, referred to normally as ferrous sulphate.

Fertilisation During conception union takes place between sperm and ovum impregnation of ovum by sperm, It can be natural or *in vitro*.

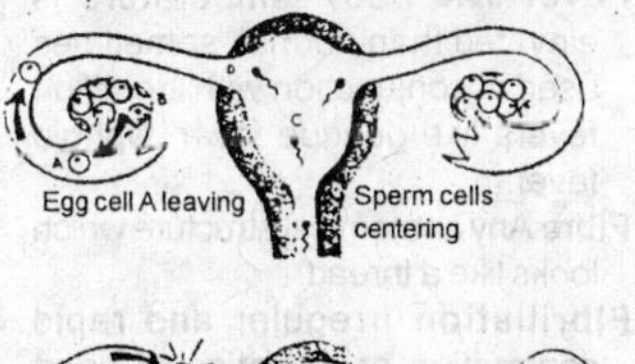

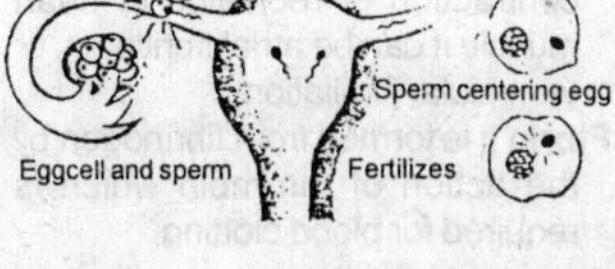

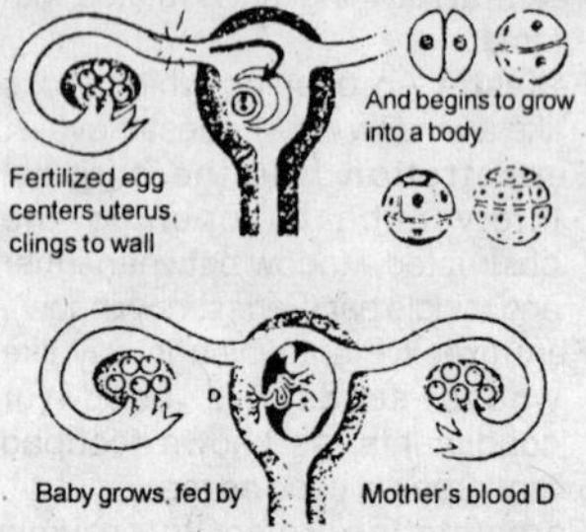

Fertilisation

Fertility It is the ability to become fertile or pregnant , it is child-bearing among women of 15-45 age group, uninterrupted marriage life and no contraception can allow a woman to bear 8 to 10 children which is called fertility status.

Fetor Very bad and offensive smell.

Feudal society Depending on possession or non-possession of land, people are ordered in a strict hierarchy.

FEV$_1$ Forced Expiratory Volume measured in one second, reduction indicates obstructive lung diseases.

Fever The body temperature is elevated than normal, sometimes used in conjunction with identified fevers like dengue fever, typhoid fever.

Fibre Any anatomical structure which looks like a thread.

Fibrillation Irregular and rapid contraction or recitation of heart muscle it can be atrial fibrillation or ventricular fibrillation.

Fibrin It is formed from fibrinogen by the action of thrombin which is required for blood clotting.

Fibrinogen It is precursor of fibrin, as such a soluble protein.

Fibroblast It is connective tissue cell.

Fibrocystic disease of pancreas It is the other name for cystic fibrosis.

Fibroid That which has fibroid tissue, uterine fibroid.

Fibroma Benign tumour of connective tissue.

Fibrosis A post inflammatory change to form a scar, fibrous tissue formation formation of fibrous tissue is called fibrosis.

Fibrositis Inflammation of fibrous tissue.

Fibula Slender bone on the outer side of the leg from knee to ankle.

Field of vision It refers to the area which is seen visible, when the eyes are fixed we can see from all angles to the given extent , what we can see during surgical procedure, covered area for focussing in a camera.

Field An open space, group of factors playing role in the development of organism, field of vision, field of operation.

Fight for sight It is an organised effort to prevent blindness which started all over the world in 1946 with the purpose to stimulate and finance research in eye care and related sciences, objectives of fight for sight by the Government and NGO are:

- Detection of blindness.
- Prevention of blindness.
- Treatment of blindness.
- Cure of visual disorders.
- Cure of impaired sight.

- Cure of incipient blindness.
- Cataract operation for cataract blindness.

Figure of eight bandage During first aid through bandaging, the figure of eight bandage is used for the part increasing in thickness, and used for the ankle and the hand.

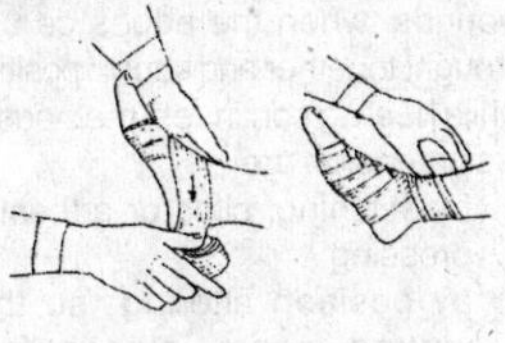

Figure of eight bandage

Figure To get a formation, to get a shape by development or metamorphosis, seen as prominent in a set of structure or object.

Filament Minute thread like structure which is delicate in nature.

Filaria One of the genus under nematode, that which causes elephantiasis.

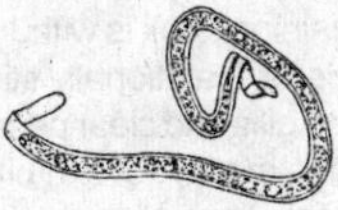

Filaria worm

Filarial Caused by a filaria.

Filariasis Filarial infection caused by *W.bancrofti* or *B.malayi* , elephentiasis.

Film badge This is called dosimeter which is put by X-ray technicians, radiologists to check the extent of exposure to ionisation in their occupation.

Filter Filter is a device to separate out certain elements, water filter, X-ray filter, I V filter.

Filters I.V. I V filters are attached to infusion tubing to ensure that a particulate matter does not enter patient's bloodstream, very fine filters which can filter the matter of the size of 0.22 μ are available, care must be taken to avoid clogging.

Filtration Process of filtering smaller particles , process of filtering X-ray particles.

Fimbria Meaning thread-like projection, a fringe, such as fimbria of fallopian tube.

Finger bandage By using inch-wide bandage continuous finger bandage is done leaving base of thumb free to move, enabling patient to use the hand to a large extent, first aid measure.

Finger sucking Habit of the baby or child, suction pressure of this can produce vomiting and unhappy babies.

Finger Referable to digit of the hand, thumb, fore finger, middle finger, ring finger, small finger etc., pathologically some of the types are known which are:

- Webbed finger.
- Trigger finger.
- Hammer finger.
- Clubbed finger.

Fingernails They are indicators of health of a person, brittleness or pallor indicate illness, they are objective manifestations.

Fingerprint Ridges on the surface of the fingertips which form whorls and the patterns are called fingerprints, used for identification purpose.

Firearm Gun and other hunting material which cause accidents, require safety procedure at home and in fields.

Fireman's lift It is useful method of carrying a patient unable to walk but must only be used when the patient is not too heavy for the first aider. It has the advantage that the first aider has one hand free.

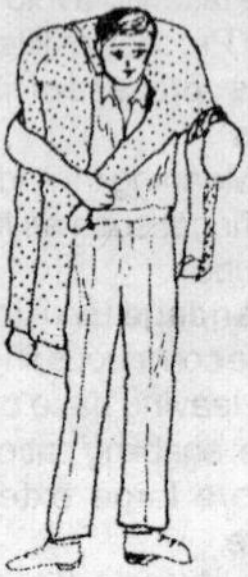

The Fireman's lift

Fires Common cause of burns in medical practice, fire burns can produce shock, objectives of first aid in fire burns are:
- Prevent shock.
- Prevent contamination.
- Control pain.

In extensive burn by fire, nursing care require
- Place the cleanest available cloth material over all burned areas.
- Have victim lie down.
- Call physician and keep patient lying till he comes.
- Place head and chest of patient lower than body.
- If conscious give fluids to drink.

First aid Immediate attention and immediate action in case of emergencies like
- Disasters.
- Medical emergencies.
- Heart attack.
- Insect bite.
- Snake bite.
- Head injuries.

First intention This word is used in repair of wound for quick healing, one of the method of wound healing is first intension , it occurs in incised wounds, when the edges can be brought together and kept in position while healing continues, methods of first intension are:
1. by stitching, clips or adhesive dressing.
2. by position altering so that wound come closer first intention is possible in healthy wounds which takes about 5 to 10 days.

Fish hooks It is a common accident that a person is hooked with fish hook who need the following nursing attention:
- Do not pull the hook backwards.
- If you pull barb will cause injury.
- Barb is cut off.
- Remaining hook is withdrawn.

Fish hygiene Traditionally stiffness, bright red gills and clear permanent eyes are known to exhibit good eatable fish, tinned fish should have following condition for fish hygiene:
- No rusting.
- No leakage.
- No evidence of tampering.
- No bloom out phenomenon at opening.

Fission Used with meaning of splitting or division, reproduction of bacteria by dividing into equal halves (Binary fission), nucleus of an atom splitting giving release of high energy (nuclear fission)

Fissure Anatomically it is a narrow split such as anal fissure.

Fissured fracture Common variety of fracture which is simple in nature but the bone is cracked and not completely broken.

Fissured fracture of clavicle and small bones in nondependent part do not cause concern,

Fissured fracture of long bones should be dealt with care.

Fistula That which connects two cavities of two organs, abnormal passage formed between surfaces, common fistulae are:

- Rectovaginal fistula.
- Vesicovaginal fistula.
- Tracheo-oesophageal fistula.
- Faecal fistula.
- Biliary fistula.
- Anal fistula.

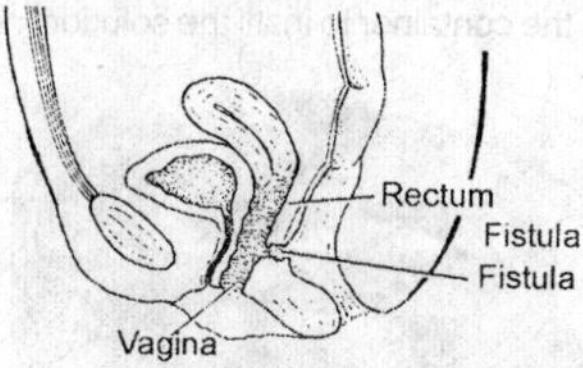

Rectovaginal fistula

Fit Convulsions occurring due to epilepsy, eclampsia, hysteria, it is paroxysmal motor nerve discharge leading to sudden involuntary compulsive rigorous movement.

Fitness This word is used when a person has a sense of well being, when a person has the ability to perform maximum limit of all physical and physiological activities and actions.

Fixation When a structure is immobilised, when a bone is immobilised, it is the process of making not mobile, when there is no psychological development, eye fixation in ophthalmology.

Flaccid Soft and flabby, refers to flaccid paralysis.

Flagella A mobile whip like process from unicellular organism which is used for its motility.

Flagyl Trade name of a pharmacological preparation of metronidazole which is commonly used as amoebicidal.

Flail chest When many ribs are fractured, or a rib is having multiple fractures state of flail chest is produced, paradoxical movement like inner movement with expiration and outer movement with inspiration are noticed.

Flammable That which is likely to get burnt.

Flank This refers to the part of abdomen which is between the rib cage and ilium.

Flap Tissue taken from one place for grafting to other place, it is mass of tissue taken for plastic surgery.

Flatfoot Because of sunken medial longitudinal arch of the foot, because of weakening and degeneration of ligaments and tendons flat foot occurs which is called Pes planus.

Foot – showing normal and flat sole

Flatulent Gas formation due to indigestion and fermentation occurring in stomach and intestine.

Flatus tube It is inserted into rectum and above to relieve distension

Requirements are:

1. A rubber rectal tube which has thick wall and the eye at the end (nurses to note that a catheter has a lateral eye).
2. A glass connection attaching the rectal tube to a length of rubber tubing with a glass funnel at other end.
3. A bowel of water.
4. Petroleum jelly or any lubricant and swabs.
5. A receiver for soiled swabs.
6. A mackintosh square and pad to protect the bed.

Nursing procedure for passing a flatus tube for the relief of istension; Rectal tube is lubricated and passed into the rectum for about 2 inches. The funnel is placed under the surface of the water in the bowl which is placed at bedside to observe the bubbles of gas when it start escaping from the funnel

Flatus Air passed through rectum or anus, fried food, milk and legumes produce more gas, the gases which are passed in flatus are:

- Hydrogen.
- Methane.
- Skatole.
- Indole.
- Carbon dioxide.
- Nitrogen.
- Small quantity of oxygen.

Fleas Cause known zoonotic diseases which can be prevented by eliminating them from dogs, cats, pets, beddings and homesurroundings

Rat flea is know to cause bubonic plague.

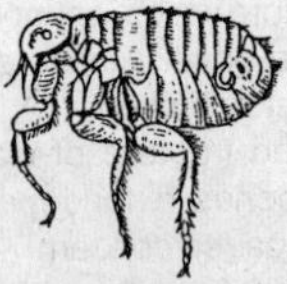

Adult female rat flea

Fleets enema It is a type of retention enema, it is a commercially prepared enema commonly known as fleets enema which is available in a plastic container for instilling the solution. Nursing instructions separate patients buttocks and gently insert the prelubricated tip of container into the anus. Then raise the base of the container to avoid instilling air to rectum. Then squeeze the container to instil the solution.

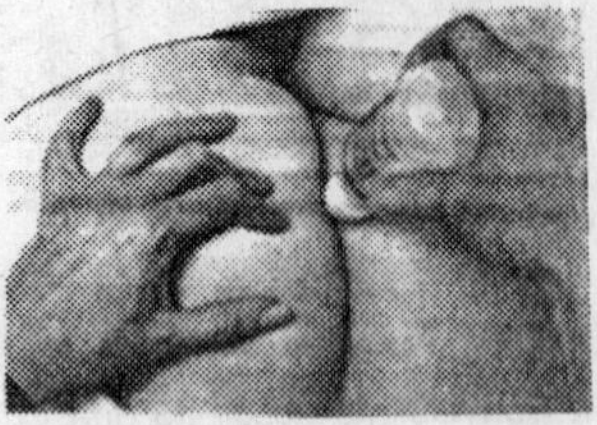

Fleets enema

Flexion The act of bending of leg, arm or back.

Flexor The muscle which bends a joint, opposite of extension.

Floaters Ageing and collapse of vitreous cause some visible strands with the eye.

Flocculation It is a chemical process where adding a coagulant like alum brings about changes by gathering smaller particles to larger visible particles, the process helps in settling sediments.

Flooding Repeated exposure treatment in phobia, severe loss of blood from uterus.

Flora plant Life of a geographical area is described as flora, intestinal bacterial content is termed as intestinal flora.

Florence Nightingale Pioneer of Modern Nursing who set standards of practical nursing and hospital administration which still serves as a model.

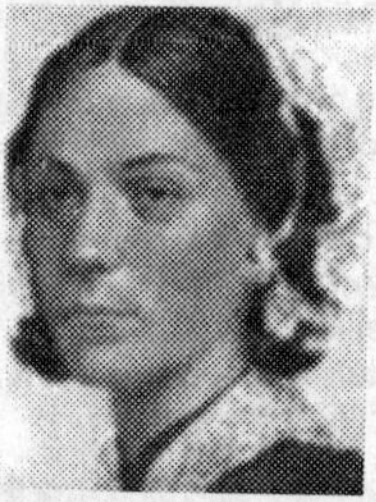

Miss Florence Nightingale

Born on 12th May 1820
Died on 13th Aug 1910

Florid Face appearance which show flushing and reddening.

Flotation pads This is used in assisting the patient with positioning and mobilisation, gel like inner substance molds to the patient's body to help minimise pressure over the bony prominences, sizes are made available for beds and for wheelchairs.

Fluctuation Movement felt as in the case of palpation of soft tumour or abdomen, variation in the structure of an organism.

Fluid balance Water, electrolytes and non-electrolytes are within normal in the human body, internal environment "Milieu Interior" is well protected.

Fluid Refers to liquid status available in our body, common reference made are:

- Interstitial fluid.
- Amniotic fluid.
- Cerebrospinal fluid.
- Body fluid.

It also refers to the replacement of fluid in cases of dehydration.

Fluke Refers to lung fluke, liver fluke and intestinal fluke which belong to trematodes under helminths.

Fluoridation Fluoride is a natural constituent of water; but when it is deficient addition of minute amounts of fluorides can supply the deficiency which is a process called fluoridation.

Fluoride Fluorine as salt is a normal ingredient of natural source of water.

Fluorine Non-metallic gaseous element belonging to halogen group.

Fluorescence Having the property of reflecting back the light waves or which is capable of producing fluorescence.

Fluorescent That which produce fluorescence.

Fluoridation It is adding fluorine to drinking water as a community health measure to protect the community from caries.

Fluoroscope Radiological instrument for observing internal organs by using contrast media.

Flush Feeling of heat and skin

reddening of the face and neck.

Flushing The blood vessels in the skin account for the reddening of the skin when we blush and we call flushing.

Flutter It is referred to irregular heart beat.

Fly They are two winged insects under dipterous, common flies of Public health importances are:
- House fly.
- Sand fly.
- Tsetse fly.
- Black fly.

Focus Localised area of infection in the body, ability of eye to focus for an object either at nearer point or farther.

Focusing Visual acuity adjusted by altering the lens focal point.

Foetal circulation The circulation which is seen in foetus through umbilical cord and placenta which differs from adult circulation.

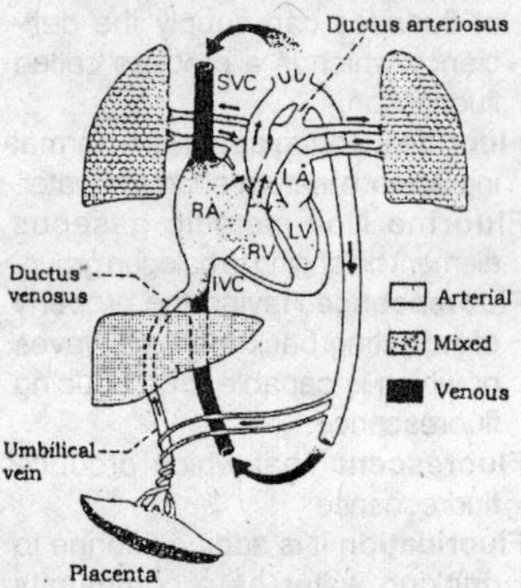

Foetal circulation

Foetal heart tone It is called FHT which is tried after ascertaining foetal position.

Normally it is best heard between umbilicus and symphysis pubis.

Upto 20 weeks of gestation it is heard by foetoscope.

FHT has to be heard after assessing the foetal position which is dependent on position and presentation.

Foetal Related to foetus like foetal mortality.

Foeticide Foetal death occurring by reasons known or by artificial means of killing foetus which is criminal in nature.

Foetoscope It is an obstetrical instrument used to hear foetal heart tone.

Foetus The growing baby inside the womb, intrauterine life of man.

Fogging Method of spraying insecticide from atmosphere to the ground method of testing astigmatic error denotes density of X-ray film due to chemicals

Foley catheter This is used to perform catheterisation with an indwelling catheter called Foley catheter, it is indicated in irrigation, instillation, drainage

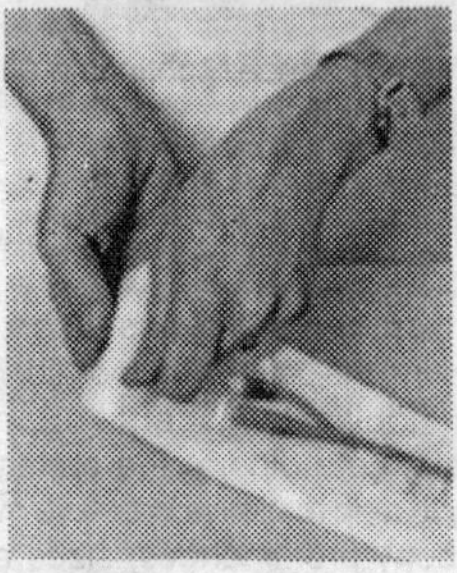
Foley (Indwelling) catheter

Folic acid One of the water soluble vitamin present in greens, liver and yeast, it corrects megaloblastic anaemia, chemically it is pteroyl glutamic acid, $C_{19}H_{19}N_7O_6$.

Folk society Rural societies in which everyone knows everyone else.

Folklore In early centuries people used to go for traditional healing which had established folklore (medical folklore), some of the examples are:

- Apollo is the originator of the healing art.
- Soothening the God who is angry to cure ill.
- Old Wives' tale.

  For backache do somersault as whippoorwill calls.

  Treat whooping cough by passing patient through a horse collar three times.
- Food fallacies.

Follicle Small gland or sac like hair follicle or Graafian follicle.

Follicular tonsillitis During the process of infection of tonsil, follicles are formed on the surface of the tonsil which may get inflammated, pus filled follicles on the tonsils which show inflammatory change.

Follicular Related to or pertaining to follicle.

Folliculosis Abnormal increase in follicle and its manifestations.

Fomentation surgical Nurse when does the surgical dressings, she may be given orders by the surgeon a fomentation for septic wound (note: wet dressing is not commonly used nowadays)

Requirements:

1. Sterile bowls, dissecting forceps, dressings in the troley.
2. A piece of lint double the size of the area to be fomented.
3. Protective material such jaconet or oiled silk large enough to cover the lint when folded.
4. Sterile cotton wool to cover lint and to overlap about one inch all round.
5. A wringer made of linen towelling or of strong cotton.

Nursing procedure for fomentation in surgical dressing:

The fomentation brought is transferred to a sterile bowl, wrings it to dry, unfolds to expose the lint. The nurse picks up the lint with sterile forceps, shakes it to allow the steam to escape, applies it to the wound, covers the lint with the protective and then with the layer of cotton wool.

Many tailed bandage is preferred to roller bandage

Fomentation Application of worm and moist dressing in surgical practice.

Fomite Non-living material which can transmit infection by getting contaminated. Any object other food that may harbour and transmit pathogens.

Fontanelle Under nursing care palpating anterior fontanelle and posterior fontanelle by fingers to get a built-in tape measure.

Anterior fontanelle is 2 to 3 cm in width, 3 to 4 cm length and is diamond-shaped

soft = normal, full or bulging = indicate increased Intracranial pressure

Posterior fontanelle is small, triangular

closure is within 12 weeks in case of posterior fontanelle and within 18 months in case of anterior fontanelle

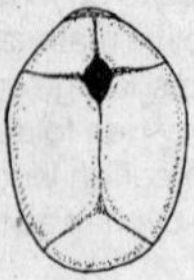

Anterior fontanelle

Food additive They are chemicals used to increase shelf life of food, improve taste to change texture, to give a colour,

Junk foods like biscuit, cake, confectionery, jam, jelly, coke and ketchup contain food additives.

Food adulteration Food when mixed with hazardous substances which are invariably for commercial purposes is called food adulteration

Asfoetida (Hing)	-	Resin, gum, grit
Butter	-	Starch, animal fat
Black pepper	-	Papaya seed
Cereals	-	Soapstone bits
Chilli powder	-	Brick powder
Coffee powder	-	Chicory, Tamarind husk
Dhal	-	Kesaridhal
Dhania powder	-	Cow dung powder
Ghee	-	Vanaspathi
Haldi	-	Lead chromate powder
Ice cream	-	Starch, cellulose
Milk	-	Water, starch
Mustard seed	-	Argemone seed

Table Common Food Adultrants

Food allergy By eating certain foods, people show sensitive reactions in the body which may be mild, moderate or severe in nature, common observation of food allergy is seen with milk, egg fish, certain fruits.

Food and Drug Act The Food Act and The Drug Act are Central Acts which regulate standard of food and drugs in the country. The Food Act was enacted in 1954. The Drug Act was enacted in 1940. Both were amended at a later dates.

The Food Act makes provisions for prevention of adulteration of food. The Drug Act envisages the regulation of import, manufacture, distribution and sale of drugs.

Food enrichment Restoration of nutrient value of a food to its normal level, vegetable oil is enriched with vitamin A and D at the source of distribution.

Food fortification Reinforcement of nutrients with additional supplies to prevent deficiency, this helps to improve the quality of diet of a community, examples are:

- Fluoridation of water.
- Iodisatin of salt.
- Vitamin A and D to vanaspathi.
- Vitamin A and D to milk.
- Iodine in salt.
- Iron in salt.

Food hygiene With the under-standing of germs, protection of food from contamination by pathogens resulted in an aware-ness of food hygiene food hygiene includes the following:

- Milk hygiene.
- Meat hygiene.
- Fish hygiene.
- Egg hygiene.
- Hygiene of fruits and vegetables.

Food poisoning It is an acute gastroenteritis by bacterial toxin, chemical toxin, plant toxin or by animal toxins.

Food poisoning occurs by:

- Staphylococcal food poisoning.
- Bacillus cereas poisoning.
- Poisoning by *Cl.perfringens*.
- Poisoning by *Cl.botulism*.
- By plant toxin.
- By chemical toxin.
- By Norwalk like agents.
- Salmonella poisoning.

Food toxin food toxins are common causes of food poisoning,common toxins are:

- Epidemic dropsy.
- Aflatoxin.
- Ergot.
- Neurolathyrism.
- Endemic ascites.
- Fusarium toxin.

Food Eatables in the form of diet which give calories, which protect infection and which help in body building.

Foot candle Expression of light at one foot of a candle, one lumen per square foot.

Foot drop Paralysis of lateral popliteal nerve produces plantar flexion of foot, paralysis of muscles in anterior compartment of leg.

Foot drop among bedridden patients is preventable. Three ways are suggested under nursing procedures;

By supporting the feet at a right angle to the legs by means of a firm pillow padding, a board or by the use of sandbag.

By ensuring that the top bedclothes are never tightly tucked over the patient's feet.

By encouraging patient to move his legs at regular intervals.

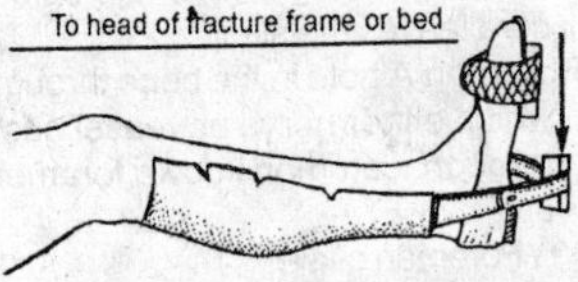

Method of prevention of foot drop

Foot support They are used to maintain dorsiflexion, prevent plantarflexion, prevent external rotation of hips, etc.

Foot supports are used with fleece, a blanket, a towel etc., to prevent formation of decubiti on the soles of the feet.

Foot Anatomical portion below the ankle up to toes which has plantar arch to carry or bear the body weight.

Football hold This is recommended to mothers who have had a caesarean delivery, because it enables them to support the infant's weight off their abdomen. The infant is held supine along the forearm with the head supported by the mother's hand; the infant's weight can be supported by a pillow.

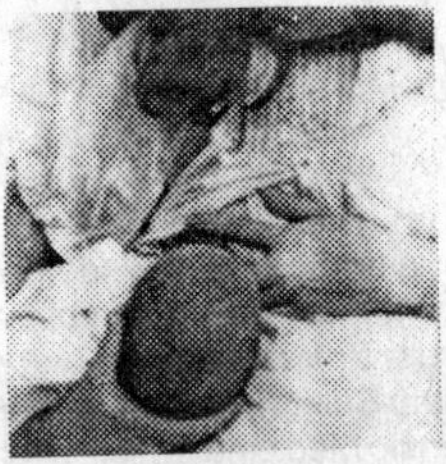

Football hold

Foramen magnum It is a large opening present in the floor of the cranium through which the spinal cord leaves the skull.

Foramen A hole in the bone through which either nerve or vessel pass through, common known foramen are:

- Foramen ovale.
- Optic foramen.
- Foramen magnum.
- Obturator foramen.

Forceps A surgical instrument for lifting , holding, or compressing a structure during operation

Fore and aft carry This method of patient carrying is undertaken when space does not permit the use of ordinary hand seats, used to carry through door through narrow corridor.

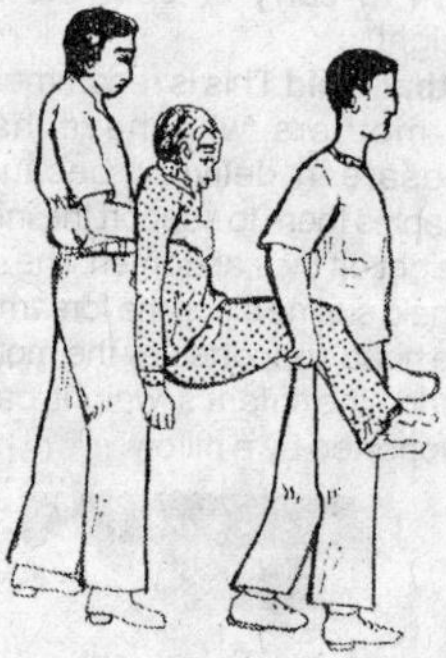

Fore-and-aft carry

care must be taken to see not to make patient uncomfortable and difficulty in breathing.

Forensic Related to legal medicine, Forensic Medicine, which is relied on Medial witness.

Foreskin Other name for prepuce

Formaldehyde It is a disinfectant used to disinfect utensils and excreta, it is a requirement's in toxoid preparation.

Formic acid Wood alcohol when oxidised we get formic acid, oxidation of formaldehyde, this is injected in stings and insect bites which can produce pain and swelling at the site of sting.

Formula A procedure followed to get a result, chemical formula, referable to infant feed.

Formulary Pharmacopial manual giving set of commonly used drugs Handbook of an R M P who prescribes drugs for treatment.

Fornix A structure which is arch or vault like shape, uterine fornix, conjunctival fornix.

Fossa Small pit on a bone like iliac fossa, cubital fossa, etc.

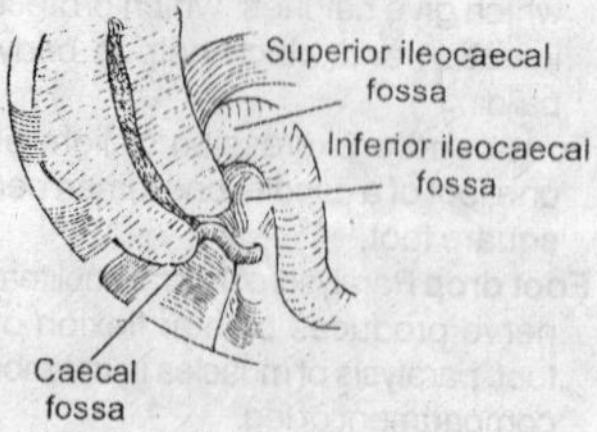

Fossae

Foster children Children who are adopted by parents who do not have children.

Foster parents Parents who adopt other children when they are infertile.

Fothergill's operation Gynaecological surgery developed by W.E. Fothergill a British gynaecologist (1865-1926) which include the following to treat prolapse of the uterus:

- Cervical amputation
- Anterior colporrhaphy
- Posterior colporrhaphy.

Four hand seat This first aid transport method is used when the patient is able to assist by using one or both of his arms and does not require support for either of his lower limbs.

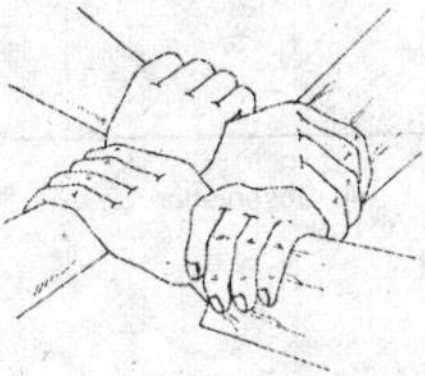

Four hand seat

Fourchette It is a band which is spread transversally in posterior commissure of vagina, anatomical fold at the perineal end of the vulva.

Fovea It denotes a small depression of the cornea which contains cones, anatomical depression in the centre of the retina from where the optic nerve leaves the eye to the brain, *Fovea is a blind spot.*

Fowler's position Angulation of upper body at 60° which gives semi-sitting position.

Fractional test meal Free HCl and total HCl examination of stomach content.

Fracture bedpan It is required for patient who is bedridden due to traction for a fracture, to position the fracture bedpan the patient has to flex the uninvolved knee and to press down with the foot to lit the buttocks.

Fracture board In case of spinal injury special stretcher is prepared by strengthening by placing fracture boards across the framework, main purpose of providing transverse board (fracture board) is to protect spinal injury patient from further injury.

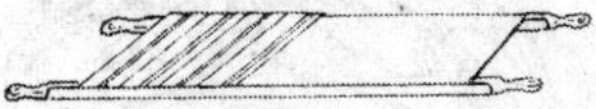

Fracture board

Fracture It is due to trauma or fall, bone is broken which can be of different types as under:

Simple fracture	=	bone is not exposed to outside
Compound fracture	=	bone is exposed to outside
Greenstick fracture	=	bone is bent and splintered on one side
Comminuted fracture	=	bone is shattered to pieces

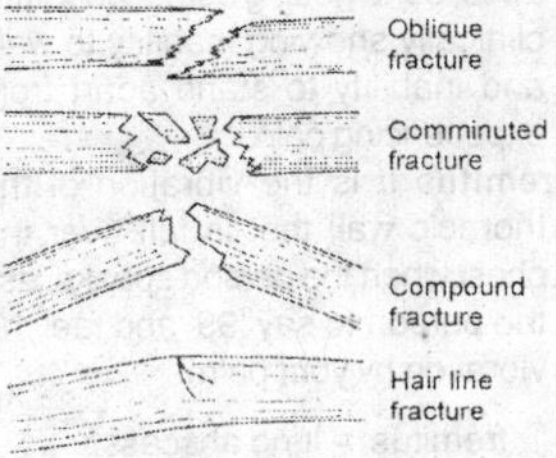

Fracture of bones

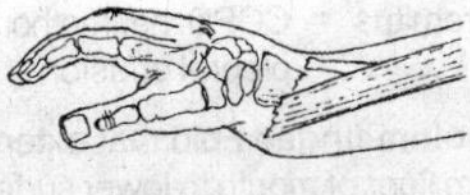

Colles' fracture

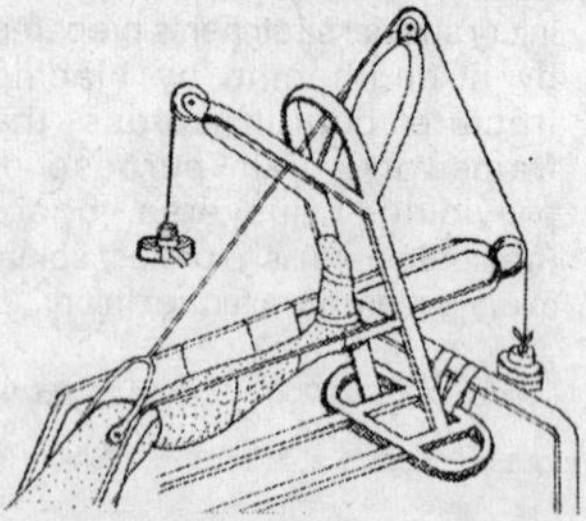

Treatment of femur fracture

Fragility It expresses brittleness, fragility of RBC.

Frame Rigid structure to immobilise a part or a bone.

Freckle They are caused by small areas of melanin pigment, they fade in winter and become prominent in summer.

Frei's test It is a skin test for the diagnosis of LGV.

Freiberg's disease Second metatarsal bone getting osteochondritis, clinically showing inability to walk and inability to stand apart from experiencing pain.

Fremitus It is the vibration of the thoracic wall that is felt over the chest when the person speaks, ask the person to say '99' and feel the vibration by your palm.

↑ fremitus = lung abscess, pneumonia consolidation

↓ fremitus = COPD, neumothorax, pleural effusion

Frenulum lingae Fold that extends from floor of mouth to lower surface of tongue along midline.

Frequency curve When number of observations are large and groups are more, the frequency polygon tends to loose its angulations and it forms a smooth curve called *Frequency curve*.

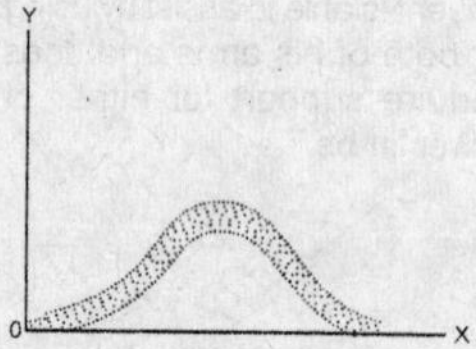

A: Observation on axis

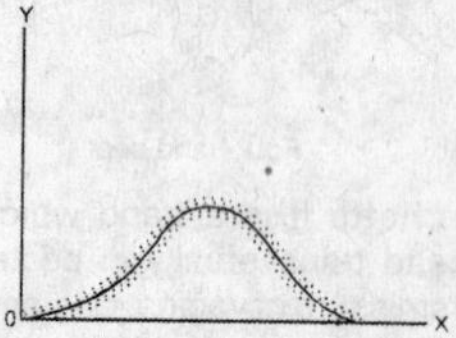

B: Frequency curve

Freud Freud Sigmund, an Australian psychologist.

Friction burn This is a special type of burns which can occur under following circumstances sudden contact with a moving surface like a grindstone or a rope can produce heat which cause burn.

Friction rub When you are auscultating the abdomen you may hear friction rubs which sound like sand paper rubbing together, they are best heard during deep respiration particularly over diseased liver, diseased spleen or diseased gallbladder.

Friction When objects or organs rub each other.

Friendlander's bacillus *Klebsiella friedlanderi* causing rare form but severe form of pneumonia in man.

Frigidity Commonly it means cold or coldness and always refers to sexual indifference experienced by females.

Frolich's syndrome It is a pituitary pathology which cause varied and different clinical manifestations like
Adiposity of higher magnitute
Atrophy of genital organs
Development of feminine characteristics.

Frontal lobe In front of central sulcus of cerebrum four convolutions, frontal lobe of cerebrum.

Frontal sinus Hollow space in side the frontal bone above orbit, it is air filled.

Frontal Forehead bone with its hollowness in side, it is a bone of the skull.

Frostbite Severe exposure to cold and chills, devitalisation due to severe cold leads to numbness, gangrene.

Frozen section A Quick examination of living tissue from a patient who is on the O T table which help, to decide the immediate course of action on Operation Table by the Surgeon.

Frozen shoulder Painful shoulder of unknown aetiology which show capsulitis of shoulder joint giving rise to stiff and painful shoulder.

Fructose intolerance Person who not in a position to digest fructose due to absence of aldolase enzyme, fructose consumption produces clinical features like nausea, vomiting, sweating, tremor and hypoglycaemia.

Fructose It is the name given to fruit sugar which is monosaccharide, chemically it is $C_6H_{12}O_6$.

Fruit stain removal In regular nursing practice, fruit stain is removed by rubbing with salt and then wash in cold water. This is followed by wash with boiling water.

Frusemide A pharmacological agent used as a diuretic.

Frustration When a person cannot achieve suggested goals he goes to a state of severe depression called frustration, personal goal is not achieved
When man is unable to meet his needs and desire he ends up with frustrations. External causes are failure, defeat, unemployment etc. this leads to drug abuse and alcoholism
When man is unable to meet his needs and desire, he ends up with frustrations which is normally by failure, defeat, unemployment, poor health, low I Q etc.,

FSH Follicle Stimulating Hormone.

FTAABS Lab test for Syphilis, Fluorescent Treponemal Antibody Absorption Test.

Fulcrum It is a fixed point for the operation of a lever, point against which a lever functions.

Fulminating When a disease has an acute onset and show a course of rapid progress in course or in its natural history of disease.

Fumigation A type of disinfection where a space or an item is exposed to disinfecting fumes, Rat hole fumigation during plague epidemic ship disinfection for quarantine purpose.

Function Natural action of a tissue, of an organ, of a part, of a bone, refers to physiological action of any organ.

Functional When we cannot demonstrate any changes in an ill person, in a patient the disease is not accompanied by demonstrable changes.

Fundoscopy clinical examination of fundus of eye by using this instrument in eye department.

Fundus It is the measurement of uterine size in pregnant women for assessing the growth of foetus, Distance from symphysis pubis up to fundus is measured by a tape up to the start of III trimester, tape measure in cm will correlate to gestational age in weeks (e.g., 24 cm = 24 weeks of gestational age) During III trimester following formula is used:

$$\text{McDonald's rule} = \frac{\text{Fundal height in cm}}{3.5}$$

Illustration of calculation of gestation age in lunar months;

Fundal height is 28 cms

Gestational age is 28 ÷ 3.5 = 8 months

Fungicide Drug which is used to destroy or kill fungus, drug used in fungal infection, it can be local or systemic administration.

Fungus It is the name of one group of plants; some fungus produce disease (Actinomysis), some fungus help to overcome infection (penicillium).

Funicular process It covers the spermatic cord which is called tunica vaginalis.

Funiculus It refers to any one of the following:

- The umbilical cord.
- The spermartic cord.
- Divisions of white matter on each side of spinal cord.
- A fascicle of nerve fibre in peripheral nerve.

Funnel chest Dternum showing depression, ribs showing inward curvature, costal cartilage showing inward curvature are seen in a condition which is a developmental anomaly.

Furley stretcher Variety of stretchers that are used to transport patients are named after the late Sir John Furley, common types are:

a. Ordinary.
b. Telescopic.
c. Metal.

parts of Furley stretcher are:

- The bed.
- The poles.
- The traverses.
- The runners.
- The slings.
- and the straps.

Furrow Anatomical groove is called furrow.

Furuncle Other name for boil which is manifested due to staphylococcal infection

Occur due to staphylococcal infection on the skin.

Furuncolosis Secondary changes due to furuncle or boil.

Fusiform Any anatomical structure which show a shape of spindle.

Fusion When two adjacent structures unite each other.

When two objects for image of two eyes merge on each other.

G

GI tract Literary meaning that the lumen from stomach through small intestine and large intestine which is gastrointestinal tract,colloquially meaning that the alimentary trace from mouth to anus, this is meant for digestive system under nutrition.

GAD Abbreviation for Generalised Anxiety Disorder, it is characterised by persistent anxiety expressed by tachycardia, choking, dry mouth dyspepsia, urinary frequency and body pain.

Gag reflex When back of the mouth is touched or irritated it produces vomiting sensation (posterior aspect of pharynx = Fauces).

Gag An appliance made soft in the outer side but solid inside which is kept in the mouth to see that no biting occurs during fits in a patient, throat reflex when the throat is touched

Giant cell They are megakaryocytes of bone marrow, cells in tuberculosis lesion, in infectious granuloma and in foreign body reactions, they have many nuclei and are very large in size.

Gait It tells how a man walks, some of the common gaits described in clinical conditions are:

- Ataxic gait.
- Spastic gait.
- Cerebellar gait.
- Four point gait.

Galactocele A tumour occurred by occlusion of milk duct in breast, condition where milk like fluid is present in hydrocele.

Galactogogue Any substance which promote the secretion of breast milk.

Galactokinase It is an enzyme which transfer high energy phosphate groups known to come from a donor.

Galactometer Instrument used to measure specific gravity of milk.

Galactorrhoea Breast milk production which is more than expected, when excess of milk is produced in the breast.

Galactosaemia It is an inborn error of metabolism which is an autosomal recessive genetic disease.

Galactose It is an isomer of glucose converted to glycogen in liver, it is a monosaccharide, galactose is present in lactose and cerebrosides of brain tissue.

Galactosuria A clinical condition where galactose is excreted in urine

Galactosaemia It is a metabolic defect present since birth in a baby which cannot take milk due to intolerance, they also show mental retardation.

A chemical birth defect which causes mental retardation in babies when they drink milk,

Nursing management include stopping milk feeding and avoiding foods containing galactose or lactose

Galen's vein They empty to straight vein after forming venacerebra magna in choroidal plexus.

Galen Famous Greek Physician in the history of medicine who has written on medicine, natural science and logic.

Gall Gall is the name given to digestive fluid of liver which is stored in gallbladder which is colloquially called as "bile".

Gallbladder It is an anatomical structure below the liver which helps to store bile.

Gallstone Concretion formed of oxalate, phosphate or urate in the gallbladder which leads to pathological disorders

Galvanisation Medical treatment with galvanic current.

Galvanometer A physical instrument in electricity to measure current, it detects the strength of current flowing in a line.

Gambusia Type of fish particularly Gambusia affinis which is larvivorous used in malaria control measure as larval control.

Gamete Name give to spermatozoa and ovum, combination of male and female gametes produces zygote, from which an organism develops

Gametocyte When a sex cell is undergoing the state of gametogenesis.

Gametogenesis It is the biological process where gonads produce gametes.

Gamma amino butyric acid It is a neurotransmitter commonly known as GABA.

Gamma globulin A protein substance in blood serum which is concerned with body immunity against infection.

Gamma rays They are electromagnetic waves which have short wave length emitted by radioactive substances, they have greater tissue penetration power.

Gamma It is represented as γ which is a common prefix in language usage like:

- Gamma rays.
- Gamma globulin.
- Gamma camera.
- Gamma benzene.

Unit of intensity of magnetic field where γ = 0.0001 gauss

It is an expression of degree of photo development.

Ganglion It is a collection of neurons and fibres, they form subsidiary nerve centre within a main nerve system, it is also a swelling on a tendon.

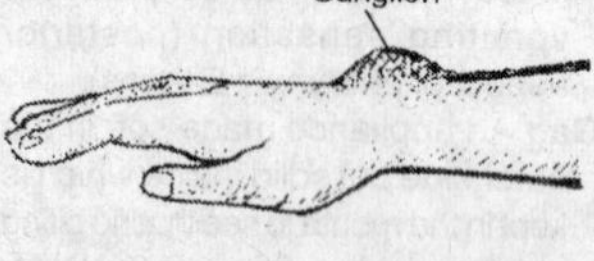

Ganglion of wrist

Gangrene Denotes tissue death due to severe infection or by cut off of vascularity, common clinical types are:

- Dry gangrene.
- Moist or wet gangrene.
- Gas gangrene.
- Diabetic gangrene.
- Arteriosclerotic gangrene.

Gargle Mouth rinsing solution, throat cleansing agent, mouth gargle.

Gargoylism It is a known congenital birth defect manifested with following defects:

- Mental retardation.
- Kyphosis.
- Dwarfism.
- Other skeletal deformities.

Garlic It is an edible root which has strong smell due to allicin, garlic is known to have antithrombotic property.

Gartner's duct It is a persistent mesonephric duct and is called a vestigial structure.

Gas exchange This occurs in arteriovenus plexus for receiving oxygen and release of carbon dioxide, alveolar area is the main place for gas exchange.

Gas Chemical substance which is in vapour form, many are poisonous and some are neutral in nature, most of the chemicals are in the form of gas like hydrogen gas, nitrogen gas, etc.

- Nitrous oxide with air in anaesthesia is called analgesia gas
- Only nitrous oxide gas is called laughing gas
- Methane is called marsh gas
- That gas which produces sneezing is called sternutatory gas
- Police use tear gas

Gasoline It is a petroleum product, It may contain some of the toxic items like tetraethyl lead or tricresyl phosphate which are toxic to tissues.

Gastrectomy Surgical removal of stomach in total or partial as surgical therapy,

When lesser curvature and pyloric portion removed it is called Bill Roth technique of gastrectomy:

- When first part of duodenum is removed it is called Polya technique of gastrectomy
- When distal portion of stomach is surgically removed it is called partial gastrectomy

Gastric analysis It evaluates the amount of acid produced by the parietal cells when the stomach is in a state of rest.

Gastric juice Juice secreted by stomach, they are:

- Hydrochloric acid.
- Pepsin.
- Mucin.
- Inorganic salts.
- Intrinsic factors.

Gastric juice is acidic in nature with pH of above 0.9.

Gastric lavage Washing out the stomach is indicated in pyloric stenosis, intestinal obstruction immediately before operation and in the treatment for poisoning when a poison is swallowed

Requirements:

1. Oesophageal catheter, adult size is 18 to 20, for child size 8 to 14, infant a soft catheter of size 8.
2. A glass connection.
3. 4 feet length of rubber tubing.
4. Large glass funnel.
5. Jug containing wash out solution which contain water, sodium bicarbonate, normal saline all at body temperature
6. A pint measure.
7. Pail to receive wash out.
8. Receiver for rubber tube.
9. Old linen.
10. Lubricant.
11. Protecting clothes.
12. Gag for an unconscious patient.

Procedure:

Nursing procedure is followed in gastric lavage: Conscious patient can swallow the tube, in between allowed breathe, lip to cardiac orifice is l6 inches, when it is 18 inches it will be in stomach, pint measure is filled with solution and allowed to flow in, when funnel is empty it is inverted over the pail and the fluid siphoned back, process is repeated till the fluid is returned clear or until the prescribed amount of the solution has been used.

Gastric ulcer This refers to ulcer formation in the linings of stomach.

Gastric When a thing is related to stomach such as gastric juice, gastric bypass, gastric lavage, gastric ulcer, gastric flu, gastric analysis.

Gastrin Gastrin is a hormone secreted by parietal cells of stomach wall which help to digest the food when it is in stomach, it stimulates HCl secretion and affects secretory activity of pancreas and small intestine.

Gastritis Inflammation of lining of stomach.

Gastrocnemius Major flexor of ankle joint and knee joint being a major muscle of calf of the leg.

Gastroduodenostomy Connecting link created between stomach and duodenum as a drainage procedure, following trunkal vagatomy as a surgical treatment for gastric ulcer (Bill Roth I procedure).

Gastroenteritis Inflammation of lumen of stomach and intestine due to stress, food allergy, poisoning and infection.

Gastroenterology It is the scientific study of diseases of alimentary tract, their diagnosis and line of management.

Gastroenterostomy When a connecting link is created surgically between stomach and intestine.

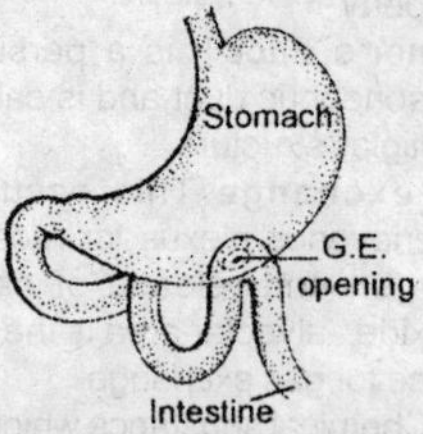

Gastroenterostomy

Gastroileac When it is related to stomach and ileum.

Gastrointestinal Referring to stomach and intestine, pertaining to stomach and intestine.

Gastrojejunostomy Commonly adopted surgical procedure in cases of persistent gastric ulcers, gastric malignancy (Bill Roth II procedure).

Gastrostomy When swallowing is impossible, an opening into stomach is created in cases of oesophageal pathology where swallowing is impossible.

Gastrotomy Incision is made in the stomach during an operation.

Gastrula It is the beginning stage of a fertilised ovum studied in embryology.

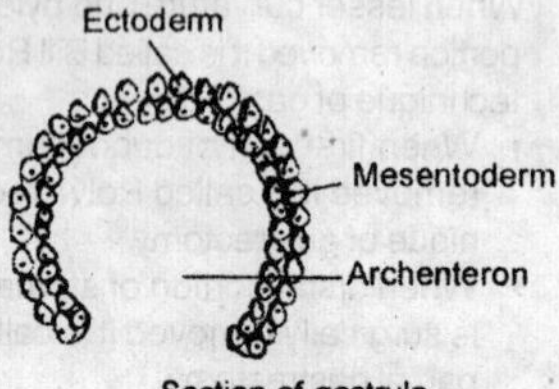

Section of gastrula

Gastrocolic Refers to gastrocolic reflex, anything related with stomach and colon.

Gaucher cell They are large R E cells with eccentric nucleus present in Gaucher's disease.

Gaucher's disease Splenomegaly and anaemia due to deposits of fats in R E cells. It is a known genetic disorder and runs in families (familial).

Gauss sign In the beginning of pregnancy if unusual mobility is seen with respect to uterus it is called Gauss sign.

Gauze restraint They are used in paediatric practice to restrict the movement of kids at treatment in the cot, commercially available restraint are avoided and gauze made restraint with gauze pads and a strip of gauze roll at least 125 cm (50 inches) in length is used, first wrist is pad around with a double thickness of gauze padding then gauze roll is tied round the bed frame which is easy to untie in emergency.

Gauze It is an open mesh material used in dressing the wound.

Gavages feeding liquid diet directly into stomach as a forced act to maintain nourishment of patients.

GB syndrome Guillain-Barre syndrome, paralysis of peripheral nerves following an acute viral infection, an acute infective polyneuritis.

GE Abbreviation for Gastro Enteritis,

Gelatin It is a protein from collagen, major uses are in capsule making and X-ray films.

Gel It is a colloid in a gelatinous form, firm but contains liquid.

Gemini It means twins.

Gene map It is the genetic map of man called genome.

Man has more than 120,000 genes which are aligned through adenine, guanine, thymine and cytosine viz., amino acid structure of protein which are species specific and man specific.

Gene splicing This word is used in molecular biology, splicing of DNA to another gene is a substitution procedure in molecular biology.

Gene therapy In the correction of genetic disorder, normal gene is inserted for a change in the form of a cure.

Gene transfer To correct inherited defects, gene is transferred to a recipient from a normal person.

Gene It is basic unit of heredity which are found in chromosomes.

General flea index It denotes number of flea per rat which is used in entomological survey, it is one the major flea index.

General practitioner Is a physician who attends to the health need of a family , treats common ailments, gives health guidance, gives health counselling and refers the case when need arises to a specialist.

General sepsis If virulent pathogens gain access to a wound and if the resistance of patient is poor, we can expect severe complications such as septicaemia or blood poisoning which can endanger life

Generation The gap which is seen from parents to their offspring, When a new organism is produced it starts as new generation.

Genesiology The study of science which deals with conception and reproduction.

Genetic engineering It is a procedure to isolate a specific DNA fragment from a genome of an organism, to determine its base sequence and to assess its function.

Genetic That which is related to genetics such as genetic counselling, genetic code, genetic mutation.

Genetics Scientific study of diseases of hereditary or genetic disorders in man.

Genetics The science that deals with genetic inheritance, genetic disorders, birth defects, eugenics, euthenics and genetic counselling for preventing congenital anomalies.

Geniculum This anatomical term describes the knee like bend in a nerve or in an organ.

Genitalia This refers to the organs of reproduction.

Genitourinary Related to genitals and urinary system.

Genius If mental ability and creative capability is more and if I Q is more the person is called a genius.

Genotype This refers to genetic characteristics of man.

Gentamicin Broad-spectrum antibiotic which is found effective against gram-negative organisms, used in the specific treatment of pseudomonas and *Staph aureus.*

Genu Latin word meaning knee, knock knee is genu valgum, bowleg is genu varum, any structure which is bent like knee.

Genupectroral It refers to position of knee chest supine position.

Genus In Zoology and Botany we do grouping and classification of genus and species taxonomically.

Geographic tongue Denuded areas of dorsal surface of tongue gives the pattern of geography and hence the name, clinically it is non-specific.

Geriatric nursing Nursing care of the elderly in hospital, health centre, old age home. Elderly people in their home calls for nursing care from Nursing profession, along with clinical rehabilitation, home visiting is demanded by the community.

Geriatrics This is the speciality which deals with diseases and disorders of old age and their line of management.

Germ A seed from which germination can occur,

Pathogens are called germs because most of them are microscopic.

German measles Rubella, a viral infection which cause fever and rashes on the body.

Germicide A chemical which can kill pathogens, refers to antibiotics.

Germinal epithelium In the embryo, on the surface of the genital ridge there is lining of epithelium which is germinal epithelium.

Germination In plants, it is sprouting of spore, in animals, it is development of fertilised ovum.

Germinoma Cancer of testes, cancer of ovaries.

Gerontology Initiative of geriatrics which deals with ageing process in man.

Gestation It is the period of fertilisation to full development of living organism, it is the period from conception to birth usually 280 days

Types of gestations are:
- Normal uterine.
- Ectopic gestation.
- Interstitial gestation.
- Secondary gestation.

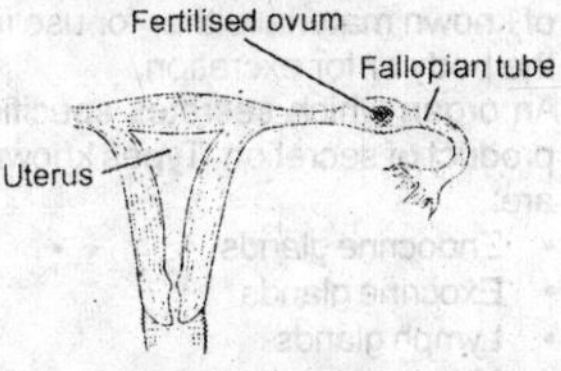

Ectopic gestation

Gestational age There are many methods of assessing gestational age, clinically following are used in nursing care for the newborn:
a) soles of the feet for creases are inspected, if the creases do not cover the sole, the infant is probably less than 38 weeks of gestational age
b) it is done by measuring breast tissue, breast tissue is compressed between thumb and index finger and the tissue is measured in cm, at normal gestational age, the tissue should measure between 0.5 to 1.0 cm.

Absence or decrease breast tissue is often indicative of prematurity of newborn who is small for gestational age.

Gesture It refers to body language, body movement is helpful in expression.

Ghon focus Healed lesion of tuberculosis as seen in radiograph as calcification. First time infection of tuberculosis in the body which is called as primary lesion.

Giardia Protozoal parasite which is flagellate which harbours intestine and produce intestinal pathology.

Giardiasis It is a common parasitic infection causing acute diarrhoea affecting children, tourists and immunosuppressed individuals, infection caused by *Giardia lamblia*.

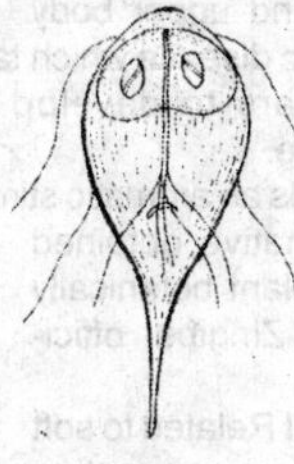
Giardia lamblia

Gibbus It is an angular deformity of collapsed vertebrae, which can occur with osteoarthritis or Pott's disease (TB of spine) Latin word meaning a hump.

GI Abbreviation for Gastro Intestinal.

Giddens British sociologist who developed structuration theory.

Geiger counter It is a biological instrument for detecting radioactivity, Radioactive isotopes are recognised very easily in selective organs e.g., radioactive isotope I^{131} can be measured with thyroid gland.

GIFT This is one of the methods of in Vitro Fertilisation and Embryo transfer (IVP-ET)

Gamete intra fallopian tube transfer.

Gigantism Hyperpituitary action leading to high growth in the body, late fusion of bones are seen which is eunuchoid gigantism.

Gillams's operation Surgery indicated for retroversion of the uterus where shortening of round ligament is done with ventrosuspension.

Gilles de la Tourette's disease A disease of unknown aetiology which is characterised by tics on face and upper body, a known chronic disease which takes 15 to 20 years to develop as adult disease.

Ginger Is an aromatic stimulant and carminative obtained from plant botanically called Zingiber officinale.

Gingival Related to soft tissue or connective tissue around teeth.

Gingivectomy Surgical correction of gum in case of hypertrophy leading to pathological conditions.

Gingivitis infection and inflammation of the gums.

Ginseng Chinese medicine for chronic diseases including impotence.

Girdle Anatomical structure which resembles a belt such as pelvic girdle, shoulder girdle.

Gitter cell When lipid granules are deposited in the cell this looks like honey combed cell which is called gitter cell.

Glabella Above the root of the nose and in between two super ciliary arches space in front of frontal bone is called glabella.

Glacial That which resembles ice and which is hard and cold.

Gland An organ meant for secretion of known material either for use in the body or for excretion,
An organ which secretes specific product of secretion. Types known are:

- Endocrine glands.
- Exocrine glands.
- Lymph glands.
- Mucous glands.

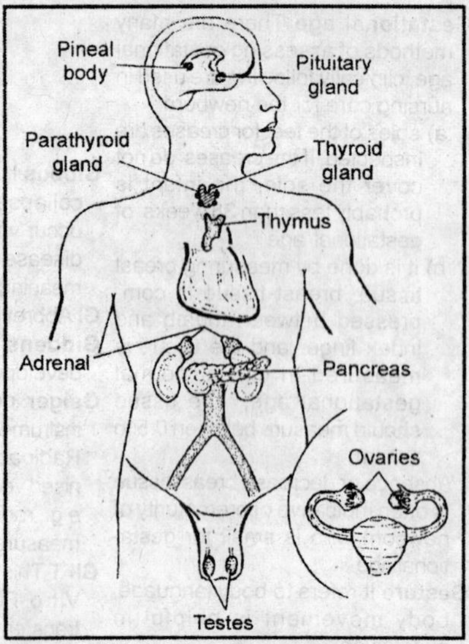

Endocrine glands

Glanders A horse disease which can affect man which is caused by a bacteria called *Pseudomonas mallei*.

Glandular When it is referred to glands such as glandular fever (infectious mononucleosis).

Glans This is the tip or end portion of penis in male or clitoris in female.

Glasgow Coma Scale To monitor level of consciousness in adults this scale is used,
Used in cases of brain malaria, meningitis and head injury and if score is 10 it is unrousable coma, it has to be done repeatedly to assess improvement or deterioration, 7 or less = coma

Eyes open	Spontaneously	4
	To speech	3
	To pain	2
	Never	1
Best verbal response	Oriented	5
	Confused	4
	In appropriate word	3
	In comprehensible sound	2
	None	1
Best motor response	Obeys commands	5
	Localises pain	4
	Flexion to pain	3
	Extension to pain	2
	None	1

Table: Glasgow coma scale for adults

Glasses contact lens Direct fixing lens for refractive error or for eye colour change,
Easy to wear and have become popular in recent years, with precaution it can be worn for 10 to 12 hours.

Glaucoma Clinical condition which show increased intraocular pressure,
There is interference with normal circulation of the eye fluids which cause hardening of the eyeball

Types can be	Primary glaucoma
	Secondary glaucoma
	Open angle glaucoma
	Closed angle glaucoma.

Gleet Mucous discharge in cases of urethritis specifically due to Gonococcal infection (STD).

Glenoid cavity It is a shallow socket at the outer angle of scapula bone, into which the head of the humerus fits, forming the shoulder joint.

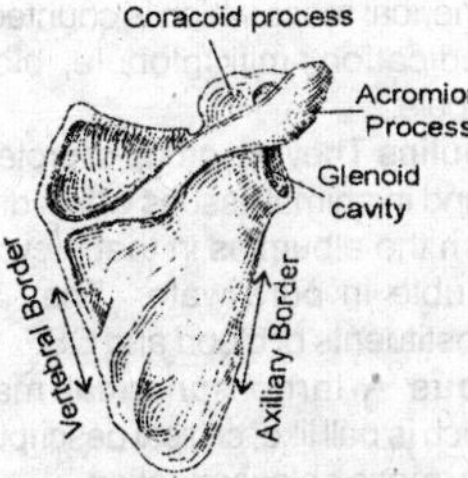

Scapula showing glenoid cavity

Glenoid fossa In the temporal bone, the fossa or cavity which receives the condyle of the mandible to form temporomandibular joint.

Glenoid That which resembles a hollow socket such as glenoid cavity.

Glia It refers to connective tissue of brain and spinal cord.

Glioblastoma It is a cancer of brain or tumour of the brain.

Glioma Tumour of neuroglial cells in brain and spinal cord.

Gliosis A pathological condition where gliomas are present in neuroglial tissues.

Global village An idea of mass communication by film and TV.

Global warming Emission of green house gases to atmosphere mainly CO_2 can bring about rise in global surface temperature, rise in sea level and extreme climatic events like cyclone, heat wave and draught. This affects global ecosystem.

Globin It is a protein fraction required in the synthesis of or formation of haemoglobin.

Globule Small pellicle pellet or spherical mass which is counted in medication, milk globule, blood globule.

Globulins They are group of proteins found in animal tissues which differ from the albumins in that they are soluble in pure water. They are constituents of blood and CSF.

Globus A large spherical mass which is ball like, clinical description of a mass on examination

Glomeruli It is the functioning unit of kidney.

Glomerulitis Infection and inflammation of glomeruli of kidney.

Glomerulonephritis Disease affecting the glomerules which perform the main kidney function Probably immune origin leading to inflammation of glomeruli and kidney causing acute and/or chronic clinical condition.

Glomerulus Tufts of capillaries in nephron meant for filtration work.

Glossal Anything which is related to tongue.

Glossina They belong to biting flies called tsetse flies which transmit sleeping sickness.

Glossitis Inflammatory disease of the tongue.

Glossopharyngeal nerve It is 9th cranial nerve which carries taste sensation from posterior third of tongue, it also supplies pharynx, meninges, parotids and ears.

Glossopharyngeal When a structure is related to tongue and pharynx such as glossopharyngeal nerve.

Glottis Anatomically it is the space in vocal cords, colloquially it is the part which produces voice, vocal apparatus of the larynx which has an opening and vocal folds.

Gloves They are used in patient's treatment particularly in surgical treatment. Firstly they protect the nurse from infections,

Second they minimize the potential for the wearer to transmit microbe to patient,

Third they minimise cross-infection in the hospital

Indicated in:

- Touching blood.
- Touching secretion.
- In AIDS patient treatment.
- In infectious disease treatment.

Glucagons They are produced by pancreas to help in the breaking down of glycogen, it is known to rise blood pressure,

Known hyperglycaemic glycogenolytic factor.

Glucocorticoid Synonym with cortisone, corticosterone or hydrocortisone which is responsible in raising liver glycogen level, they are adrenal hormones useful in carbohydrate metabolism, they are released during stress conditions.

Glucometer It is an electronic meter to measure and monitor blood glucose, in addition to this meter, following items need to be procured in the blood collecting procedure:
1. skin puncturing device.
2. alcohol sponge for skin reparation.
3. squeeze bottle filled with tap water.
4. reagent strip for the meter.
5. a lint free paper towel.

Gluconeogenesis Liver and kidney help in this metabolic activity in the body.
It is the production of glucose from non-nitrogen portion of amino acids after deamination.

Glucose tolerance test This is done for the diagnosis of prediabetic and hyperinsulinaemia state,
Procedure: Glucose powder is given orally at the dose of 1.5 gram per kg body weight in empty stomach
Blood sample is collected every 30 minutes for 2 hours.
Blood sugar is found out in each sample and interpreted.

Glucose Grape sugar, one of the simpler chemicals belonging to the group monosaccharide, commonly called D glucose, it is primary fuel of the body.

Glue ear Common in school age children to see accumulation of wax in middle ear giving rise to hard of hearing, ear syringing clears it.

Glue sniffing This is common among drugs addicts who use airplane model glue for sniffing, glue sniffing by adolescents lead to serious physical results, this leads to big and strong "kicks".

Glutamic acid It is an amino acid produced during protein digestion.

Glutamic oxaloacetic transaminase It is cardiac muscle enzyme and also liver enzyme,
Serum level measurement (SGOT) help in the diagnosis of cardiac disease or liver disease (particularly MI and cirrhosis of liver).

Glutamic pyruvic transaminase It is liver enzyme, serum level measurement (SGPT) help in the diagnosis of liver disorders.

Glutathione It is helpful in tissue respiration, it has glutamic acid, cystine and glycine (tripeptide).

Gluteal Any thing that is related to buttock such as gluteal muscle.

Gluten free diet When wheat, barley, rye and oats are avoided in the diet, it becomes therapeutic diet called gluten free diet.

Gluten Normally it is referred to wheat protein, protein of wheat which gives tough elastic character.

Glutin Viscid substance from wheat called gluten-casein.

Glycerine It is a chemical of the alcohol group, obtained from fat or fatty oils, it is an emollient in all skin preparations, glycerine mouth wash and glycerine suppository are commonly known.

Glyceryl trinitrate It is sublingual preparation for angina pectoris, also known as nitroglycerine.

Glycine An amino acid which come under non-essential group.

Glycogen storage disease It is an inherited disorder where abnormal glycogen storage in liver occurs, There are 7 types of glycogen storage disease. They are:

S.N.	Type	Deficiency	Remarks
I	Von Gierke's disease	Glucose 6 phosphatase	
II		Lysosomal alfa glucosidase	
III		Debranching enzymes	
IV	Anderson's disease	Brancher enzyme	hepatic failure
V	McArdle's disease	Muscle phosphorylase	
VI		Liver phosphatase	liver enlarged growth retarded acidosis & hypoglycaemia
VII		Muscle phosphor fructokinase	weakness cramps

Glycogen Starch stored in the body to be converted into sugar when need arises in the body, animal starch, common site of store is liver and body muscles.

Glycogenesis Biochemical process of formation glycogen from blood glucose.

Glycogenolysis Biochemical process of breaking down of glycogen as calorie.

Glycoside Fermented sugar or the produce of a plant yield glucoside and glycoside respectively, crystalline body in plants when acts with acid (laboratory) or ferments (naturally) produce sugar.

Glycosuria One of the objective manifestation of diabetes where sugar in the urine is found at pathological level.

Gnat They are sand flies, black flies and midgets which are smaller than mosquitoes.

Gnathic Anything that is related to upper jaw or lower jaw.

GNC Abbreviation for General Nur-sing Council.

Goblet cell They are mucous secreting cells in the intestinal epithelium.

Going steady This is good for a socialisation among adolescent boys and girls, parents and counsellors may be troubled when young teenagers begin to "go study", go study can be good or bad depending on the social circumstances.

Goitre Thyroid gland seen visible when enlarged, common clinical goiterous conditions are:

- Toxic goitre.
- Exophthalmic goitre.
- Colloid goitre.

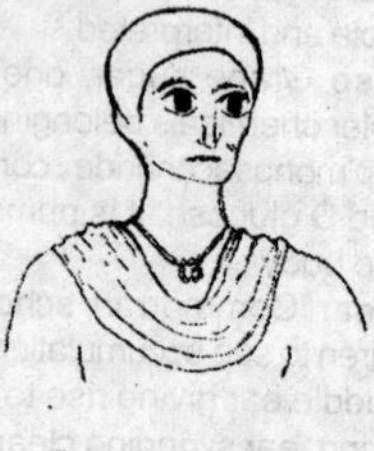

Exophthalmic goitre

Gold standard A standard which is standardised and time tested with which all other tests can be compared and evaluated.

Golgi apparatus Intracytoplasmic biological part seen nearer the nucleus of a cell.

Gonad Refers to testicle or ovary which are reproductive organs.

Gonadal dysgenesis Otherwise called Turner's syndrome with abnormal genetic pattern of 45 × O, congenital non-functioning of ovaries, clinical features include
- Amenorrhoea.
- No secondary sexual characteristics.
- Short stature.
- Neck webbing.
- Cubital valgus.

Gonadotrophic One which stimulates the gonadotrophin.

Gonadotrophin Hormone which stimulate gonads, they are:
- Follicle stimulating hormone.
- Luteinising hormone.
- Gonadotrophic hormone of placenta.

Gonion Lower jaw midpoint is called gonion.

Gonioscope An ophthalmic instrument which is used to measure and examine angle of the anterior chamber of the eye.

Goniotomy Surgical correction procedure in case of glaucoma which is an ophthalmic clinical condition.

Gonococcus It is a diplococci called *Neisseria gonorrhoeae* which causes
Gonorrhoea (STD).

Gonorrhoea It is STD caused by *N.gonorrhoeae* infecting genital tract, causing discharge and pain during urination.

Gooch's splinting It is corrugated wood splinting, which may be cut to any size required, may be used as a "first aid" support for a fracture, it is sometimes used to prevent movement of child's arm in nursing care.

Gossypol It is derived from cotton seed seems to have male contraceptive effect (male pill).

Gouge Surgery instrument which looks like a curved chisel used to scoop dead bone.

Gouley's catheter Surgical instrument which is grooved on its inferior surface used with a guide through a urethral stricture.

Goundou Present in native of South Africa who show bone exostoses on the sides of the nose,
Osteoplastic periostitis of the nose.

Gout A general disease where body cannot handle protein foods containing purin bodies,
Major clinical manifestations are in the joints of the extremities,
Excess uric acid in blood causing swelling and inflammation of toes and fingers.

Gowns It refers to sterile gown, when the nurse is to wear gown for procedures in which surgical asepsis is necessary ; she should wash her hands, she should put on hair cover, she should put on a mask, then open the sterile gown to wear as per the learnt O T procedure.

GP A doctor who can render primary health care in the community, often they are family physicians.

GPI Abbreviation used for General Paralysis of the Insane.

Gracile Thin build person with slender extremities.

Gracilis A muscle on the medial side of thigh which is slender and long.

Gradient Whenever we come across a slope or graded areas we refer to it as gradient.

Graduate In a measuring vessel when markings are done to measure, person who is given a degree from a University.

Graefe's sign It is a sign of Graves' disease, when eyeball moves downward the upper eyelids do not move downwards.

Graafian follicle It is ovarian follicle which is matured and ruptures to give rise to ovum, in this ruptured ovarian follicle corpus luteum develops that secretes oestrogen and progesterone when both help in implantation of fertilised ovum Ovarian follicle which matures during menstrual cycle and rupture to give ovum for fertilisation.

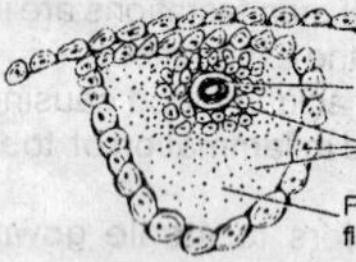

Graafian follicle

Graft Any tissue which is used for transplantation,
Major issue in plastic surgery or reconstructive surgery. Types are :

- Full thickness graft.
- Homologous graft.
- Corneal graft.
- Autogenous graft.
- Pedicle graft.

Graham's law This physical law states that the rate of diffusion of a gas is inversely proportional to the square root of its density.

Grain Seeds of cereal plant, 1/20th of a scruple which is 0.065 gram.

Gram's stain Common microbiological stain which can classify bacteria into two group
(a) Gram-positive.
(b) Gram-negative.

Grand mal It is major epilepsy or major seizure.

Grandiose When a psychic patient show manifestations of unrealistic and exaggerated symptoms e.g.,

- Very poor tells that he has amassed wealth.
- Both legs amputated telling he comes first in long jump.
- Illiterates telling he can take a lecture class.
- Beggar telling that he is the prince of the nation.

Granular Refers to urinary casts which show small granules, particle containing small particles.

Granulated eyelids Eyelid inflammation in which there are scales and crusts on the edges of the lids and around the eyelashes.

Granulation Changes seen in healing of wound or ulcer, it also refers to conversion of hard big particles into small finer particles.

Granule Small grains or small particles.

Granulocyte When granules are present in the cytoplasm of the cell, such as in certain types of WBC which are granulated.

Granuloma Tumour due to foreign body reaction or by chronic infections.

Granulomatosis Granuloma produced by chronic infections, common types are:

- Malignant granulomatosis.
- Lipoid granulomatosis.

Grasp reflex It is tested under "caring for the newborn". By stimulating the newborn's palm with our fingers we can assess the grasp reflex. The newborn should grasp our fingers tightly enough to be lifted up off the surface on which is he lying, Weak grasp suggests the possibility of CNS damage.

Graves' disease Thyrotoxicosis or exophthalmic goitre.

Gravel Tiny sand particles, in clinical lesions it refers to tiny calculi formed in urinary bladder or in the kidney.

Gravid One which is pregnant or one who is pregnant.

Gravity Gravitation force which gives the weight to a substance, actually it means weight.

Gray matter Cortex of the brain is called gray matter:

- The substance forming the outer part of the brain.
- The substance forming the inner part of the cord.
- All these contain specialised nerve cells which perform known physiological functions.

Gray It is a unit used in radiation therapy and expressed in SI units, it tells the quantum of radiation absorbed in the body.

Greenstick fracture It refers to orthopaedic situation where the bone is injured and has a crack but not actual fracture, it is like breaking a green twig where cracking will occur but not complete severance of the part.

Grey matter They are present on the surface of the cerebrum, which is thrown into a number of ridges called convolutions, which greatly increase the amount of grey matter.

Grief Is a common situation in life associated with failure, divorce, death, and loss of health, stages of grief are:

- Shock.
- Emotional release.
- Utter depression, loneliness and sense of isolation.
- Physical symptoms of distress.
- Panicky.
- Guilty about everything.
- Hostility.
- Unable to return to his usual activities.
- Begin to overcome.
- Readjust our lives to reality.

Griseofulvin A drug used in the treatment of ringworm infection of skin.

Groin Crease and junction where thigh and abdomen join, inguinal region.

Grooming Is a personal neatness which is essential for life of an individual

It is called "good grooming and order" in real life.

Groove Shallow linear depression found in embryos or on bones.

Ground itch When larva of hookworm enters the skin of lower limb, the skin gets inflamed.

This is called ground itch.

Ground substance Normally cartilage and bone which occupies the intercellular space in its connective tissue are called ground substance.

Group behaviour Interaction and social behaviour of an individual in a group,

This can lead to progressive reformation of society or can lead to civil unrest.

Group counselling It helps in realising family potential or group potential to help themselves as contrasted to helping them,

Following are the requisites in group counselling :

- The setting.
- Group acceptance of a problem.
- Building self confidence.
- Should modify destructive emotional state.
- Should attack fear component.
- Take off group inhibition.
- Nurse should effect counselling to group maturity level.
- Tackling disbeliefs of group.

Group discussion It is a face to face interaction between nursing tutor and nursing students of a batch of 20. It is informal and democratic which allow good interaction, its advantages are:

- All can participate.
- They gain insight.
- It allows synthesis of ideas.

Group dynamics This is a character of good leadership in nursing profession, it allows 'telling, consulting and joining with each others' and is called group dynamics.

Group health insurance It is the purchase of health insurance through organised groups of any organisation, any industry or any institution.

Group morale It is an attitude where organisational or professional prestige is given importance over the leadership or activity performance,

It is one of the influencing characters that build group dynamics and understanding others.

Grouping Classification of people on any given set of traits which are shared by them such as social grouping, blood grouping, etc.

Growth and Development Growth is the increase in physical size of the body. Development is the increase in skills and functions.

Age (year)	*Male child Mean weight kg*	*Female child Mean weight kg*
1	8.1	7.8
2	10.1	9.6
3	11.8	11.2
4	13.5	12.0
5	14.8	14.5
6	16.3	16.0

I.C.M.R Standard for weight (Boys and Girls)

Age (year)	*Male Mean hight (cm)*	*Female Mean height (cm)*
1	8.1	7.8
2	10.1	9.6
3	11.8	11.2
4	13.5	12.0
5	14.8	14.5
6	16.3	16.0

I.C.M.R Standard for height (Boys and Girls)

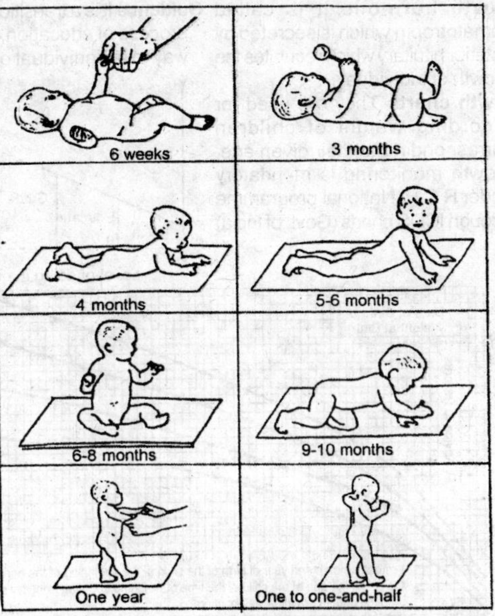

Milestone

6 wks	smiles, recognises
3 mths	holds object deliberately
4 mths	holds head without support
5-6 mths	lifts head turns to see
6-8 mths	sits without support
9-10 mths	crawls
1 year	stands with support
1- 1 ½ yrs	stands without support

Table: Motor developments

6-8 wks	looks and smiles
4-5 mths	recognises mother
6-8 mths	enjoy hide and seek
9-10 mths	suspects stranger

Table: Major Sociopersonal developments

4-5 mths	reaches for object
6-8 mths	transfer objects hand to hand
9-10 mths	releases objects
12-14 mths	builds the shape

Table: Major Adoptive dents

6-8 mths	experiments, with noise
9-10 mths	high sounding noise
10-11 mths	first word "ma ma"
18-21 mths	joins words

Table: Major language developments

Growth hormone It is called somatotropin which is secreted by anterior pituitary which regulates the growth of individuals.

Growth charts They are used for recording weight of children corresponding to their given age, growth monitoring is mandatory under R C H National programme through ICDS charts (Govt. of India)

Guidance It is a transitional unit in the process of education, it is to help a way to an individual or a group.

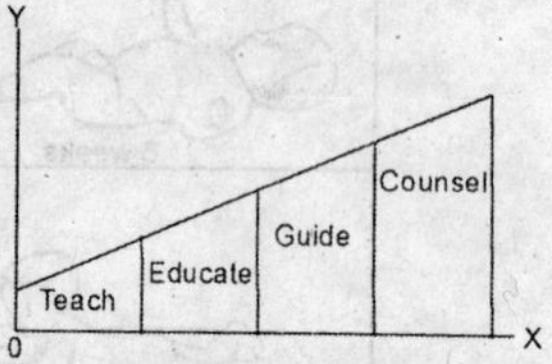

Level of doing in guidance

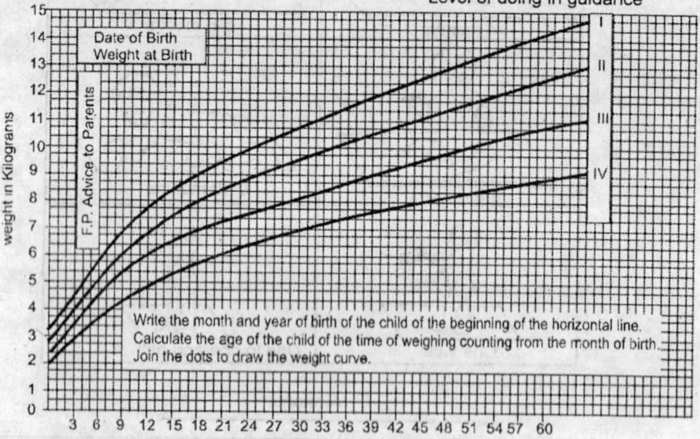

ICDS growth chart used for growth monitoring

Growth Refers to progressive physical development of the body.

Guaiacum test This test is done for blood pigment which is an indirect test for blood in the urine test.

Guanethidine An adrenergic blocking agent used in the treatment of hypertension.

Guanidine It is a protein product.

Guanine One of the constituent of nucleic acid which is purine base.

Gubernaculum An anatomical part which guides other parts, that which is prominent for description of neighbouring parts.

Guillotine Traditionally refers to instrument used to cut the head under punishment, but now this is the name of surgical instrument used in excision of the tonsils.

Guilt It is sixth state of grief where the person begins to feel guilty about everything related to his loss Handicapped and habits like masturbation lead to guilty in an individual.

Guinea pig Commonly used experimental animal in research, a small rodent.

Guinea worm It is longest nematode Dracunculus medinensis which causes Drucunculosis.

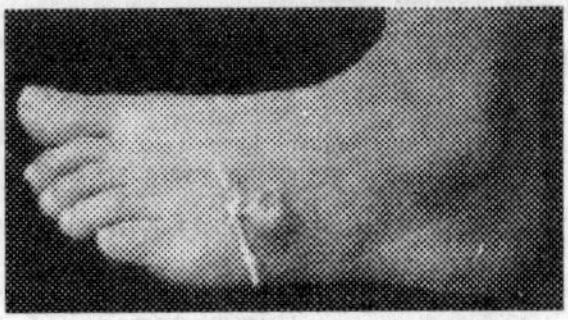

Traditional removal of guinea worm

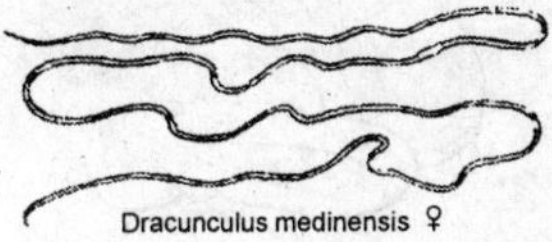

Adult guinea worm

Gullet Oesophagus is called gullet into which the food bolus is passed through. This is a long thin tube which connects the pharynx to stomach.

Gumboil This is the infection of the root of a tooth which drains through the gum.

Gum Soft tissue overlying the teeth which gets easily infection called gingivitis or inflammation of the gums.

Gumma It is tertiary syphilis involving brain, bone and other internal organs. Gumma refers to soft degenerating swelling of organs in syphilis.

Gums Soft portion into which teeth are fixed which is a special region susceptible for lacerations and bleeding in some of the known oral pathology.

Gut Colloquially it means intestine.

Gymnastics Most popular recreational activities which involve some degree of exercise and which are suitable for men and women of all ages.

Gynaecoid One which resembles women, feminine in its characteristics.

Gynaecologic technique Performing routine gynaecologic techniques, refers to the examination of following female reproductive system:

- Breast examination.
- Breast self-examination.
- Post-mastectomy exercises.
- Providing perineal care.
- Cervical uterine radiation implants.

Gynaecological examination A nurse should learn the preparation of patient for gynaecological examination for

a) P V exam.

b) Douching.

c) Vulval toilet.

d) Vaginal pessary, etc.

Preparation of patient for gynaecological examination:

Rectum should be empty

Bladder should be empty (not necessary when urethral examination is imminent)

Adjustment of external clothing to facilitate exam

Requirements like gloves, receptacles, lotion, swabs, swab holding forceps, vaginal specula

Requirement for smear taking like platinum wire loop, slides, spirit lamp, label.

Gynaecologist Person who is a consultant and specially trained in dealing with the diseases of women.

Gynaecology The discipline that deals with occurrence, diagnosis, treatment of diseases among women

Medical speciality which deals with diseases of women,

Study of science which deals with women's diseases.

Gynaecomastia Breast developed in male which is usually a hormonal imbalance.

Gypsona plaster bandage It is required for the making of the plaster splint or plaster of Paris splint, they are available in required length.

Gypsum It is calcium sulphate colloquially called plaster of Paris, Dehydrated calcium sulphate used in dental casting.

Gyrate Spiral shape which is twisted in a ring.

Gyrus Convolution seen in cerebral cortex, enfolding of cerebral cortex which are separated by the fissure or sulcus.

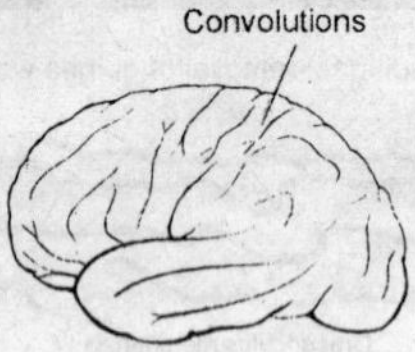

Gyrus on brain

H

Haasim This is the nickname given to some of the clinical conditions among children, such as:

- Bleeding disorders.
- Stoppage of breathing.
- Lung collapse.
- Severe sepsis.
- Syphilis manifestations.
- Severe jaundice.
- Meningial irritations.

Habilitation Process of improving ability to function better in society by training and education to persons with disabilities.

Habit They are accustomed way of doing things. They are acquired through repetitive act and are automatically exerted.

Types are:

- Good habits.
- Bad habits.
- Healthy habits.

Habit formation depends on the following principles:

- Starts from early childhood.
- Frequently repeated.
- Occurs in due course of time.
- Emotions create habits.
- They are under human control.

Habituation When a person becomes accustomed to the use of a drug, which in due course can affect normal functioning of the physiological function.

Slow adaptation to the environment.

Frequent use makes a person accustomed or dependent.

Habitus When the tendency to become ill is gauged by physical appearance.

Habit Frequent repetition that produce involuntary act and further that can produce a *reflex action*.

Hacking cough Dry and non-productive cough which is recurring frequently.

Haematoma Due to injury or a low bleeding under the skin occur although no actual wound has been caused, soft swelling formed thus is haematoma.

Haemangioblastoma Brain tumour with proliferated blood vessels.

Haemangioma Benign tumour of blood vessels, common types are:

- Simple haemangioma.
- Capillary haemangioma.
- Congenital haemangioma.
- Cavernous haemangioma.

Haemophysalis It is a group of ticks which transmit tick fevers.

Haemarthrosis Blood collection in the joint commonly due to injury.

Haematemesis When patient vomits blood usually due to gastric conditions. Vomiting of blood which is dark in colour and acid in reaction.

Haematin Iron portion of haemoglobin

Haematocele When blood is oozed out and gets collected to produce a swelling.

Haematocolpos Accumulation of menstrual blood in vagina usually due to imperforate hymen.

Haematocolpometra Accumulation of menstrual blood in uterus and vagina.

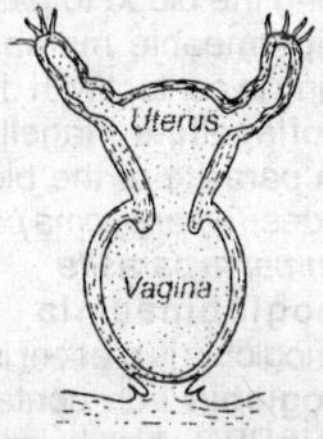

Haematocolpometra

Haematology Scientific study of diseases of blood in man from physiological to pathological changes.

Haematoma Collection of blood in tissues which is circumscribed, blood clot.

Haematometra Accumulation of menstrual blood in uterus usually due to imperforate hymen.

Haematosalpinx Blood getting accumulated in fallopian tubes.

Haematocrit It is also called packed cell volume which is found out by Wintrobe'stube, average value is 45%.

Haematuria Blood in the urine either by injury or by disease.

Haemochromatosis Very high level of iron in serum leading to skin pigmentation and hepatic dysfunction, colloquially it is called bronze diabetes.

Haemoconcentration Circulating fluid when gets reduced in the blood it leads to increased viscosity and raised RBC.

Haemocytoblast Stem cell of bone marrow which differentiates to blood component.

Haemocytometer Counting RBC or WBC in known volume of blood is done by this instrument.

Haemodialysis With the help of artificial kidney blood is purified by making the blood to pass through semipermeable membrane after coming in contact with dialysate.

Haemoflagellate Flagellate protozoan parasite of the blood which includes *Trypanosoma parasite* and *Leishmania parasite*.

Haemoglobinaemia More of haemoglobin is present is plasma

Haemoglobin Iron containing pigment in RBC which helps in carrying oxygen to the tissues, colouring matter of RBC.

Haemoglobinometer This is used to measure HB percentage.

Haemoglobinopathy Haemoglobin production is not proper in some of the haematological conditions like, thalassaemia, sickle cell anaemia and some of the hereditary disorders.

Haemoglobulin Red colour material in RBC which is responsible for the transport of oxygen to the tissues.

Haemagogus In South America, mosquitoes of genus Haemagogus are the primary vectors of yellow fever viral infection.

Haemogram It is the laboratory examination for differential blood count.

Haemolysis Poisoning and infection can cause disintegration of RBC that may cause anaemia.

Haemolytic Substance which is able to destroy RBC.

Haemopathology Scientific study of diseases of the blood, pathology of blood disorders.

Haemophilia It is a hereditary hypoprothrombinaemia which cause bleeding tendencies among males who inherit the disease from their mothers, Majority are Haemophilia A type, Minority suffer from Haemophilia B which is deficiency of factor IX (Christmas disease) In Haemophilia A we see deficiency of factor VIII.

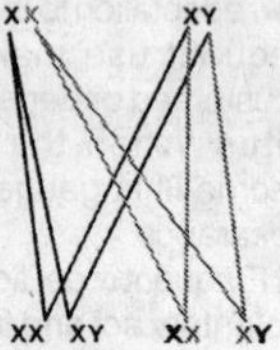

Haemophilia transmission from mother to son

Haemophilus ducreyi Organism that causes soft chancre which is like a rod and gram-negative.

Haemophthalmia Due to injury bleeding into the vitreous of the eyeball.

Haemopneumo thorax Due to injury air and blood is present in pleural cavity.

Haemopoiesis It is the process of blood cell formation in bone marrow

Haemopoietic That which is related to blood cell formation in the body.

Haemopoietin Is an *extrinsic* factor present in food which when combines with *intrinsic* factor of gastric juice produces *antianaemia* factor. This antianaemia factor is stored in the liver and carried to bloodstream and on to the bone marrow where it brings about maturation of erythrocytes.

Haemoptysis Bright red and frothy blood is coughed out from lung and bronchi which is due to lung pathology like cancer of the lung,

Either blood stained sputum or blood in sputum, clinically we come across following types of haemoptysis in nursing management:

- Parasitic haemorrhage.
- Endemic paragonius haemo rrhage.
- Vicarious haemorrhage.
- Vardiac haemorrhage.
- Telangiecticbleeding (Goldstein's)

Coughing blood from the lung which is bright red and frothy.

Haemorrhage Bleeding either internal or external due to rupture of vessels.

Common types of haemorrhage are:

- Traumatic haemorrhage.
- Cerebral haemorrhage.
- Antepartum haemorrhage.
- Postpartum haemorrhage.
- Intracranial haemorrhage.
- Concealed haemorrhage.

Haemorrhagic fever Group of arbo viral infection which cause fever and bleeding such as KFD and yellow fever.

Haemorrhagic Related to the bleeding from a vessel.

Haemorrhoidectomy Surgical removal with cutting and ligation of haemorrhoid.

Haemorrhoids Varicosity of rectal veins, colloquially called piles at or above the anus.

Distension and dilatation of rectal vein which is colloquially called "piles"

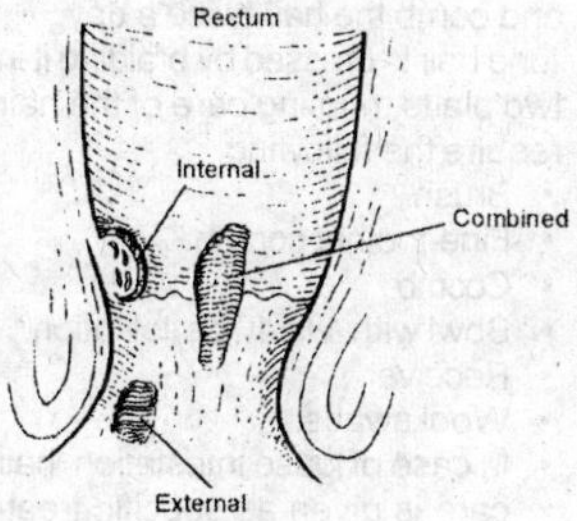

Haemorrhoids

Haemosalpinx Surgical and gynaecological conditions where bleeding occurs in fallopian tube.

Haemosiderin Disintegrated red cells liberate this iron containing pigment.

Haemosiderosis In certain conditions such as haemolytic diseases repeated blood transfusion pro-

duces deposition of iron in R E cells of liver.
Haemolysis of RBC produces iron deposits in tissues.

Haemostasis Method of making the bleeding arrest.

Haemostatic That which checks the flow of blood, Surgeon's ferric chloride (Martin's haemostatic), Dental haemostatic containing formaldehyde solution and gelatine (Wright's haemostatic),
Drug to arrest bleeding.

Haemothorax Injury like chest cage injury which cause blood in thorax.

Hageman factor It is a blood coagulation factor, Hageman factor helps in Kinin production.

Hahnemann Founder of Homeopathy (1755 to 1843).

Hair care Hospital patients shall brush and comb the hair twice a day,
long hair is dressed by braiding it in two plaits, nursing care of the hair require the following:

- Brush.
- Fine-toother coomb.
- Coomb.
- Bowl with 1 in 40 dettol lotion.
- Receiver.
- Wool swabs.
- In case of louse infestation, hair care is given as specific treatment.

Halogens Non-metallic elements like chlorine and iodine have disinfection property,chief halogen (chlorine compound) are Eusol, Dakin's solution,
chloramine and sodium hypochlorite.

Hair follicle Is an epidermal invagination from where hair shoots,
Arrector pili muscle and sebaceous glands are attached to these hair follicles.

Hair loss This is the first sign after radiation injury,
Hair loss occurs in post-cancer therapy with anticancer drugs
Alopecia may be localised or total is usual clinical condition.

Hair transplantation It is the treatment for alopecia where skin from different place containing hairs are transferred to the required place.

Hair Epidermal element which grows from the skin.

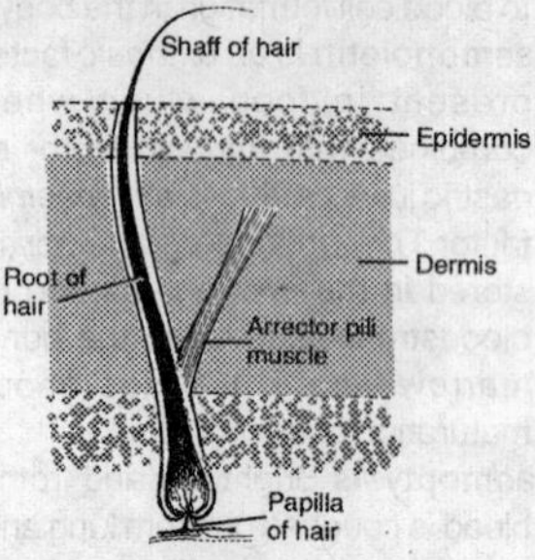

Structure of hair

Hairball It is also called trichobezoar when hair accumulation occur in stomach.

Hairy tongue In fungal infections by *Aspergillus* or *Candida* hair like papilla are projected from tongue.

HALE Health Adjusted Life Expectancy is an indicator estimating the expectation of equivalent years of good health, It is also called healthy life expectancy.

Half-life In case of radiological half-life, it is the time taken by radioactive substance to come to its half energy,
In case of Biological half-life, it is the time taken by a drug to get half inactivated in human body.

Halibut liver oil Derived from fish which yield rich source of vitamin A and vitamin D.
Animal source of fat soluble vitamins.

Halibut oil Oil from liver of halibut used for vitamin A and D supplementation.

Halitosis Clinical condition which give rise to bad breath or unpleasant breath.

Hallucination Seeing, hearing or experiencing a thing which is not there in the true sense
Common causes are:
- Mental illness.
- Drug induced.
- Due to alcohol.
- Brain tumour.
- Old age due to atherosclerosis
- Severe exhaustion.

Hallucinogen A substance which gives false sense of well being,
Common known substances are:
- Peyote derived from mescal weed used in India on the occasion of religious ceremonies.
- A derivative from jimson weed
- LSD 25 and Cannabis.

Hallux It is the other name for big toe- it refers to great toe, displaced great toe can gives rise to either Hallux valgus or Hallux varus.

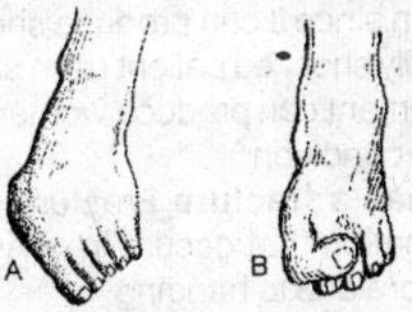

Hallux valgus

Halo effect Final outcome by a treatment, management, counselling or intervention.

Halo vest A metallic ring (halo) surrounding the head attaches to the skull with four pins, each penetrating thrugh the skin and into the skull approximately 30 mm (1/ 8th of inch),
It is used for patients with scoliosis, cervical fractures and fusions, torticollus and rheumatoid arthritis.

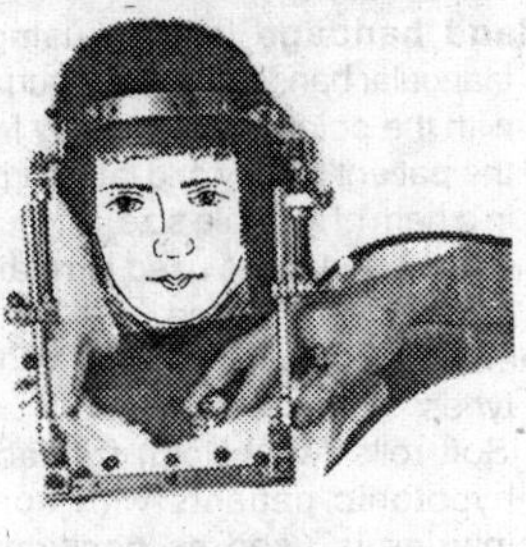
Halo vest

Halogen One of the group in chemicals which include chlorine, iodine, bromine and fluorine.

Halothane Used in general anaesthesia, it is a halogenated phenolic ether.

Halotraction Traction by using Halo vest which allows early mobility and which reduces potential for circulatory, respiratory and neurological complications.

Ham, test This is a lab test for haemoglobinuria where red cells are lysed in acid medium.

Hamate One of the carpal bones of the wrist.

Hammer finger Flexion deformity of the distal joint of a finger due to tendon avulsion.

Hammer Refers to percussion hammer which is used for eliciting tendon reflexes.

Hamster It is a laboratory experimental animal which looks like rat.

Hamstrings They are flexor of leg and adductors of thigh, muscles on the posterior aspect of thigh viz., semimembranous muscle, semitendendinosus muscle and biceps femoris muscle go to form hamstrings muscle.

Hand bandage It is by using a triangular bandage on a flat surface with the point directed away from the patient's body and later turned in a hem of suitable size,

Hand bandage is used to retain a dressing on the hand.

Hand rolls Hand rolls are of two types;

Soft rolls (washcloth) for flaccid hypotonic patients with spinal injuries is used as positioning device,

This will help in keeping hand, wrist and fingers in a position that maintain a functional grasp

Hard rolls(Metal cone) for spastic hypertonic patients to press muscles to inhibit spasticity.

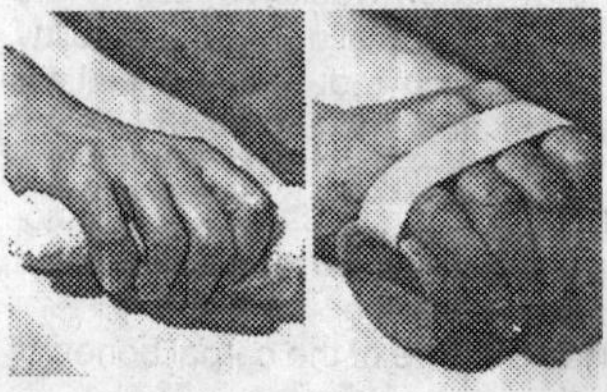

A: Soft roll B: Hard cone

Handball This sports develops speed and endurance primarily, although it develops muscles of the legs and shoulders.

Hand Part below the wrist which contain carpal bones, metacarpal bones and phalanges and other structures on dorsal and palmar aspects

Clinically we have claw hand and cleft hand.

Handicap Person with defects which prevents his normal doings or physiological functions, refers to both physical and mental handicap.

Handicapped children The term refers to the presence of an impairment or other circumstances that are likely to interfere with normal growth and development or with the capacity to learn.

Handicapped	*Impaired*	*Disabled*
Cannot perform a social role	Abnormal structure and function	Unable to perform an activity

Table: Handicap differentiated from impairment and disability

Handicrafts Making things of beauty or utility is a satisfying hobby,

Crafts can be by wood, metal, leather, plastics or other materials.

Handling patient Careful handling of patient is a requisite in first aid, Unnecessary handling of patient is avoided; support is given in cases of pain since it can produce shock, In badly shocked patient even slight movement can produce worsening of the condition.

Hangman's fracture Fracture and dislocation that occurs in cervical vertebra due to hanging.

Hangover After effects of alcohol consumption or after effects of antidepressants which cause fatigue and irritability.

Hansen bacilli Bacteria which was discovered by Hansen which cause leprosy.

Hansen's disease A chronic bacterial disease caused by *Mycobacterium leprae*

It was discovered by Hansen who lived during 1841-1912.

Haplo It means a simple and that which can combine easily to form one.

Haploid Single set of chromosome which is present in gamete, that which has one complete set of chromosomes.

Hapten Portion of antigen which determines specific immunity.

Hardey's lotion Liquid preparation for washing, it contains:

- Corrosive sublimate in alcohol.
- Zinc sulphate.
- Lead acetate.
- Water.

Hardness Refers to hardness of water which may be temporary or permanent,

Temporary hardness is due to bicarbonates and permanent hardness is due to chlorides and sulphates,

Type of hardness of water	*hardness level*
Soft	less than 1.0 mEq per litre
Moderately hard	1 – 3 mEq per litre
Hard	3 – 6 mEq per litre
Very hard	Above 6 mEq per litre

Table: level of hardness in water

Hard Tick They belong to ixodidae group that transmit some of the insect borne diseases such as KFD.

Harelip This is a special case where mouth feeding in nursing care is important, infant with harelip are unable to sucks naturally and are fed with a spoon or a pipette or by nasal catheter.

Harpoon instrument with hook used to scoop out tissues in surgery.

Harrison's groove This is a visible finding of Rickets in the lower border of thorax at the level of diaphragm.

Hartman's solution Each 100 ml contains.

Used in I V therapy which contains:

- NaCl 0.6 grams.
- KCl 0.03 grams.
- $CaCl_2$ 0.02 grams.
- Sodium lactate 0.31 grams.

Harvey William Harvey who first described human blood circulation.

Hashimoto's disease An autoimmune disease leading to hypothyroidism.

Hashish Cannabis or Indian hemp seen in drug abuse.

Hassal's corpuscle These bodies are present in thymus which are spherical in shape, they also show central area of degeneration.

Heating pad When nursing care is given with heating pads, care be given on wiring, continuous use for children and old people is not recommended.

Hats safety Safety hats should be worn on certain jobs especially around overhead work or where there might be falling objects.

Haunch It is a colloquial term which denotes hips or buttocks.

Haustra Pouches that are formed in colon because of its shorter longitudinal bands.

Haversian canal Openings in bone which connect themselves by transverse branches which are needed for providing nutrition to bone.

Havérsian system Histological observation of bone tissue which consists of canals described by Havers, Intracellular matrix around this gives the appearance of cylinders.

Haversian It denotes the name of a structure which is named after Dr.Havers, an English Anatomist who lived during 1855-1932.

Hay fever Allergic manifestation due to grain dust which affect nasal mucosa and conjunctiva, also called grain dust fever.

HCG Abbreviation for **H**uman **C**horionic **G**onadotrophin.

HCl Chemical formula for hydrochloric acid.

Head bandage This is used for fixing a dressing to the head by using 2 roller bandages and sew or pin the ends together.

Head rolling Unsightly head movements usually start from some irritative cause like rickets, this should not be attributed to teething, hunger or some other vague condition.

Headache Pain in head due to many causes which include stress, emotion, refractive error and brain pathology.

Heaf test By using Heaf's gun, tuberculin is injected into skin as a diagnostic test.

Healing From illness or from inflammation, the condition returning to normalcy.

Surgical healing is described in three different types. They are:

Healing by first intension healing without granulation of incised wound edges.

Healing by second intension healing with granulation of wound.

Healing by third intension repair of wound after few days by surgical suturing.

Healing The edges of wound can be brought together by the following method:

- By stitching.
- By clips.
- By adhesive dressings.
- By position.

Healing It refers to cure of illness or disease which depends on the following:

- Competence.
- Goodness and human touch.
- Treating with dignity.
- Ethics of Trust.

Health education Creating health awareness by health professionals, of an individual, and of the community through traditional and modern methods of health education. A process that informs, motivates and helps people to adopt and maintain healthy practices and lifestyles, advocates environmental changes as needed to facilitate this goal and conducts professional training and research to the same end.

Health foods Word used by food faddists and food promoters, Scientifically we cannot use the word because we do not have health foods.

Health for all Attainment of a level of health that will enable every individual to lead to socially and economically productive life.

Health indicator In order to evaluate the effectiveness and efficiency of a health treatment, health programme or health service, the extent of achievement of targets and objectives etc., we need the yardstick called *Health Indicators*.

Health insurance Insurance against expenditure of medical, surgical and hospital care such as Mediclaim and other health insurance schemes.

Health legislation Law governing health practice in India include The Central Acts,
The State Acts and The Municipal Acts, They are amended from time to time.

Health museum In India many health exhibitions are conducted through museum which can inform public about themselves for their better health.

Health service Health services include medical care and community health care through organised effort, through organised heath care system.

Health spectrum At the given point of time, we come across all category of people in varying state of health which is called health spectrum.

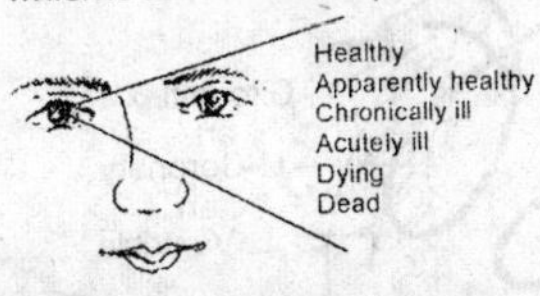

Health Spectrum

Health visitor Health visitor male and health visitor female at Primary Health Centres who play role in primary health care and in the preventive health care of the community.
MPW male and female who work under the supervision of HS male and female have been assigned with job responsibilities to coordinate National Health Programmes.

Health Problematic nature of concepts both health and disease "not merely the absence of disease and infirmity, but complete physical, mental and social well-being"
We look for positive health in a community
Health is a state of complete physical, mental and social well being and not merely an absence of disease or infirmity,
It is characterised by
- Sense of well being.
- Ability to work efficiently and with enthusiasm.
- Cheerfulness.
- Self-confidence.
- Self-control.
- Absence of illness.
- Conducting better in society.
- Good mental attitude.
- Absence of anxiety.

Hearing aid An ENT aid which is used by people with impaired hearing that can amplify the sound.

Hearing assessment Auditory function assessment is done by the following methods:
- Whispering at a distance of 60 cm.
- Performing the watch test.
- performing the Weber and Rinne test.

Hearing Sound waves are received and transmitted to CNS in the form of nerve impulse which is a special sense in human beings.

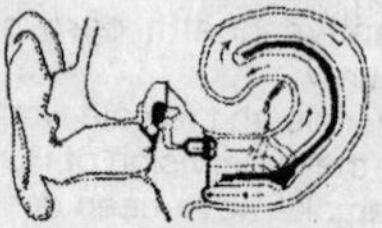

Hearing to show sound conduction

Heart block There is an interruption in AV node which leads to independent beating of auricles and ventricles,
It is also called Adams-Stokes disease.

Heart This is the centre of the circulation which is made of muscles that pump blood to all parts of the body, ♥ shaped organ is situated in thorax behind sternum and towards left side of the body
Common related terminologies used are:

- Heart sounds.
- Heart murmurs.
- Heart attack.
- Heart failure.

Heartburn In stomach when more of gastric juice is secreted with HCl, which when regurgitate to food pipe a sense of burning sensation occurs in epigastric region,
Burning sensation in the stomach
Symptom of peptic ulcer.

Heat application Heat applied locally is prescribed to some of the patients which will be by hot water bottle, a heating pad, radiant heat from an electric heater, hot wet pack, etc. They must be watched closely.

Heat exhaustion When a person collapses due to overexposure to heat. Symptoms are pale, clammy skin, rapid and weak pulse, weakness head-ache and nausea, it is controlled by first aid procedures, prevention of hazards by physical agents are prescribed.

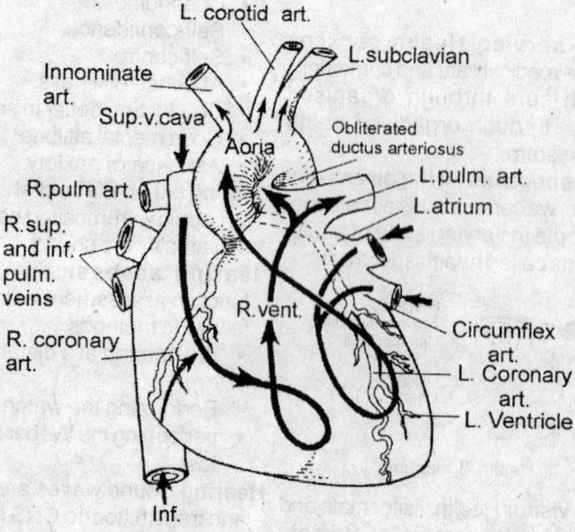

Structure of heart

Heat flash They are thermal radiation which produce flash burns, common cause is nuclear explosion,
It is one of the hazards of a nuclear explosion, other hazards are fire, blast and radioactivity associated sickness and syndrome.

Heat illness This is general term which is more common among unacclimatised persons working in hot environments,
These heat illnesses are:
- Heat stroke.
- Heat exhaustion.
- Heat syncope.
- Heat cramps.

Heat stroke It is severe form of reaction to exposure of man to hot climate,
Flushed hot skin, rapid and strong pulse are common,
If immediate first aid is not given, one can expect mortality.

Heat Raised temperature in an area, in the surrounding or in the body,
Fire and electricity are common source of heat,
Physical hazards due to heat could be:
- Heat stroke.
- Heat exhaustion.
- Heat syncope.
- Heat cramps.

Heating system They are normal source for home accidents, camp accidents,
Care must be exerted in maintaining safe heating system.

Heaves Clinical condition of pulmonary emphysema where elasticity of bronchioles and alveoli are seen and there will be forced expiration ,
Heaves indicate respiratory disturbances.

Hebephrenia Clinical psychiatric disturbance which comes under Schizophrenia,
Common manifestations are:
- Hallucinations.
- Delusions.
- Thought disorder.
- Emotional incongruity.

Heberden's node It is a condition of phalangeal bone osteoarthritis causing deformity of terminal finger joints.

Hegar's dilator Gynaecological instrument called cervical dilators which are in different numbers from lower to higher order.

Hegemony Simultaneous consent by masses to the type of society imposed upon them by the dominant group in society.

Heimlich manoeuvre It is an emergency manoeuvre for Foreign Body in Trachea, steps are:
1. Body of the patient is made to hang forward by holding the person with arms around him
2. Fist of one hand is grasped with other hand
3. With both fist hand forceful blow is given on the abdomen with upward thrust (this thrush shall be on the space between umbilicus and below the rib cage)
4. Repeated several times to clear the air passage

In case of unconscious patient, he is turned on to his back and the manoeuvre is done as described above.

Helicobacter This Gram-negative bacteria is responsible for progressive gastritis and gastric ulcer, common species is *H.pylori*.

Helix Outer rim of the external ear, Spiral twist of DNA

It is the margin of pinna of the ear.

Hellin's law This law states that multiple pregnancy is related with existing infertility modalities in the world,

Suppose prevalence of twins is 1 in 100, then it progreses in geometric progression for increasing multiple pregnancies as under;

Twin pregnancy	=	one in 100
Triplet pregnancy	=	one in 100^2
Quadruplets pregnancy	=	one in 100^3.

Helminthiasis Intestinal infection with helminths like cystode, trematodes and nematode which are due to poor personal and environmental hygiene.

Hemi canes They are used by the patients who have the use of only one upper limb and they give more security than a quad cane.

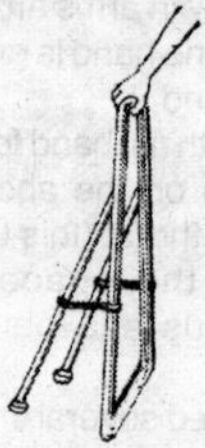

Hemi cane

Hemianopia Blindness in one half of the field of vision which can be in one eye or in both the eyes, Common clinical types are:

- Complete hemianopia.
- Bilateral hemianopia.
- Bitemporal hemianopia.
- Binasal hemianopia.
- Crossed hemianopia.

Hemicellulose They are high molecular carbohydrates which are soluble and get composted, They contain hexose, pentose and uronic acid.

Hemicolectomy Surgical removal of ascending colon and part of transverse colon followed by ileotransverse colostomy, (Hemi=half, removal of half of colon in a surgical intervention).

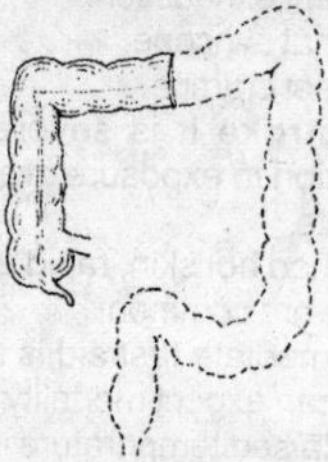

Showing part of colon which is removed in hemicolectomy

Hemiparesis Weakness and nonfunctioning of half of the body which is called Hemiplegia occurring due to stroke.

Hemiplegia One side of the body is paralysed due to cerebral haemorrhage.

Hemisphere Any one side of the brain, half of the brain say left or right sided.

Hemizygote One who has one chromosome or single chromosome which is unpaired, X chromosome in male (XY) is hemizygous.

Henle's loop Uriniferous tubule of the kidney which is U-shaped.

Heparin lock It is a male adaptor plug called heparin lock for intermittent infusion therapy.

When continuous infusion therapy has been discontinued for patient who has an indwelling over-the-needle catheter, one can insert a male adaptor plug (MAP) into the catheter to convert it to a heparin lock

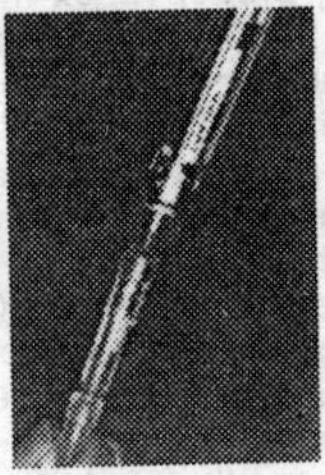

Heparin lock

Heparin It is an inhibitor of prothrombin to thrombin conversion, Chemically it is a polysaccharide from mast cells of liver,

Natural heparin is produced in liver and circulates in blood,

Thrombosis is treated with heparin

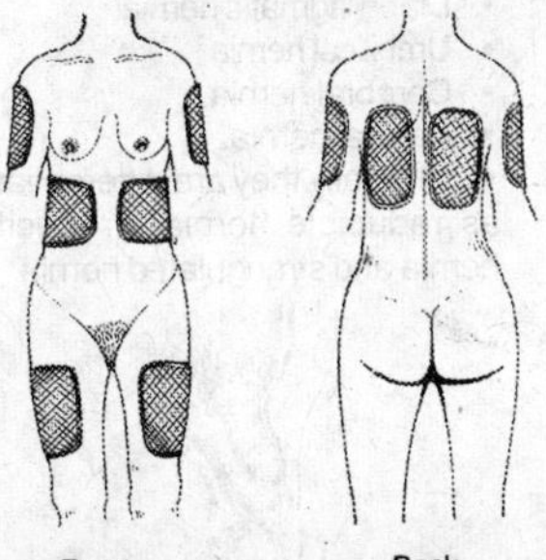

Sites used for heparin subcutaneous injection given repeatedly.

Hepatic coma Acute and severe liver disorders lead to impaired central nervous function, clinical characteristics which a nurse shall note are:

- EEG changes are present.
- Flapping tremor .
- Sweet disagreeable smell at the entry to ward.

Hepatic Any thing that is related to liver such as hepatic coma, hepatic flexure, hepatic vein.

Hepatitis B vaccine A recombinant DNA yeast derived vaccine 20 micrograms initially and later at I month and 6 months interval give good protection

Formalin inactivated subunit viral vaccine for I M 1.0 ml dose in 3 doses (0, 1, and 3 months).

Hepatitis Infection and inflammation of liver by different types of viruses and by toxic agents including alcohol, Hepatitis include a range of viral pathogens that are:

- Hepatitis A (HAV) RNA enterovirus
- Hepatitis B (HBV) DNA hepadna
- Hepatitis C (HCV) RNA flavivirus
- Hepatitis D (HDV) RNA incomplete virus
- Hepatitis E (HEV) RNA calicivirus
- Hepatitis G (HGV) RNA flavivirus
- Major ones like cytomegalovirus and Epstein Barr
- Minor ones like Herpes simplex
- Rare ones like chickenpox, measles, rubella and HIV

Amoebic hepatitis is also common in India.

Hepatojugular reflex In congestive cardiac failure, a pressure on right upper abdomen causes a rise in jugular venous pressure (JVP).

Hepatolenticular degeneration Low level of ceruloplasmin in an autosomal recessive genetic disorder; copper is deposited in liver, cornea, kidney and brain.

Hepatolenticular When a condition is related with liver and lentiform nucleus.

Generally refers to hepatolenticular degeneration.

Hepatomegaly When liver is enlarged and palpable on palpation.

Hepatosplenomegaly When liver and spleen are enlarged and palpable on palpation.

Hepatotoxic Any substance and any drug which is toxic to liver.

Herbal medicine It is used in traditional medicine such as Ayurveda where plants and plant extracts are used in the treatment of diseases.

Herbart's approach It is one of the approaches to lesson plan.

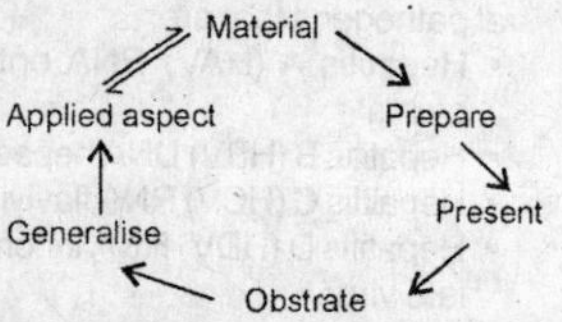

Herbart's approach of presentation

Herd immunity Body resistance seen among population for certain infections,

Since susceptible are very less a disease cannot occur in the community,

It is obtained by immunisation programme such as vaccination against Diphtheria, whooping cough, tetanus, tuberculosis, measles, polio under National programmes.

Hereditary Anything that is inherited or got from previous generation through genetic transmission.

Heredity and environment They can influence individual difference like colour vision, rate of memory, learning, deducing and reasoning, Group differences are influenced by environmental factors.

Herring Breuer reflex It is reflex inhibition of breathing by the stimulation of lung receptors following lung inflation.

Hermaphrodite If a person possesses both testes and ovary (True hermaphrodite)

If a person is of one sex (physical appearance of genitalia) but histologically of opposite sex (Pseudohermaphrodite).

Hermaphroditism A person with male and female sex organs, one can demonstrate both ovarian and testicular tissue in them.

Hernia In a weak body structure, organs are pushed into areas where they do not belong such as:
- Inguinal hernia.
- Femoral hernia.
- Diaphragmatic hernia.
- Umbilical hernia.
- Cerebral hernia.
- Vaginal hernia.
- Clinically they are differentiated as reducible hernia, irreducible hernia and strangulated hernia.

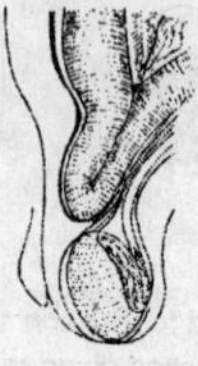

Inguinal hernia

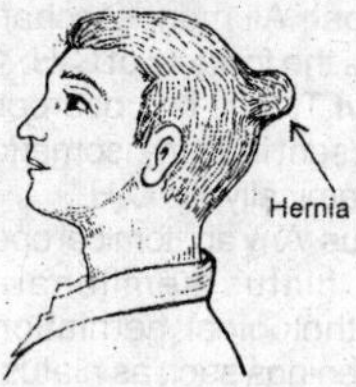

Cerebral (brain) hernia

Hernioplasty After reducing a hernia, repair of the abdominal wall is done.

Herniorrhaphy Surgical removal of hernial sac and repair of abdominal wall is done.

Herniotomy Surgical procedure of removal of hernial sac.

Heroin A drug derived from opium which is diacetate of morphine which has euphorial effects and makes an individual dependent for pleasure, following are the slang used in society:

- Brown sugar consumption.
- "H" consumption.
- Smack to fellowship.
- Shooting up when injected subcutaneously.
- Mainlining when IV taken.
- Chasing the Dragon when smoked.
- After the Dragon when snuffed.

Herpangiana This is coxsackie virus infection which is manifested with fever, inflamed and vesicular throat and hypersalivation.

Herpes simplex Herpes simplex (genital) by HSV-1 or HSV-2 are known STD infection which is characterised by irritable vesicles which rupture and ulcerate on genitalia.

Herpes Skin eruptions by herpes viral infection commonly occurring in mucocutaneous junction of lip and vagina.

Other types of herpes are:

- Herpes zoster commonly on forehead and eye(Shingles).
- Herpes simplex encephalitis in the brain.
- Type I Herpes infection is common in children who do not show any symptoms.
- Type II Herpes infection is common in adults which is associated with their sexual activities; which may end up with aseptic meningitis.

Herd immunity It means the immunity developed and demonstrated in a group of people against a disease, this gives protection to an individual in that group by virtue of being a member of that group.

Hertz Noise level is measured in hertz as unit of sound frequency in terms of cycle per second.

Hess's test It is a diagnostic test for purpura,if a tight pressure is exerted by BP cuff it produces raised pressure and rupture of capillaries (Purpuric spots).

Hesselback's triangle It is an anatomical triangle created by the following anatomical structures:

- Poupart's ligament.
- Outer border of rectus sheath.
- Epigastric artery.

Heterogenous This is made of different items or diverse constitutents.

Heteronomous ethics Heterogenous ethics deals with desirability of a thing particularly useful in health practice which is subject to

Extrnal Law examples:

1. Terminal cancer patient need good attention.
2. Newborn with defects need available care.
3. Girl and woman not married cannot have sterilisation.

Heterosexual Great interest bestowed on opposite sex, between male and female.

Heterozygous Inherited characteristics are intermixed when transmitted by parents to offspring , Dominant character from one parent and recessive character from other parents are derived.

Hetrazan Drug used in filaria infection, Chemically it is 1-diethyl-carbamyl-4-methyl-piperzine dihydrogen citrate.

Hexachlorophane It is present in soap and many skin preparations, used as detergent and antiseptic.

Hexokinase This is an enzyme present in muscle tissue and yeast which is a catalyst in phosphorylation of glucose.

Hexose All monosaccharide which has the formula of $C_6H_{12}O_6$.

Hexyl This is hydrocarbon which is present in many isomeric forms , chemically it is C_6H_{13}.

Hiatus Any anatomical opening such as hiatus semilunaris or any pathological herniation into the openings such as hiatus hernia.

Hibernation Animals keeping themselves asleep and inactive during winter season.

Hiccough Sharp inspiratory cough which follows the closure of glottis and spasmodic contraction of diaphragm.

Hiccups Spasms of the diaphragm usually due to irritations in upper abdominal area usually by overeating.

Hickman catheter They are semi-permanent indwelling central lines that are inserted into right atrium via cephalic, subclavian or jugular vein and is indicated in:

- Frequent venipunctures.
- Hyperalimentation.
- Chemotherapy.
- Intermittent blood transfusion.
- CVP monitoring.

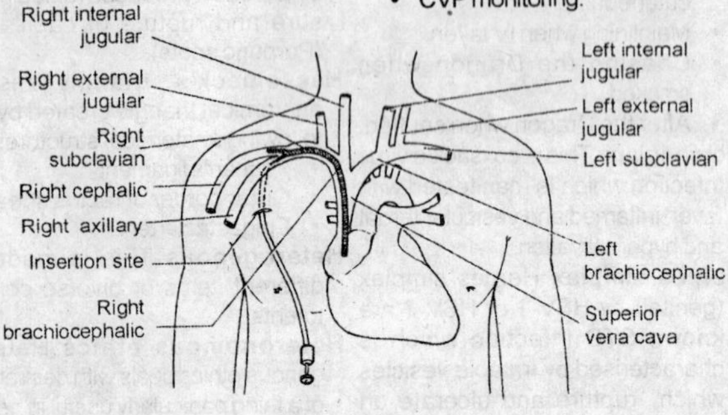

Managing Hickman catheter

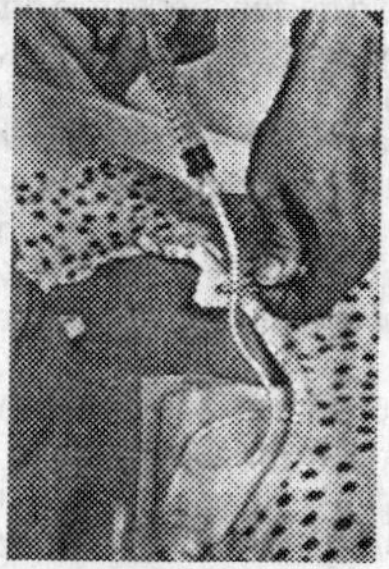

Hickman catheter in use

Hierarchy That which is in the order of importance.

Hierarchy of needs This is Maslow theory which describes physiological needs such as food and shelter safety, and security love, companionship and affection self-esteem and the esteem of other, self-actualisation (i.e., realising one's potential to the fullest).

High culture Opera, ballet, sculpture and such arts patronised by elite in society, to reach different audience.

High residue diet It is a hospital diet for colorectal disease, diabetes and obesity, the diet contains minimum of 30 grams of cellulose or fibres per day.

Hiking Hiking and camping i.e., living in the woods is one of the most enjoyable and relaxing vacations, Precautions against potential health hazards is necessary in hiking and camping.

Hilton's law The law states that a nerve supplying a muscle also supply the joint which has the movement by that muscle and simultaneously the same nerve also supplies the skin overlying the insertion of that muscle.

Hilton's sac This is the external portion of vocal cord which is in the form of pit.

Hiltons' line A white line at mucocutaneous junction of anal mucosa and skin of perineum.

Hind gut Ileum colon and rectum which are developed from caudal portion of entoderm.

Hinge joint When only flexion and extension is possible in one axis.

Hip bandage It is a method of first aid bandaging in hip management. Narrow bandage round the lower part of the abdomen is tied so that the knot is on the injured side, second knot also is tied in line with other and placed along the middle of the outer side of the limb

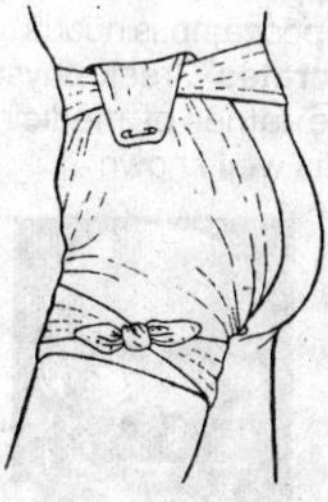

Hip bandage

Hip Evaluation of hip is done by Thomas test to identify flexion contracture.

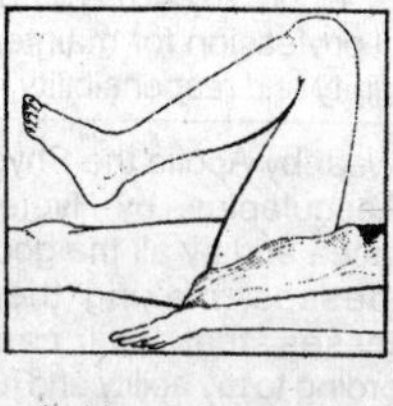

Opposite hip remain extended as the other flexes (normal)

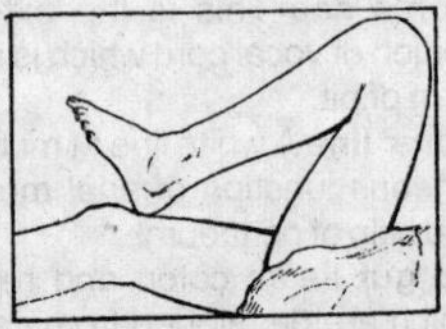

Opposite hip also flexes (Positive Thomas) indicate flexion contracture

Hippocampus Meaning of the word is Sea Horse,

It is the anatomical curved structure on the floor of the middle horn of lateral ventricle,

Anatomical description of Hippocampus includes:

- Hippocampus major.
- Hippocampus minor.
- Hippocampus nudus.

Hippocrates Greek physician who is the father of medicine whose oath is well known.

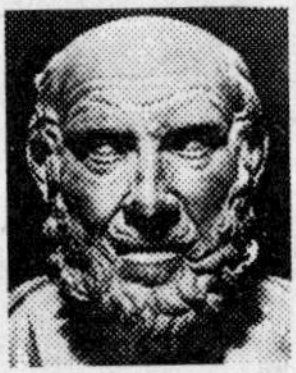

Hippocrates

Hippocratic oath this noble code of ethics adopted by all medical men in their profession for maintenance of dignity and responsibility.

" I swear by Apollo the Physician, by Aesculapius, by Hygieia, by Panacea and by all the gods and goddesses, making them my witnesses, that I will carry out according to my ability and judgement, this oath and this indenture. To hold my teacher in this art equal to my own parents; to make him partner in my livelihood; when he is in need of money to share mine with him; to consider his family as my own brothers, and to teach them this art, if they ant to learn it, without fee or indenture; to impart precept, oral instruction and all other instruction to my own sons, the sons of my teacher, and to pupils who have taken the physicians' Oath, but no nobody else. I will use treatment to help the sick according to my ability and judgement, but never with a view to injury and wrongdoing.

Neither will I administer a poison to anybody when asked to do so, nor will I suggest such a course. Similarly I will not give to a woman a pessary to cause abortion. But I will keep pure and holy both my life and art. I will not use the knife, not even, verily, on sufferers from stone, but I will give place to such as are craftsmen therein. Into whatsoever houses I enter, I will enter to help the sick, and I will abstain from all intentional wrongdoing and harm, especially from abusing the bodies of man or woman, bond or free. And what-so-ever. I shall see or hear in the course of my profession as well as outside my profession in my inter course with men, if it be what should not be published abroad, I will never divulge, holding such things to be holy secrets. Now if I carry out this oath, and break it not, may I gain for ever reputation among all men for my life and for my art; but if I transgress it and forswear myself, may the opposite befall me"

The Hippocratic oath

Hippocratic As described by Hippocrates the father of medicine, relates to Hippocratic oath.

Hippus Common symptom in multiple sclerosis where pupillary contraction and dilatation occurs alternatively.

Hirschsprung's disease Megacolon and absence of mesenteric plexus in rectosigmoid area of colon.

Hirsute Tuft of hair present in an individual.

Hirsutism Large tufts of hair all over the body is present,
Term often denotes presence of hair in women in unwanted place.

His bundle The conduction bundle which starts from AV node and ends in ventricle.

Histamine It is an amine present in animals and plant tissue which is a vasodilator, used in gastric studies, chemically it is beta imidazolylethyl amine,

$CH.NH.CH{:}N.C.-CH_2.CH_2NH_2$

|==========|

Is a substance released in the body during allergic reactions.

Histidine One of the essential amino acid from which histamine is derived

Histamine headache Headache induced by consumption of food containing histamine or after effects of histamine injection by certain insects.

Histochemistry Study of chemistry of cells and tissues by:

- Light microscope.
- Electron microscope.
- Special chemical tests.
- Tissue stains.

Histogram Data collected is represented in the form of a graph or bar chart, or when data is represented in the form of column or rectangle,

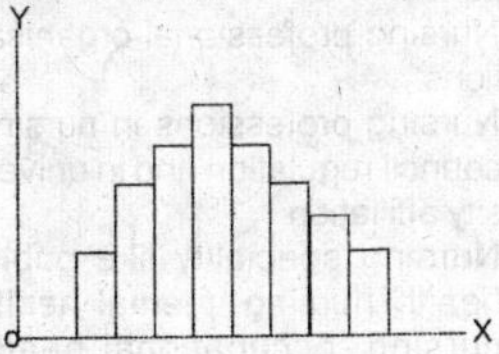

Histogram

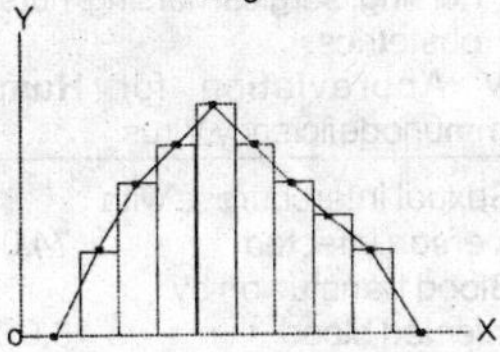

Histogram with frequency polygon

Histoid When a structure resembles like a tissue.

Histology It is the scientific study of cells and tissues under microscope for understanding their structure and composition.

Histoplasmosis Tuberculosis like disease which is caused by Histoplasma capsulatum (a fungal infection).

History of nursing History of nursing is studied with the bifurcation of past, present ages with the evolution of nursing care in illness treatment:

- Nursing history is studied under the following headings.
- Nursing profession in past ages.
- The Christian era of nursing.
- Nursing care by the Sisters of Charity.
- English nursing in dark ages.
- Pre-Nightingale period where reforms took place.

- Nursing profession in Nightingale period.
- Nursing professional organisations.
- Nursing professions in nursing council regulation and in university affiliation.
- Nursing speciality like public health nursing, mental health nursing, occupational health nursing, surgical nursing, nursing obstetrics.

HIV Abbreviation for **Human** Immunodeficiency Virus

Sexual intercourese with person infected	74.0%
Blood transfusion by infected blood	8.0 %
Drug users by common syringe use	7.0%
Non-specific mode (Includes mother to child transmission)	11.0%

HIV transmission cycle

Hives Due to allergy from food and from emotional upsets, bumps in skin which appear and disappear often.

Hoarseness Voice change due to chronic laryngitis which are commonly due to vocal cord infection, vocal cord palsy or secondaries of vocal cord.

Hobbies Good hobby help to better emotional health, but not a cure of ill,
Game, sports, social service, attending to sick are examples of hobbies,
It gives satisfaction, relaxation and contentment to one who practices it.

Hodge pessary During post-operative care of correction of retroversion of uterus
Hodge pessary is used to maintain the position of the uterus.

Hodgkin's disease A malignant disease with proliferation of lymphoid tissue associated with fever, lymphadenopathy, liver enlargement and spleen enlargement, diagnostic biopsy show Sternberg's giant cells,
With cytotoxic drugs and radiotherapy it has good prognosis.

Hoffman's sign This is positive in pyramidal damage, the test show the flexion of other fingers of same hand by flicking the terminal phalanx of finger.

Holdger Nielsen resuscitation This method of artificial respiration was introduced in Denmark,
This is recommended by British Red Cross society,
Essential movement of pressing and arm raising not only ventilate the lungs but also stimulate the heart.

1

1a

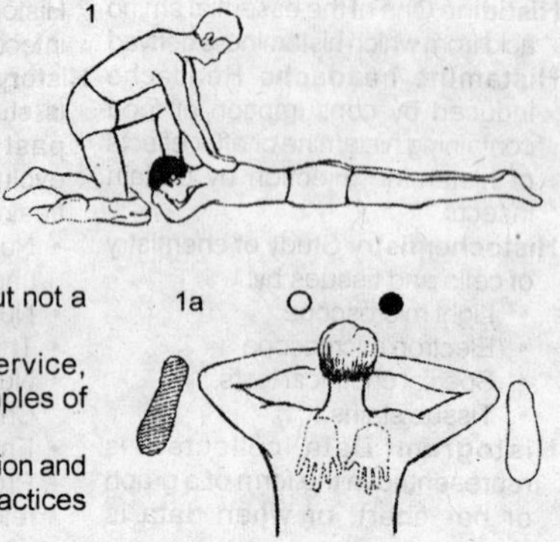

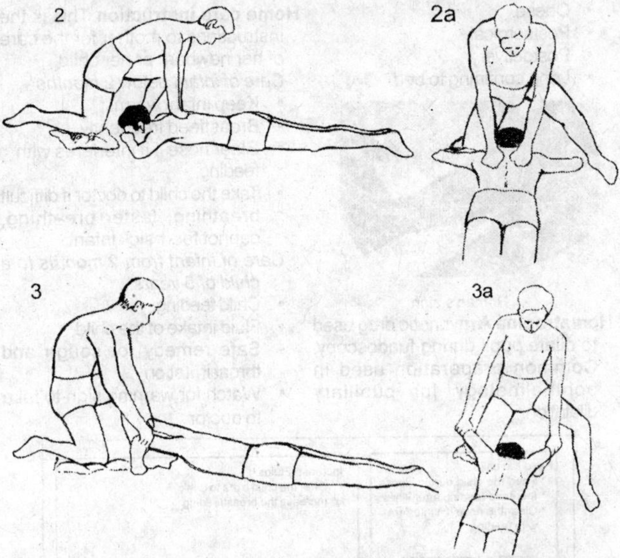

The Holdger Nielsen method of artificial respiration (1, 2, 3, side view 1a, 2a, 3a aerial view)

Holistic Consideration of all aspect and both internal and external environment is seen in Holistic approach,

Case management is person oriented and not disease oriented.

Hollister urinary collection system It is external collection device called condom catheter used in case of patients for whom the prolonged use of indwelling catheters is contraindicated.

Holoendemic It denotes that a disease is present at all time in all the population,

Malaria is common example for Holoendemic.

Holter monitor This instrument is used in ICCU for continuous recording of ECG of patients under treatment for M I and for arrhythmias.

Homan's sign This sign is positive in venous thrombosis where patient experiences pain of calf muscle when the foot is dorsiflexed.

Homan's sign Pain elicited in calf during dorsiflexion is positive Homan's sign who needs further evaluation for deep vein thrombophlebitis,

The test is done on the following conditions:

- Pain, tenderness, redness in lower limb.

- Obese.
- Postsurgical.
- Postdelivery.
- Long confining to bed.

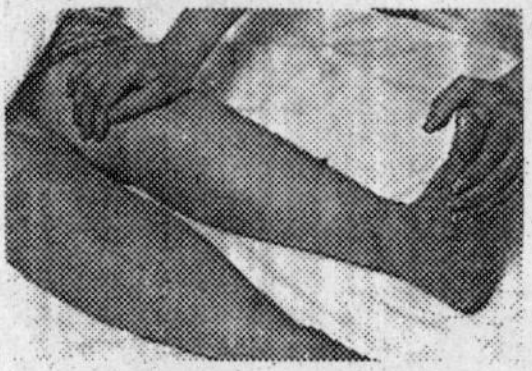

Homan's sign

Homatropine A mydriatic drug used to dilate pupil during fundoscopy, Common preparation used in ophthalmology for pupillary dilatation.

Home care instruction This is the instructions to mother for the care of her newborn or her child,

Care of infant below 2 months:
- Keep infant warm.
- Breastfeed frequently.
- Clear nose if it interferes with feeding.
- Take the child to doctor if difficult breathing, faster breathing, cannot feed sick infant.

Care of infant from 2 months to a child of 5 years:
- Child feeding
- Fluid intake of the child
- Safe remedy for cough and throat irritation
- Watch for warning sign to take to doctor

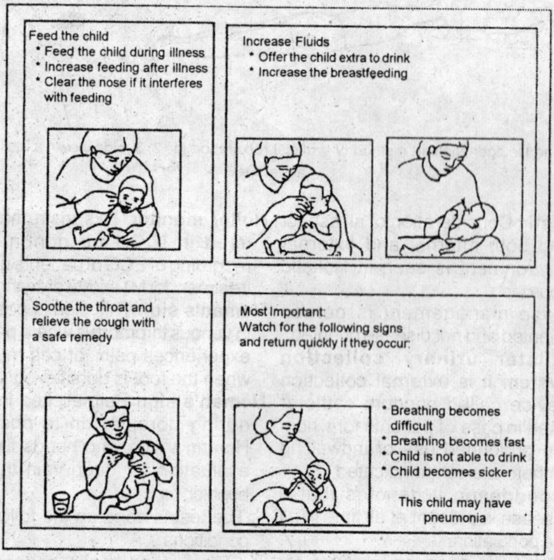

Home care instructions for children aged 2 months upto 5 years with acute respiratory infections

Home delivery As domiciliary MCH services, Home delivery is instituted by PHC and subcentre activities by the health worker female in rural and urban areas,

Trained traditional birth attendant assures best service in home delivery.

Home made solution In case of emergency due to acute diarrhoea, GE and cholera

Home made solution is given to child which is prepared as under;

Table salt ..... Thumb and 2 finger pinch

Water/Orange juice/Tea ... ½ litre.

Home nursing Public health nursing leads to the care of the sick at home by the special nurse who attends to him in their surroundings, in case of communicable diseases, Parkinson's diseases, stroke, cancer, and certain chronic disorders need home nursing care.

Home safety Safety at home is by common sense and hence better be visualised,

Falls, fire, home heating system, automotive, gas poisoning, electricity, poisoning, cuts, use of cutting implements, firearms, power tools in garden, are to be attended in home safety.

Home visiting In public health nursing, nurse visits home to give advice which will promote mental and physical well being of all the members of the family and reinforce the stability of the home,

Objectives of home nursing care are:

- To carry out nursing care at home.
- To prevent diseases among members.
- To promote health of all members.

Home Home has the family which constitute the centre of human being, health begins at home.

Homeopathy Remedy in Homeopathy is " like cures like",

Hahnemann who is father of homeopathy found small dose administration of drug can produce symptom of disease to be cured.

Homeostasis Body adjustment to internal and external environment for survival, maintenance of stability in biological system

Milieu Interior or internal environment of human body which is maintained at equilibrium status for best physiological function.

Homicide Criminal offence of killing others,

Literarily it means killing of human being, types of homicide are:

- Culpable homicide which is actually crime and murder.
- No culpable homicide which is lawful execution.

Homogenous Items those are similar in their characteristics,

One which is dissolved in another, Clear like water.

Homologous Developmentally items are from same embryo but perform different functions,

Chemically items having same chemical structure

Genetically same identical DNA pattern.

Homosexual person getting attracted with the same sex, male to male relation,female to female relation with respect to sexual habits When reference is made of a person with the person of the same sex.

Homozygous In genetic inherited character, identical pair of genes are possessed.

Honey From bees it has the traditional inclusion in medical preparations for palatability, it is a natural solution of sugar.

Hookworm One of the nematode which is responsible for hookworm anaemia in India,

Ankylostoma duodenale and *Necator americanas* are two common-species known to produce pathology.

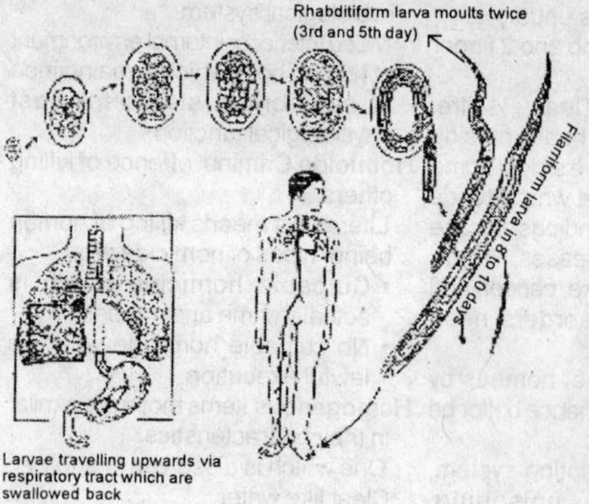

Life cycle of hookworm

HOPE project It is one of the People-to-people Health Foundation initiated by USA, Little later it got a component called people-to-people Health component in the form of Project called HOPE project (Health Opportunity for People Everywhere).

Hordeolum Infection and inflammation of sebaceous glands of eyelash which is called *Stye*.

Hormone Generally a biological substance which is produced in an endocrine gland and gets circulated to different site for its action.

Horner's syndrome It is a sympathetic nerve lesion in cervical region producing following symptoms:

- Ptosis.
- Enophthalmos.
- Pupillary contraction.
- Loss of sweating.

Horn Skin outgrowth with full of keratin, Outgrowth or projections of brain also are common terms such as anterior horn, posterior horn, horn of Ammon, etc.

Horny layer Outer skin layer which is less sensitive which protects the true skin.

Horrock's apparatus An apparatus used to find out the chlorine demand of a sample of water , a test conducted in the field before actual chlorination,

Inference drawn will be *Bleaching powder in grams per 100 gallons of water which is tested.*

Horse power The term used in physical dynamics to depict energy which is the of power equivalent to 550 ft.Lb per second or (745.7 watts).

Horseshoe-shaped kidney It is one of the congenital defect of the kidney where lower poles of kidneys are united.

Horseback riding It mainly exercises the legs, forearms and wrists, it is not much help for heart and lung.

Hospice This is the concept of giving care of patient with his family members where emphasis is laid on emotional, spiritual and medical problems and are attended throughout their period of ill health,

Hospes is root word for hospital which was originally was shelter of the homeless and for entertainment of travellers.

Modern hospitals chief function has been the care and treatment of the sick which work on socioeconomic and political framework of society.

Hospital acquired infection Infections that are acquired during the stay of patient in the hospital, They are called nosocomial infections.

Hospital disinfections It is the procedure followed in disinfection at hospital,

Faeces, urine	2 hour contact by Phenol 10% Formalin 10% Bleaching powder 8% Cresol 5%
Sputum	Burning Autoclave(20 min 20 Lb) Cresol 5%.
Room	Soap water wash Cresol 2.5% Phenol 5% Formalin 10% Formalin + $KMNO_4$ in water(200G/half Ltr)
Linen	Boil Steam Cresol 2.5%
Dead body, covered sheet	Formalin 10% Phenol 5%
Instruments	Boiling
Glove, dressing	Autoclave
Rubber catheter, plastic catheter	Boiling
Gum elastic catheter	Formalin vapour
Cystoscope face mask	Pasteurisation
Catgut suture	Lugol's iodine
Other suture	Autoclaving
Polythene tubing	Gamma radiation
Urinals	Hypochlorite solution
Bedpans	Lysol
Blanket	Hot formalin vapour

Table:Hospital disinfection procedures

Hospital insurance Social insurance has entered Hospital services which makes a citizen to insure against illness and the insurance company takes care of the expenditure on treatment, surgery and other expense towards illness,

Medicare, group insurance, are examples.

Hospital organisation It has a structure with board of directors who direct administration,

Function is unique in human service through medical care,

Nursing care, surgical intervention, emergency care, preventive care and rehabilitation care

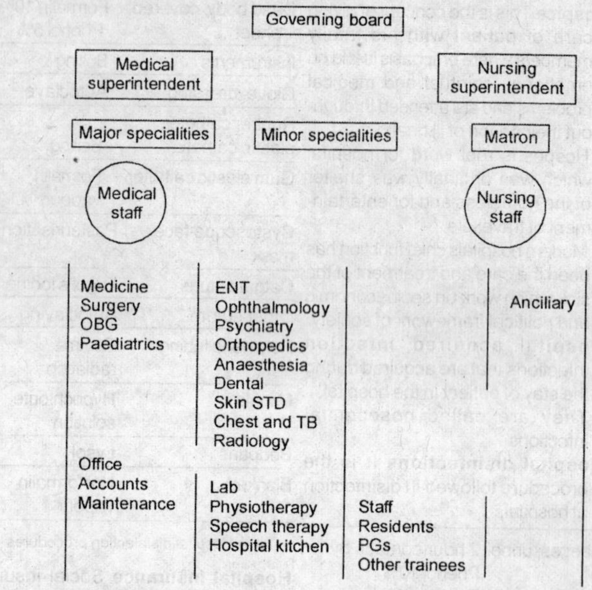

Organisation of a hospital

Hospital standardisation Construction, organisation and practice that serve as standards have been recommended from time to time, minimum standard can classify them under fully approved, provisionally approved or not approved.

Hospital It is a professional organisation or institution which takes care of admitting, diagnosis, investigation and treatment of illness or injury, types of hospitals are given below (table)

Public health sector hospitals	Civil hospitals (district hospitals) Teaching hospitals attached to medical colleges ESI hospitals CGHS hospitals Defence hospitals Railway hospitals
Private sector hospitals	Private hospitals Nursing homes

Indigenous systems of medicine hospitals	Ayurveda hospitals Sidda hospitals Unani hospitals Tibbi hospitals Homeopathy hospitals

Table: Types of hospitals

Recent introduction of hospitals are	General hospital Children hospital Maternity hospital Infectious disease hospital Orthopaedic hospital Hospital for chronic sick Hospital for nervous disorder Hospital for plastic surgery Hospital for cardiac surgery Hospital for neuro-surgery Cancer hospital Tuberculosis hospital Leprosy hospital Eye hospital ENT hospital

Table: Recent entry of hospitals

Host When parasites live and multiply in an organism that organism is called host, definitive host and intermediate host are used to denote presence of sexual stage and non-sexual stage of parasites
Person who harbours the disease.
Animals or organisms which nourish the parasites,
The person who receive organ transplantation
In parasitology terms like definitive host and intermediate host are used to denote Asexual and sexual development of parasites.

Hostility It is one of the manifestation of depressive psychosis where person shows anger, animal behaviour and attacking on others

Hot applications They are external applications for relieving pain and congestion, Benefits are:

- Increase local blood supply.
- Through leucocytes remove. waste and inflammatory.
- Exudate.
- Eelax the muscle.

Common clinical hot applications are:

- Fomentation and stupes.
- Turpentine stupe.
- Kaolin poultice.

Common hot baths are practiced as hot application therapy, this will include medicated baths like:

- Mustard bath.
- Alkaline bath.
- Saline bath.
- Bran bath.
- Starch bath.

Hot packs are ordered to promote sweating in cases of renal diseases and paresis and paralysis.

Hot water bag Rubber container with hot water is used in clinical practice to keep the area of the body warmer and also to keep moist applications warm.

Hot water bottles It is common method of hot applications.

Hotels Common area for food and lodging for travellers and vacationers.

Hotline It refers to telephone connections which works without any stop.

Hour glass contraction In case of gastric ulcer or cancer stomach when the stomach is contracted in the centre, it gives the appearance of hour glass, when there is a contraction in the middle of hollow organ (say stomach or uterus) it gives hour glass appearance.

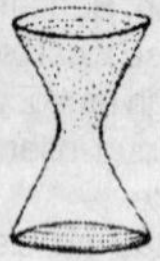

A. Hour glass

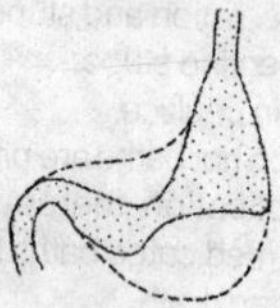

B. Hour glass stomach

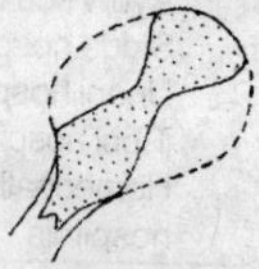

C. Hour glass uterus

House calls Attending the sick at home by doctor or by a nurse,
It is done for medical care, attending emergency care and for required referral of patients.

House dust Mixed dust due to atmospheric pollution which cause allergic conditions like asthma.

House fly They are non-biting common house fly called *Musca domestica*
Their density is an index of poor sanitation, they transmit
Typhoid, diarrhoea, cholera, GE and trachoma.

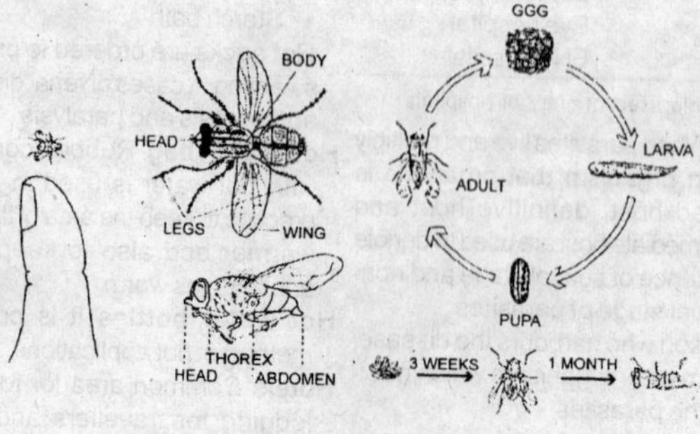

Life cycle of house fly

Household Individual or group have same address and share meal and living accommodation.

House physician He is a resident under the supervision of a consultant or senior staff who is responsible for patient care in a hospital.

Housemaid knee Chronic inflammation of bursa in front of patella which is swollen with serous fluid

Housing It is a physical structure where unit of society the, family lives, but the concept is slowly changing to *Human settlement* which allow the extended outlook of a house, where people live.

Human volunteer research It is a study design where healthy individuals participate in research/ drug trial/ clinical trial/ preventive trial, Based on type of group study design, research ethics has given a code of conduct specially applicable to human volunteer research.

Human behaviour It is human response to his surroundings. Stimulus determines human behaviour, for example

- See a snake we run away.
- See a coin we pick up.
- Hit a person who spit on us.
- See a girl show attachment.

Housing

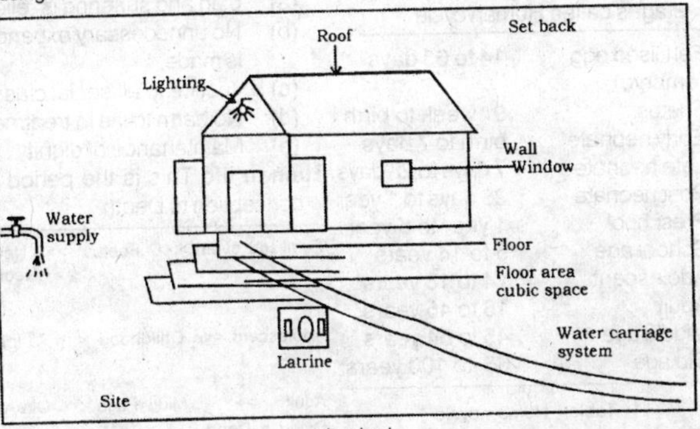

standards

Hoyer lift It is a mechanical lift that is used to lift and transfer immobile patient and is contraindicated in spinal injury.

Huhner's test Indirect method of investigation for infertility when husband fails to cooperate in investigation,
Within one hour of coitus vaginal content is aspirated for sperm motility and sperm pathology

Human chorionic gonadotrophin Hormones which stimulates gonads, FSH and LH are secreted by anterior pituitary gland.

Human crutch This is the mode of transport of the sick and injured when patient is suffering from a slight injury to one leg only,
With the help of first aider patient can place light weight on the injured

foot and by supporting himself against the first aide's body

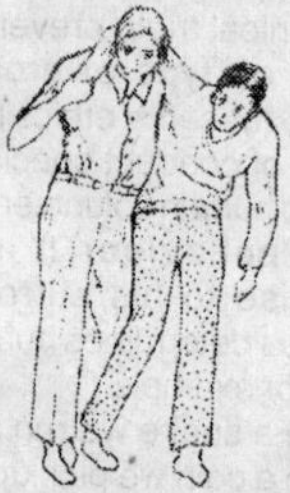

The Human crutch

Human cycle It is intricate human development through different stages called Human cycle

Fertilised egg (embryo)	14 to 63 days
Foetus	9th week to birth
Early neonate	birth to 7 days
Late neonate	7 days to 28 days
Post neonate	28 days to 1 year
Preschool	1 year to 5 year
School age	5 to 14 years
Adolescent	14 to 18 years
Adult	18 to 45 years
Middle age	45 to 64 years
Old age	65 to 100 years

Table: Human cycle

Human experimentation experiment or trial on human beings are regulated through medical codes of conduct such as:

(a) Guide lines from CIOMS and WHO 1982.
(b) Guidelines from ICMR 1980.
(c) Declaration of Helsinki modification 1975.
(d) Declaration of Helsinki 1964.
(e) Code of Nuremberg 1947.

Human factors Medical help for the poor, not practicing for the sake of money,

Doing doctors' job out of compassion constitute the area of human factors under ethical issues Some of the major human factors from the great list are:

- Social status.
- Trust.
- Privacy.
- Sex preselection.
- Euthanasia.
- Fund donation (money).

Human fulfilment This is composed of

(a) pain and suffering is relieved.
(b) No unnecessary expenditure is made.
(c) Justice to all social class.
(d) No harm to life in treatment.
(e) Maintenance of dignity.

Human life This is the period from conception to Death.

Fertilised ovum >>> Foetus >>> Newborn >>> Neonate
↓
↓
Adolescent <<< Childhood <<< Infancy
↓
↓
Adult >>> Middle age >> Old Age >> Dying > Dead

Diag: Human cycle

Human insulin With the help of recombinant DNA technology prepared insulin.

Human organ transplant Act Main Act is Human Organ Transplant Act 1989 U.K. which is following National level Acts in India and Turkey for Organ transplantation to save the life of patients.

Common organs used in transplantation are:
- Kidney.
- Cornea.
- Blood.
- Liver.
- Foetal brain tissue.
- Bone marrow.
- Heart.

Human sexuality It has certain norms in our society for our protection and for progeny, Unaccepted sexual behaviour are punishable. Common sexual offences are rape, exhibitionism, necrophilia.

Human stretcher This is a useful method of carrying the sick and injured particularly when patient is unconscious,
Patient is carried in the lying down position.

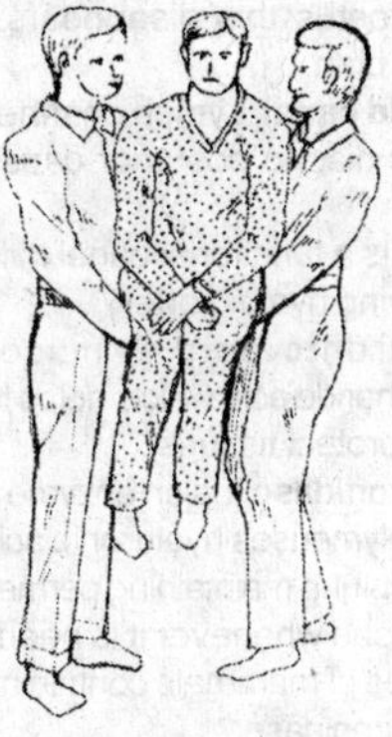

Human stretcher

Humectant It is a skin preparation which is meant to preserve moisture of the skin.

Humerus Bone of the upper arm.

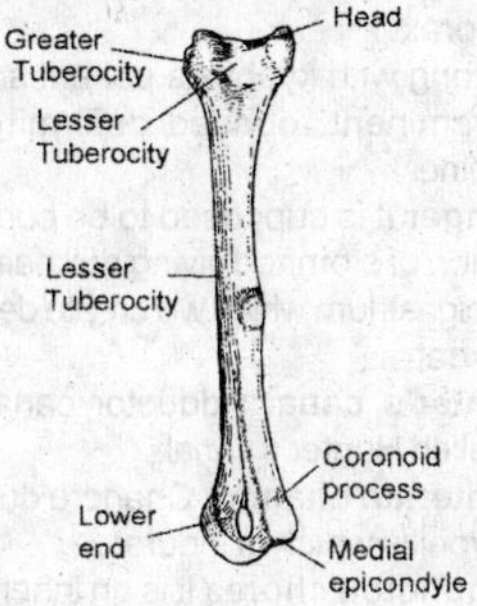

Humerus

Hum Any soft continuous sound on auscultation.

Humidification It is setting up of oxygen system with humidification by using humidifier.

Humidity Humidity is the water content of the air or the moisture content of the air,
Types of humidity are *absolute humidity* and *relative humidity*
Humidity therapy is the therapeutic use of water in hospital which is indicated in:
- Oxygen administration.
- Respiratory tract irritation.
- Aspiration of mucous secretion
- At sputum collection for examination.

Humour It refers to blood and lymph in human body,
Natural fluid present in some of the anatomical places such as:
a) Vitreous humour.
b) Aqueous humour.

Humpback It is the other name for kyphosis.

Hunchback It is kyphosis which is an abnormal roundness of the thorax
Along with kyphosis patient show prominent rounded deformity of spine.

Hunger It is supposed to be contraction of stomach giving dull pain in epigastrium which will create desire to eat.

Hunter's canal Adductor canal is called Hunter's canal.

Hunterian chancre Chancre due to syphilis which is indurated.

Huntington chorea It is an inherited disorder of nervous system which give rise to dementia,
Degenerative inherited disorder of the brain which is mainly manifested in the form of dementia and chorea.

Hurler's syndrome Synonyms is Gargoylism which is a genetic disorder with the deposit of large quantity of mucopolysaccharide in the brain causing loss of learning abilities in children.

Hutchinson's teeth One of the sign in congenital syphilis in which notching of border of incisor teeth is noticed.

Hyalase Is hyaluronidase an enzyme that catalyzes the hydrolysis of hyaluronic acid the cement substance of the tissues,
It is found in snake venom, leech venom, spider venom, in cancerous testes.

Hyaline cast These casts are present in nephropathy which are transparent and have rounded ends.

Hyaline membrane disease A disorder of the newborn where the newborn cannot breath properly and cannot have gas exchange process.

Hyaline membrane This name is given to 3 different anatomical areas, they are:

- Hyaline membrane of lung.
- The basement membrane.
- The membrane between the outer root sheath and the innerfibrous layer of a hair follicle.

Hyaline Name of translucent cartilage like thyroid cartilage
Histological section stained with haematoxylin and eosin gives pink glassy appearance of a cell
Associated terminologies are hyaline degeneration and hyaline membrane disease.

Hyaloid artery Artery present only in foetal life which supply lens in the foetus this disappears soon after birth.

Hyaloid canal Lymph channel from optic disc to posterior capsule of lens,
This is a functional canal in foetus carrying hyaloid artery.

Hyaluronic acid A mucopolysaccharide acid which helps to bind and protect tissues.

Hyaluronidase It is an enzyme which depolymerises hyaluronic acid that is helpful in maintaining permeability of tissue whenever it is needed
Testes of mammals contain natural hyaluronidase.

Hybrid Modified or changed characteristics of succeeding generation from its parent generation,
New generation.

Hybridisation Cross-matching in plants and in animals in order to get hybrid generation.

Hydantoin Chemically it is glycolyl urea which is a base.

Hydatid Cyst of *Echinococcus granulosus* which is seen within an organ such as brain, lung and liver.

Hydatidiform mole When chorionic villi degenerates within uterus they transform to cysts in uterus.

Hydatidiform That which resembles hydatid cyst.

Hydragogue Sulphates of calcium and sulphates of magnesium are hydragogue which when given produce watery evacuation.

Hydraulic society Survival depend on, appropriate irrigation where ancient culture depended on access to water.

Hydrate It is a chemical compound having the element of water.

Hydrocele In tunica vaginalis when fluid accumulates it is called hydrocele

Depending upon the nature and placement they can be:

- Congenital hydrocele.
- Encysted hydrocele.
- Cervical hydrocele.

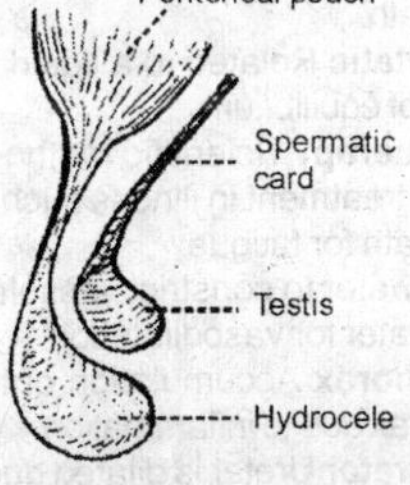

Hydrocele

Hydrocephalus Developmental anomaly due to

(a) Increased CSF content.
(b) Decreased CSF absorption.
(c) Block in CSF circulation.

Skull enlargement due to accumulation of CSF.

Hydrochloric acid A chemical compound containing hydrogen and chlorine which is present in gastric juice that help in food digestion.

Hydrochloroquine Drug used in the treatment of arthritis.

Hydrochlorothiazide Drug used as diuretic in hypertension and in oedema.

Hydrocortisone Adrenocorticoid mainly glucocorticoid secreted by adrenal gland,

Main medical uses of hydrocortisone are:

- Asthma.
- Shock.
- Collagen disease.
- Severe inflammation.
- Hypersensitivity.
- Cancer treatment.

Hydroculator pack It is moist heat applied to arthritic patients to relieve pain

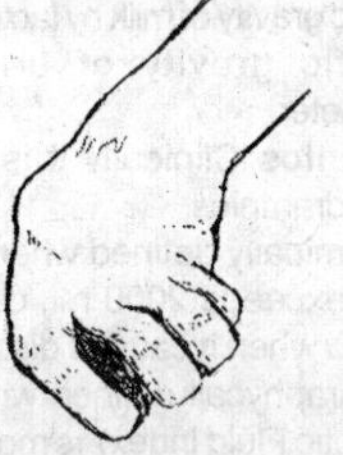

Hydroculator pack in arthritis

Hydrogen ion concentration Hydrogen ion concentration determines acidity or alkalinity of any body fluid. Normally blood pH is around 7.35, pH of below 7.0 is acidic and above 8.0 is alkaline.

Hydrogen peroxide Used as an antiseptic solution by using 10 volumes diluted in equal quantity of water.

Hydrogen peroxide Chemically greasy liquid and irritating odour , It is germicide, antiseptic and cleansing agent, its formula is H_2O_2.

Hydrogen sulphide It is a harmful gas with pungent odour, its formula is H_2S.

Hydrolase It is an enzyme which is responsible for hydrolysis.

Hydrol This is also known as Hydrone which is produced in the manufacturing process of glucose from cornstarch, it is liquor form.

Hydrolysis By utilising water, a salt is split into simpler substance, Chemically it can be represented as under:

Salt + Water → an acid.
Salt + Water → a base.

Hydrometer It is used to measure the density of a liquid, such as specific gravity of milk by lactometer, specific gravity of urine by urinometer.

Hydramnios Clinically it is called polyhydramnios,
Anatomically defined when liquor amnii exceeds 2000 ml, clinically defined when it causes discomfort Sonographycalli defined when AFI (Amniotic Fluid Index) is more than 20 cm.

Hydronephrosis Because of obstruction of urine, fluid is collected in renal pelvis which cause renal parenchymal atrophy
Urine collected in pelvis of kidney which forms a cyst,
Hydronephrosis leads to distension of kidney and later to atrophy of kidney.

Hydrophobia Rabies, painful spasm when seeing water in Rabies viral infection,
Fear to drink water a symptom in rabies infection.

Hydrops Clinically it is called dropsy where serous fluid is accumulated in body cavity (oedema), common clinical entity are:

- Ascites.
- Hydramnios.
- Hydrops of antrum of Highmore.
- Hydrops of joint.
- Beriberi.
- Meniere's syndrome.
- Hydrops of foetus.
- Hydrops of Graafian follicle.
- Angioneurotic oedema.
- Hydrosalphynx.

Hydrostatic test In this test, lung tissue of dead newborn is put to water, if it sinks it is inferred that newborn has not breathed before its death.

Hydrostatic Related to a liquid in a state of equilibrium.

Hydrotherapy Scientific method of water treatment in illness such as
Hot bath for fatigue
Cold water to constrict vessels
Hot water for vasodilatation.

Hydrothorax Accumulation of fluid in thorax due to inflammation.

Hydroureter Ureter is dilated due to some obstruction.

Hygiene Science that helps to keep physically and mentally fit through cleanliness of body and mind

Following types of hygiene are met with in the course of nursing activities:

- Personal hygiene.
- Environmental hygiene.
- Industrial hygiene.
- Mental hygiene.
- Oral hygiene.
- Community hygiene.

Hygienist Person technically trained in the principles of healthful living such as dental hygienist, industrial hygienist.

Hygroma A distended sac, a distended cyst or a distended bursa which is filled with fluid,

Common clinical entities are:

- Cystic hygroma.
- Subdural hygroma.

Hygrometer It is the instrument used to measure moisture of the atmosphere.

Hygroscopic That which absorbs water, such as glycerine suppository where glycerine helps to moisten stool for proper evacuation.

Hygroscopy It is the estimation of amount of moisture in the atmosphere.

Human behaviour It is human response to his surroundings

Stimulus	*Responses*
Snake	run away
Coin	pick it up'
Spits on face	hit him

Table: Human behaviour

Hymen It is a mucous membrane which closes vagina in virgins,

It perforates at the start of menstruation.

Hymenectomy Surgical excision of the hymen.

Hymenolepis One of the tapeworm called Hymenolepis nana which is called short tape worm.

Hymenorrhaphy Repair of ruptured hymen by plastic surgery.

Hymenectomy Surgical excision of hymen in case of imperforate hymen.

Hyoglossus This muscle is retractor of tongue and also draws sides down,

Its origin is hyoid bone and insertion is dorsum of tongue.

Hyoid Any anatomical structure which is shaped like "U"

Refers to hyoid bone above the hyoid cartilage which is attached to the tongue.

Hyoscine It is an anticholinergic drug used in premedication during anaesthesia, it has the property of antispasmodic

Common sea sickness remedies like Quells and Mothersils contain hyoscine hypobromide which is quick acting and effective.

Hyperacidity Excessive secretion of acid in gastric juice a symptom of gastric ulcer, can also be a psychosomatic disease.

Hyperaemia When a part or organ gets more blood supply, commonly due to vasodilatation.

Hyperalimentation In indicated cases of Gastroenteric pathology parenteral administration of nutrients is done,

Synonyms are total parenteral, nutrition and total parenteral alimentation.

Hyperalimentation technically mean total supplementary nutrition
Hyperalimentation procedurally do not mean and do not involve excessive quantity of feeding.

Hyperbaric oxygen Oxygen with very high pressure which is used in the following clinical conditions:
- Gas gangrene.
- Decompression sickness.
- Carbon monoxide poisoning.
- Air embolism.
- Chronic non-healing ulcers.

Hyperbaric Refers normally to atmosphere pressure which will be more than normal.

Hyperbilirubinaemia Raised level of bilirubin in the blood.

Hypercalcemia Raised level of calcium in the blood.

Hypercapnia Raised and abnormal level of carbon dioxide in the blood produce hypercapnia by stimulating respiratory centre.

Hypercholesteraemia High level of cholesterol in the blood leading to atheroma and gallstone.

Hyperemesis Vomiting which is more than our expectation,
Vomiting in pregnancy, also it is called hyperemesis gravidarum.

Hyperesthesia Very high perception, very high sensitiveness of skin,
Types of hyperesthesia are:
- Acoustic hyperesthesia.
- Auditory hyperesthesia.
- Cerebral hyperesthesia.
- Gustatory hyperesthesia.
- Olfactory hyperesthesia.
- Optic hyperesthesia.
- Sexual hyperesthesia.
- Tactile hyperesthesia.

Hyperextension In orthopaedic correction forced extension of limbs is done.

Hyperflexion Forced flexion of limb done which is little more than normal.

Hypergamma globulinaemia Clinical conditions where gamma globulin are increased in the blood level.

Hyperglycaemia Clinical conditions where blood glucose level is raised above the normal level as per the criteria fixed for fasting blood sugar or PPBS.

Symptoms of diabetes mellitus
Random blood sugar above 11.1 mmol per litre
Fasting plasma glucose above 7.0 mmol per litre
Two hour plasma glucose above 200 mg/dL by GTT

Table: Criteria for diagnosis diabetes

	Normal	*Hyperglycaemia*
	Impaired Glucose Tolerance	Diabetes Mellitus
FPG ‹ 110	110 – 125	≥ 126
2-h PG ‹ 140	140 – 199	≥ 200

Table: Glucose spectrum (Homeostasis)

FPG = fasting plasma glucose in mg/dL
2-h PG = 2 hour plasma glucose in mg/dL

Hyperglycaemia Glucose level in the blood is more than normal and is pathological.

Hyperhidrosis Too much of perspiration than expected in a patient.

Hyperkalaemia High quantity of calcium circulating in the blood which is deleterious to heart condition.

Hyperkeratosis Thickening of the skin described as hypertrophy of horny layer.

Hyperkinesis General term for hypermotility or hyperactivity of a person.
Refers to increased motor activity in general.

Hyperalimentation To achieve good growth, excessive intake of food or fluid therapy which contain all nutrients.

Hypermetropia Other name for long sightedness,
Image fall behind retina since rays entering eye converge beyond retina,

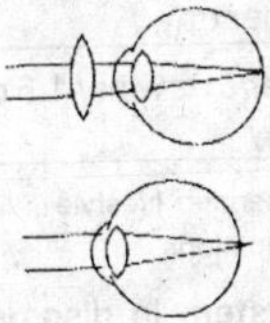

hypermetropia above picture under this is with correction by Convex lens for Hyperme-tropia, Below picture under this is before correction showing rays focussed behind retina.

Hypermotility Too much of movement of an organ such as intestinal hypermotility, gastric hypermotility.

Hyperostosis It refers to bony growth or excess bone growth which is felt as thickening of the bone.

Hyperparathyroidism Over activity of parathyroid gland leading to calcium drainage that result in fragility of bone and subsequent fractures.

Hyperpituitarism Over activity of pituitary gland leading to pathological conditions.

Hyperplasia Formation of normal cells are formed in excess leading to thickening of tissue or organ
When there is an increase in multiplication of normal cells giving rise to more number of cells in normal arrangement in tissues
Common clinical entities are:
- Endometrial hyperplasia.
- Inflammatory hyperplasia.
- Lipoid hyperplasia.
- Polar hyperplasia.
- Swiss cheese hyperplasia.
- Cement hyperplasia.

Overgrowth in numbers of tissue cells.

Hyperpnoea Increased rate of breathing which leads to hyperventilation.

Hyperpyrexia High body temperature to the level of 106^0 F (above 41^0).

Hypersensitivity Too much of reaction to foreign body or an antigen, Allergy and anaphylaxis conditions, Common types are;
- Immediate hypersensitivity.
- Delayed hypersensitivity.
- Contact hypersensitivity.

Hypersplenism Spleen enlargement which causes destruction of RBC and platelets.

Hypertension High blood pressure which is usually pathological,
In an individual if BP is persistently high at supine arterial systolic greater than 140 mm Hg and diastolic is greater than 90 mm Hg (when resting and taken on three consecutive days in early morning) hypertension is diagnosed.

Category	*Systolic BP*	*Diastolic BP*
Normal	‹ 120 mm Hg	‹ 80 mm Hg
Prehyper tension	120 – 139	80 – 89
Hypertension stage I	140 – 159	90 – 99
Hypertension stage II	≥ 160	≥ 100

Table: Classification of hypertension

Sleep apnoea
Drug induced or drug related
Chronic kidney disease
Primary aldosteronism
Renovascular disease
Cushing's syndrome
Steroid therapy
Pheochromocytoma
Coarctation of aorta
Thyroid disease
Parathyroid disease

Table: Identifiable causes of BP

Obesity BMI ≥ 30 kg/m²
Dyslipidaemia
Diabetes mellitus
Cigarette smoking
Physical activity
Microalbuminuria GFR ‹60 mL/min
Age above 55 men, above 65 women

Table: Risk factors of BP

Life style modification	*Recommendation*
Weight reduction	to maintain normal body weight Body mass index 18.5-24.9 kg/m²
DASH eating plan	Adopt a diet rich in fruits, vegetables and low fat dairy products with reduced content of saturated and total fat
Dietary sodium reduction	Reduce dietary sodium intake to ≤100 mmol per day (2.4 g sodium or 6 g sodium chloride)
Aerobic physical activity	Regular aerobic physical activity (like brisk walk)at least 30 min/day most days of the week
Moderation of alcohol consumption	Men ≤ 2 drinks* per day Women ≤ 1 drinks* per day

1 drink = 12 oz beer/5 oz wine/ 1.5 oz 80-proof whiskey

Table: Recommended lifestyle modifications

Hyperthermia system In disorder of hypothalamus, too much variation in body temperature occurs which is to be regulated with the help of Blanketrol which can keep the body temperature in required level.

Hyperthermia Raised body temperature,

Clinically at GA when high body temperature is noticed it gives signal to bad prognosis (Malignant hyperthermia).

Hyperthyroidism Hyperactivity of thyroid gland giving rise to clinical conditions which include thyrotoxicosis.

Hypertonic saline bath Hypertonic saline baths, 3 pounds of salt to 30 gallons of water may be ordered in the treatment of septic skin conditions.

Hypertonic Refers to high tone of muscle and vessels,
When a liquid has high osmotic pressure it is called hypertonic solution.

Hypertrichosis Abundant hair seen on the body or on any part of the body.

Hypertrophy The word denotes enlargement such as muscular hypertrophy,
Increased tissue growth leading to increase in size of an organ,
Sometimes equivalent to hyperplasia.

Hyperventilation Other word for hyperpnoea where prolonged and deep breathing occurs,
More of air in the lung field.

Hypervitaminosis This refers to consumption of large quantity of vitamins A and D leading to certain clinical manifestations.

Hyphaema An ophthalmic condition where bleeding into anterior chamber of the eye occurs.

Hypnosis The artificially created state which makes the individual to respond to any command, this is found useful in minor surgery normal childbirth and tooth extraction.

Hypnosis It is a state of suspended consciousness produced by the process of hypnosis by hypnotist

Hypnotic A substance that induces sleep or a state of suspended consciousness.

Hypnotism It is the traditional practice of hypnosis.

Hypocalcaemia Low level of calcium in the blood which give rise to certain clinical conditions.

Hypocapnia When carbon dioxide level is lowered in the blood.

Hypochlorite It is hypochlorous acid salt which is used as disinfectant and germicide.

Hypochondria Preoccupied mind which thinks a condition which really do not exist, a type of anxiety syndrome.

Hypochondriac Person who is afflicted with hypochondria.

Hypochondriac Obsession where a person imagines that he is ill and diseased.

Hypochromic Item which is less colour of its nature and deficient in pigmentation.

Hypocrine It refers to endocrine hypofunction.

Hypodermic Drug introduction just below the skin,
Subcutaneous injection by hypodermic needle.

Hypogastrium Lower middle area of abdomen which is just below umbilicus.

Hypoglossal nerve This 12th cranial nerve function can be tested by asking the patient to extend his tongue, if tongue quivers excessively or deviates to one side suggest nerve impairment.

Hypoglossal This mean that a structure is below the tongue, Usually refers to hypoglossal nerve which 12th cranial nerve.

Hypoglycaemia The patient with insulin shock is treated as emergency case,
After attending emergency protocol hypoglycaemia is treated by oral orange juice, dextrose, sugar.

Hyperkalaemia Low potassium level in the blood which is usually due to dehydration.

Hypometropia It refers to short sightedness.

Hyponatraemia Low sodium level in the blood.

Hypoparathyroidism Very less secretion of parathyroid gland leading to tetany which is as a consequence of low calcium level in the blood.

Hypophysis An outgrowth of an anatomical structure such as Hypophysis cerebri.

Hypopituitarism Low secretion of anterior lobe of pituitary gland causing Frolich's syndrome.

Hypoplasia Incomplete development of an organ due to dysgenesis.

Hypopnoea Patient who has shallow breathing.

Hypoproteinaemia Low level of protein in blood, established in frank starvation and severe malnutrition.

Hypospadias A birth defect where urethra opens below penis or on perineum
A condition in which the urethral meatus appears on the underside of the penis.

Hypostasis Sediment noticed in a liquid,
Congestion of a part due to poor circulation.

Hypotension Low arterial blood pressure of a patient,
Common clinical conditions are;
- Induced hypotension.
- Orthostatic hypotension.

Hypothalamus Anatomically floor and lateral wall of the third ventricle,
Hypothalamus includes the following:
- Optic chiasm.
- Mammillary bodies.
- Tuber cinereum.
- Infandibulum.
- Neurohypophysis.

Hypothermia system In case of lesion of hypothalamus where body temperature varies body temperature has to be maintained with the help of Blanketrol system.

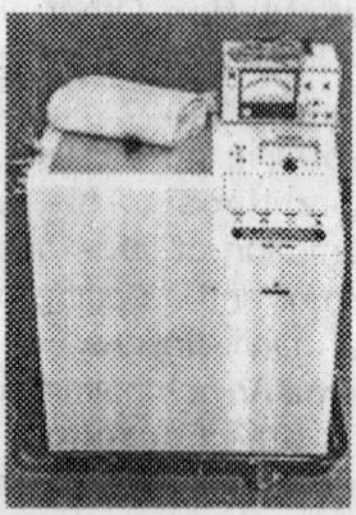

Blanketrol system

Hypothermia Very low body temperature of a patient in terminal illness,
Because of sudden exposure of newborn after birth to low temperature which is hazardous.

Hypothermia Is due to fall in body temperature since ambient temperature to which they are born is always by several degrees cooler than temperature in the womb, Newborn baby's body temperature is

99.5^0 F and hypothermia occurs if room temperature is below 97.5^0 F

---

1. After birth baby is quickly dried with clean cloth and wrapped with cotton clothing (Turkey Towel) (Two Towel method)
2. Skin to skin contact with mother at breastfeeding is allowed
3. Avoid bath to newborn for one week

Table: Hypothermia prevention

Hypothesis Assumption based on reasoning and experimentations in science,
Postulating hypothesis is the basis of medical investigations.

Hypothyroidism Deficiency of thyroid secretion leading to myxoedema in adults and cretinism in children.

Hypotonia It refers to reduced intraocular tension, it also refers to low muscular tone.

Hypoxemia If oxygen is below normal physiological level in the blood of a person.

Hypoxia If oxygen level or quantity is reduced in tissues.

Hysterectomy Surgical removal of uterus,in gynaecological intervention, we have the following types of hysterectomy

- Total hysterectomy.
- Subtotal hysterectomy.
- Vaginal hysterectomy.
- Abdominal hysterectomy.
- Wertheim's hysterectomy.

Hysteria Lack of control over acts and emotions called psychoneurosis,
Conversion of mental or emotional illness to physical symptoms,
It *should not be* confused with *hysterical.*

Hysteric chorea Hysteria with uncontrolled movements.

Hysterical fit Hysteria is manifested in the form of fit among young women which simulate epileptic fit,
Rigid muscle followed by violent jerky movements and without any stages, woman will be conscious and there is no incontinence of urine or faeces.

Hysteropexy Surgically fixing the uterus which is displaced,
According to the place of fixation it can abdominal hysteropexy or vaginal hysteropexy
Common gynaecological operation is called Manchester type operation which include:

- Ventral suspension of uterus.
- Shortening of round ligaments.
- Shortening of sacro-uterine ligaments.
- Shortening of endopelvic fascia.

Hysterotome A surgical instrument which is used to incise uterus.

Hysterotomy Caesarean section done to remove the foetus in obstructed labour,
Uterus is cut open to take out the foetus in cases of foetal distress and in maternal distress.

I

I P P breathing Intermittent Positive Pressure Breathing will assist patient in achieving deep long inflation while also promoting expectoration of secretions,

To facilitate lung expansion patient is assisted in Fowler's position unless it is contraindicated.

I Q It is a measure of a person's intelligence by a test.

Iatrogenic Infections, new reactions, side effects and psychological distress because of complications, rare medicaments, drugs and activities of health professionals are called iatrogenic effects,

Drug induced illness.

ICD It is the classification of diseases and causes of mortality by WHO which periodically revises as necessary,

The current 10th revision issued in 1992 is currently used, ICD is a member of family of WHO.

ICDS Integrated Child Development Services.

Ice bag poultice It is one of the local applications called cold application to relieve pressure and prevent swelling, it also causes increase of muscle tone

Ice skating It is now made a sports and are available in places where indoor ice rinks around the country is made available, can be all round season sports or seasonal sports depending upon ice availability.

Ice Water in the liquid state used clinically as ice bag applications.

Iceberg of disease Like an iceberg, presymptomatic and what health professional cannot see is exceedingly high and this is called iceberg of disease.

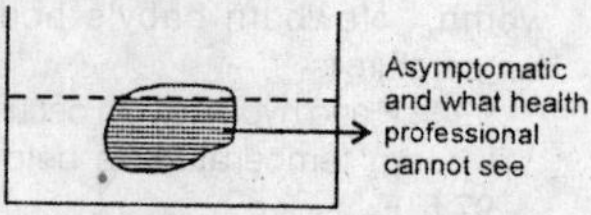

Iceberg of disease

Ichor Discharge from an ulcer which foul smells.

Ichthammol It is a cold tar product used in skin ointment.

Ichthyosis Dry, thick and horny layer of skin seen in a congenital abnormality of the skin.

Ichthyosis Xeroderma or fish skin disease characterised by rough, dry and scaly skin.

Icons Signs and pictures representing some meaning in a society

Examples:

Om = Hindu.
Moon = Muslim.
Cross = Christian.

ICSH Abbreviation for Interstitial Cell Stimulating Hormone.

Ictal Acute epileptic attack.

Icterus Clinical condition called jaundice, pregnancy jaundice and neonatal jaundice are common nursing care situations which need attention in hospital nursing care.

ICU Abbreviation for Intensive Care Unit.

Id It is in the state of unconsciousness the need that arises in a person.

Idea A conceptual idea of the mind, common types of ideas are:

i. Referred idea.
ii. Fixed idea.
iii. Compulsive idea.
iv. Dominant idea.

Identical Items those look alike such as twins.

Identification It is a state of mental mechanism through which the person points out to the correctness or adopts to an attitude
Person or a thing is identified by existing common characters,
Mole, scar, finger prints and other anthropometric values are used in identification of a person, dental charts and radiographs identify a person.

Identity Personality of self concept which can be differentiated, if this is lost we have identity crisis
Physical and mental characters which help to recognise a person.

Ideology It is the study of ideas and thoughts.

Idiopathic This refers to the clinical condition for which the cause cannot be ascertained.

Idiosyncrasy Susceptible to reactions of drugs or substances by a person, physical and mental status of an individual which is specific and peculiar to the given person.

Idiot Person with very low I Q which reflects severe mental deficiency.

Idoxuridine An iodine preparation which is used in certain clinical conditions such as
a) Keratitis
b) Dendritic corneal ulcer
c) Herpes infection.

Ig Abbreviation for immunoglobulin, common immunoglobulins are:
- IgA(milk, saliva, intestinal secretions, tears).
- IgD.
- IgE(mast cells).
- IgG.
- IgM.

IgA Immunoglobulin A which protects against mucosal invasion by pathogens.

Ill effects of iodine Iodine deficiency disorders are manifested in the form various disorders,
Since it is endemic, National Programme is taking care of it.

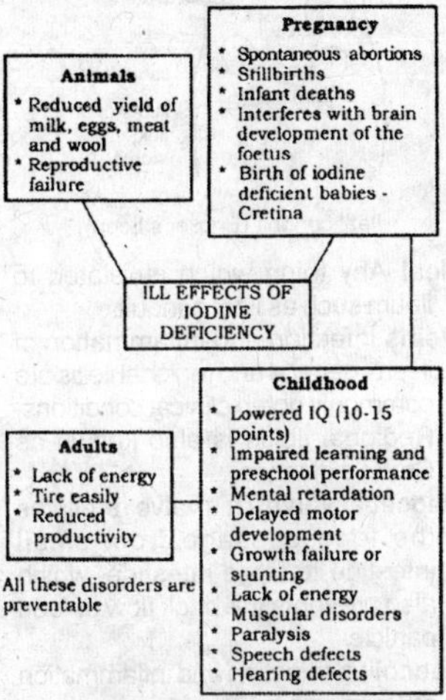

Ill effects of iodine deficiency

Immunochemistry It is the chemistry of antigen, antibody and antigen-antibody reaction.

Ileal by-pass Surgical anastomosis of small intestine with another portion of small intestine to reduce the absorption of nutrients and it is indicated in obesity.

Ileal conduit It is also called ileal loop, Bricker's loop or ileal bladder
A type of urinary diversion indicated in the following clinical conditions:
- Congenital anomalies.

- Bladder malignancy.
- Chronic urinary tract infections.
- Neurogenic bladder.
- Intractable incontinence.

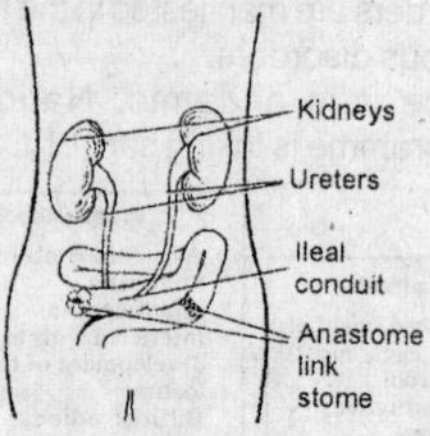

Ileal conduit (Bricker's Loop)

Ileal Any thing which is related to ileum such as ileal conduit.

Ileitis Infection and inflammation of ileum, general and regional ileitis are commonly noted clinical conditions, Regional ileitis is also known as Crohn's disease.

Ileocecal valve This valve regulates the food passage from small intestine to large intestine, which also prevents the back flow of food particle.

Ileocolitis Infection and inflammation of ileum and colon.

Ileocolostomy Surgical intervention to produce connection between ileum and some part of the colon Surgical anastomosis between ileum and colon.

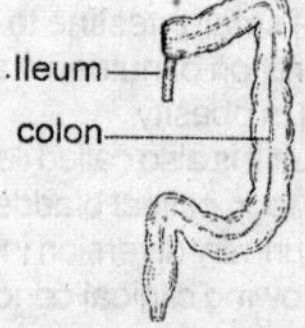

Ileocolostomy

Ileorectal That which is connected with both ileum and rectum such as ileorectal anastomosis.

Ileostomy Surgical creation of a stoma or an opening of ileum to the surface of the abdomen for the purpose of evacuation, temporary and permanent ileostomies are known

Surgical indications for ileostomy are:

i. Ulcerative colitis.
ii. Crohn's disease.
iii. Cancer.
iv. Trauma.
v. Familial polyposis.

Ileum Terminal portion of the small intestine which ends at caecum which form 3/5th of small intestine from jejunum to ileocaecal valve.

Ileus When there is no peristalsis this word is used, common causes are intestinal obstruction, peritonitis, Ileus is the common cause of shock and dehydration in surgical patients.

Iliac crest The upper portion of the pelvis on both sides is made of flat portion and this flat portion of the ilium which ends in a broad ridge is called iliac crest that can be felt close under the skin.

muscles of abdominal wall are attached to this iliac crest

Upper free margin of innominate bone.

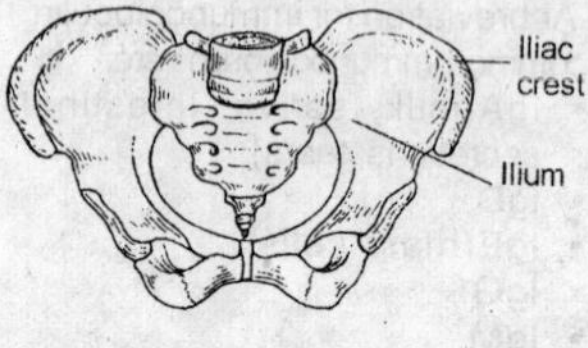

Pelvis showing iliac crest and ilium

Iliac fascia It is the transversalis fascia on the anterior surface of iliopsoas muscle.

Iliac region It lies on either side of the hypogastrium on inguinal region.

Iliac spine Spines of the ilium which can be any one of the following:
- Anterior superior iliac spine.
- Anterior inferior iliac spine.
- Posterior superior iliac spine.
- Posterior inferior iliac spine.

Iliac Anything that is related to ilium such as:
- Iliac artery.
- Iliac crest.
- Iliac vein.
- Iliac fossa.

Ilium This is the part of hip bone which has haunch appearance and the word is derived from the haunch bone.

Illness Person who is sick, there is deviation from physiological status to pathological status.

Illusion To believe an item which as such does not exist,
Mistaken perception of mentally ill patient.

ILO **I**nternational **L**abour **O**rganisation.

Image Referred to the image that is transmitted to brain by optic nerve,
Mental imagination of a person which is called recall phenomenon.

Imaging By using resonance (magnetic), ultrasound or X-ray image of an object is produced.

Imbalance When there is no balance in biological system such as:
- Muscular imbalance.
- Electrolyte imbalance.
- Endocrine imbalance.

No balance between opposing forces in the body such as: sympathetic and parasympathetic, vasodilatation and vasoconstriction

Imbecile Mentally defective and feebleminded person whose mental age is 2 to 7 years.

Imipramine A pharmaco therapeutic agent which is used in depression as antidepressant.

Immature It refers to any thing that is not well developed such as
- Mentally immature.
- Immature cataract.
- Immature behaviour.

Immiscible Those which do not mix with each other such as oil in water.

Immobilise Common term for keeping a part, organ or limb motionless through plaster of Paris or splints,
Postfracture treatment modality is immobilisation.

Immune response It is the response in human body for primary immunisation and for re-immunisation which are called primary and secondary immune response,
Immunological memory is developed by primary immune response
Booster immunisation is secondary immune response.

Immune response

Primary	*Secondary*
Long latent period	Short latent period
Slow antibody production	Rapid antibody production
Antibody titre is less good response seen for short time	Antibody titre is more Good response seen for long time
Binding capacity of antibody is less	Binding capacity of antibody is more

Table: Difference between primary and secondary immune response.

Immune When a person is immunised with selected active immunising agents.

When a person has the body resistance that he do not develop illness

Great tolerance.

Immunisation Development of body resistance through schedule of active and passive immunisations by vaccines.

Immunise By giving active immunising agent a particular disease can be prevented, Passive immunity can also be obtained by immunising with passive immunising agents.

Immunity When a person is not susceptible to disease,

It is the body resistance present in an individual to protect himself or herself from disease

Capability to overcome the response by an antigen, an infectious agent, by a toxic substance or by any foreign body

The capacity of the body to resist infection,

T cells and B cells are important for the establishment of immunity.

Immunoassay This is the method of quantitative analysis of protein in the blood serum which are responsible for the body immunity such as albumin, globulin, their ratios and immunoglobulins.

Immunoassay With the help of antigen-antibody reaction immunity is assessed.

Immunodeficiency Deficiency of the body immunity mechanisms.

Immunodiagnosis Immune response is used in the diagnosis of clinical conditions.

Immunofluorescence Examination of fluorescence in labelled antibodies with the help of fluore-scent microscope.

Immunoglobulin Mainly gamma globulins constitutes immunoglobulins.

Ig	*Source and actions*
IgA type I & II	Antiviral property Colostrum has secretory IgA Breast milk has secretory IgA Serum Useful in local immunity
IgD	Serum B cell surface receptor Has undermined immunity
IgE	Serum in allergy reaction increased Called reaginic antibody
IgG	Found abundant general immunity Cross placental barrier
IgM	Intravascular Primary antibody response

Table: Immunoglobulin highlighted

Immunology Science that deals with body immune mechanism and body defence mechanism in terms of antigen antibody reaction.

Immunopathology Tissue changes that occur as a consequence of allergy are studied.

Immunosuppressant Substance that reduce body immune response, that are useful in cases of autoimmune diseases

Immunosuppression Immune mechanism where formation of antibodies to antigens is not found, Important in transplantation of organ and tissues.

Immunotherapy Substance given to produce immunity in the body, Treatment with immunisation on man, usual in passive therapy and in leukaemia therapy

Immunotherapy Treatment given to enhance body immunity.

Impacted fracture Fragments of a fractured bone may be driven into each other and wedged into each other and wedged firmly together, Common example is the fracture of upper end of humerus.

Impaction Accumulated or wedged condition such as faecal impaction and dental impaction.

Impairment Usually referred to vision and hearing, if structural and functional changes in an organ, Psychological abnormality, loss of structure or function or both

Loss of structural and functional aspect with regard to anatomical, physiological and psychological abnormality.

ImpalpableThat which is not palpable, Refers to an organ or tumour on clinical examination such as spleen not palpable or cystic tumour not palpable.

Impedance Word meaning resistance offered by any matter such as sound wave impedance, current impedance.

Imperative When there is need, obligatory, when action take to place involuntarily.

Imperforate That which is not perforated or no opening is made, Always this refers to defects found in case of

- Imperforate hymen.
- Imperforate anus.

That which is not having opening such as Imperforate anus, imperforate hymen.

Impermeable Refers to cellular membrane which do not allow fluid flow or the movement of molecule.

Impervious That which cannot percolate, when there is difficulty for penetration.

Impetigo Highly contagious superficial skin infection caused by staphylococci and streptococci which is manifested in the form of pustules and scabs.

Implant Non-reactive substance is grafted to the tissue as a part of therapy, hormone pellet is implanted as contraceptive, IOL is implanted after cataract surgery, silicone is implanted in plastic surgery of breast

To graft or to insert or to implant a prosthetic device.

Implantation In natural sense fertilised egg getting implanted in the uterus, implants are put in therapy for cancers or for contraceptives, Healthy tissues are implanted after removing damaged tissues.

Implementation Is an administrative word in nursing profession where the nurse proceeds with defined nursing intervention and nursing goals.

Importance One which has greater relevance, One which has good association and dependence with another.

Impotence It usually refers to absence or failure of sexual function in male.

Impregnation Semen deposited for the purpose of fertilisation in human beings, sexual intercourse leading to pregnancy.

Impression tray It is dental tray to carry material required for taking impression to hold in opposition to teeth, Impression taking material in a tray for preparing denture.

Improvident maternity It is said to occur to a woman when the childbirth occurring to that women who has already given birth to three children of whom one is alive, This is about 42.8% in India.

Improvised splints In an emergency when regular splints are not available, they must be improvised from any suitable articles which are at hand,umbrella, walking stick, billiard cues, broomstick, rolls of card board, etc. Can be improvised splints.

Improvised stretchers It is easy to improvise a stretcher in case of emergency where door, board, window shutter etc., can be used, Most satisfactory improvised stretchers are:

Two overcoats with their sleeves turned inside out are spread out with their backs on the ground, long poles are threaded through the sleeves over which buttons are buttoned to made a suitable bed. Blanket or rug are used to carry a patient for a short distance through short step movement by carrying persons.

Impulse Pushing force in biological sciences, sudden involuntary act, Along with nerve fibres when electrochemical activity is transmitted it is called nerve impulse,

Heart beat causing the movement of chest wall is called cardiac impulse,nerve conduction that occur to produce muscle action or a stimulus, mind incitement.

IMR Abbreviation for **I**nfant **M**ortality **R**ate.

In coordination muscle movements cannot be coordinated , clinical conditions where muscular movements cannot be coordinated effectively.

In situ Latin word meaning the organ or a structure in its original position.

In vitro Experiment or study or reactions observed outside the body, opposite to *in vivo*, such as test tube babies, laboratory experiments.

In vivo Experiment or study or reactions observed within the body, opposite to *in vitro*, such as drug trial in human beings, experiment on human volunteers.

Inarticulate One who is not able to speak with articulated words, items that are not joined together.

Incarcerated that which is fixed in a localised area by other structures, such as uterus fixed in sacral brim and not moveable, such as hernia which is strangulated and cannot be reduced.

Incarnation Originally it refers to rebirth, in professional care it refers to growth of any tissue, organ or biological matter such as.

Conversion of material to flesh,

Nail growth particularly toe nails.

Incentive spirometer This instrument is used for a goal oriented and measurable exercise for breathing exercise which helps patients to increase their inspiratory volume while also inflating their alveoli.

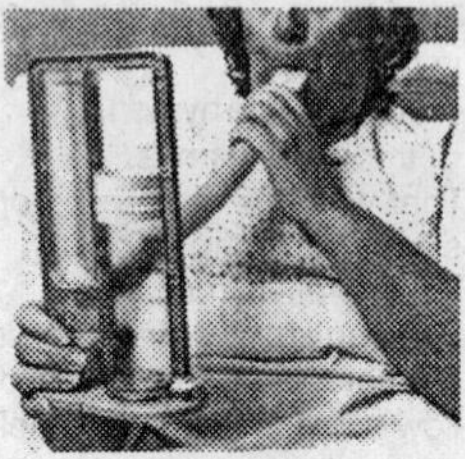

A : Incentive spirometer

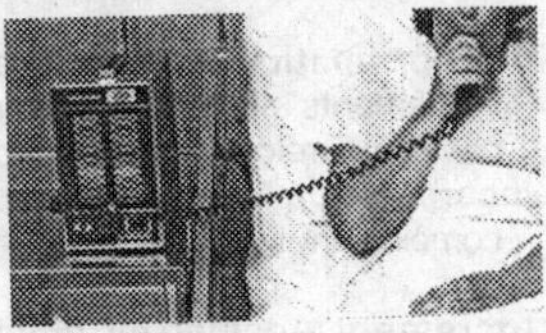

B: Incentive spirometer

Inception It refers to the meaning of from the beginning.

Incest One of the sexual offence where brother and sister indulge in sexual intercourse which is socially prohibited.

Incidence It is the events occurring in a population over a period of one year, particularly it refers to new events.

Incipient Made available in the given situation, the one which exists and starts existing or made available.

Incised wound A blow, sharp knife cut produce incised wound which show sharp edges which are well defined, they bleed profusely, they can be cleaned satisfactorily and heals with little scar.

Incise Cutting the skin, tissue, organ or any surgical procedure with surgical knife.

Incision Surgical cut by the knife during the course of an operation, incised wound by homicide situations, to cut the skin and soft tissue.

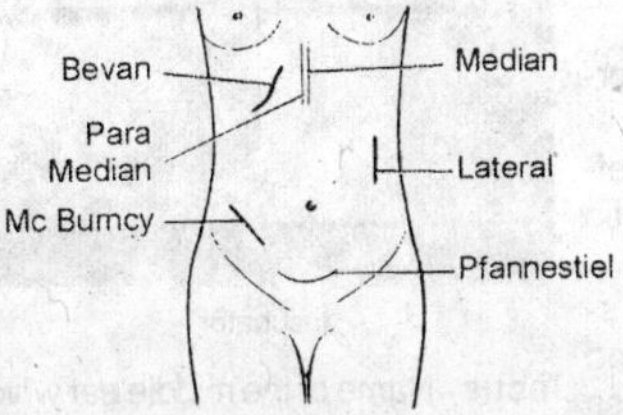

Various types of incision

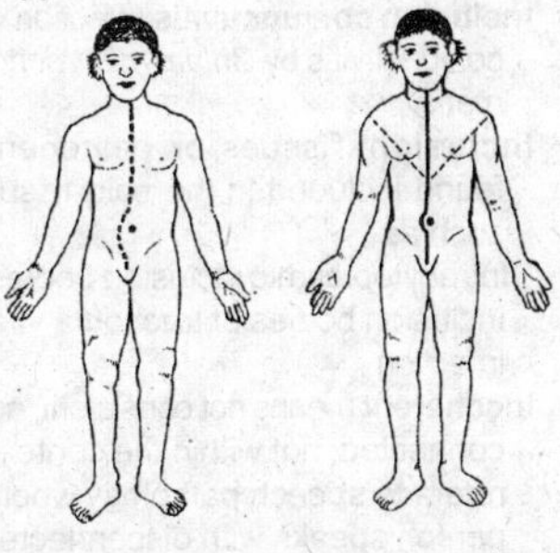

A : " I " Shape primary incisions at autopsy

B : " V " Shape primary incisions at autopsy

Primary incisions

Incisor It refers to front two teeth of upper jaw and front two teeth of lower jaw.

Incisura Presence of an indent at the edge of a structure such as stomach

Incisura(Indentation at the edge of distal end of lesser curvature).

Inclination To incline is to bend away from a vertical curvature or vertical line

In nursing profession usual reference is to an inclined tooth, inclined spinal column.

Inclusion bodies They are granular eosinophilic or basophilic accumulation within the cytoplasm or nucleus of cell such as representing the remnants of pathogens or substances eg.,

- Negri Bodies (Rabies)
- Mallory bodies (Alcoholichepatitis)
- Councilman bodies (Acutehepatitis)
- Russel bodies (Proteinaceoussubstance).

Inclusion conjunctivitis Infection of conjunctivitis by *Chlamydia trachomatis*.

Inclusion Tissues or pathogens found included in the said tissue such as

Intracytoplasmic inclusion bodies, inclusion bodies of trachoma viral infection.

Incoherent means not consistent, not connected, not within the context, refers to speech pathology where person speaks with disconnected speech

Not understandable speech.

Incompatibility It refers to blood incompatibility where one person's blood may not match with other person's blood,

Within the body when two substances antagonise each other,

When a mixture of drugs show antagonising property on each other.

Incompatible Not adjustable, not harmonious such as Rh incompatibility.

Incompetence That which is not efficient, such as aortic incompetence and mitral incompetence

When heart valve show inefficiency in regulating blood flow.

Incontinence Not able to control bowel movement (Faecal incontinence)

Not able to control urination (Overflow incontinence)

Not able to control urination or defecation in nerve paralysis (paralytic incontinence).

Incontinence During unconsciousness, apoplexy, epilepsy and infantile convulsion patients pass urine or motions involuntarily.

In coordination No coordinated movements in muscles present in certain neurological disturbances.

Incorporation To incorporate or to combine any two materials to make one.

Increment Addition of number, addition in size or addition of extent of an organ, tissue or cell,

Usually refers to growth and development in human life cycle.

Incubation Development of embryo or pathogens,

Period taken for this development is called incubation period.

Incubator A contained space with regulated temperature and humidity for a premature baby,

A contained space with regulated temperature and humidity for the growth (culture) of organism.

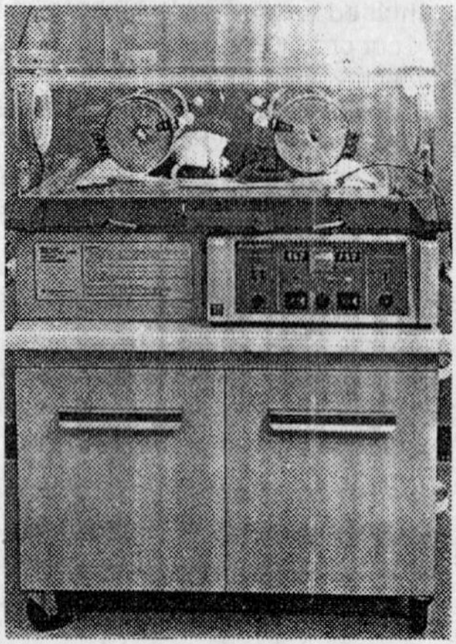

Incubator

Incus Name of the middle ear which is also called auditory ossicle.

Index case In investigations, we survey first case which is the initial case which can lead to further investigation.

Index of quality of life There are 2 indices, They are:

- PQLI (**P**hysical **Q**uality of **L**ife Index) which considers.
- IMR, Life expectancy and literacy which varies from 0 to 100.
- HDI (**H**uman **D**evelopment **I**ndex) which considers life expectation.
- Literacy and income which varies from 0 to 1.

Indian Red Cross Society There are many branches across the country executing relief work during earthquake, floods, drought and disease epidemics.

Indicator of RCH They indicate the status of health of mothers and children,
Main indicators are:

- MMR.
- Foetal deaths.
- Stillbirth rate.
- Perinatal mortality rate.
- Neo natal mortality rate.
- Postneonatal mortality rate.
- IMR.
- Child death rate.
- Child mortality rate (Under 5 mortality).
- Child survival index.

Indicator Chemical substance which show or indicate the appearance or disappearance by a chemical reaction, chemical substance that indicate pH at which it produce a change in colour,
Used in the qualitative analysis of a chemical substance
Name given to the index finger because it indicates,
Name given to the extensor muscle of the index finger because it is the extensor muscle of the index finger.

Indicators of class Both by objective and subjective, an individual's exact class position is ascertained.

Indigenous dais They are called TBA (Traditional Birth Attendant), They are trained by giving 1 month training with 300/- stipend, after training they are provided with a delivery kit, she gets 10/- for every registered case of pregnancy and 3/- for every registered infant.

Indigenous Normally occurring in a locality as a natural phenomenon such as malaria fever, monkey fever.

Indigestion Digestive upset due to various reasons, dyspepsia.

Indirect standardisation Standard mortality ratio is more common and useful form and is calculated by

$$SMR = \frac{\text{Observed deaths}}{\text{Expected deaths}} \times 100$$

Indole Product of tryptophan which is due to bacterial decomposition present in human faeces
A product derived from Indigo,
Chemically it is

$$\underline{|\ C_6H_4CH{:}CH.NH\ |}$$

Indolent Refers to chronic ulcer of skin ulcer which do not heal, slow growing and painless.

Indomethacin Anti-inflammatory drug used in gout and arthritis.

Induction Those which initiate common terminology in nursing practice are:

- Induction of abortion.
- Induction of labour.
- Induction of anaesthesia.
- Electromagnetic induction.

Induration Hardened tissue or hardened organ,
This is observed after 72 hours of giving test dose which confirm early introduction of an antigen (in case of Mitsuda reaction, Fernandez reaction, tuberculin test, other skin tests).

Industrial health Recognising the importance of preserving the health and safety of workers many industries have organised safety programmes and preventive industrial health programmes.

Industrial nursing Nursing care is a requisite in factories where more than 500 workers are employed, Care of the sick, injured, first aid, safety crèche, rehabilitation and nursing administration are the main nursing care activities in an industry.

Industrial poisoning Certain chemicals employed in industry are liable to produce harmful effects among workers, skin changes, dermatitis,
General signs of poisoning are common,

Chemicals, inorganic	Lead, arsenic, phosphorus, mercury, chromic acid, radium
Chemicals, organic	Aniline, trinitrotoluene, asbestos
Poison gases	1. CO and CO_2 which are asphyxiants 2. Ammonia and nitrous fumes hich are irritants 3. Volatile solvents which give away toxic vapours

Table: Harmful industrial chemicals

Industrial safety It is on-the-job safety, they include engineering devices,
Medical care to workers, provision of protective devices, and welfare schemes and legal protection to the workers.

Industrial Pertaining to an industry such as Industrial Act, industrial hazard.

Indwelling catheter Performing a catheterisation with a Foley or indwelling catheter need following nursing considerations:
a) Coil and secure the drainage tubing to the bed linen.
b) Keep the drainage bag below the level of patient's bladder.
c) One indwelling catheter in one ward minimises cross-infection.
d) Encourage fluid intake if patient is not a cardiac case or renal failure case.
e) Hand irrigation only when obstructed.
f) Check for urinary infection signs.
g) Inspect and cleanse perineal are a during bath.

Inebriation Reaction of a person who has take too much alcohol.

Inert Silence and that which do not react such as inert gas.

Inertia Slow and sluggish, a common term used in slowed down delivery is uterine inertia.

Infant care Health care given to the newborn during the period of first one year to see that it will not be afflicted with any illness,
This includes immunisation, nutritional care and other family welfare activities.

Infant feeding Early months of life baby gets breast milk which is it's staple food,
Breastfeeding up to 4 to 6 months followed by weaning and supplementation for good growth and development are the requisites of infant feeding.

Infant mortality This is the best index of RCH care or MCH care in the community
The rate is expressed per thousand live births,
Majority of causes are preventable.

Infant parasite rate This is one of the main malaria measurement in the community,
It is the percentage of infants who show M.P.smear +ve.

Infant Child between the age of 0 to 1 year,
Associated terminologies are infant feeding and infant mortality.

Infanticide Child is killed between the age of 0 to 1 year,
Killing of an infant.

Infantile paralysis This is the colloquial name for poliomyelitis a viral infection in the community which produce paralysis among infants.

Infantile Childishness or related to infant such as infantile paralysis.

Infarct Area of necrosis in the heart due to blocking of blood supply, haemorrhagic infarcts are red in colour, *'White infarct'* is used in the case of very poor blood supply producing paleness.

Infarction It refers to the formation of an infarct,
Common types in nursing practice are:

- Myocardial infarction.
- Pulmonary infarction.

Infarction Usually refers to heart attack, Here an area of tissue death occurs due to blockage of circulation.

Infection Entry, development and tissue damage by pathogens,
Associated terminologies are:

- Aerobic infection.
- Anaerobic infection.
- Air borne infection.
- Droplet infection.
- Hospital acquired infection.
- Iatrogenic infection.
- Cross-infection.
- Resistant infection.
- Severe infection.
- Mixed infection.
- Secondary infection.
- Sexually transmitted infection
- Subclinical infection.

Infection Introduction and development of illness by microbes like bacteria, virus, rickettsia and parasites.

Infectious mononucleosis One of the acute communicable disease transmitted as droplet infection or by direct contact probably a viral origin.

Infectious Diseases that are communicated to others through infection examples are diphtheria, whooping cough, measles, mumps, german measles, chickenpox, etc.

Infective That which is infected or a person who is infected and harbours pathogen thereby is responsible for producing infection.

Inferior Anatomically specify that it is lower such as inferior vena cava.

Infertility Not fertile, one who cannot produce offspring, unable to become parent (father or mother).

Infestation Parasite infecting on the surface of the body like lice, mites.

Infiltration Fluid percolating to the cell

or tissue which are not their original place.

Inflammation Reaction of cell or tissue to injury or infection, marked by redness,pain, swelling and heat, Common types of inflammation are:

- Acute inflammation.
- Chronic inflammation.
- Diffuse inflammation.
- Suppurative inflammation.
- Traumatic inflammation.
- Catarrhal inflammation.

Inflatable splints Common item in ambulance, it takes up little storage space and is easy to apply and comfortable for the patient.

Influenza A group of viruses which produce Flu or Coryza in man which is manifested as upper respiratory infections.

Informed consent Professional ethics to obtain a sort of permission or consent by patient by informing him or her about the nature of treatment being given,

Formal acceptance by the patient for treatment, surgery or any type of intervention

Real, adequate information or knowledge about research in understandable language when given to human volunteers in human volunteer research constitutes INFORMED CONSENT.

Infrared They are the rays beyond the red end of the light spectrum, They are useful as heat sources in medical treatment in the form of U V rays.

Infundibulum Latin word meaning funnel, refers to funnel like passage such as:

- Renal infundibulum.
- Hypothalamic infundibulum.
- Ethamoidal infundibulum.

Infusion pump They are indicated for patients who need accurate and carefully monitored flow rates as well as those for whom positive pressure is required for the delivery of highly viscous solutions,

Abbott life care model 3 pump are commonly used as infusion pumps.

Infusion Slow introduction of glucose, dextrose or other medicamentation through vein with the help of gravity, extraction of ingredients by soaking them in water by infusion method.

Ingestion Act of food eaten, Act of consuming the drug.

Ingrown nail Nail edge grows deep into soft tissues giving rise to clinical symptoms such as inflammation and pain.

Inguinal canal Anatomical canal which provides passage for round ligament in females and spermatic cord in males is about ½" long,

This is a weak point that cause inguinal hernia and undescended testis.

Inguinal ligament This is Poupart's ligament that extends from anterior superior iliac spine to public tubercle which is a fibrous band.

Inguinal region Anatomically on either side of pubes the iliac region form inguinal region.

Inguinal That which is related to groin such as inguinal ligament, inguinal canal, etc.

INH Abbreviation for **I**so **N**icotinic **H**ydrazide or Isoniazid.

Inhalant medication For pulmonary disorders nebuliser is used to administer an inhalant solution, Nebuliser medication.

Inhalation of vomit This is very important in case of asphyxia where resuscitation is done, When breathing has stopped action is taken for artificial respiration by mouth to mouth respiration is given and when once the breathing has started patient is gently turned over into the *recovery position* to *avoid risk of inhaling* vomit which is dangerous.

Inhalation Air drawn by inspiration to the lung, drug used in the form of nebuliser or aerosols.

Inhaler An apparatus used for inhalation of drug in the form of aerosols.

Inherent A character that is natural to a person by nature, an innate characteristic of man specific and peculiar to him.

Inheritance Qualities acquired from parents and grand parents by a person.

Inhibition Arrest of a biological process such as growth inhibition, Involuntary restraining of an instinct by a person.

Injectable hormone Women who use this method receive injections to prevent pregnancy, common preparations are:

a) DMPA (**D**epot **M**edroxy **P**rogesterone **A**cetate).

b) NET-EN (**N**or **E**thisterone **En**antate).

Injection Giving medicamentation to a person by route other than mouth, Types of injections are:

- Subcutaneous injection.
- Intradermal injection.
- Intravenous injection.
- Hypodermic injection.
- Depot injection.
- Intrathecal injection.

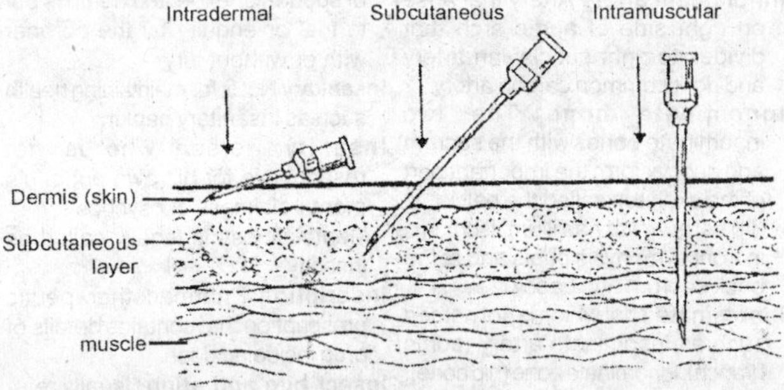

Routes of injections

Injury Damage that occur to cell, tissue or organ.

Ink stain removal In nursing care ink removal from linen are as under:

1) Soaking the linen in cold water for 24 hours.
2) Soaking the cloth in milk for 24 hours.
3) Rubbing a paste of salt and lemon juice on the ink and allowing it to dry in sun.
4) Ball pen ink is removed by the application of methylated spirit.

Inlay Tissue defect if replaced by a nonreactive material as therapeutic measure such as metal cast to fill the hole in the tooth.

Innate Any character that is present since birth or that which is inborn.

Innervations It refers to the nerve supply to an anatomical part or structure.

Innocent In nursing practice the word means that a tumour is benign or that which is not cancerous.

Innocuous Refers to material or drug which is harmless to the human body.

Innominate artery Artery that arise on right side of aortic arch that divides to right subclavian artery and right common carotid artery.

Innominate bone The two innominate bones with the sacrum and coccyx form the important part of the skeleton called the pelvis,

Hip bone which has ilium, ischium , in front symphysis pubis and at the back sacrum and coccyx.

Innominate That which is not named such as innominate artery (aortic branch), innominate bone (hip bone).

Inoculation For producing body immunity introduction of vaccine to man,

For culture of pathogens suspected material is introduced into the media.

Inorganic Substance which is not derived from animal or from vegetable.

Inositol Simple sugar from plant or from muscle which do not have the property of sugar, but has the formula of sugar

Part of B complex group of vitamins.

Inotropic Beta blocking agents are called inotropic because they affect the heart muscle contraction.

Inpatient Patient who is admitted to a hospital for treatment of ailments.

Input output analysis Input like nursing manpower, money, material, time spent and output like lives saved, transfusion done, first aid provided,injections given etc., are accounted, Here we can analyse "X" input which yield "Y" output and correct the fallacies in nursing device administration.

Inquest In forensic science, enquiry of sudden unexpected death is put to trial or enquiry by the coroner with or without jury.

Insanitary Not fit for maintaining health such as insanitary napkin.

Insanity Person who is not responsible for his own act in his mental sickness or psychosis,

Mental illness is legally called as insanity.

Inscription Pharmacotherapeutic prescription that contains details of drug including dose.

Insect bite and sting Usually referred to bee, vasp and biting insects which produce hypersensitivity reactions.

Insect repellent Dimethylphthalate or Dibutyl phthalate which are used as insect repellent to avoid the bite of mosquito and other insects,
It helps to discourage the bite of insects,
Commonly it refers to mosquito repellent.

Insecta This is the major group of phylum arthropoda which have common morphological characters like head, thorax, abdomen, 2 pairs of wings and three pairs of legs.

Insecticide Chemical compounds that are used to kill insects such as DDT, BHC, malathion, etc.

CHEMICAL CONTROL OF ARTHROPODS OF PUBLIC HEALTH IMPORTANCE

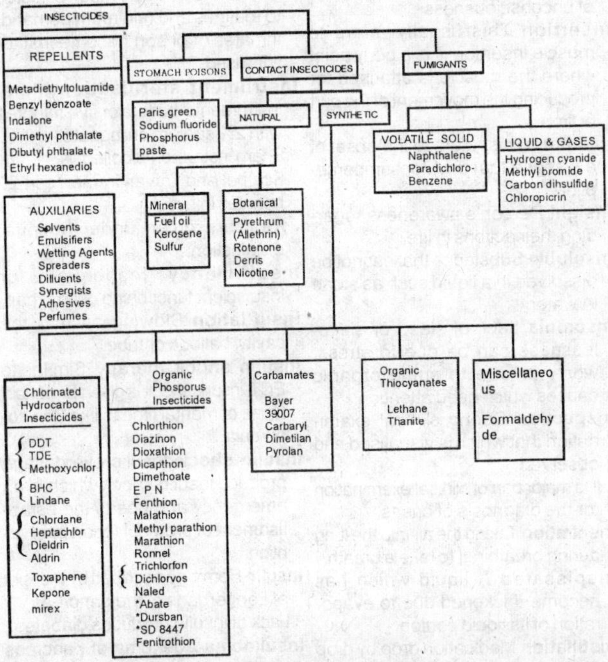

Insecticides commonly used

Insemination Introduction of semen into vagina at orgasm during the act of intercourse which is called natural insemination,

Artificially when semen is introduced into vagina forms artificial insemination which may be by using Husband's semen or by using Donor's semen which are called AIH and AID respectively.

Insensible When sense of perception is lost this happens in the state of unconsciousness.

Insertion This usually refers to muscle insertion, it is a bony point where the muscle is attached for producing the movement of the part or limb.

Insidious This refers to the onset of a disease that develops imperceptibly.

Insight Person's awareness regarding their actions in life.

Insoluble Substance that cannot be dissolved in a liquid such as stone in water.

Insomnia Lack of sleep or sleeplessness can be due to stress, worry or due to some organic causes which need attention.

Inspection During clinical examination that which is visualised and observed

It is major part of clinical examination for the diagnosis of cases.

Inspiration Taking the air into the lung during breathing, to take a breath.

Inspissated A liquid which has become thickened due to evaporation of its liquid portion.

Instillation Medication drop by drop either to eye or to the ears.

Instincts Human body is endowed with many feelings which protect life, and are called instincts, common ones are:

a) Fear.
b) Sex.
c) Hunger.
d) Pain.
e) Death.
f) Group action (Herd).

Institutionalisation After having stayed in an institution, person does not like to leave the institution since he has become very much adjusted to routines and minimum demand, inmates of prison become institutionalised.

Instrument sterilisation Metal instruments boiled for five minutes with 2% sodium carbonate

Sharp instruments boiled

Scalpel and knives immerse in 20 minutes in Lysol

Rest are given under hospital disinfection.

Insufficiency Inadequate or insufficient functioning of an organ.

Insufflation Blowing air into the cavity, balloon or tube.

Insulin shock therapy Similar to ECT, insulin shock is given for certain types of mental illness like Schizophrenia.

Insulin shock Insulin overdosage produce insulin shock which is an emergency and needs the establishment of protocol for an intervention.

Insulin Hormone secreted by the islet of Langerhans of the pancreas,

Lack of insulin produces diabetes.

Insulinoma Adenoma of pancreas which produce hypoglycaemia.

Insult Mental trauma or physical trauma by injury.

Integrated vector control Following are the major measures through integrated vector control:
a) Residual spray.
b) Antilarval measures.
c) Personal protection.
d) Control of breeding places by intermittent irrigation and source reduction.

Integument Tissue that covers the body of an organ, usually it refers to skin.

Intelligence Good mental ability to understand, It is measured by a quotient,

$$I.Q. = \frac{\text{Mental age}}{\text{Chronological age}} \times 100$$

Level of Intelligence	*IQ*
Genius	140 and above
Very superior	120 to 139
Superior	110 to 119
Normal	90 to 109
Low normal	80 to 89
Borderline	70 to 79
Moron	50 to 69
Imbecile	25 to 49
Idiot	0 to 24

Table : Level of Intelligence

Intensive care unit An established unit for the treatment of critically ill, Here special equipment and trained medical personnel are made available including emergency treatment.

Intention This refers to healing which can be primary or secondary by definition.

Intercellular Refers to structure between cells such as connective tissue and fluid.

Intercostals Means that an item or structure is between ribs.

Intercourse This refers to interchange of ideas and to sexual intercourse.

Interdisciplinary Joint effort by Medical profession, Nursing profession and other para medical professions,
Refers to planned team work.

Interferon Viral infection produces interferon which is a protein, Interferon inhibits the invasion of virus.

Intergluteal Anatomical position to express that which is in between two buttocks.

Interlobular Refers to between lobules such as interlobular vein

Intermammary Anatomical position to express that which is in between two breast.

Intermenstrual Event that occur in between two menstruation cycle

Intermission Refers to fever which stops in-between to recur again.

Intermittent That which occurs at a given interval,
Common clinical examples are:
- Intermittent fever.
- Intermittent claudication.
- Intermittent positive airway ventilation.
- Intermittent mandatory ventilation.

Intermittent fever Fever followed by normalcy and again fever, Fever which has in between absence of symptoms between paroxysms.

Intermittent infusion therapy is done by intermittent infusion set which is an indwelling reservoir in the vein for intermittent infusion therapy when continuous infusion therapy is not indicated.

Intermittent positive pressure This is adopted when patient needs deep lung inflation and there is a need for promotion of expectoration of secretions.

Internal bleeding Usually refers to GI bleeding and brain haemorrhage in clinical practice.

Internal ear Innermost part of ear (sensory organ) which contain Cochlea, semicircular canals and vestibule.

Internal medicine It refers to general medicine, treatment through clinical diagnosis and through therapeutic agents, non-surgical in nature.

Internal respiration Type of respiration or a portion of respiration that takes place inside an organism.

Internal secretion It refers to the secretions of ductless glands, hormones.

Internal skeleton Bony framework of human body, which also grows along with other tissues.

Internal Situated inside or occurring inside such as internal haemorrhage
Internal secretion.

International code of medical ethics In 1963 this was made available which is the guideline in medical and nursing profession, It depicts the following:
- No judgement on behalf of the patient.
- No self advertisement unless permitted by law.
- Referral done for fee is prohibited
- Dignity in discharging duty as a doctor.
- Safeguarding the patient's confidence.
- Using only professional channels for discovery.
- Act only in the patient's interest.
- No certification without verification.
- Loyalty, confidentiality and humanitarian on duty.
- Respect for professional colleagues.

International code It refers to international code of medical ethics which is based on WHO proposed guidelines.

International Council of Nurses Popularly known as ICN which is conglomeration of associations of nurses across the world,this was founded in 1899 which is now a corporate organisation.

Intern Young doctor who has just graduated but needs practical training of clerkship under senior doctor to get final degree,
Final experience gaining in a hospital after passing a degree.

Internist Doctor who has specialised in internal medicine.

Interphase Phase between cell divisions at which time chromosomes are not seen.

Intersex Person who displays male and female personality,
Birth defect with anatomical features of male and female are present.

Interstitial Structure in between tissues such as:
- Interstitial fluid.
- Interstitial keratitis.
- Interstitial cell stimulating hormone.
- Interstitial nephritis.

Intertrigo Moist skin surfaces chafing produce eczematous eruptions.

Intertrochanteric That which is situated between greater trochanter and lesser trochanter.

Intervention Procedures and measures adopted to bring back the patient to normalcy by different modes and at different levels

By taking appropriate action normalcy is regained in patients.

Primary		*Secondary*	*Tertiary*	
Health Promotion	Specific Protection	Early diagnosis and Treatment	Disability limitation	Rehabilitation
* Health education * Life style change * Use protected water * Mosquito control *Food fortification	* Immunisation * IFA prophylaxis * Chemoprophylaxis * Seat belt, helmet * Food safety	* TB patient * Leprosy case * Hypertension case * Cancer cervix case * Severe malnutrition	* Physiotherapy polio case * IV fluid to severe dehydration * Bed rest, sedation to IHD * IV therapy in severe malaria * IV therapy in meningitis	* Artificial limb to limbless * Gardener job to leprosy cured * Family restoration of TB cured * Brill schooling to blind * Reconstructive surgery to leprosy patient

Examples of intervention therapy in prevention

Intervertebral disc The bodies of vertebrae are separated by thick pads of cartilage called intervertebral discs which are liable for injury and common clinical condition is *disc prolapse*.

Intervertebral Refers to as between the vertebra such as intervertebral disc.

Interview Interviews are done to collect information, they are also done for the purposes of counselling which can be directive type and non-directive type.

Intestinal Which refers to intestinal or which pertains to intestine

Intestinal juice This refers to maltase, lipase, peptidase and sucrase that are secreted in the intestine, they are enzymes required for food digestion.

Intestinal obstruction Intestinal lumen is blocked by various pathological and functional reasons such as:

- Stricture.
- Worms.
- Fibrous bands.
- Foreign body.
- Stones.
- Hairs.
- Faecalith.

Intestinal tube They are commonly used in the following conditions:

- Gavage.
- Decompression.
- Medication instillation.
- Splinting of the small bowel after anastomosis.

Common intestinal tubes that are used in surgical practice are:

- Single lumen type.
- Double lumen tube.
- Jejunostomy tubes.

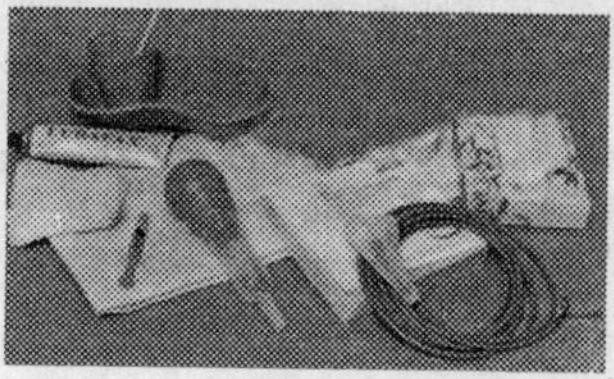

Intestinal tube

Intestine Part of GI system that contains part from stomach to anus, This is divided into 2 portions

Small intestine - Contains duodenum, jejunum, ileum about 6 meters in length

Large intestine - Contains caecum, ascending colon, transverse colon, descending colon and rectum about 2 meters in length.

Intima On transverse section what we see as innermost layer of an artery or of a vein.

Intolerance In nursing practice, we use the word idiosyncrasy where person cannot tolerate certain drugs, May be effect of some drugs on an individual.

Intoxication Intoxicated with excess of alcohol,

Toxic reaction by poisons consumed by a person.

Intra-abdominal That which is within the abdomen.

Intra-articular That which is within the joint capsule such as intra-articular injection of cortisone.

Intra atrial That which is within the atrium of the heart such as intra-atrial thrombosis.

Intracerebral That which is within the brain such as intracerebral haemorrhage.

Intracranial pressure The pressure by CSF within the sub-arachnoid space and ventricles of the brain.

Intracranial It refers to an item within the skull such as:

- Intracranial pressure.
- Intracranial aneurysm.
- Intracranial abscess.

Intradermal Is the type of injection of medication or test drug to the body, common intradermal injections are Mantoux test and allergy testing,Most frequently ventral aspect of the forearm is selected though there are many located sites for intradermal injection.

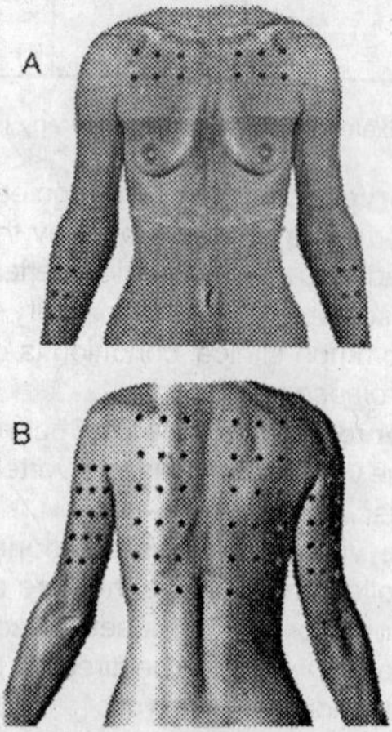

Intradermal injections site

Intracapsular Refers to within the capsule of a joint such as intra-capsular extraction.

Intracellular Refers to within the cell such as intracellular fluid.

Intractable Relief, cure or control cannot be obtained.

Intradermal Medicamentation given in between the skin layers.

Intradural Refers to within the dura mater such as intradural haemorrhage.

Intragastric That which is within the stomach.

Intrahepatic That which is within the liver.

Intralobular That which is within the lobule.

Intramedullary That which is within the bone marrow or within the medulla oblongata.

Intramuscular Medicamentation given to the muscle mass commonly to deltoid or gluteal muscles.

Intranasal That which is within the nose.

Intraocular That which is within the eyeball.

Intraorbital That which is within the orbit of the eyeball.

Intraosseous That which is within the bone tissue.

Intrapartum Events that occur during childbirth.

Intraperitoneal That which is within the peritoneal cavity.

Intrathecal That which is within the meninges of spinal cord which refers to subarachnoid space.

Intratracheal That which is within the trachea, endotracheal.

Intrauterine That which is within the uterus, common nursing terminology are:

- Intrauterine life.
- Intrauterine growth retardation.
- Intrauterine douche.
- Intrauterine contraceptive device.

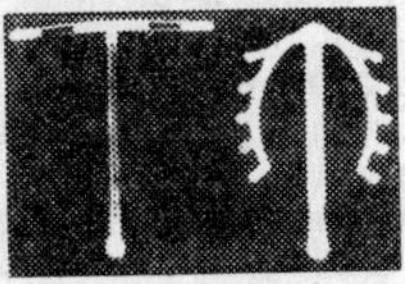

Copper T and multiload MLCu 375

Intravenous Method of giving drug or medicamentation through vein, Emergency medication method, Method of giving nutrition to patients.

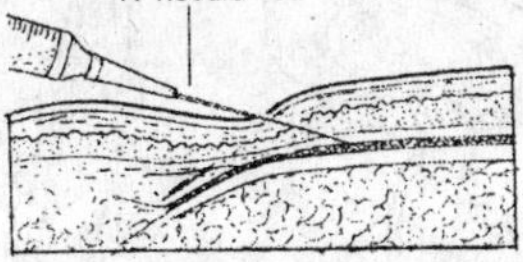

I V needle in position

Intraventricular Within the ventricle of the heart or ventricle of the brain.

Intercurrent One disease superimposed on another, occurring simultaneously.

Intrinsic Internal such as intrinsic factor, essential nature of a thing.

Introitus Refers to the opening into a hollow organ, common term for vulva or introitus vaginae.

Introversion Loss of interest with the external world,
An organ turning to within itself.

Introvert Opposite to extrovert which means person who do not give outwardly reaction,
Person who keeps everything to himself.

Intubation Introduction of a tube to the air way, Done during anaesthesia or at the time of emergency airway creation in asphyxia.

Intuition Knowing a thing that can occur ahead of a time,information in advance, spontaneously in advance.

Intumescence Inflammatory reaction and swelling of nasal mucosa in catarrh.

Intussusception Collapsing of one part of intestine into the lumen of adjacent part of intestine causing intestinal obstruction

Invagination.

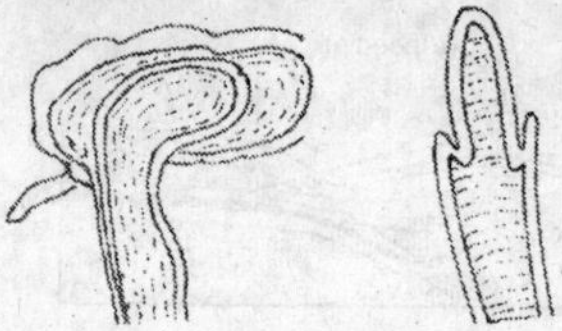

Intussusception

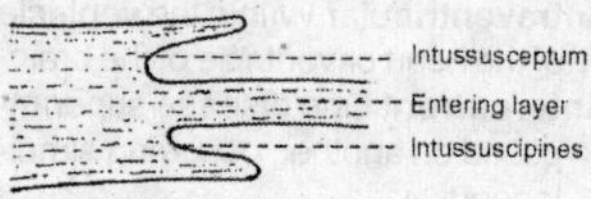

Parts of intussusception

Inunction Application of skin preparation on to the skin as therapy,

Rubbing of medicine externally for absorption through skin.

Invagination Inword folding of a structure such as intussusception forming a pouch.

Invasion Entry of pathogen or parasite to human body causing illness.

Invasive Refers to diagnostic technique in medicine where incision and introduction of diagnostic instrument is inserted inside an organ or a tissue.

Inventory management Without inventory management nursing profession cannot render good professional service, right drug supply, the equipment be at right place, at the right time and in the right quantity in order that nurse can deliver nursing care,

Regular indent, daily indent, maintain stock, proper store, proper use comes under inventory management.

Inversion Refers to turning of an organ upside down such as inversion of uterus,

When male to male sex or female to female sex occurs which is abnormal in nature.

Invert sugar Inversion of sucrose produce levulose and dextrose in presence of invertase.

Invertebrate Lower animals which do not have spinal or vertebral column.

Investigation of epidemic During epidemic, which sometimes beyond our imagination,procedure followed to examine, observe and analyse the disease occurrence is called epidemic investigation,

Following actions are taken:

a) Diagnosis is confirmed.
b) innumerable cases occurring are confirmed.
c) Geographic area is mapped.
d) Contact search of cases done.
e) Data analysis for time, place and people done.
f) Cause is suspected (Hypothesis).
g) That cause is tested.
h) After report, measures to check is taken.

Involucrum Changes in chronic osteomyelitis where new bone is formed around dead bone.

Involuntary muscle They are smooth muscles of the body, which are unstriated muscle tissues which act independently of the will, they help to function for automatic physiological functions.

Involuntary That which is not within the control of will such as involuntary muscle contraction in the body.

Involution Turning back or going back to original status such as involution of uterus after delivery,
Also refers to degeneration of organs as part of senescence.

Iodine non-metallic element obtained from seaweed which has the following uses:
- In radio contrast diagnostic radiology.
- Treatment of hypofunction of thyroid gland.
- Essential micronutrient to human body.

Iodised salt Under National Iodine Deficiency Disorder Control Programme, iodised salt is made available where salt contains 100 mg of sodium iodide per gram.

Iodamoeba It is a genus of amoeba present in gastrointestinal tract

Ion Atom that contains either cation or anion which are electrically charged
Substance that forms ions are electrolytes.

Ionisation When current is passed through electrolytic solution electrically charged particles are formed by breaking of molecules,
When radiation is deposited in the tissues it is ionisation.
Acid, base or salt gets dissociated to their constituent ions.

Ipecacuanha Obtained from shrub from Brazil,
In small dose is an expectorant and in large dose it is emetic.

IPPI (pulse polio) Intensive Pulse Polio Immunisation.

IPPV Abbreviation for Intermittent Positive Pressure Ventilation.

Ipsilateral That which occurs on the same side,
Refers to paralysis or paresis due to nervous origin where the lesion occurs on the same side of the injury or infection.

IQ Refers to Intelligence Quotient.

IRDS Abbreviation for Infant Respiratory Distress Syndrome.

Iridectomy It is done for the surgical treatment of glaucoma,
Removal of part of iris by surgery, by cutting.

Iridencleisis It is a procedure done for the treatment of glaucoma,
Providing a drain out of a part of the iris.

Iridocyclitis Infection and inflammation of iris and ciliary body.

Iris bombe Clinical condition where iris is bowed forward by the collection of aqueous humour between the iris and lens in total posterior synechia.

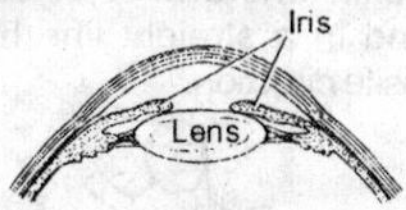

Iris Bombê

Iris Colour layered part of the eye which surrounds the pupil, This is visible behind the cornea
Circular pigmented membrane behind the cornea.

Iritis Infection and inflammation of iris, common manifestations are:

- Pain in the eye.
- Photophobia.
- Pupillary contraction.
- Colour change in the iris.

IrradiationTreatment of cancerous growth by electromagnetic radiation such as Cobalt therapy.

Irreducible Refers to not reducible hernia or of a fracture.

Irrigation of bladder It is commonly ordered for cystitis where the bladder may hold only 1 or 2 ounce of fluid, but as the condition improves and inflammation subsides its capacity increases and a note should be made of the amount every time the treatment is carried out.

Irrigation Wound washes or washes of a cavity with a stream of water or lotion.

IrritableThat which reacts violently to a stimulus such as irritable bowel syndrome.

Irritant A substance that causes irritation or stimulation.

Irritation Nervous excitement due to abnormal sensitiveness such as cerebral irritation.

Ischaemia Blood supply is deficient as in the case of M I.

Ischiopagus Double monster joined at ischia where axes of bodies extend in a straight line but in opposite direction.

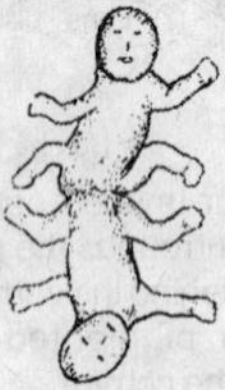

Ischiopagus

Ischiorectal Connected with ischium and rectum such as ischiorectal abscess,

Ischium It is lower posterior bone of the pelvic girdle or innominate bone.

Ishihara chart Chart devised by a Japanese Ophthalmologist Dr.S.Ishihara who lived during 1879 to 1963,

Chart contains patterns of dots of the primary colours on similar background which a normal man can see where as a colour blind cannot see them.

Islands of Langerhans They are clusters of cells in the pancreas which produce and supply insulin required for carbohydrate metabolism, they are described by German Pathologist r.P.Langerhans

Isoaglutination RBC agglutination of a person by agglutinin of another person's blood.

Isocarboxazid Drug used in depression illness, it is a monoamine oxidase inhibitor.

Isogel Prepared from husks of mucilaginous seeds for the use in chronic constipation, Is a laxative.

Isoimmunisation This refers to Rh incompatibility,

Rh–ve woman immunise herself against her foetus which leads to malformation or mortality.

Isolation attire This is an isolation precaution, gown is worn to prevent soiling of clothing when caring for patients

Isolation attire applying include in nursing profession are:

- Applying a gown.
- Applying a mask.
- Applying gloves.

Isolation Selective separation of infectious person from healthy person.

Disease	*Isolation for*
Cholera	Until 2 days of antibiotics or culture negative
Chickenpox	6 days after rash development
Diphtheria	Until 2 days of antibiotics or culture negative
German measles	Do not expose pregnant in first trimester
Hepatitis A	3 weeks from onset
Herpes	6 days after rash
Influenza	3 days after onset
Mumps	Till mumps swelling subsides
Meningococcal meningitis	6 to 8 hours after effective antibiotic therapy
Poliomyelitis	15 days for adult and 50 days for children
Shigella and salmonella infection	Till 3 stool sample is negative
Streptococcal haryngitis	6 to 8 hours after effective antibiotic therapy
Tuberculosis	Till sputum is negative which takes about 3 to 4 weeks of therapy
Whooping cough	One month or till paroxysm ceases

Table: Isolation recommended

Isolette Otherwise called incubator a self-contained clear unit with access partholes for giving nursing care to deliver 60% of oxygen Used for premature infants and infant isolations.

Isoleucine One of the essential amino acid which is required for normal health.

Isomerase Enzyme that catalise isomerisation of its substrate.

Isomerism Two compounds with same formula, Each molecule possessing an identical number of atoms of each element but in different arrangement.

Isometric exercise Isometric exercises are taught to patient to minimise muscle atrophy in the affected limb,isometric means muscle setting exercises on the unaffected limb so that patient can adapt the exercise to the casted limb Muscles of fixation do not contract themselves, those that pull without shortening (by exercise or physiotherapy) is isometric in nature.

Isometric Term means equal dimension.

Isoniazid It is called Iso**N**iazid Hydrazide (INH) which is used in the treatment of tuberculosis.

Isoprenaline One of the sympathomimetic drug used in the treatment of asthma.

Isosorbide dinitrate Drug used in the treatment of angina pectoris, A short acting vasodilator.

Isotonic exercise By teaching muscle exercise or physiotherapy muscles are made to contract is isotonic in nature.

Isotonic That which has uniform tension or osmotic pressure that is equal to other fluid which is under comparison, blood plasma and Normal saline are isotonic in nature.

Isotope Different forms of element with same atomic number but with different atomic weights.

Isotopes Usually refers to radioactive isotopes which are chemicals that are tagged with a radioactive charge,they are used for diagnosis and treatment of certain malignant conditions.

Isthmus Refers to a narrow connecting link such as thyroid lobe isthmus.

Itch mite Sarcoptes Scabiei which causes scabies.

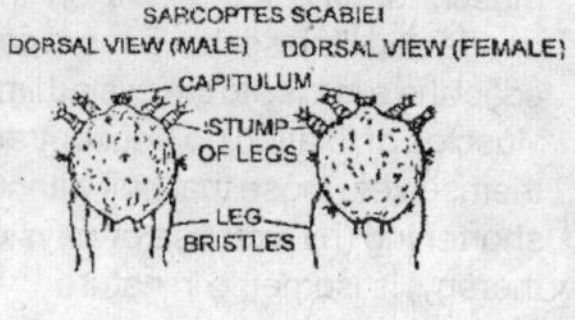

Dorsal view of itch mite

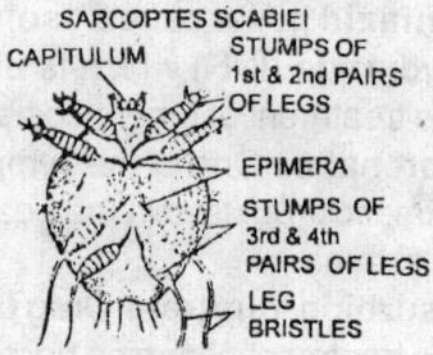

Ventral view of itch mite

Itch Irritation by skin eruption which may be due to many causes such as:

- Itch by itch mite.
- Itch by Dhobi itch.
- Itch by barbers itch.
- Itch by washerwomen's itch.
- Itch by baker's itch.

Item analysis Measurement used in data collection is scientific based when it follows set of rules and scientific basis.

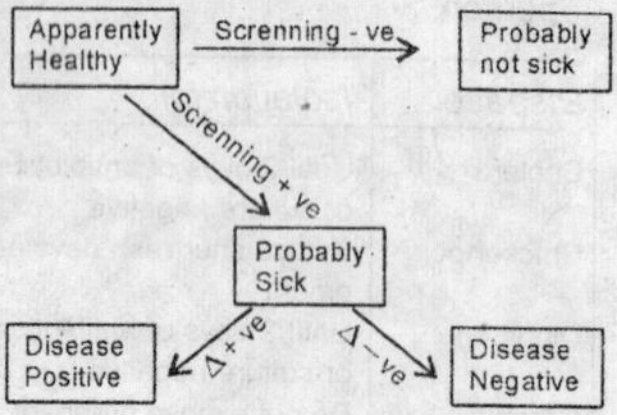

Item analysis in the measure of screening test

ITP Abbreviation for Idiopathic Thrombocytopenic Purpura.

IUD Abbreviaion for Intra Uterine Device for Contraception.

IVF In Vitro Fertilisation colloquially called 'test tube babies for infertile couples who has very many medical and bioethical problems.

step1 -	Hormone is given to induce ovulation
step 2 -	Oocyte is brought out by the suction method
step 3 -	Oocyte removed is mixed with male gamete
step 4 -	Oocyte and male gamete mixture is cultured
step 5 -	The cultivated embryo is transferred to the uterus for implantation

Table: steps in IVF

IVP Abbreviation for Intra Venous Pyelography.

IVU Abbreviation for Intra Venous Urography.

Ivy method It is a laboratory procedure to estimate bleeding time.

J

Jacket Jacket to immobilise the trunk

Jackscrew Screw used in expansion of dental arch.

Jackson safety triangle Triangle space bounded below by lower end of thyroid cartilage, apex in suprasternal notch sides the inner edges of the sternomastoid muscle.

Jacksonian epilepsy Focal epilepsy.

Jacobson cartilage Cartilage lying along anterior inferior border of nasal septum.

Jacobson's anastomosis The anastomosing part of the tympanic plexus.

Jacobson's retinitis Retinitis of syphilis.

Jacquemier's sign A violet coloured spot on the mucous membrane of the vagina just below the urethra seen after the fourth week of pregnancy.

Jactitation Restless condition of acutely ill patient tossing to and fro of a patient in acute disease.

Jaffe's test Qualitative test for creatinine, with trinitrophenol and sodium hydroxide a red colour is produced.

Jakob's disease Spastic pseudosclerosis.

Jamaisa vu Familiarity is lost in a condition of temporal lobe epilepsy

James fibre Fibres which bypass AV node which connect atrium to distal bundle of His.

Janet disease Clinical condition called psychasthenia.

Janeway lesion Clinical manifestation of red blue macular lesion on palm and sole in bacterial endocarditis.

Jargon Words used in medical speciality or any other speciality, nonsense talk by an insane unfamiliar words in a speech or in writing.

Jarvis's snare Snare used for removal of nasal growth.

Jatrophine An alkaloid, a purging nut.

Jaundice Bile pigment in the blood and tissues giving them a yellow appearance, liver disorders, icterus, types are physiological **j.** obstructive **j.** hepatocellular **j.** haemolytic **j.**

Javal's ophthalmometer Ophthalmic instrument which is used to measure refractive power and defect by measuring the sizes of the images reflected from the cornea and lens.

Jaw Upper and lower jaw with teeth for mastication, for mouth movement.

Jaccoud's fever Fever with slow and irregular pulse in TB meningitis.

Jeffersonia A herb used for tonic diuretic expectorant and emetic.

Jejunostomy An opening made into the jejunum is used for feeding in a similar manner to the gastrostomy in conditions like cancer growth of stomach, very large ulcer or stomach intolerance.

Jejunostomy feeding Special type of feeding, artificial feeding.

Jejunostomy tube For gavages the tube is surgically inserted into jejunum and sutured into place; after 2 weeks it can usually be removed and reinserted as necessary for feedings.

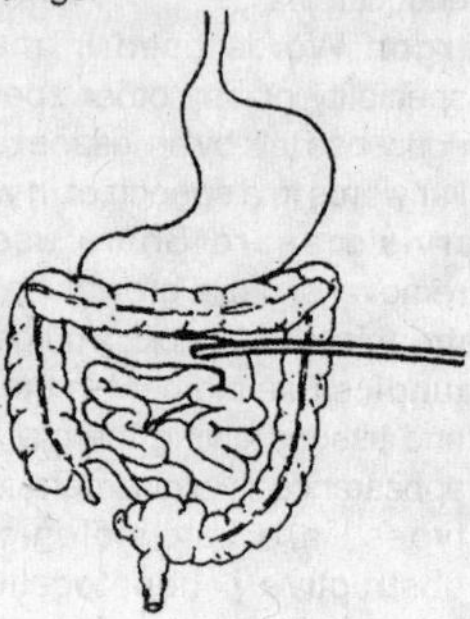

Jejunostomy tube

Jejunum Portion of intestine from duodenum to ileum which runs to 240 cm.

Jelly Gelatinous thick semisolid substances, types are petroleum **j.** Wharton's **j.** contraceptive **j.**

Jendrassik' maneuver A procedure for emphasising the patellar reflex, the patient hooks his hands together by the flexed fingers and pulls apart as hard as he can.

Jenner's stain A staining method of demonstration of blood cells.

Jenner Edward Jenner who discovered vaccination.

Jensen's classification Classification of bacteria depending on the nutritive characteristics of the organism.

Jerk Sudden muscular movement sudden involuntary movement, sudden reflex knee **j.** ankle **j.**

Jhin jhinia An epidemic condition called neuromimesis, tingling sensation of toe, pressure in head and trembling of whole body are seen.

Jigger fleabite It is caused by the intracutaneous attachment to man by Tunga penetrans called sand flea or jigger flea.

Jigger Sand flea bite which burrow into sole causing irritation.

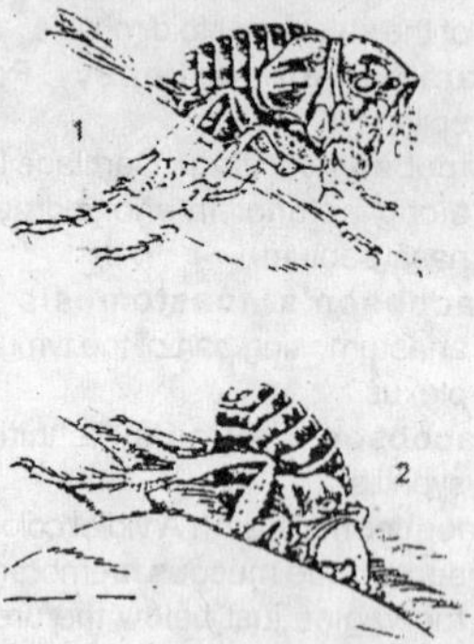

Sand flea female (shown as 1) piercing and penetrating skin of man (shown as 2)

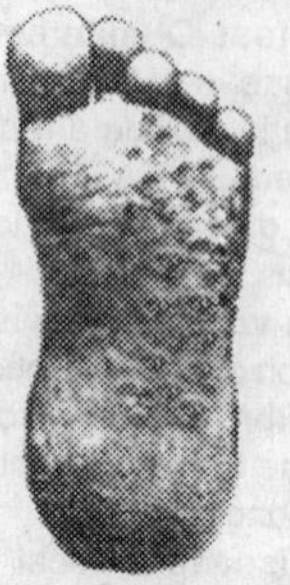

Jiggers in sole

Jimson weed A weed from which a drug is derived which gives a false sense of well being.

Job responsibilities Refers to duties and responsibilities of student nurse, staff nurse or tutor nurse in case of nursing profession.

Jogger's heel Irritation of fibrous and fatty tissue of heel in joggers

Joint capsule Sac to enclose articular ends of bone, has an inner synovial layer apart from outer fibrous layer.

Joint exercise Musculoskeletal exercises when casts are put, when skeletal traction is put as traction care.

Joint Articulation point of two or more bones for body movement.

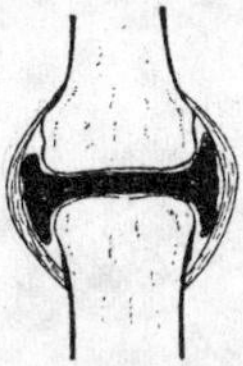

Joint

Jolly's body Howell's body

Jones criteria Used in the diagnosis of acute rheumatic fever

Jones criteria

Major criteria	minor criteria
carditis	fever
polyarthritis	Arthralgia
chorea	past history of hreumatic fever
erythema marginatum	abnormal ESR
subcutaneous nodule	C reactive protein
	leucocytosis prolonged PR interval (ECG)

Table: Jones criteria

Jones' nasal splint Splint for the fracture of nasal bone

Joule Energy spend in one second by current of one ampere against a resistance of one ohm a unit work of energy, 10 million ergs, SI unit of energy

Judgement Ability of nurse to estimate a situation to arrive at reasonable conclusion for a decision to the course of action

Jugal Yoke like connection, cheek

Jugate Locked together, marked by ridges

Jugular foramen Jugular notches of occipital and temporal bones go to form an opening called jugular foramen

Jugular process Occipital bone projection towards temporal bone

Jugular vein its pressure is assessed in monitoring the CVS

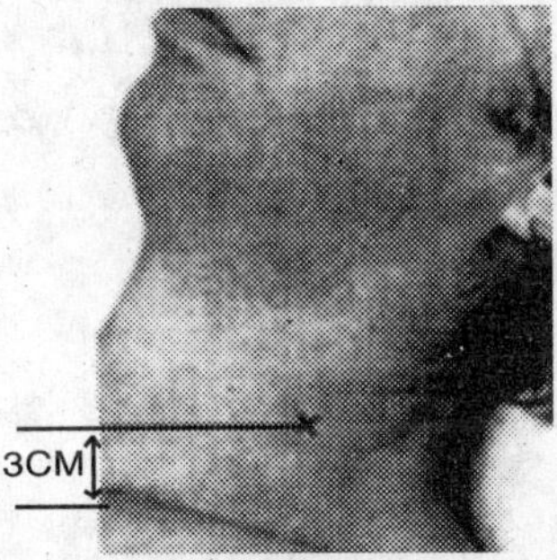

Inspecting jugular vein

Jugular Connected with throat, related with neck, jugular vein

Jejunitis Infection and inflammation of jejunum

Julliard's mask Mask for administering ether in anaesthesia

Junction Where two parts unite

Jung's method Method of psychoanalysis

Junk food Fast food, junk food, opposite of traditional food

Jurisprudence Forensic medicine the science of law and medical jurisprudence

Jury mast Upright bar to support head in Pott's disease, head supporter in spinal conditions

Justice Justice in ethics, social and distributive justice to one and all with a view to serve the sick and fairness equity and impartiality

Jute Fibre of a plant formerly used in surgical dressing

Juvenile delinquency Disorder and disruption caused by young in a society,

Juvenile Related with childhood, related to young

Juxta-articular Very near to a joint

Juxtaglomerular Near to the glomerulus of the kidney

Juxtaposition In apposition

Juxtapyloric Situated near the pylorus

Juxtaspinal Close to the spinal column

K

Kader's operation Surgical procedure to insert the feeding tube.

Kahn's test An immunological test for syphilis.

Kala azar Tropical leishmania infection transmitted by sand fly.

Kallikrein An enzyme, activated enzyme acts as vasodilator.

Kamala An East Indian herb used as purgative, used in the treatment of tapeworm and roundworm also.

Kamaline An alkaloid from kamala herb.

Kanamycin Antibiotic used against Gram-negative bacilli.

Kaolin Aluminium silicate powder used in diarrhoea, for poultices and as dusting powder native hydrated aluminium silicate employed in skin diseases, used for ointment, fine clay of China, adsorbent in diarrhoea.

Kaolin poultice Basis is China clay and glycerine, menthol, methyl salicylate used for external application as analgesic as well as heat retaining poultice, *cataplasma kaolini*.

Kaposi's sarcoma Skin cancer associated with AIDS disease, malignant reticulosis.

Kapseal a sealed capsule.

Karman catheter Catheter used in suction curettage of uterus.

Karnataka Nursing Home Act Amended in 1976 in Karnataka State, it specifies services to be provided in terms of accommodation, staff and facilities in nursing homes, it has enumerated 438 medical surgical and obstetrical procedures listed with specific amount to be collected.

Kartar Singh committee Committee on Multi Purpose Worker in the year 1973, ANM was redesignated as. **MPW** female by this committee, Health supervisor Female to supervise 3-4 MPW female by this committee, a mile stone in the history of public health nursing administration in India.

Karyocyte Early normoblast, a nucleated cell.

Karyo It denotes a nucleus, represents a nut, related to nucleus.

Karyosome Knots in the chromatic net, false chromatin, chromatin nucleolus, clumps of nondividing chromatic.

Karyotype During metaphase of cell division we can see the pattern of chromosome according to length of their short arm, photomicrograph of one cell during metaphase to show descending order of their size.

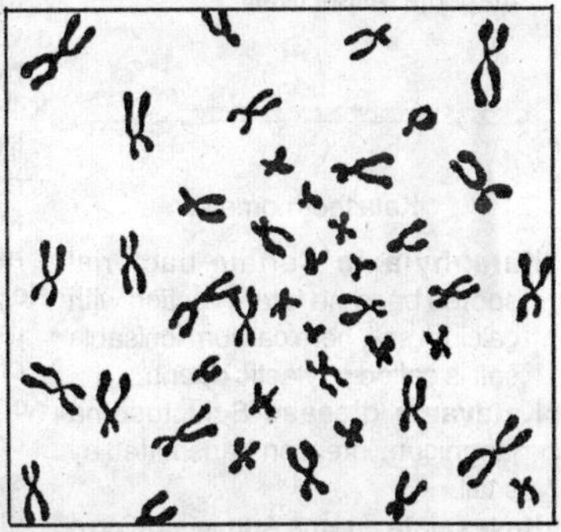

(A Spread out chromosome)

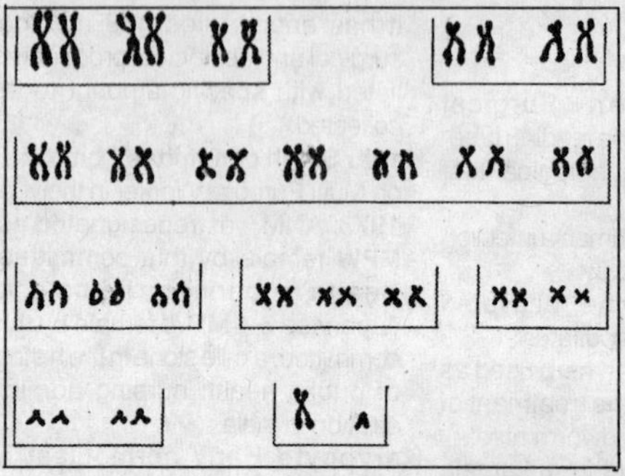

B Denver-London system of karyotyping of human chromo-some

Karyotype A and B

Kata thermometer A meteorological instrument to determine *cooling power of the air* measured in millicalories per square cm per second types are Standard kata, High temperature kata and Extra high Temperature kata, According to colour they are red, dark blue and magenta respectively.

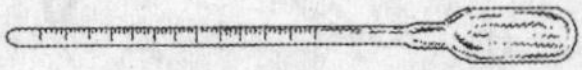

Kata thermometer

Kataphylaxis Certain bacterial spores become fatal infection with calcium salt, here calcium ionisable salt is called phylactic agent.

Katayama disease Schistosoma japanicum infection transmitted by snail.

Kayexalate enema Administrating a sodium polystyrene sulphonate enema given to patients suffering from hyperkalaemia, it is frequently given with sorbitol which because of its hypertonicity induces diarrhoea, this facili-tates expulsion and prevents reabsorption of the potassium.

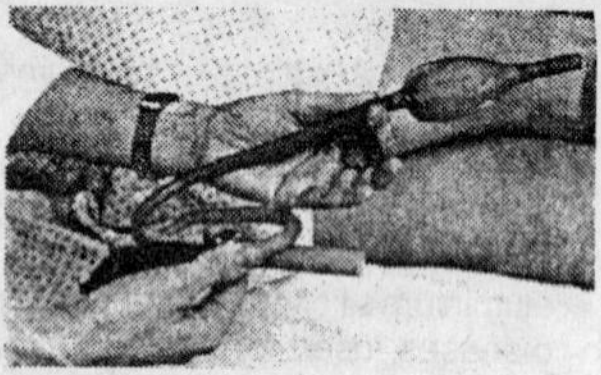

Administration of Kayexalate enema

Kcal Kilocalories.

Kegel exercise Exercise for stress incontinence in women, pelvic vaginal muscle exercise developed by Dr.Arnold H Kegel.

Keloid Meaning tumour form, trauma like burn or injury causes whitish ridges nodules and plates of dense tissue, scar, common in dark people, healed wound.

Kelp Seaweed, promoted far beyond its limited usefulness as a source of iodine in the diet.

Kempner diet A diet consisting of only rice, fruit juice, sugar and supplemented with vitamin and iron, therapeutic diet for renal disease and B.P.

Kenny treatment Physiotherapy like massaging, oil massaging, hot pack application, muscle exercises in the physical treatment of polio.

Keratectasia Postinflammatory protrusion of cornea, eye complication due to infection.

Keratectomy Excision of portion of the cornea.

Keratic Pertaining to cornea.

Keratin Principle component of all horny cells, it is an albuminoid substance.

Keratinise To become horny.

Keratitis Infection and inflammation of cornea.

Keratocele Horny growth of skin, protrusion of Descemet's membrane in a corneal ulcer.

Keratoconjunctivitis Infection and inflammation of cornea and conjunctiva.

Keratoconus Cone-shaped deformity of the cornea.

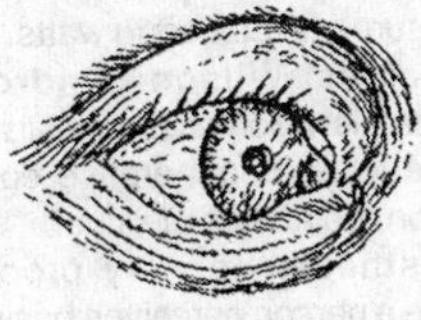

Keratoconus

Keratoderma Skin becoming hard and horny, keratodermia.

Keratolytic Capable of dissolving keratin the hard substance of the hair and nails.

Keratoma A growth or tumour of horny tissue.

Keratomalacia Softening of the cornea in vitamin A deficiency, cause of preventable blindness.

Keratome Knife used to do incision on the cornea.

Keratoplasty Corneal grafting, eye surgery.

Keratoscope Instrument called Placido's disc used to detect Keratoconus.

Keratosis Horny tissue growth on the skin wart, callosity, a horny growth.

Kernicterus Severe form of neonatal jaundice associated with erythroblastosis foetalis, pigmentation of brain and spinal cord by bile pigments; icterus neonatorum, icterus gravida neonatorum.

Kernig's sign A positive sign of meningitis; patient is unable to straighten leg at knee joint when his thigh is supported at right angles to the trunk.

Kerosene Petroleum product, inflammable fuel, causes pneumonitis.

Ketogenic The one which is capable of converting into ketone bodies.

Ketone bodies Acetone, acetoacetic acid and beta hydroxyl butyric acid produced during fat metabolism.

Ketone Metabolic product of fat metabolism.

Ketonuria Urine showing the presence of ketones.

Ketosis More ketone bodies in the blood causing acidosis.

Ketosteroid Androsterone, isoandrosterone, estrone, corticosterone are called ketosteroid, a steroid which possess ketone group on functional carbon atom e.g., 17 ketosteroid.

KFD Kyasanur Forest Disease prevailing only in Karnataka State, monkey fever, transmitted by hard tick.

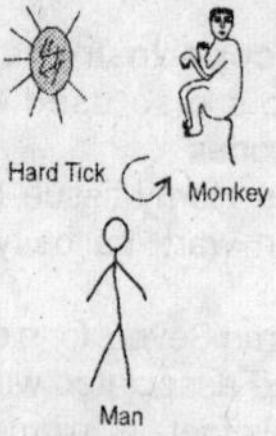

Diag: K F D

Kick chart Method of foetal kick counting by the mother, highlight foetal distress, Less than 10 kicks per 12 hours–mother contacts midwife No kicks in a day–mother to contact hospital doctor.

Kidney failure Loss of kidney function due to kidney diseases, acute or chronic kidney renal failure.

Kidney palpation A comprehensive assessment by palpation of kidney to assess for difference in size, absence of kidney, mass, nodule and for the discomfort.

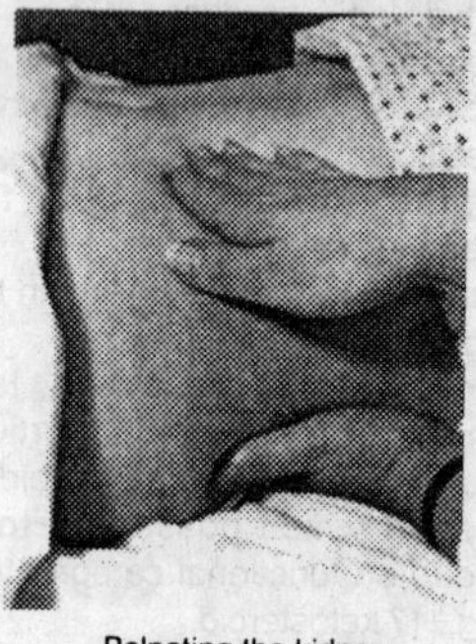

Palpating the kidney

Kidney stone Urate, oxalate or phosphates of calcium stone present in renal parenchyma, gout and hyperfunction of para thyroid usually stimulates kidney stone formation.

Kidney Two excretory organs situated in lumbar region which help in purification of blood and in secretion of urine.

Kilocalorie A unit of energy which indicates one thousand calories.

Kilocycle Electrical term denoting one thousand cycles.

Kilogram Weight measure denoting one thousand grams.

Kilohertz Similar to electrical conduction in one thousand cycles.

Kilojoules It is also food energy unit indicates one thousand joules.

Kilometre Equivalent to 0.6 miles, measures 1000 meters, equivalent to 3281 feet length.

Kilowatt Electric energy which measure one thousand watts.

Kimmelstiel Wilson Syndrome intercapillary glomerulonephritis due to diabetes, degenerative complication of diabetes mellitus.

Kinaesthesia Sensory process where a person perceives position, weight and muscle movement.

Kinanaesthesia Sensation of body movement is lost.

Kinase They are enzyme activators, enterokinase, thrombokinase.

Kinesiology It is the study of body movement and body muscles.

Kinetic Related to motion or movement of the body.

Kinetoplasm Most highly concentrated part of cytoplasm of cell.

King's evil Neck TB which was though to be cured by the touch of The King.

Kinin Naturally occurring polypeptide which is a vasodilator.

Kink A bend or a twist seen in an organ or part of an organ.

Kinship An anthropological term indicating relationship in human beings.

Kirschner wire Thin wire used in bone traction developed by Dr.Kirschner, orthopaedic wire.

Kiss of life Nickname for mouth to mouth respiration, a first aid procedure.

Kite apparatus Physiotherapy instrument to give exercises to forearm, wrist and finger muscles, physiotherapy by Kite in contractures.

KJ Kilojoules.

Klebs-Loffler bacillus Diphtheria causing bacteria.

Klebsiella Enterobacteria, Gram-negative bacteria.

Klepto Word meaning the act of stealing, word used in psychiatry.

Kleptomania A depressive psychosis which causes a person to steal any thing though that object is not required by him.

Klinefelter's syndrome Affected men have physical development of a woman, sex chromosome pattern will be XXY instead of XY in the person.

Knapp's forceps Forceps used in eye surgery for trachoma granulations' expression.

Kneading Massage treatment which include pressing, rolling, lifting, grasping, wringing.

Knee bandage Bandaging of knee as in first aid.

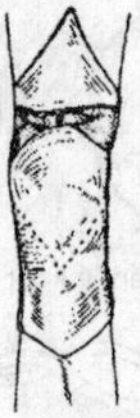

Knee bandage

Knee chest position Surgical posture for sigmoidoscopy and repositioning of uterus.

Knee exercise Exercising the hips and knees to assist the patient with positioning and mobilisation of knee joint.

Knee jerk reflex Knee reflex test for testing pyramidal lesion, contraction of quadriceps on tapping ligamentum patellae when legs are loosely kept.

Knee Joint between thigh and leg,, major joint of body for locomotor activity, a big synovial joint.

Kneecap Patellar bone.

Knife Cutting instrument used in dissection and surgery.

Knot Done in surgical suture, done in bandaging.

Knots for bandage Reef knot, granny knot and surgeon's knot are well known.

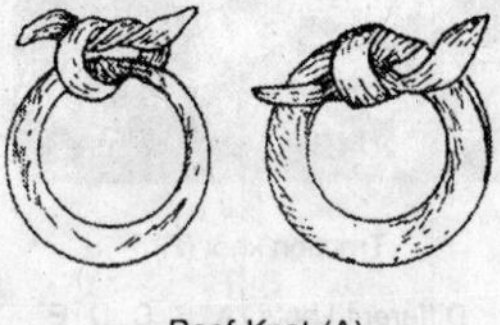

Reef Knot (A)

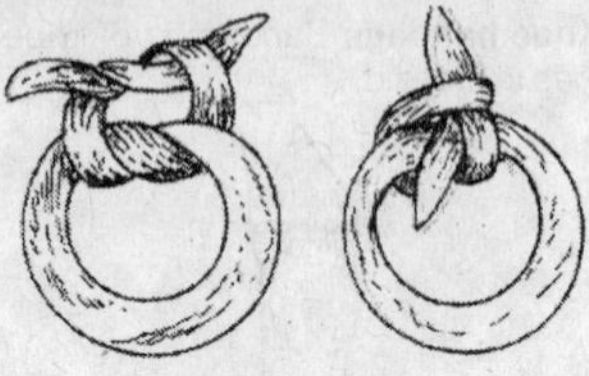

Granny knot (B)

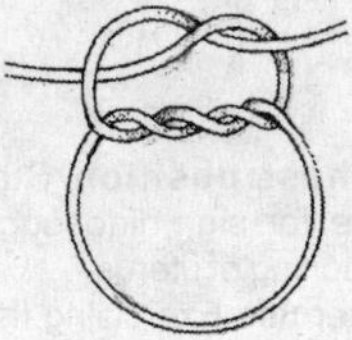

Surgeon's knot (C)

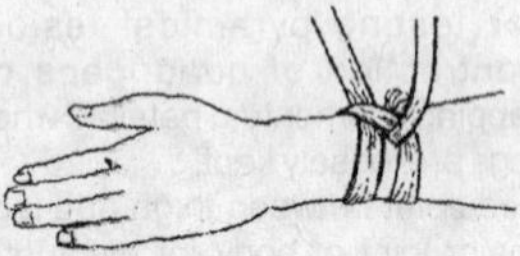

Clove-hitch knot (D)

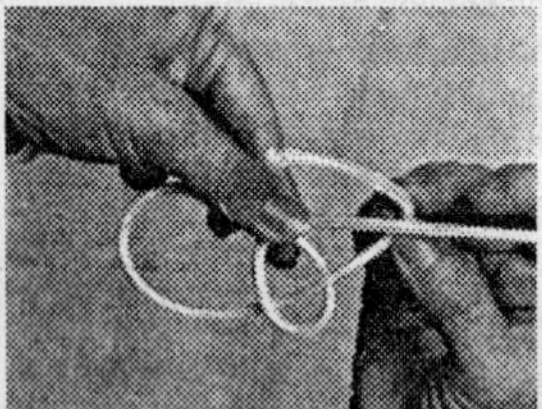

Traction knot (E)

Different knots A, B, C, D, E

Knuckle Dorsal aspect of phalangeal Joint, loop of bowel in hernia.

Koch Weeks' bacillus Haemophilus bacteria of Koch and Weeks.

Koch's bacillus The causative organism of tuberculosis.

Kocher's reflex Contraction of the abdominal muscle on compression of the testicle.

Kock pouch It is called continent ileostomy, done for ulcerative colitis and familial polyposis, it is contra indicated for patients with Crohn's disease.

Koilonychia Brittle spoon-shaped nail in iron deficiency anaemia.

Koplik's spots Its presence is pathognomic of measles, spots on internal buccal mucosa.

Korotkoff's sound When inflated cuff is tied on the arm; sound is produced in artery which can be listened by stethoscope, which help in assessing systolic and diastolic blood pressure of a person.

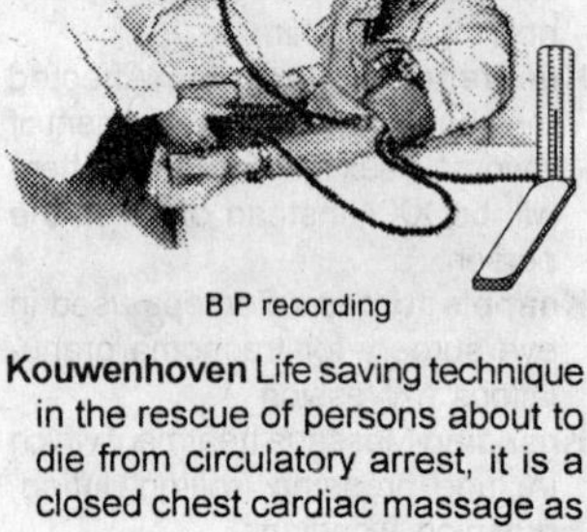

B P recording

Kouwenhoven Life saving technique in the rescue of persons about to die from circulatory arrest, it is a closed chest cardiac massage as first aid in cardiac arrest, described in 1960 by Dr.Kouwenhoven.

Kramer's wire splinting First aid in fracture, Kramer's wire is cut to a required length and easily bent to support a limb in any desired position, mouldable wire splint for fracture of limbs.

Krebs cycle Cycle showing aerobic oxidation of pyruvic acid under carbohydrate metabolism.

Krypton Inert gas found in the atmosphere.

Kupffer's cell Liver cells which produce bile from haemoglobin, phagocytic R E cells of liver.

Kuru Viral infection causing fatal encephalopathy, cannibalism is associated encephalitis.

Kussmaul's breathing Acidosis, deep and gasping respiration in acidosis.

Kveim test An intradermal test for sarcoidosis.

Kwashiorkor local name of Africa 'golden boy', P E M, underprivileged children protein deficiency disorder.

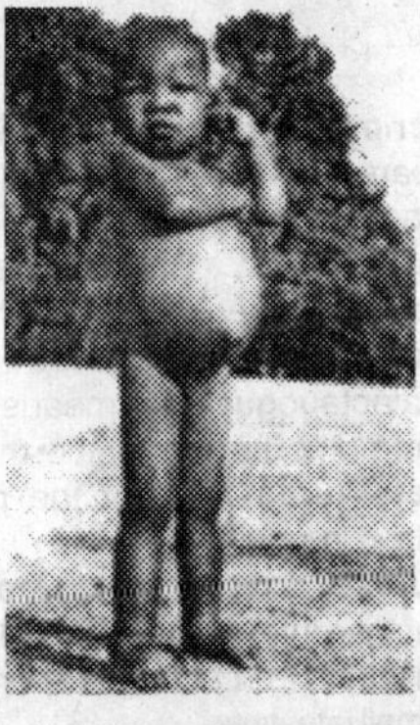

Kwashiorkor

Kyllosis Foot deformity, club foot.

Kymograph Instrument to record the variation of blood flow in an artery.

Kyphoscoliosis Forward and sideward displacement of spinal curvature.

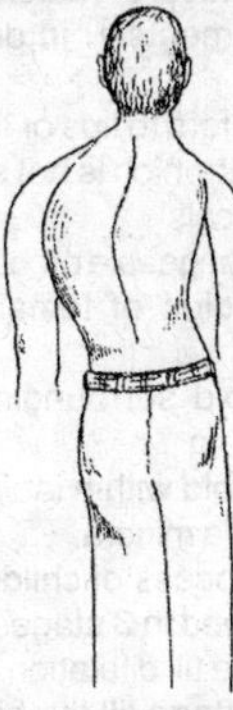

Kyphoscoliosis

Kyphosis Humpback, posterior bent of spinal curvature, abnormal roundness of the thorax called hunchback appearance.

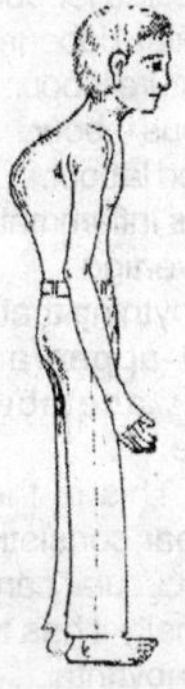

Kyphosis

L

Lagophthalmos Complete closing of eyelid is not possible as in facial palsy.

Labelling It is a procedure of labelling by a chemical or radiological label in experiments or in diagnosis of illness.

Labial It refers to lips or labia.

Labile That which is not stable such as chemicals
Easily changeable emotions.

Labium Folds of female external genitalia,
Larger fold surrounding vulva is labia majora
Smaller fold within labia majora is called labia minora.

Labour Process of childbirth which is described in 3 stages:
First stage till dilatation of cervix
Second stage till the birth of child takes place
Third stage till placenta is expelled
Common types of labour in nursing care services are:

- Normal labour.
- Obstructed labour.
- Precipitate labour.
- Premature labour.
- Spurious labour.
- Induced labour.

Labrinthitis Inflammation of labyrinth causing vertigo.

Labrum Anything that is like lip in its physical appearance such as labrum acetabulare, labrum glenoidale.

Labyrinth This is the structure in internal ear consisting of cochlea and semicircular canals
Anatomically it has two parts:
1) Bony labyrinth.
2) Membranous labyrinth.

Lacerated wound In lacerated wound edges are jagged irregular and often bruised.
It is caused by a blow with a blunt instrument or by a fall on to a surface, gunshot wound is a lacerated wound.

Laceration Torn and ragged edges when present in a wound it is called lacerated.

Lacrimal apparatus It is tear producing apparatus which consists of:

- The lacrimal gland.
- Two fine canals called canaliculi.
- The lacrimal sac.
- The nasal duct.

It produces clear watery fluid which naturally wash eyeball and remove specks of dust.

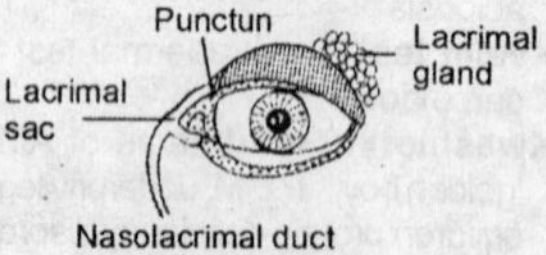

Lacrimal apparatus

Lacrimal Any thing that is related to tears such as Lacrimal apparatus, Lacrimal gland.

Lacrimation When there is excessive secretion of tears.

Lactagogue It is also called galactagogue that means which promotes the secretion of milk.

Lactalbumin One of the protein albumin in milk.

Lactase Enzyme which converts lactose into glucose and galactose in intestine, Lactase is secreted in small intestine.

Lactate dehydrogenase It is a tetramer enzyme consisting of 2 types of chains:
α LDH — present in heart muscle
β LDH — present in skeletal muscle
It helps in anaerobic glycolysis.

Lactate Substance that promote lactation
Also mean salt of lactic acid lactate dehydrogenase (LD or LDH) is present in kidney, liver, myocardium, LD has 5 isoenzymes viz., LD_1 LD_2, LD_3, LD_4, and LD_5
In acute M.I. LD_1 level is higher (Flipped pattern).

Lactation amenorrhoea Woman uses lactational amenorrhoea method (breastfeeding) when
- her baby gets little or no other food or drink except breast milk, and she breastfeeds often, both day and night
- her menstrual periods have not returned
- her baby is less than 6 months old.

Lactation Milk secretion by breast, It is a period where mother breast-feeds the newborn after childbirth

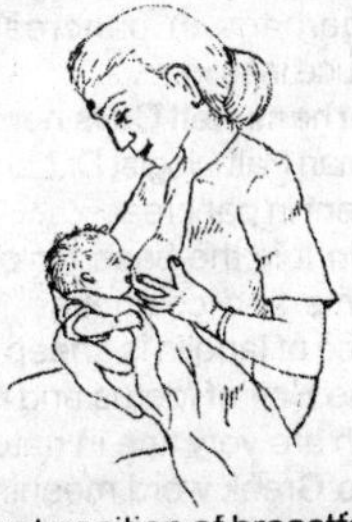
Correct position of breastfeeding

Lacteal That which contain milk,

Lactic Related to milk such as lactic acid.

Lactiferous That which secretes milk.

Lactobacillus Rod-shaped Gram-positive bacteria that produce fermentation.

Lactobutyrometer It is an instrument used to measure the proportion of cream in milk.

Lactoferrin Iron binding protein seen in milk, tears, saliva and bile which show bactericidal activity and colony formation inhibitor.

Lactogenic That which stimulates the production of milk.

Lactometer This is used to measure the specific gravity of the milk.

Lactose A sugar found in milk.

Lactosuria Presence of lactose in the urine.

Lacuna Deficiency or depression or defect in any structure or organ.

Lacunae Space naturally available between cells or in between structures.

Laënnec's disease Alcoholic cirrhosis described by French Physician Dr.Laënnec during 1800.

Laerdal resuscitator This a manual resuscitator which is called Ambu resuscitator or
Laerdal resuscitator which is attached to the source of oxygen during the management of routine tracheostomy care and at suctioning the patient with a tracheostomy,
Used to oxygenate the patient with 3 to 5 deep lung inflations to help compensate for the oxygen

which will be removed during the suctioning process.

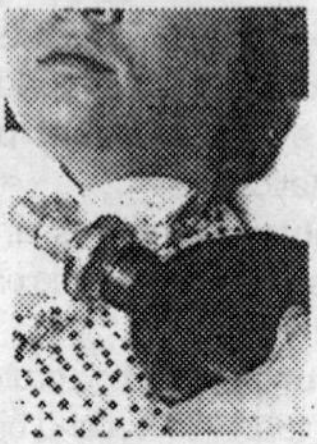

Manual resuscitator (Laerdal)

Laevulose It is fructose popularly known as fruit sugar.

Laking The word denotes that haemolysis of RBC has culminated releasing haemoglobin.

Lallation Immature talk, childish way of speech which is colloquially called as babbling.

Lamaze method Lamaze method of preparing for natural childbirth is a technique of giving training to mind and body for modifying perception of pain at labour and delivery. French obstetrician Dr.F.Lamaze described the method during thirties of past century.

Lambda λ is a Greek alphabet ,
It is the suture junction between sagittal and lambdoid sutures.

Lambdoid It represents the Greek letter lambda – λ
Any item or structure which is shaped like this Greek letter such as Lambdoid suture.

Lambliasis Short form of *Giardia lamblia* infection or giardiasis.

Lamella It represents a thin layer or a thin membrane,
It also represent a disc of gelatin applicator to the eye
Thin sheet of compact bone.

Lamina It denotes a layer or a bony plate such as lamina propria. Thin sheet of plate like material seen anatomical structures.

Laminaria They are seaweeds which are used as sources of alginates.

Laminectomy Surgical intervention in spinal cord compression where excision of posterior arch of vertebra is undertaken.

Lancefield's group Beta haemolytic streptococci are classified based on serological action into many groups, group A are found to cause most of the human infections.

Lancet Pointed and two edged surgical knife,
Surgical blade used for incision and drainage.

Landry's paralysis It is acute ascending polyneuritis described by Dr.Landry French Physician.

Landsteiner's classification It is the system of blood groups where the group consists of
Group A, Group B, Group AB and Group O.

Langerhans He is a German pathologist who described Islet of Langerhans in pancreas which produce insulin.

Langerhans'cell Cells named after German Pathologist Dr.Langerhans present in pancreas.

Lanolin It is the base for ointment, creams and cosmetics and the source of lanolin is sheep's wool.

Lanugo Hair of foetus and newborn which are very fine in nature.

Laparo Greek word meaning flank, Combining form to relate loin or flank, Sometimes loosely used for abdomen.

Laparoscope An endoscope devised for abdominopelvic organ examination.

Laparoscopy Examination and surgical intervention through abdominal wall by using an endoscope through abdominal wall Sterilisation is done by using laparoscope, Abdomen is inflated with nitrous oxide tubes, when tubes are accessible clips are put, and tubes are occluded, this is done only in 2nd month after delivery, postoperative observation is done for 48 hours,

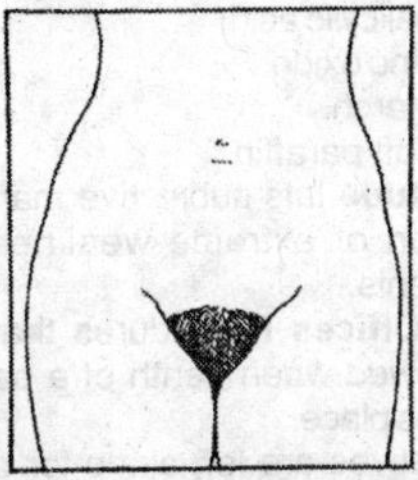

Laparoscopy for female sterilisation, note small incision just below naves

Laparotomy Entering abdominal cavity through abdominal incision for exploring the possible cause of surgical condition ,
Indicated in emergency abdominal conditions and for final diagnosis.

Lapidus airfloat mattress This mattress changes its pressure points over the body every 15 seconds, It aerates the skin through tiny air holes in the mattress,
Helps in rapidly circulating air in a wavelike fashion,
Main uses are:

- to prevent decubiti.
- to absorb perspiration.
- to prevent skin maceration.
- to stimulate peripheral circulation.

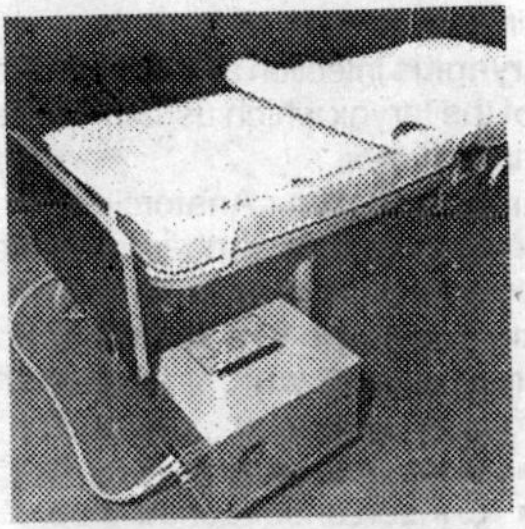

Lapidus Airfloat system with mattress

Larva Motile developing stages of worms, maggots .

Larva migrans Random wandering of larva in the body which show migratory phase of life cycle of helminths in a host,
Depending on the site of wandering they are classified as cutaneous larva migrans or visceral larva migrans.

Larvicide Medications to kill larval form of worms to prevent parasitism.

Larviparous Deposition of hatched larvae in parasites or insects, they do not lay eggs.

Larvivorous That which feed on larvae such as Gambusia fish eating mosquito larva.

Laryngeal That which is related to larynx.

Laryngectomy Surgical excision of larynx for therapeutic purpose
Removal of voice box for the cure of cancer of larynx,
The person who has had his voice box removed is called laryngectomy.

Laryngismus Spasmodic contraction of the larynx, which sometimes is an ENT emergency.

Laryngitis Infection and inflammation of the larynx which usually causes harsh voice.

Laryngopharynx Anatomically it is lower portion of pharynx which connects the larynx.

Laryngoscope It is an endoscopic instrument which serves the following purpose:
- to insert bronchoscope.
- to insert endotracheal tube.
- aids ENT surgeon to examine larynx.

Laryngospasm Laryngeal muscle contraction which commonly occurs during the insertion of endotracheal tube.

Laryngotomy It is the other name for tracheostomy, an emergency opening made on the trachea for easing breathing.

Laryngotracheal That which is related to larynx and trachea.

Larynx The organ of voice situated at the front of the neck, beginning below the base of the tongue and being continuous with the windpipe; the air breathed passes through it

It is contained within the thyroid cartilage or Adam's apple, It opens into the pharynx above and below it is continuous with the trachea or windpipe

It is both cartilaginous and muscular structure which is lined by a lining mucous membrane

Laser (LASER) Abbreviation for **L**ight **A**mplification by **S**timulated **E**mission of **R**adiation,This is equal to concentrated beam of light which can cut metals, Treatment of clinical cases are done in the case of:
- Cancerous tumour.
- Retinal detachment.
- Degeneration of macula.
- Skin conditions.
- Diabetic retinopathy.

Lassa fever A viral infection which is a known zoonotic condition, It is prevalent in West Africa in which rats are found to act as reservoirs of infection,Mode of transmission have been rat bite, person to person and by accidental inoculation.

Lassar's paste It is a soothening agent used in skin disorders, common ingredients are:
- Salicylic acid.
- Zinc oxide.
- Starch.
- Soft paraffin.

Lassitude It is subjective manifestation of extreme weakness of patients.

Last Offices Procedures that are followed when death of a patient takes place,

Relatives are left alone for some time, death certificate is issued,

Notification is done to the concerned higher officials,

Required cloth is left removing the remaining clothes

Mouth is cleaned and then closed with jaw bandage

Requirements for the preparation of dead body after death:
- A gown and clean sheets.
- Washing bowl with warm water, soap, flannel and towel.
- Brush comb cotton wool.
- Dissecting forceps and Spencer Wells forceps.
- Name card.
- Cotton wool to plug external.
- Rifices.
- Screens for cleaning the body and for dressings.

Latent That which is hidden and not seen or which is not manifested, Common professional terminologies are:

- Latent period.
- Latent heat.

Lateral Anatomically the one which is situated away from the centre of the body, situated sideward such as thumb is lateral to index finger.

Lateroversion When an organ turns to one side as in the case of uterus.

Lathyrism A paralytic disease caused by consuming contaminated non-edible pulse "Lathyrus sativus" (Kesaridhal), The toxin identified is BOAA (**B**eta **O**xalyl **A**mino **A**lanine).

Laughing gas An anaesthetic gas nitrous oxide.

Laurence Moon Biedl syndrome It is a syndrome characterised by the following:

- Obesity.
- Hypogenitalism.
- Retinitis pigmentosa.
- Mental deficiency.
- Skull bone effects.
- Syndactylism.

Lavage colonic Is done for sigmoidoscopy or barium enema examination

Requirements to be procured by the attending nurse are:

- Rubber catheter (14 size) or rectal tube.
- Length of rubber tubing.
- A tubing clip.
- Glass connection to fit the rubber tubing and the catheter.
- Lubricant and swabs.
- Jug containing the washout fluid (water or normal saline).
- Irrigation can.
- Large bedpan.
- Receiver for swabs and catheter
- Water or lotion (prepared at 105°F and used at 100°F

Procedure: Patient lies on left side with the knees flexed and the catheter is passed into the rectum for a distance of about 3 inches. The clip is released and fluid is allowed to flow slowly. When one pint is given, turn patient into knee chest position while a further pint is allowed to run in steadily, then patient sumes right lateral position while the third pint is given. The tubing is then clipped, the catheter is removed, patient is placed on the bedpan and allowed to return the wash-out fluid.

Lavage gastric This is stomach wash indicated in cases of :

- Pyloric stenosis.
- Intestinal obstruction immediately before operation.
- In the treatment for poisoning when the poison has been swalowed (narcotic poisoning, acute alcoholic poisoning).
- Poisoning by caustic substance

Requirement in nursing preparation:

1) Jacques's oesophageal catheter, adult 18 to 20 sizes, child 8 to 14 sizes, infant soft 8 size.
2) Glass connection.
3) Rubber tubing (3 to 4 ft).
4) Glass funnel.
5) Jug containing tap water, sodium bicarbonate 1 drachm to water 1 pint, (or normal saline 6 pint) prepared at 100°F.
6) Pint measure.
7) Pail for washout receiving.
8) Tray to receive the tube.
9) Mouth wash.

10) lubricant like glycerine.
11) Mackintosh to protect bedclothes.
12) Gag if patient is unconscious

Procedure: Sitting upright position if patient is conscious and prone position if unconscious
Tube is marked 18"
Chilled tube is passed over the tongue slightly to one side of midline towards the pharynx and the patient (directed to swallow if conscious,)
Patient is allowed to breathe in between
When 18" have been swallowed the tube will be in stomach (distance between lips and cardiac orifice)
One pint solution is allowed to flow in later inverted over the pail and the fluid siphoned
Tube is compressed and with drawn quickly
Mouth wash is given
Doctor performs in case of poisoning.

Lavage In nursing care, wash given to a hollow organ such as stomach or colon which are called as gastric lavage and colonic lavage respectively.

Law An accepted rules made by the society leaders following of which is mandatory in life,
In professional care in nursing, they become time tested phenomenon
Uniform principle in life.

Lawn movers They are common injury producing instruments and is considered under safety in the home,
Not in gear at start, keep chain shields in place, keep blade shields in place, mow crosswise, disconnect spark plug before repair etc., are advocated signals to prevent injury.

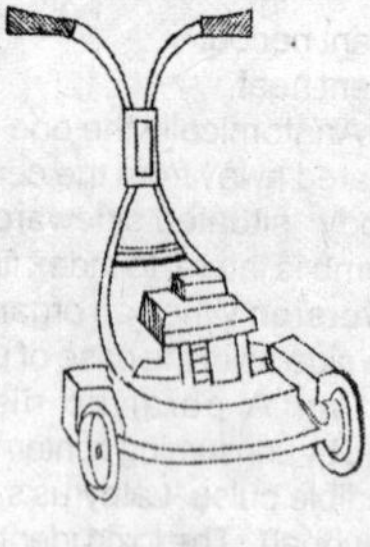

Lawn mover

Laxative These are commonly used for constipation, but are dangerous if used when a patient has appendicitis or an intestinal obstruction
Long-standing constipation should consult doctor than taking self-medication like laxative
That which helps in evacuation are classified into 3 categories depending on mild, moderate and severe effects of evacuation as aperient, cathartic and purgative.

Lead poisoning Poisoning with organic or inorganic lead are known, industries like battery, glass, ship building, printing, potteries, rubber are known to cause lead poisoning, non-occupation sources like gasoline use, lead paint on toys, water running through lead pipes are common in present societies.

Lead A chemical which is a common source of occupation hazard producing lead poisoning, battery, automobile industry, hair dyebatteries are known industrial source, it is a metal, an element.

Leads ECG leads used as chest leads.

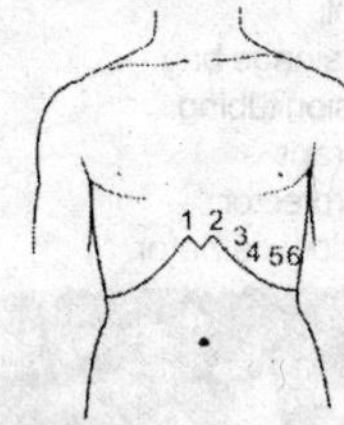

Precardial leads (chest leads)

Leadership Whenever nursing profession embark on a joint project some form of leadership is required, In case of play or conversation where no specific purpose exist one person assumes leadership, Sometimes leader is appointed.

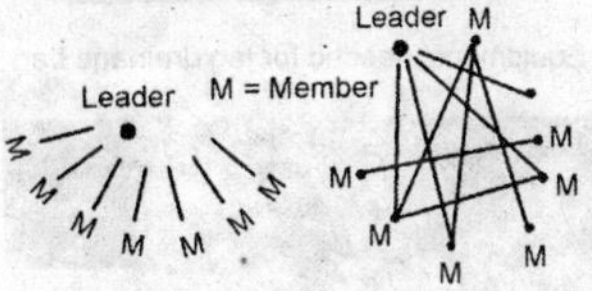

A. Dictate type B. Interact type

Leadership types

Learning Learning is a psychosocial process that is required for survival and human progress, It is to acquire knowledge, skills, habit formation and perception development.

LEC Abbreviation for Leprosy Elimination Campaign, Elements of LEC are:

- Capacity building measures for local health workers to improve MDT.
- Increasing community participation.
- Diagnosis and curing leprosy patients.

Lecithin They are phospholipids that are responsible in fat metabolism, They are present in tissues Origin is from yolk of the egg and this Greek word means Mono Amino Mono Phosphatide (CH_2 (R). CH (R') where R and R' are fatty acids, As therapeutic properties of phosphorus it is given in:

1) Rickets.
2) Dyspepsia.
3) Neurasthenia.
4) Diabetes.
5) Anaemia.
6) Tuberculosis.

Lecture Lecture is a careful presentation of facts with organised thought and ideas by a qualified sister tutor.

Advantage	*Disadvantage*
Live	Low reception
Personal means	Do not stimulate
Economical	Concentration doubtful
Gives latest	Self-learning possible
Can give clarification	Slow learners have difficulty
Big batch is taught	

Table Advantage and disadvantage of lecture

Leech They are present in water and are blood sucking worms, since they secrete hirudin at blood sucking they are called Hirudo worms. Hirudin is an anticoagulant, Leech was used in ancient medicine to let blood from selected patients (Hirudo medicinalis was used).

Leech bite They are invertebrates with 3 jaws and 2 suckers, With sucking blood they present as dark bloated objects, Aquatic leeches are common.

Leg cramps In nursing practice, this is commonly found among pregnant women who experience painful muscle spasms in their legs during their third trimester when circulation is impaired in the lower limb, Other cause is also by the weight of uterus which presses on the nerves in their legs,

Leg cramps are precipitated when pregnant woman is recumbent and when she extends her feet,

Leg cramps in pregnant woman is relieved by the following procedure

- By straightening the leg with one hand as the nurse dorsiflexes the foot with her other hand, It is better if this technique is taught to the husband of pregnant women

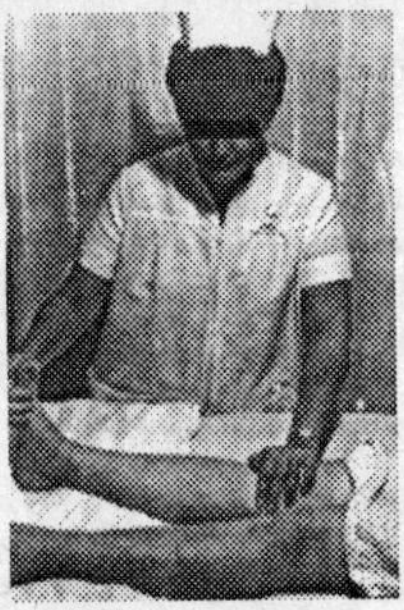

Counter pressure to relieve leg cramps

Leg drainage bag This is used in external urinary device for caring the patients with renal urinary disorders, Leg drainage bag application needs the following equipment:

- Leg drainage bag.
- Extension tubing.
- Leg straps.
- Skin protector.
- A condom catheter.

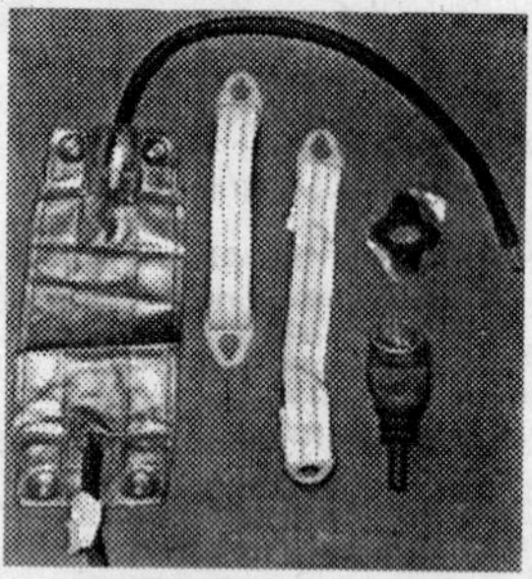

Equipments needed for leg drainage bag

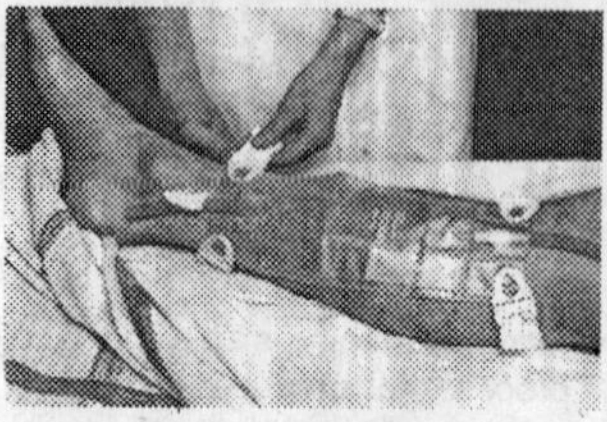

Leg drainage bag in position of a patient

Leg exercises This is to assist patient with positioning and mobilisation of lower limb by exercising following leg points:

a. Exercising the hips and knees.
b. Exercising the ankles and toes.

Usually passive range of motion exercises are advocated (ROM) by following known range of motions:

- Passive range of motion.

- Active range of motion.
- Assisted range of motion.
- Abduction.
- Adduction.
- Extension.
- Flexion.
- Hyperextension.
- Opposition.
- Radial deviation.
- Lateral deviation.
- Medial deviation.
- Rotation.

Leg Anatomical structure from knee to ankle, various types of legs are used in clinical practice are:
- Bow leg (Genu varum).
- White leg (Phlegmasia alba dolens).
- Scissor leg (Cerebral diplegia).
- Barbados leg (Elephentiasis).

Legonnaires' disease Lung infection caused by *Legionella pneumophila.*

Legislation of health It refers to public health laws which are enacted and amended from time to time to protect the health of people, They are The Central Health Acts, The State Acts and the Municipal Acts.

Legumes They are rich sources of protein for vegetarians which on an average give 20% of proteins in available form.

Leiomyoma Fibroid uterus, a smooth muscle tumour.

Leishmania A parasitic infection by Leishmania causing Kala Azar.

Leishmaniasis This consists of group of parasitic infection by genus Leishmania.

Leisure society Is a predicted automation which help to enjoy leisure activities as their central life interest.

Lemberts' suture French surgeon developed this type of suture for intestinal suturing.
At suturing the suture edges are turned inwards by keeping the contact of peritoneal surface.

Lemniscus It denotes a band or ribbon, A bundle containing axons such as lateral lemniscus, medial lemniscus, trigeminal lemniscus.

Length Measurement of distance or length, distance from one end to another.

12 inches	=	1 foot
3 feet	=	1 yard
22 yard	=	1 chain
10 chains	=	1 furlong
8 furlongs	=	1 mile

Table: Units of length

Lens It is the structure which allows rays of light to fall on retina to produce images which we see from our eyes, If lens become opaque it is called cataract which needs removal of lens and replacement by IOL or by external lens for the purpose of focusing the image on to the retina
Lens is a crystalline body, convex on either side like a magnifying glass, lies towards the front of the eye immediately behind the iris and is held in position by tiny ligaments running to the walls of the eyeball

Alternation in the size of the lens is brought about by the action of a muscle situated within the eye In case of artificial lens to be worn it will be spectacles for wearing from outside or contact lens which is fitted directly over the cornea as a measure to correct refractive errors

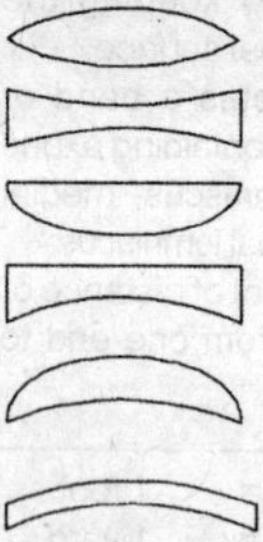

Lenses

Lentiform Anything which looks like a lentil or lens of the eye.

Lentigo Small local pigmentation of the skin, a nevus or a freckle.

Lentivirus Name is derived from its meaning "slow" and retroviruses including HIV are slow progressive diseases.

Leopold's maneuvers This is performed to determine foetal position, hands at examination is made warmer and maneuver is done inbetween uterine contractions which can either be labour contractions or Braxton Hicks contractions

Leopold's maneuvers are described in four stages for methodical examination to determine foetal position

1. Bilateral palpation of upper abdomen
2. Bilateral palpation of sides of abdomen
3. Palpation of lower abdomen above pubic symphysis
4. Bilateral palpation by curving downward towards and immediately above the pubis.

Performing Leopold's maneuvers

Leopold's maneuvers are performed to determine fetal position. Make sure your hands are warm, and perform the assessment between contractions, whether Braxton Hicks or labor contractions.

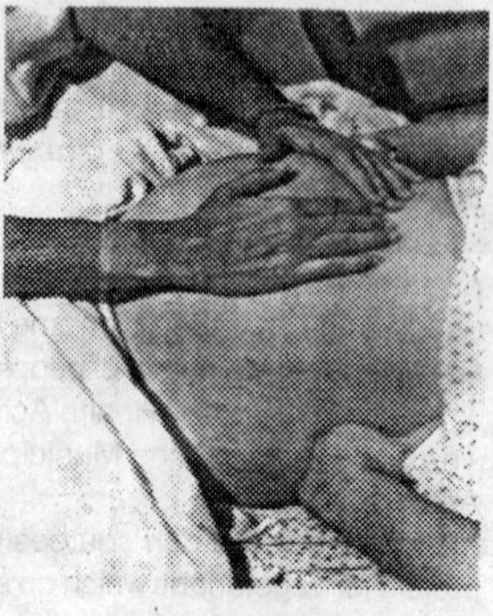

A: First maneuvers

First maneuver: Face the client and bilaterally palpate the upper abdomen. This will help you determine which of the fetal parts is in the uterine fundus. The breech is large, soft, and asymmetrical; the head is round, hard, and it moves freely.

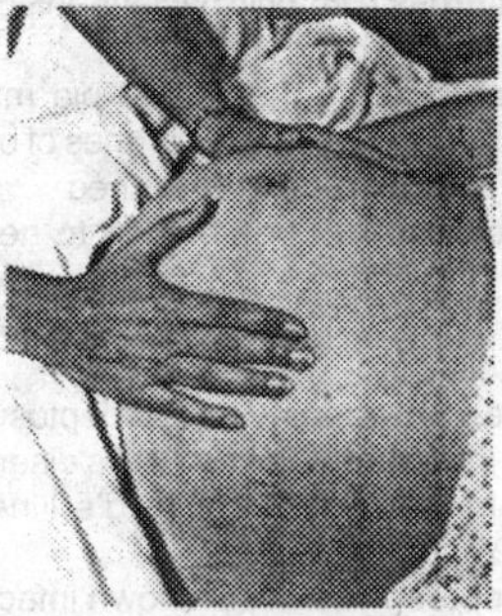

B: Second maneuver

Second maneuver: Continue facing the client, and place each hand along the sides of the abdomen. Gently but firmly palpate with your palms and fingers. Assess one side and then the other to determine the side on which the fetal back lies. One side should feel smooth and quite firm—the fetal back; the other side should be indentable and less resistant—the extremities on the opposite uterine wall.

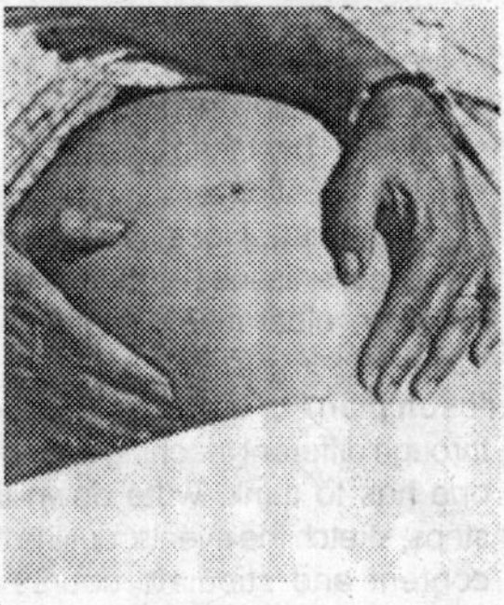

C: Third maneuver

Third Maneuver: While still facing the client, position your dominant hand over the lower abdomen just proximal to the symphysis pubis, and firmly palpate with your thumb and index finger. Explain to the client that this maneuver may be uncomfortable. This maneuver helps to confirm the data gathered in the first maneuver. Again, the head will be round, hard, and ballotable (moveable) if it has not already engaged. The breech will feel soft and asymmetrical. (This assessment will be much more difficult if the presenting part has already engaged.

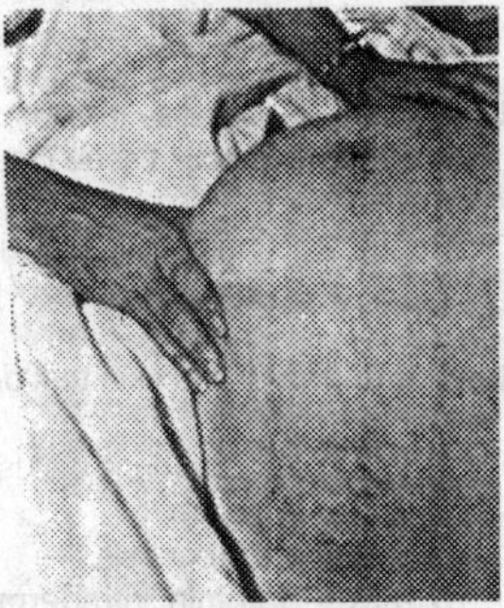

D: Fourth Maneuver

Leopold's maneuvers for foetal position

Fourth maneuver : Face the client's feet and position your hands on both sides of the abdomen with your fingers curving downward toward, and immediately above, the pubis. This maneuver will help you locate the cephalic prominence, which is the most prominent portion of the fetal head. Press deeply with your fingertips because you will need to palpate through several layers of tissue, muscle, and fluid. The cephalic prominence is located on the side in which your fingers meet the greatest resistance. If it is located on the side opposite the back, the head is extended and a normal delivery will probably ensue. If it is located on the same side as the back , the head, the face or brow will probably present, again, the greater the engagement, the more difficult the assessment.

Lepra Greek word meaning leprosy.

Leprologist An expert who can diagnose and treat leprosy.

Leproma A characteristic lesion in the form of granulomatous nodule in leprosy.

Lepromin Sterilised saline suspension of lepromatous tissue for skin test,

Lepromin test helps in recognition , classification and prognosis of leprosy.

Lepromin test It is a skin test done in leprosy for

a) Evaluation on immune status.

b) For classification.

c) To estimate prognosis.

0.1 ml of lepromin intradermally injected to inner aspect of forearm and the reaction is read at 48 hours and on 21st day as under:

Fernandez reaction: if induration and redness is more than 10 mm at 48 hours, it is positive and is called early reaction

Mitsuda reaction: on 21st day a nodule of more than 5 mm is positive and this is late reaction.

Leprosy A chronic bacterial infection caused by Lepra bacilli.

Leptomeningitis When pia mater and arachnoid membranes of brain and spinal cord is inflamed.

Leptospira They belong to genus spirochaetes, *Leptospira icterorohaemorrhagica* causes Weil's disease.

Leptospirosis Group of leptospiral infections such as Weil's disease, Mud fever, Swineherd's illness, Autumn fever etc.,

Leptospirosis It is known infection among swine, Reservoir in India are rats,

Other names are infectious jaundice, swineherder's disease

Rat bite fever , rat bite jaundice, fever, jaundice and kidney diseases are common features.

Lesbianism Homosexuality among women.

Lesch-Nyhan syndrome X-linked hereditary disorder of purine metabolism which show following manifestations :

- Cerebral palsy.
- Kidney dysfunction.
- Mental handicap.
- Self mutilation tendency.
- Physical handicap.
- Body spasticity.

Lesion Structural loss or functional loss of cells, tissues or organs such as ulcer, ulcerative tumour, skin sores, eczema, etc.

Lesson plan For carrying out lesson through different teaching methods one has to think, write down the steps, sketch the events, outline the content and stipulate course of action which constitute lesson plan

LESSON PLAN
Acute Respiratory Infections

Sl.No	Time	Content	Method/Media
1	5 minutes	Clinical conditions involving respiratory infections by virus and bacteria	a) blackboard b) Narration
2	10 minutes	* cough, fever, ear discharge, fast breathing * Stridor at rest,drowsiness, fits,cyanosis * URI sinusitis, pharyngitis, ASOM, tonsillitis, epiglossitis, laryngitis * LRI broncho pneumonia, bronchitis , asthma * Complications like emphysema, pneumonia,lung abscess, collapse of lung	a) slide b) OHP c) explanation
3	5 minutes	Common pathogens Virus and bacteria	a) chart b) OHP c) narration d) illustration
4	10 minutes	Agents- virus, bacteria Host – age, sex and immunity Environment – physical, biological and social	a) chart b) OHP c) Narration
5	5 minutes	High risk children, preterm, small for date, new born, malnutrition with measles	a) OHP b) Narration
6	20 minutes	Case management, Mild (home care), Moderate (antibiotic, homecare), Severe (referral, admission and assessment)	a) explanation b) Nursing chart c) Case sheet
7	5 minutes	Control –* health education on Nutrition, breastfeeding and immunisation *Risk child identification *Avoid trigger factor	a) derivation
8	10 minutes	Conclusion- Mortality, morbidity and ARI control programme	a) Narrate b) blackboard

Duration - 1 hour

Evaluation - by short answer questions

Follow up assignment - Nurse students to collect common pathogens of ARI in their paediatric ward

Table: Model of lesson plan on "ARI" for the nursing tutor to III B.Sc Nursing

Lethal That which is deadly or which can produce death.

Lethane oil Indicated in head louse infestation along with nits,
Lethane oil is composed of
Liquid paraffin 50 %
Lethane 384 special 50%
Procedure for application of lethane oil:
Eight partings is made in the hair, four on each side of the midline. The oil is then applied to the scalp from a teaspoon or a dropper and spread by massaging the scalp thoroughly. Following the application the hair should be combed daily to remove dead lice and nits but it should not be washed or brushed vigorously for the following eight days as the aim is to leave the oil on the scalp for sufficient time to kill the parasites. Lethane oil also kills nits.

Lethargy Pathological laziness, stupor or drowsiness.

Leucine Essential amino acid which is responsible for Nitrogen equilibrium and for growth.

Leuco Leuco meaning white such as leucocytes, leucoderma

Leucopoiesis Indicates the formation of WBC.

Leukaemia Blood cancer which is a progressive type of malignancy Colloquially it is called blood cancer, in which WBC become too numerous in the bloodstream.

Leukocyte WBC present in the blood which are of following types:

Neutrophils	
Basophils	Polymorphonuclear
Eosinophils	granular cells
	(Bone marrow cells)
Lymphocytes	Lymph gland cells
Monocytes	

contd...

Table: A general classification
I. Granulocytic series
Myeloblast
Myelocyte
Neutrophilic metamyelocyte
Stab cell
Segmented neutrophil
Eosinophil
Basophil
II. Non-granulocytic series
Lymphocyte
Monoblast
Monocyte
Plasma cell

Table:B. Another classification

Normal Leucocytes	*Abnormal Leucocytes (Precursors)*
Granular	Myelocytes
Polymorphs 65 to 72%	Metamyelocytes
Eosinophils 2 to 5 %	Lymphoblasts
Basophils 0.5 to 1.0%	Monoblasts
Non-granular	
Lymphocytes 20 to 25%	
Monocytes 3 to 8 %	Myeloblasts

Table:C. Proportions of WBC in blood and their precursors

Leukocytolysis This indicates destruction of WBC

Leukocytopoiesis This indicates the formation of WBC.

Leukoderma Other word for vitiligo or abnormal white patch on the skin by the absence of melanin pigment.

Leukonychia White patch present underneath the skin.

Leukopenia Decreased WBC count in the blood indicating some pathological conditions.

Leukoplakia Presence of white patches on gum, cheek or tongue and vulva which are due to chronic inflammatory reaction

White patches in the mouth, colloquially it is called smokers' patch.

Leukorrhoea White discharge per vagina due to certain infections.

Leukotrienes They are mediators of inflammation which are derived from arachidonic acid

Leukotriene C_4 Leukotriene D_4 Leukotriene E_4	These help in anaphylaxis
Leukotriene B_4	Chemoattractant of neutrophils

Table: Common Leukotrienes

Levamisole Pharmacologically it is l-form of tetramisole used in the treatment of roundworm, hookworm and strongyloides infestations.

Levator Prefixing for a muscle which means that which elevates structure.

Levels of health care It means care given before, during and after the illness phases:

- Preventive care.
- Primary care.
- Secondary care.
- Tertiary care.
- Restorative care.
- Continued care.

Primordial: Measures to prevent risk factors before they emerge e.g. regular exercise for CVS disease prevention, smoking regulation for cancer prevention.	
Primary: Measures taken before the onset of disease e.g., health promotion and specific protection.	
Secondary: Measure to halt the progress of disease e.g., early diagnosis and prompt treatment.	
Tertiary: Intervention in late phase of illnesseg., disability limitation and rehabilitation	

Table: Levels of prevention

Levi's disease Paraxysmal hyperthyroidism which is named after Paris endocrinologist Lêopold Levi during 1900.

Levin tube It is used in Nursing management with gastric tubes and are called single lumen tubes which are available in following types:

- 12 to 18 French (F) for adults.
- 8 to 12 F for children.
- 5 to 8 F for infants.
- 8 F for paediatric feeding.
- 30 to 40 F for common oral tubes.

Uses are for gavage, administration of medications, for lavage, for diagnostice valuation and for decompression. Nursing considerations are:

- Before insertion chill rubber tubes in icy water.
- Warm plastic tubes before insertion.
- Unless contraindicated it is nasal route of insertion.
- Stomach irritation, oesophagus irritation and nose irritation indicate that you have inserted larger lumen tubes.

Levodopa L. dopa which is used in Parkinsonism.

Levonorgestrel It is progestin, in combination with oestrogen it is used as oral contraceptive.

Lewisite A lethal war gas being a mixture of the following:
Dibetachlorovinyl chloroarsine
Betachlorovinyl dichloroarsine
Named after American chemist Dr.W.Lee Lewis during 1900.

LGV Abbreviation for **L**ympho **G**ranuloma **V**enerium , it is caused by *Chlamydia trachomatis,* one of the S T D.

Liaison Contact and communication between two units or two groups Public relation works in a network.

Libido Impulsive force in sexual drive, sexual desire.

Lice They are small wingless Ectoparasite of man which are dorsoventrally compressed and are of three types

I. Head louse (pediculus capaitis)
II. Body louse (Pediculus corporis)
III. Pubic louse (Phthirus pubis).

Lichen Papular eruption on the skin due to inflammatory process Sometimes raised flat reddish scaly eruptions develops and are called Lichen planus.

Lid Usually refers to eyelid.

Lidocaine A local anaesthetic available in the form of spray, cream and injection.

Lie Describes the foetal position in uterus which is usually longitudinal.

Lieberkühn's gland These glands are present in small intestine which was described by German anatomist Dr.J N Lieberkühn.

Lien Other name for spleen.

Life event It is a sociological term which describes events of an individual or of a family such as child birth, marriage of son or daughter, construction of a house of their own to live on, getting an appointment to earn livelihood, death of life partner etc.

Life expectancy in years This is an index that has bearing to the life expectation which can be increased by intervention,

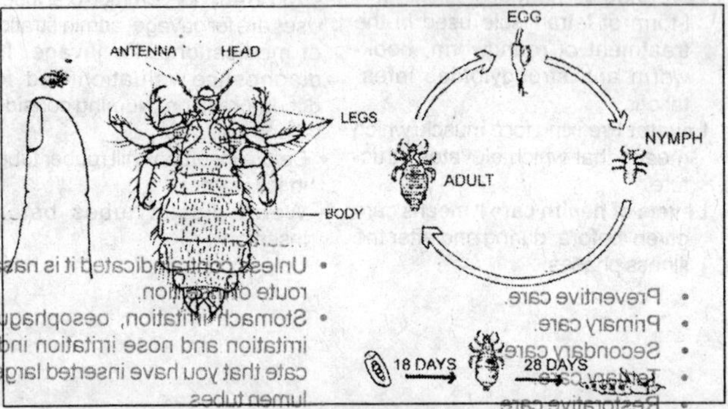

Lice morphology and life cycle

In otherwords prolongation of life by increasing life expectation is the hallmark of professional ethics Average life which depends on death trend among the community.

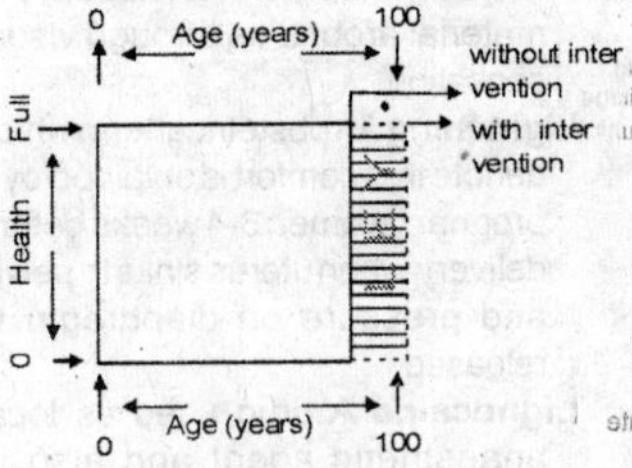

Life expectancy in years with and without intervention

Life jacket An inflated garment intended to keep a person afloat in water.

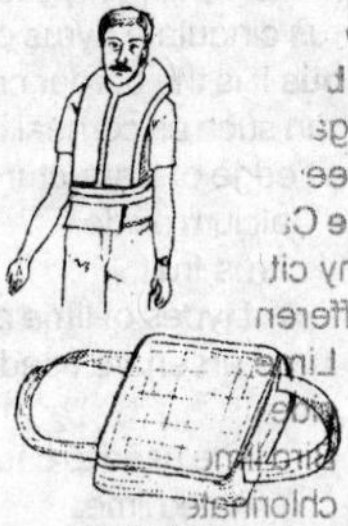

Life jacket

Life supporting system There are two types of defined deaths one is somatic death and the other is brain death (legal death), In case of somatic death life support system achieves the maintenance of oxygenated circulation through the corpse

Medical equipment used to maintain respiration and circulation without which death occurs.

Lifestyle It determines the general health of an individual, It describes the pattern of daily living of a person, a family or a society.

Ligament Fibrous tissue bands that binds bone to help function of a joint.

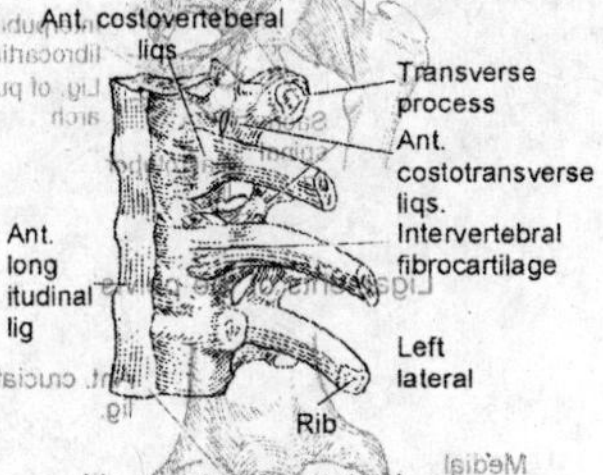

Ligaments of vertebral column

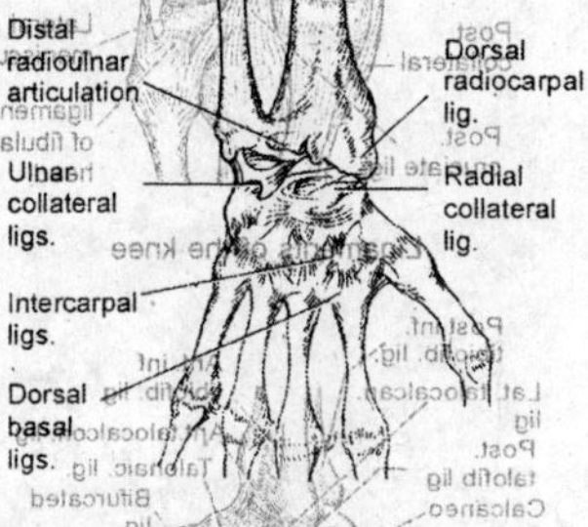

Ligaments of the hand

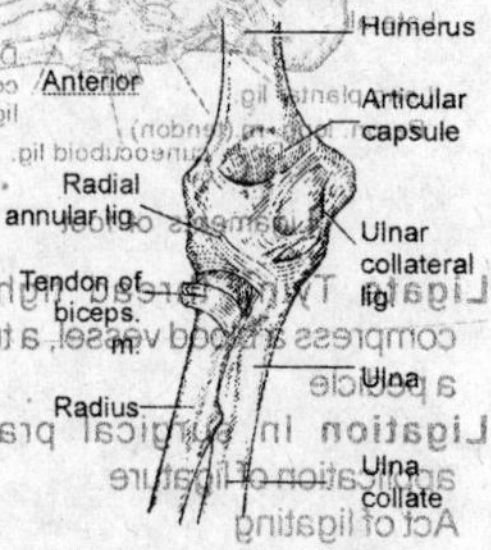

Ligaments of the Elbow

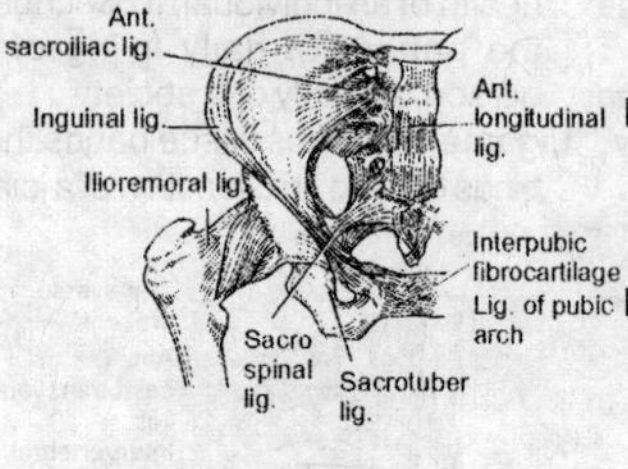

Ligaments of the pelvis

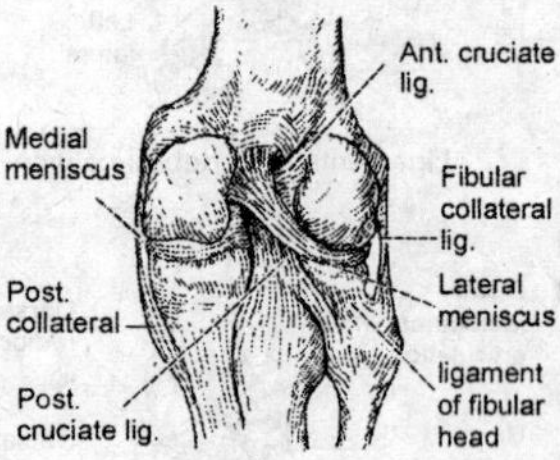

Ligaments of the knee

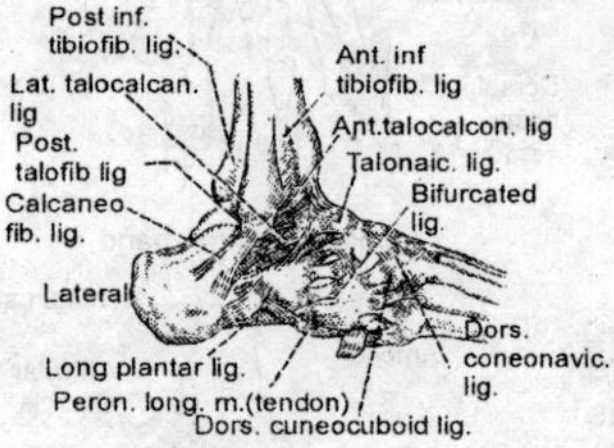

Ligaments of foot

Ligate Tying thread tightly to compress a blood vessel, a tumour, a pedicle

Ligation In surgical practice, application of ligature
Act of ligating

Ligature Any non-reactive material that can be tied to a blood vessel during surgical intervention

Light They are electromagnetic waves which help to visualise a material around us through visual sensation

Lightening An obstetrical term which denote that comfort is obtained by a pregnant women 3-4 weeks before delivery when uterus sinks to pelvis and pressure on diaphragm is released.

Lignocaine A drug used as local anaesthetic agent and also in cardiac arrhythmias.

Limbic system This is attributed for emotion, arousal, behaviour and motor function and the seat are hippocampus, amygdala, dentate gyrus cingulate gyrus of the brain.

Limbus It is the border or edge of an organ such as corneal limbus
Free edge of a structure.

Lime Calcium oxide,
Any citrus fruit,
Different types of lime are:

- Lime arsenate used as insecticide.
- Bird lime used to capture birds chlorinated lime.
- Slaked lime which is calcium hydroxide.
- Soda lime.
- Sulfurated lime.

Liminal It refers to the threshold of perception.

Lincomycin An antibiotic derived from streptomyces which is used in bone infections.

Linctus Thick viscid cough preparation.

Lindane An insecticide chemically gamma benzene hexachloride.

Line diagram It is to present the variation by line, or presenting the data on a line.

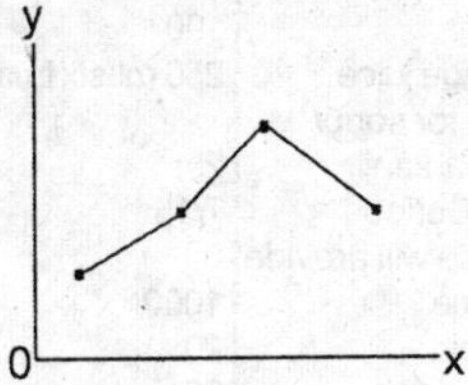

Line diagram

Linea It denotes a line such Linea alba, Linea nigra.

Linear Related to a line.

Lingual That which is related to tongue Name given to an anatomical structure that looks like a tongue when they are projecting in their natural projections.

Liniment Medicament for external application by rubbing which are usually liquid in nature.

Linoleic acid An essential fatty acid.

Linseed Used as laxative and demulcent in the form of oil.

Lip reading By observing the lip one can understand his speech at talk

Lip Fleshy margin of the mouth which has upper and lower lips.

Lipaemia Presence of lipid in blood which is more than the expectation.

Lipase Enzyme present in serum which help in digestion of fat into glycerol and fatty acids.

Lipid One of the proximate principle of food that are not soluble in water and that yield high calorie.

Lipochondrodystrophy It is called Hurler's disease where an inborn error of metabolism of fat is seen which has the following clinical features:

a) Short stature.
b) Abnormality of the face.
c) Abnormality in learning skill.
d) Bone deformities.

Lipodystrophy It is a pathological disorder of fat metabolism, sometimes it is progressive in females which is called progressive lipodystrophy.

Lipoidosis Reticuloendothelial tissue hyperplasia and occurrence of xanthoma that occurs in abnormal fat metabolism in the body.

Lipoma Benign tumour of fat cells.

Lipomatosis Patient have multiple or diffuse lipomas, When it is painful in nature it is called lipomatosis dolorosa.

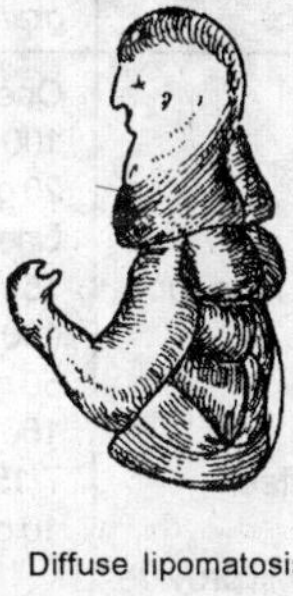

Diffuse lipomatosis

Lipoprotein Fat proteins that are present in the blood.

Liposarcoma Malignant tumour of fat cells.

Liposyn It is 10% IV fat emulsion and is indicated for patients who are deficient in essential fatty acids due to disorders such as severe burns, endstage kidney disease, ulcerative colitis and malignancies

Liquefaction Process of change to liquid form.

Liquor That which is like liquid or like watery such as liquor amnii.

Liquid diet Soft and easily digestible hospital diet given in following clinical conditions:

- All acute illness.
- Fever.
- Diarrhoea.
- Postoperative.
- Jejunostomy.
- Cancer oesophagus.
- Anorexia nervosa.
- One who cannot swallow.
- Severe burns.
- Gastric surgery.

Item	*Amount in grams*
Milk	One litre
Bread	100 grams
Butter	20 grams
Egg	One
Greens for soup	150 grams
Potato	100 grams
Sugar	50 grams
Fruit	150 grams
Tea/Coffee	7/15 grams
Salt	10 grams
These will provide:	
Calorie	1500
Protein	45
Fat	60
Carbohydrates	190

Table: Full liquid diet for all acute illness

Item	*Quantity in grams unless mentioned*
Cow's milk	500 ml
Sugar	100
Orange juice	250 ml(six fruits)
Dhal for soup/ Cereal kanji	25
Tea/Coffee	7/15
These will provide:	
Calorie	1000
Protein	20
Fat	20
Carbohydrate	180
Sodium	285 mg

Table: Liquid diet for fever, diarrhoea, postoperative cases, jejunostomy, cancer oesophagus, anorexia nervosa, patient who cannot chew, severe burns and gastric surgery.

Liquid Substance which flows readily in nature, It is one of the physical state of an object (originally solid, liquid and gas are natural status of objects).

Listeria Gram-negative bacteria which cause URI and encephalitis, was identified by British surgeon Dr.Baron J Lister during 1890.

Listerine An antiseptic solution under National Formulary.

Listeriosis Infection with Listeria group of organism.

Lithiasis This denotes the formation of calculi such as conjunctival lithiasis.

Lithopedion Dead foetus which has come stone like or putrified.

Litholapaxy Crushing calculus in the bladder and later washed out as fragments.

Lithosis Occupational pneumoconiosis resulting by the inhalation of silica dust, infection and inflammation of lung by silica dust.

Lithotomy position This is common position for gynaecological examination,
The patient lies on her back with the knees flexed and the thigh raised and separated. The buttocks are brought to the edge of the couch, the legs are supported in stirrups and the foot end of the examination couch is dropped.

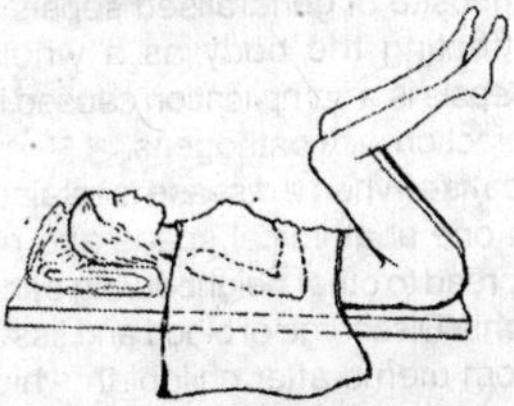

Lithotomy position

Lithotripsy Surgical intervention in the management of urinary calculi, method of crushing of calculi in the urinary bladder.

Litmus Usually litmus paper of a substance from lichen used in finding out the reactions of fluid either acidic or alkali
It has a range of pH of 4.5 to 8.3 at measure of test

Turning blue by an alkali = Red litmus

Turning red by an acid = Blue litmus

Litre Unit denoting one cubic decilitre which is SI unit for capacity.

Litter It is a stretcher for transporting the invalid or sick or injured.

Little's disease Muscular rigidity of lower limbs causing "scissor leg" deformity which is called spastic diplegia , a congenital disorder.

Liver biopsy It is required in the investigation of liver disorders where physical and laboratory examination have failed to give a diagnosis

Requirements:

1. Spirit.
2. Swabs.
3. Hypodermic syringe with needle.
4. Local anaesthetic.
5. Scalpel.
6. Gloves.
7. liver biopsy needles (Silverman's).
8. Bottle for specimen.
9. Request form.
10. Receptacle for waste.

Nursing preparation:

Blood group is ascertained, cross-matched, Hb%, bleeding time and clotting time are noted, If prothrombin content is below 70% liver biopsy is not carried out

The patient lies on his back well over to the right side of the bed, the trunk is then slightly tilted to the right by placing a pillow under his left side

After biopsy pulse chart is maintained, observed for any internal bleeding.

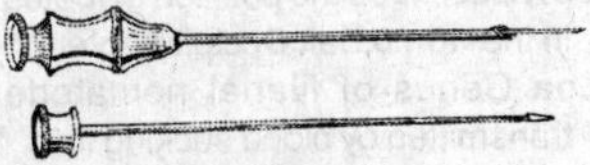

Liver biopsy needle (Silverman's)

Liver Major organ under G I system which forms following functions:

1. Regulates body metabolism
2. Maintains the blood composition
3. Help in bile production

Common associated terminologirs are:

- Liver biopsy.
- Liver cirrhosis.
- Liver transplantation.

Livid Blood congestion giving rise to bluish grey discolouration of skin.

Living will It is the declaration of a person giving future course of action with respect to the following (when incapacitated or terminally ill)

- Property distribution to living heir.
- Money distribution to living heir.
- Legal heir adoption to the property.
- On personal illness what course of action to be taken.
- For the decision on life supporting system maintenance to prolong the life.
- For action on foreseen circumstances.
- For action on unforeseen circumstances.

Leukocytosis Abnormal increase of WBC indicating infection in the body.

Loa loa It is one of the filarial infection found in Africa, colloquially called river blindness, blindness and calabar swelling are seen.

LOA Describes the position of foetus in the womb,**L**eft **O**ccipito **A**nterior.

Loa Genus of filarial nematode transmitted by blood sucking flies.

Lobar When a lesion is related to a lobe of the lung.

Lobe One identifiable part of an organ such as lobe of the lung, lobe of the brain, lobe of the liver, etc.

Lobectomy Surgical removal of a lobe of the lung.

Lobotomy Surgical operation on the brain.

Lobular When related to lobule of the lung.

Lobule Component of a lobe, many lobules go to form a lobe.

Local sepsis When sepsis is localised i.e., confined to the wound itself it is called local sepsis, opposite of generalised sepsis or affecting the body as a whole, Sepsis is a complication caused by infection with pathogens.

Localise When a disease is retained in one anatomical space and not spread to other neighbouring parts.

Lochia Discharge of blood and tissue from uterus after childbirth which lasts for 3 to 4 weeks

It is one of the major postpartum technique ,Nursing considerations are very important in Lochia assessment which are:

- Detach peri pad from woman's sanitary belt.
- Make sure to remove pad from front to back to minimise the risk of contaminating vagina with rectal discharge.
- Note amount, character, odour of discharge.
- First few days it is Lochia rubra (dark and red).
- From third day it is Lochia serosa (serous and brown).
- Clots if observed it is abnormal which is needs further examination by the doctor.

- In first 24 hours 4 to 8 saturated pads are normal.
- In caesarean amount will be excessive.
- Foul smelling indicate infection.
- Nursing observation documentation must be specific and should give clear cut picture: examples of nursing documentation are as under:
  * Lochia rubra, moderate amount, few.
  * Clots present.
  * Lochia serosa and scanty.

Lockjaw Other name for tetanus.

Locomotor Related to movement from one place to other place.

Loculated An order or tissue which is divided into many cavities or many locules.

Loculus It denotes a small cystic cavity of an organ.

Locum tenens This refers to the provision of substitute nurse for a patient over a given period of time Morning duty nurse is replaced by night duty nurse at night

This also refers to a patient who changes to a new doctor in place of old doctor (doctor who is substituted over a span of time to look after a patient).

Log roll Nursing technique of turning a reclining patient from one side to other for nursing care in nursing routines.

Logrolling It is done to the immobile patients, If patient has a neck injury or a spinal disorder, it will be necessary for the nurse to logroll the patient when the nurse changing the position of the patient so that one can maintain the alignment of patient's vertebral column during the turn.

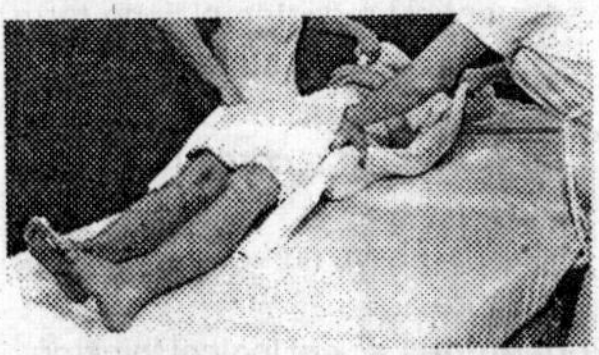

A: Log rolling the patient

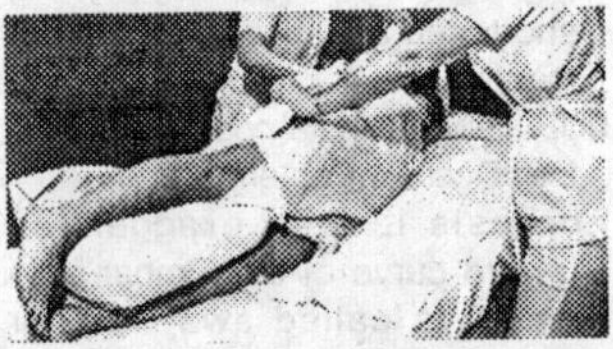

B : Log rolling the patient

Loiasis A tropical infection by *Loa loa* parasite in the conjunctiva.

Loin It refers to the area on the back between thorax and pelvis, part of the back and sides of body between ribs and pelvis.

Lomotil Pharmacological preparation containing diphenoxylate which is used as antidiarrhoeal drug.

Long sight Other name for hypermetropia.

Longevity It is the length of life, survival period

By the available immunisation, better sanitation and superior nutrition and our active participation in programmes of health, longevity or living healthy for longer time is made possible.

Longitudinal study A scientific study in medicine which is done by making observation made over a sequential time interval, long-term study to observe changes over a time.

Loop A bend in a cord or cord-like structure

A turn or sharp curve in a cord-like structure.

Loosening Lack of logical thinking, one of the thinking disorder in psychiatric illness, fragmented, shortened and disturbed ideas in thinking.

LOP Refers to foetal position in uterus Left **O**ccipito **P**osterior.

Lordosis It is an exaggerated inward curve of the lumbar area which is called swayback or lordosis,

Abnormal forward curvature of lumbar spine.

Losartan It is an angiotensin receptor blocker used in the treatment of hypertension.

Lotions Drugs used for skin afflictions and skin conditions, they have soothening effect and sometimes antiseptic property,

Common lotion in nursing practice are:

Calamine lotion

Dilute alcohol lotion

Lead lotion

Potassium permanganate lotion.

Loudness It is the intensity of noise or sound.

Loupe Used in eye examination which help to magnify the parts of eye.

Louse Common vectors in diseases transmission in developing countries

Head louse and body louse transmits vector borne diseases whereas louse do not

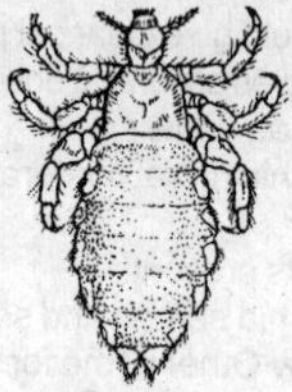

Adult head Louse

Lovibond comparator This is an instrument used for finding out total protein or pH of urine by colour matching method.

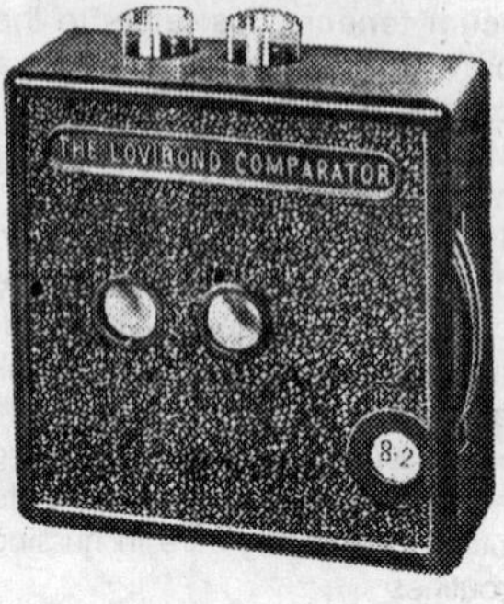

Lovibond comparator

Low birth weight When birth weight of newborn is below 2500 grams, it is 30% in developing countries.

Categories according to gestational age	*Three main of LBW*
Preterm (less-than 259 days)	Malnutrition
Term (259 to-293 days)	Infection
Postterm (294 days and above)	Unregulated Fertility

Low cost drug A model of drugs are listed by Government of India that are essential and are expected to meet the health care need of majority of people,this takes care of affordability of the community, This also helps in treatment guidelines and in National formulary.

Loxotomy Surgical amputation by means of an oblique incision.

Lozenge Medication having sweetening agent and flavouring agent for chewing to get contact to the throat.

LSD **L**y**S**ergic acid **D**iethyamide, is a hallucinogenic drug which cause auditory and visual hallucinations Commonly called Lysergide.

Lubb-dupp They are heart sounds heard through stethoscope at auscultation,
Closing of AV valve and meeting of semilunar valve respectively.

Lucid Clear cut picture of the mind, Incase of mental disorders and cerebral injury when patient is clear in his mind we use the word Lucid interval.

Lues It is a colloquial word used for syphilis.

Lumbago Common clinical condition of pain in the back due to various clinical conditions such as muscular sprain, disc prolapse, etc.

Lumbar puncture Insertion of trocar and cannula into spinal canal in lower back to draw CSF for diagnostic purposes.

Lumbar Anything that is related to loin such as lumbar puncture, lumbar pain, Lumbar vertebra, etc.

Lumbosacral Related to lumbar and sacral vertebra or regions, common terms in nursing care are lumbosacral vertebrae, lumbosacral support.

Lumbricus Intestinal roundworm which has round and circular body.

Lumen In a tubular structure the anatomical space available.

Lump Lumps are swellings or mass where it does not belong and need investigations, common lumps like lump in the breast, lump in the axilla need thorough investigations to confirm that they are harmless.

Lunacy Now the term is not used which used to mean insanity or madness.

Lunar pertaining to moon or pertaining to silver.

Lund-Browder chart The chart used in Burns unit to calculate the total surface burnt in a patient of fire injury or burn injury,
Mapping out the burn area on a map for the case management.

Lung inflation techniques Patients who have undergone lobectomy, mastectomy or gross pleural effusion will be splinting from pain, they need apical expansion exercises,

Patients who are recovering from chest surgery who inhibit bilateral chest movement need basal expansion exercises
For above both categories teaching diaphragmatic breathing helps better lung function by using their abdominal muscles and diaphragms.

Lung They are conical organs of respiration, right lung has 3 lobes, left lung has 2 lobes.

Lunula Near the root of the nail it is the semicircular white structure.

Lupus Latin word meaning "wolf", formation of brown nodules in the corium, Depending on their appearance they are termed as:

- Lupus annularis.
- Lupus butterfly.
- Lupus discretus.
- Lupus disseminated follicular.
- Lupus erythematosus.
- Lupus exfoliative.
- Lupus papillomatous.
- Lupus vulgaris.

Lupus erythematosus Inflammatory changes in skin and internal organs with plaque like area of hyperkeratosis in certain autoimmune disorders, sunlight also can cause Lupus erythematosus.

Lupus Term used to denote chronic infective and reactive disorders of the skin producing various clinical manifestations.

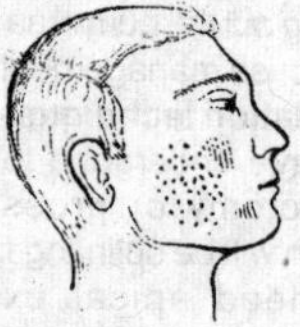

Lupus

Luteal Relating to corpus luteum of ovary.

Luteinisation Process of transformation of granulosa cells into lutein cells in the ovary.

Luteinising hormone This hormone controls the activity of the gonads which is secreted by anterior pituitary gland, Abbreviated as L H.

Luteotrophin Otherwise known as prolactin which stimulates the formation of corpus luteum and the production of milk.

Luxation It denotes the dislocation of a joint or of eyelens which are referred to as luxation of joint or luxation of lens.

Lux It is the unit of illumination which is equivalent to one lumen per square meter of area.

Lyme disease A disease caused by a spirochete is transmitted by ticks, it is a zoonotic disease, it is characterised by

i. Skin rash (erythema chronicum migrans).
ii. Arthritis.
iii. Aseptic meningitis.

Lymph nodes Small glandular organs inserted in the lymph vessels at strategic points where they can filter out infection and so protect the remainder of the body,, Lymph nodes are also called lymph glands.

Lymph A clear yellowish fluid which bathes all cells and is returned to the bloodstream from the tissues by the lymphatic vessels.

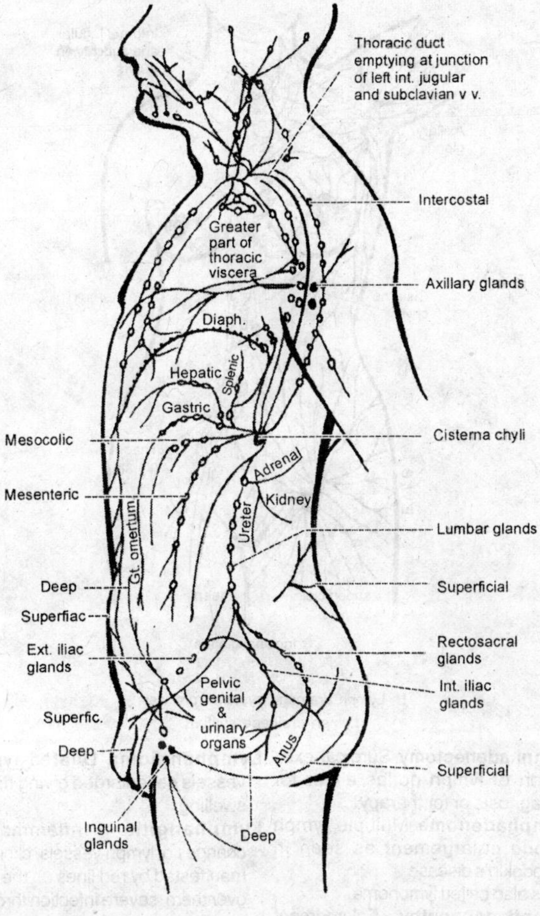

A: Lymph drainage system latereral view

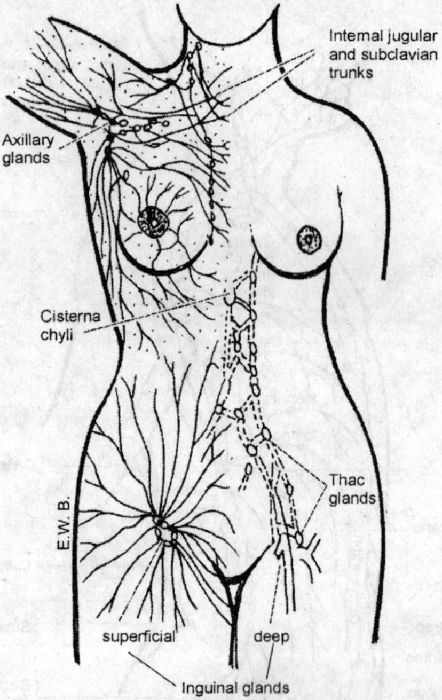

B: Lymph drainage system front view

Lymph drainage system

Lymphadenectomy Surgical excision of lymph nodes either for diagnosis or for therapy.

Lymphadenoma Multiple lymph node enlargement as seen in Hodgkin's disease
It is also called lymphoma.

Lymphadenopathy Enlargement of lymph nodes due to infective, malignant or other chronic disorders, which can be genera-lised or localised.

Lymphangioma Dilated lymph vessels get enlarged giving rise to swelling.

Lymphangitis Inflammatory changes of lymph vessels, clinically manifested by red lines on the skin over them, severe infection through the skin gives rise to lymphangitis.

Lymphatic system A circulatory network of vessels and filter glands which drain and distribute the lymph.

Lymphatic This refers to the lymph system, They refer to glands and vessels through which lymph is returned to the circulation which end in the thoracic duct and right lymphatic duct.

Lymphoblast Precursor of lymphocyte, early developmental stage of lymphocyte.

Lymphocyte WBC from lymphoid tissue,they produce immune bodies to prevent the person from infection They are lymph cells, Leucocytes formed in lymph nodes are lymphocytes (White cells)

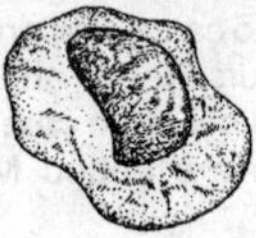

Large lymphocyte

Lymphocythaemia Depicts more lymphocytes in the blood called lymphocytosis.

Lymphocytopenia Depicts less lymphocytes in the blood called lymphopenia.

Lymphoedema Due to obstruction of lymph drainage, there will be abnormal amount of lymph in intercellular spaces giving rise to oedema.

Lymphogranuloma Usually reffered to a STD infection which is called LGV (Lympho Granuloma Venereum).

Lymphoma Malignant condition of lymphoid tissue It can be Hodgkin's or Non Hodgkin's group of diseases, Lymphoma of East Africa among children is called Burkitt's lymphoma.

Lymphoma A tumour arising from the lymphoid tissue in our body.

Lymphopoiesis Production of lymphocytes in bone marrow.

Lymphosarcoma It is the other name for malignant lymphoma.

Lymphokine Lymphocytes when they come in contact with antigen to which they are sensitised they produce hormone like factor which regulate immunological response.

Lyophilisation Stable preservation technique for plasma, serum, bacteria, virus and tissues, Biological substance preservation technique.

Lyosol A sol in which the dispersion medium is a liquid.

Lysine Is an essential amino acid that help in the digestion of protein $NH_2(CH_2)_4.CH\text{-}(NH_2).COOH$ α- ε-diaminocaproic acid first isolated from casein.

Lysis Denotes destruction of tissues,

Denotes the decrease in fever, or clinical manifestations of illness.

Lysol Solution containing aryl and alkyl phenol derivatives saponated for solubility in water, it is antiseptic and disinfectant in nature.

Lysosome It is a particle in cytoplasm which breaks down any foreign substance that enter the cell.

Lysozyme This is an enzyme present in saliva, nasal secretion and tears that has bactericidal effect

M

MI Abbreviation for **M**yocardial **I**nfarction which is colloquially called heart attack.

MRI Abbreviation for **M**agnetic **R**esonance **I**maging.

Macaca Genus of monkeys which are found to be reservoir of certain diseases. Macaca rhesus is main group in which RBC were studied by Dr. Alexander Wiener for complicated substances called Rh-Hr agglutinogens and Rh-Hr antigens Macaca rhesus helped in identifying 8 Rh factors which are rh, rh', rh", rh_y, Rh_0, Rh_1, Rh_2 and Rh_z.

Maceration When a solid is soaked in a liquid it becomes liquefied and softened such as dead foetus gets macerated in the uterus.

Mackenrodt's ligament In the pelvic cavity, uterus is supported by transverse ligaments that are called Mackenrodt's ligaments.

Mackenzie's syndrome Associated paralysis of the tongue, soft palate and vocal cords on the same side.

Machine In nursing care, machine is used for an instrument which accomplish treatment modality such as:

- Heart Lung machine.
- X-ray machine.
- Dialysis machine.
- ECG machine.
- EEG machine.
- ECT machine.

Mackintosh In nursing profession, it refers to Bed Mackintoshes. They should be thoroughly scrubbed after use with warm water and soap. If necessary, they may first be mopped with 1-20 phenol or 1-30 Lysol solution.

Bed Mackintoshes should not be folded; they are usually stored on rollers, or may be hung over rollers in a Mackintosh cup board.

Macleod 1923 Noble prize winner for medicine and physiology, Scottish Physiologist.

Macmillan nurses Macmillan who transformed the management of cancer patient and who devised Macmillan home visiting services was responsible for training programmes of training in pain relief, palliative care and emotional care support to cancer patients:

Those nurses who are trained in pain and palliative care of cancer patients are called Macmillan nurses.

Macro-sociology Large scale focus on a society with functionalism.

Macrocheilia Thick and wide lip of a person who has it since birth, described as a congenital defect.

Macrocyte Enlarged size of RBC in some form of anaemia.

Macrocythaemia Abnormal large RBC in blood; in other words macrocytosis.

Macromastia Abnormal large breast in a person.

Macronutrient Nutrients that are needed more than 100 mg per day in the diet, such as calcium, phosphorus, magnesium, pota-ssium, sodium and chlorides.

Macrophage They are abundant in inflammatory sites at connective tissues,

R.E cell which ingest debris and bacteria.

Macrophthalmia Abnormal large eye which is a congenital defect.

Macroscopic That which is seen by the naked eye.

Macrosis That which is increased in its size.

Macrostomia Abnormal big and wide mouth because of wide gap between mandible and maxilla which is a defect in embryogenesis.

Macula Discoloured patch which is not raised above the surface of the skin; sometimes called macule.

Macule Skin eruption which is not raised above the surface of the skin.

Maculopapular Patches of skin not raised above the surface of the skin and also patches of skin raised above the surface of the skin , both are seen.

Madarosis Clinical condition where eye lashes are totally disappeared

Mad Colloquial term used for mental illness, or for madness.

Madura foot Fungal infection Mycetoma of the foot.

Maduramycosis Madura foot with discharging sinuses.

Mae west Name of a life jacket, from a nautical term.

Mag sulph Magnesium sulphate is a saline purgative.

Maggots Larva of flies that are found in the wound which look like worms

Magma It is an organic matter paste, Tiny particles which is suspended in water.

- Pharmacy preparations include:
- Magma bentonite.
- Magma bismuth.
- Magma magnesia.

Magnesium sulphate enema This solution is given as an enema attracts fluid from the tissues into the bowel. It may be ordered as an evacuant and also in cases of increased intracranial tension in order to relieve the tension by causing dehydration of the tissues. For this purpose 6 to 8 fl. ozs. of a 50% solution of magnesium sulphate may be given twice a day for several days.

Magnet Iron or steel that has an effect of magnetic field, a magnet that is used to remove metallic foreign body from eye.

Magnetic resonance imaging This is an advanced radiological diagnostic tool where cross sectional images in any plane of the body is obtained for examination, Abbreviated as MRI.

Magnetism Physical property of a magnet or electricity,
Force exhibited by a magnetic field,
Attraction and repulsion of different poles of a magnet.

Magnify By using suitable lens and mirror a substance is made to look big in size or larger in size.

Maim Because of trauma or injury a person who is mutilated.

Mainlining individuality of man Colloquial term which denote drug taken by drug addicts.
A patient is an individual member of society who has rights, Privileges and immunities which would be respected regardless of his race, creed, social or economic status and personal fears and needs which usually are exaggerated by his illness
It is a social responsibility.

Major principles of medical ethics They are as under:

- Beneficence, the principle of doing good.

- Justice, social and distributive justice to one and all with a view to serve the sick with fairness, equity and impartiality.
- Self-determination and liberty, full freedom right of individuals to make choice, right to make decision for themselves.
- Fraternity, the principle of not harming patients.

Making oral fluid It is making oral fluid in nursing care. One litre glucose salt solution which contains the following proportion is readily made available:

- Sodium chloride 3.5 G.
- Sodium bicarbonate 2.5 G.
- Potassium chloride 1.5 G.
- Glucose 20.0 G.

They are measured, pre packed in aluminium foil and sealed by drug companies. They are distributed through health service network. The above packet is dissolved in 1 litre of drinking water is suitable size for use in Home visiting.

For clinic or hospitals bags or bottles containing 10 times this amount for dissolving in 10 litres of water is more practical.

Standard measure is used at dispensing. Once prepared the ORS should be used within 24 hours. Every 24 hours fresh solution shall be prepared. It should not be boiled.

Mal It is a French word denoting sickness or disease, such as grandmal, petitmal, malfunction, etc.

Malabsorption When intestine cannot absorb nutrients which occurs in deficiency diseases including PEM.

Malacia It denotes the meaning of softening of a given thing such as bone softening or eye softening which are called osteomalacia and keratomalacia respectively.

Maladjustment In psychiatric practice, this word means that a person has not adjusted to his environment.

Malaise General symptom which shows a person as ill,

Discomfort in the body which is a vague feeling.

Malalignment Displacement and lying other than its normal anatomical position as in case of (a) bone (b) teeth.

Malaria Protozoal infection caused by Plasmodium and is transmitted by Anopheles female mosquito.

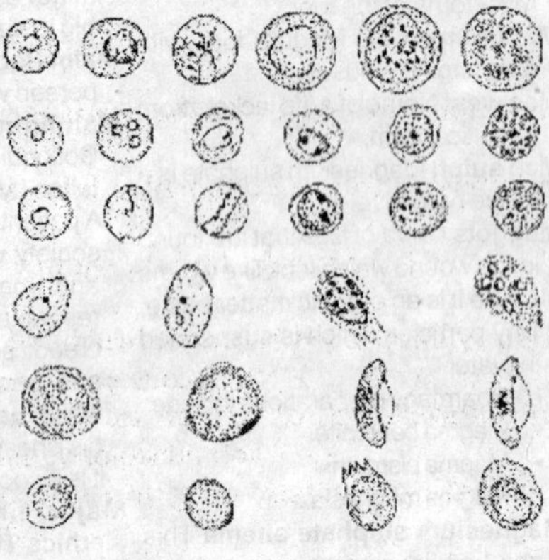

Malaria Parasite smear differentials

Malady It can be any one of the following:
- Illness or disease.
- Discomfort or uneasiness.
- Disability by injury or illness.

Male adaptor plug It is also called heparin lock which is inserted as male adaptor plug for intermittent infusion therapy, see heparin lock.

Male pill A derivative of cotton seed oil "gossypol" for 6 months orally has produced azoospermic in men. It is not in routine clinical use.

Malic acid An intermediate product of carbohydrate metabolism, malic acid is present in unripe tomato, cherry and apple.

Malignant This is referred to a tumour which progresses to worsening condition leading to death,
The tissue that has anaplasia, invasiveness and metastasis

Malingering Faking of disease which is purely intentional,
Wilful and deliberate exaggeration of symptoms of a disease.

Malta fever It is the local or native name for brucellosis, now that the clinical manifestation of Malta fever is known that in olden days this was for abortion in animal or for fever in man.

Malleolus The lower extremity articulates with anklebone and forms the inner prominence of the ankle which is called *internal malleolus*. Lower end of the fibula forms the outer prominence of the ankle which is called *external malleolus*.

Malleus It is a hammer-shaped bone attached to the inner side of the ear-drum.

Malnutrition Nourishment is not proper which indicates defective nutrition in quality and in quantity.

Malocclusion Abnormal "biting " at eating is present in dental condition where teeth do not meet properly, overlapping of bite due to malde-velopment
Depending upon excursive move-ments of the jaw for efficiency of mastication, malocclusion is classi-fied into 5 categories by Angle which is called Angle's classification of malocclusion.

Malpighian body The glomerulus and Bowman's capsule of kidney are named after Italian anatomist who was also a teacher in physio-logy and clinical medicine.

Malposition Any structure if in abnormal position in the body plane.

Malpractice It is the other name for professional misconduct where moral and ethical considerations are not taken.

Malpresentation When foetus presents face, breech, transverse etc., at birth,
Any presentation other than occiput (flexed head).

Malrotation Usually referred to G I tract which do not rotate in normal direction due to developmental failure.

Malta fever Other name for Bruce-llosis or undulant fever.

Maltase Intestine juice and panc-reatic juice which contain this sugar splitting enzyme,
That which converts maltose to glucose.

Malt Barley which contain maltose, glucose, dextrin and enzymes.

Malthusian theory This theory postulates that over population is controlled by natural calamities like volcano, earthquake, floods, epidemics, etc.

Though it is not a scientific version it can only be an antithesis of population.

Maltose When starch is reacted with intestinal enzymes maltose sugar is formed, $C_{12}H_{22}O_{11}$.

Malum Latin word meaning disease or evil condition in the body.

Malunion Refers to improper union of bones after fracture management, Faulty union of ends of fractured bones.

Mammary Any thing that is related to the breast.

Mammography It is a radiological examination by using X-ray or infrared rays.

Mammoplasty Plastic surgery on breast which is pendulous,

Plastic surgery on breast to enhance its size for feminine look.

Man midwife In late early centuries, the word 'Midwife" is heard. It was a hereditary family profession. During seventeenth century the word "Man Midwife" came to existence.

Mandible Bone of the lower jaw which joints at temporomandibular joint.

Mandle's paint It is compound pigment of iodine, which contains:

Iodine	6 grains
Potassium iodide	12 grains
Peppermint oil	3 min.
Glycerin	to 1 fl.oz.

Maneuver Skilled movement used in obstetrics such as:

- Credes maneuver to separate placenta
- Prague maneuver in breech delivery.
- Scanzoni maneuver to rotate foetal head.
- Bracht maneuver in breech extraction.
- Valsalva maneuver to ↑ lung pressure.

Mange This word is used for scabies.

Mania Mental illness where patient show extreme excitement or very much obsession

Mania is characteristic in Maniac depressive psychosis and in Kleptomania.

Maniac Refers to a person who is having serious nature of madness.

Mania Very commonly it is temporary mania in case of fits. In other organic lesion, mania is irreversible.

Manikin Human like body model used in nursing practice,

Manikin for delivery, Manikin for first aid, Manikin for dentistry.

Manipulation In nursing care, it refers to the following:

i. Hand movement for a desired movement of an organ or of a structure during surgery.
ii. Hand movement for a desired fixation of fractured bone.
iii. Hand movement for a desired change of foetus in the womb for normal delivery.
iv. Hand movement for the repair of hernia during surgical operation.

Mannitol It is a sugar alcohol used in nursing management in the following:

- Drug intoxication.
- Cerebral oedema.
- For producing diuresis.

Manometer It is used to measure liquid pressure or gaseous pressure.

Mantle It refers to a covering of a structure.

Manubrium This is upper portion of sternum where clavicle are joined from both sides through sterno-clavicular joints.

Mantoux test A form of tuberculin test where test material is injected between the layers of the skin for diagnosis purpose, PPD is given intradermally to anterior aspect of forearm and read for the reaction after 72 hours, if induration is above 10 mm it is positive for tuberculosis.

Manual method of resuscitation Advanced training is given under first aid for manual method of resuscitation which is called SylvesterBrosche .

1. The patient is placed on back and head to fall back.
2. Grasp the forearm from behind the head.
3. Draw arm upwards.
4. Sweep arm back.
5. Repeat 12 times per minute.

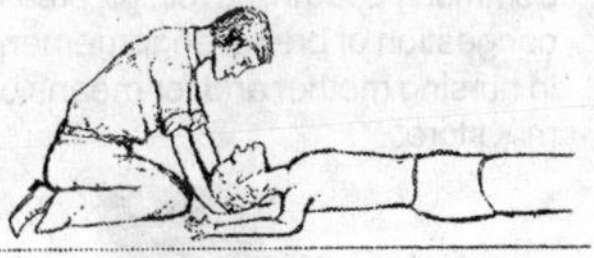

Inspiration (a)

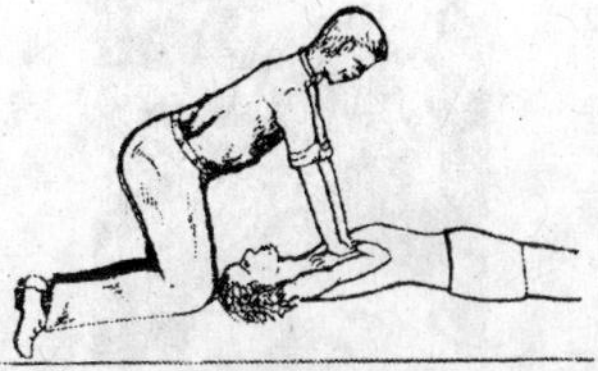

Expiraton (b)
Manual artificial respiration

Manual resuscitator It is used in the management of routine tracheostomy care and for suctioning the patient with a tracheostomy.

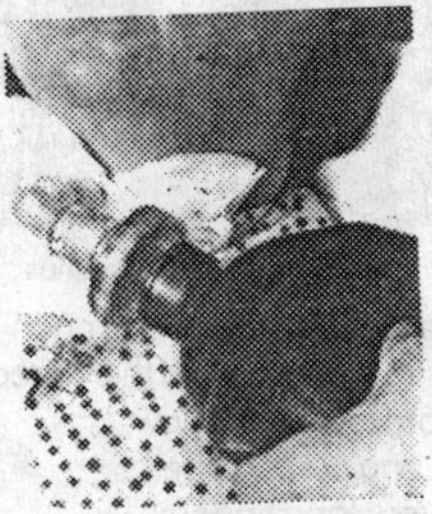

Manual resuscitator

Many tailed bandage This is a special bandage which is used for trunk dressing, for amputation stumps and for limbs dressing at painful conditions.

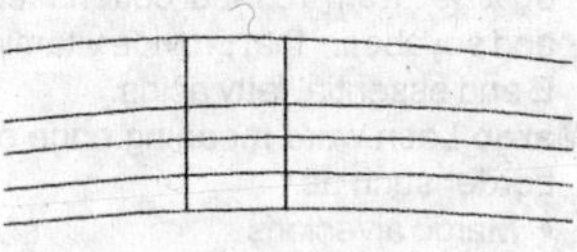

Many tailed bandage

Maple sugar urine disease It is birth defect and abnormality is seen in body chemistry.

Mapping It is a procedure to locate the position and order of gene loci on chromosome.

Marasmus It is usual manifestation of protein energy malnutrition found in infants and children, due to poor socioeconomic conditions
Skin and bony type of protein and calorie deficiency.

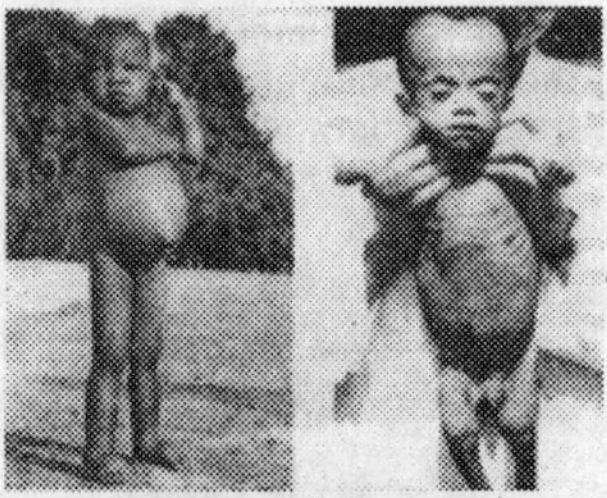

Kwashiorkor and Marasmus

Marfan's syndrome French paediatrician described this hereditary disorder which show:

- Long personality.
- Very long fingers.
- Palate is high arched.
- Hypertonic musculature.
- Dislocation of lens.
- Cardiac manifestations or diseases.

Margarine Food product containing 80% fat from refined cottonseed and soyabean that provide vitamin E and essential fatty acids.

Margo Latin word meaning edge or border such as:

- Margo alveolaris.
- Margo palpebrae.

Marijuana Age old known weed which has exhilarating effects when smoked often leads to troublesome conduct by the smoker.

Marjolin's ulcer Ulcer seated upon old cicatrix which follows the breaking down of wart tumour.

Marriage Social sanction for husband and wife to live together with each other's happiness and with learning the give and take which is the basic to the marriage relationship and to family life in general Marriage is also for procreation and maintenance of generation.

Marrison's approach It is one of the approach developed by Marrison to develop a lesson plan . This can be applied in developing a lesson plan by nursing tutor while taking classes to nurses.

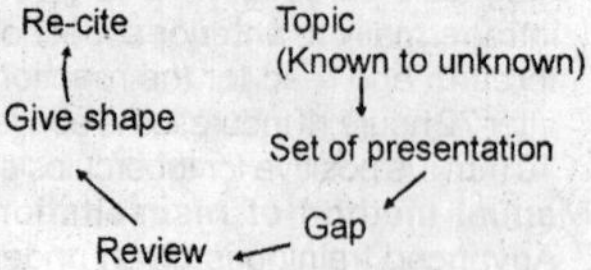

Marrison's approach of units

Marrow This is central portion of all cancellous bones,
Bone marrow.

Marshall Kaneson breast pump It is popular brand of hand pump that is used for milking from breast and later to store the milk in a plastic container,
Commonly used in the relief of breast congestion or breast engorgement in nursing mother and for means of milk store.

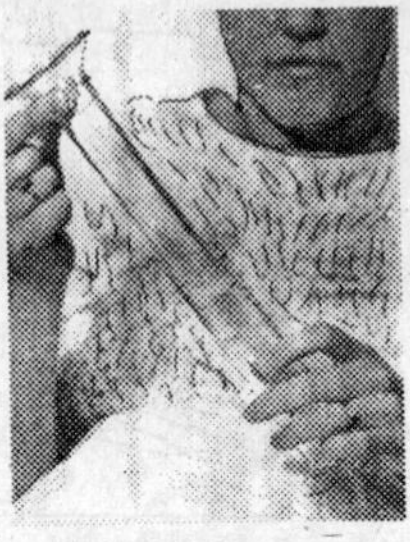

A: Marshall Kaneson pump

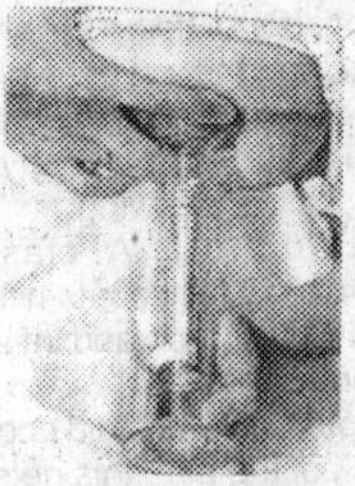

B: Marshall Kaneson pump in use

Marsupialisation The surgical procedure of stitching edges of incised sac to the edges of external incision,

The procedure to take away a cyst completely.

Martin's syringe It is one type of two-way syringe used for aspiration of the chest.

This syringe has a bayonet fitting and is supplied with a trocar and cannula and a sharp needle. A piece of rubber tubing is attached to one arm of the nozzle through which the fluid drawn up in to the syringe is ejected into the measure jug.

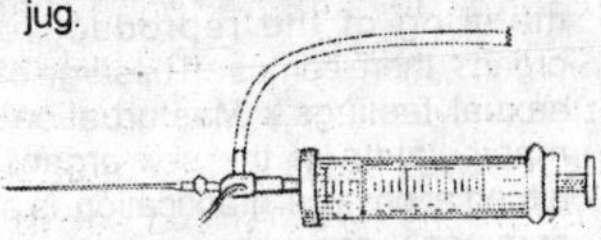

Martin's syringe

Marx A classical sociologist. His followers seized power,

Industrial sociology and class analysis emphasised.

Marzine It is used in travel sickness, This contains cyclizine which is long acting antiemetic, it produces drowsiness.

Mask non-rebreathing mask (Low flow high flow system).

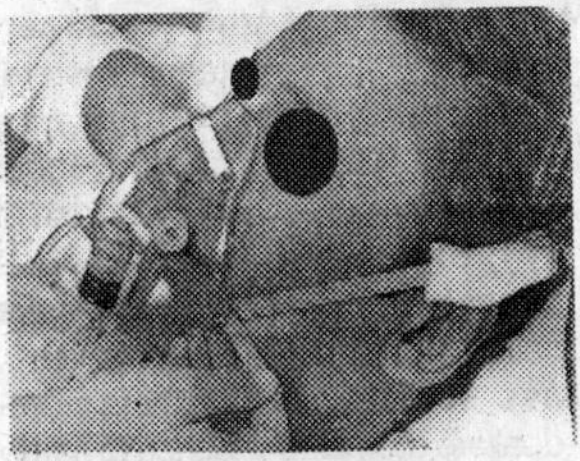

Non-rebreathing mask

Masculinisation When male secondary sexual characters develop in female.

Maslow's hierarchy of needs Human needs are given ranking by American Psychologist.

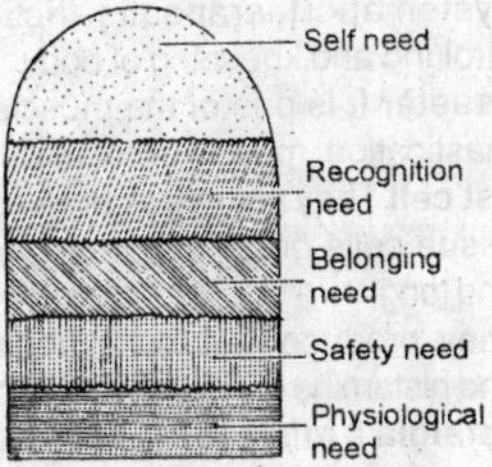

Maslow's Hierarchy of needs

Masochism It is a sexual perversion where person gets pleasure by inflicting physical pain and mental torture.

Mass Cohering particles bind together to form a mass, common words used in nursing practice are:

- Appendicular mass.
- Inner cell mass.
- Granular mass.

Mass culture Modern leisure is often provided for people in large number.

Mass media T.V.,Newspaper, Internet, Printed material, Posters, Health exhibition and folk media like Harikatha, Yakshagana, Puppet show, drama etc., are made use of in creating health awareness through mass media. All these are called Media of health education.

Mass society Society where individual are atomised attached to hardly any group between power and the group.

Massage Stroking, kneading or pressure scientifically applied by trained persons for the relief of pain or muscular stiffness or stimulate circulation or to promote sense of well being,

Systematic therapeutic friction, stroking and kneading of body.

Masseter It is one of the muscle of mastication, muscle of cheek.

Mast cell They are large connective tissue cells present in heart, liver and lung,

They produce serotonin, heparin and histamine during inflammation.

Mastalgia It refers to the pain in the breast common in inflammatory conditions.

Mastectomy Surgical removal of breast in cancerous conditions.

Masterly inactivity When a patient is seen unconscious some of the golden rules are found useful in the management of cases. They are posture, care of the mouth, maintaining the body warmth.

Masterly inactivity And *Immediate Medical advice.*

It consists of doing nothing beyond watching the patient which is very difficult in the case of emergencies.

Mastication It is the physiological process of chewing.

Mastigophora A class under protozoa which contain flagella.

Mastitis Infection and inflammation of breast tissue.

Mastoid bone Mastoid bone is at the back of the ear, this gets affected in case of untreated ear infection.

Mastoid Any structure which is breast-shaped or nipple-shaped such as:

- Mastoid antrum.
- Mastoid cell.
- Mastoid operation.
- Mastoid process.

The heavy bone at the rear of the base of the skull which contains sinuses.

Mastoidectomy This is the surgical treatment for purulent mastoiditis where mastoid bone is removed and mastoid antrum is drained.

Mastoiditis Infection and inflammation of mastoid antrum.

Masturbation Along with the maturing of the reproductive organs, there comes an upsurge of sexual feelings. Masturbation-manipulation of the sex organs aimed at physical gratification is a commonly seen phenomenon in boys and girls

Reliving strain, giving happiness reduces the incidence of masturbation

Sexual excitement by genital manipulation by the unmarried.

Matching To select similar characteristics in 2 items, matching is done as in blood matching , cross-matching of blood, etc.

Maté It is Paraguay tea, The tea leaf is got from a herb from South America, though it is folk medicine it has no medicinal value.

Materia medica It is the science that deals with the source and preparation of medicamentations and formulations that are dispensed in medical practice.

Material Physical substance from which one can make or compose another substance.

Maternal Anything that is related to mother such as maternal mortality, maternal cause, maternal nutrition, etc.,

Maternity Related to pregnancy in women.

Mating It is copulation, mating or intercourse for the purpose of reproduction.

Matrix When cells are embedded in the tissue

It is a mould or a cavity in which anything is formed

Matron Chief of nursing battalion in a hospital.

Matter It refers to a substance such as grey mater, White mater.

Mattress (egg crate) This mattress of a patient has corrugated surface, Its uses are:

- Minimises the pressure points. under the bony prominences.
- Promotes better air circulation.
- Prevents skin breakdown.

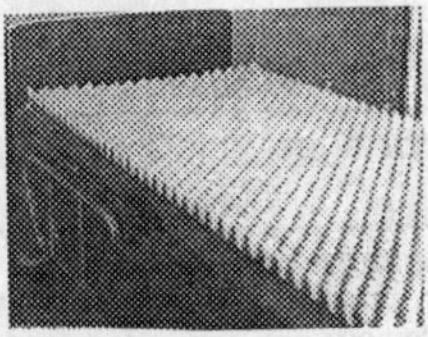

Egg crate mattress

Maturation Fully developed stage, Fully ripened stage.

Maxilla Bone that forms upper jaw.

Maxillary That is related to maxilla Name of the upper jaw bone which contains sinuses.

Maxillofacial That is related or pertains to maxilla and face.

Maza Greek term denoting placenta.

MBO Abbreviation for **M**anagement **B**y **O**bjectives,

In nursing service, different objectives are set with its own plan of action on short-term basis. Main aim of MBO is to achieve good result in nursing administration.

McBurney's point American Surgeon Dr.McBurney found out that on pressure at this point (the point midway between the anterior iliac spine and the umbilicus) elicits pain,

Tenderness in this point is diagnostic of appendicitis.

McDonald's rule It is used to estimate gestational age of pregnant woman in her 3rd trimester

If pregnant women showed the measurement as 30 cm from the fundus to the pubis, the gestational age can be estimated by using McDonald's rule as under:

$$\frac{\text{Fundal height in cms}}{3.5} = \text{is expressed in lunar months}$$

$$\frac{30}{3.5} = 8.5714 = 8.6 \text{ lunar months}$$

McGraw's ligature It is an elastic ligature used in intestinal anastomosis.

MCHC Abbreviation for **M**ean **C**orpuscular **H**aemoglobin **C**oncentration.

MCI code of ethics This has detailed guidelines on research and experiment in human beings (1980). ICMR has taken responsibility of revising from time to time, it has dealt with the following:
- Doctor to doctor relationship.
- Interprofessional relationship.
- Consultation.
- Cases of interference.
- Citizen care.
- Licence and other disciplinary action.

MDT Abbreviation for **M**ulti **D**rug **R**egimen in Leprosy

Though it involves using many drugs in therapy, major parts that are described under W.H.O "MDT" regimen are as follows:

A. Clinical grouping
B. Treatment with specified drugs
C. Leprosy surveillance.

Lesion	*PB single skin lesion(patch)*	*PB paucibacillary*	*MB Multibacillary*
Skin lesion	1	2 – 5	6 and above
Nerve involvement	No	only one	more than one
Skin smear	-ve	-ve	+ve

Table Clinical grouping in MDT regimen in leprosy

	Drug	*Dose*	*Frequency*	*Criteria for cure*
MB	Rifampicin Dapsone Clofazimine	600 mg 100 mg 300 mg	once monthly daily once monthly 50 mg	completion of 12 monthly pulses within 18 months daily
PB	Rifampicin Dapsone	600 mg 100 mg	once monthly daily	completion of 6 monthly pulses within 9 months
Single skin lesion	Rifampicin Ofloxacin Minocycline	600 mg 400 mg 100 mg	single dose	single dose treatment

Table: MDT drug regimen in leprosy

Category A	*Surveillance*
Single patch and 1 – 5 patch	Follow up once a year upto 2 years
Patches 6 or 6 +	Follow up once a year upto 5 years

Table: Surveillance in leprosy

Mean deviation This is an average deviation from the mean and is calculated by

$$\text{Mean deviation} = \sum \frac{|X - \overline{X}|}{n}$$

Measles An acute infectious disease of children caused by virus, Measles is included under National UIP programme

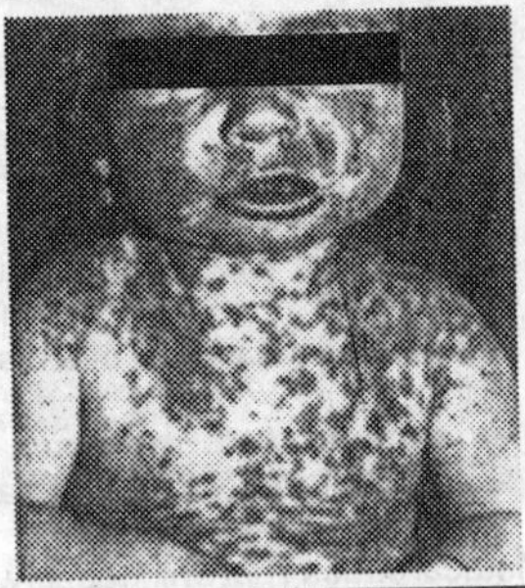

Measles rash

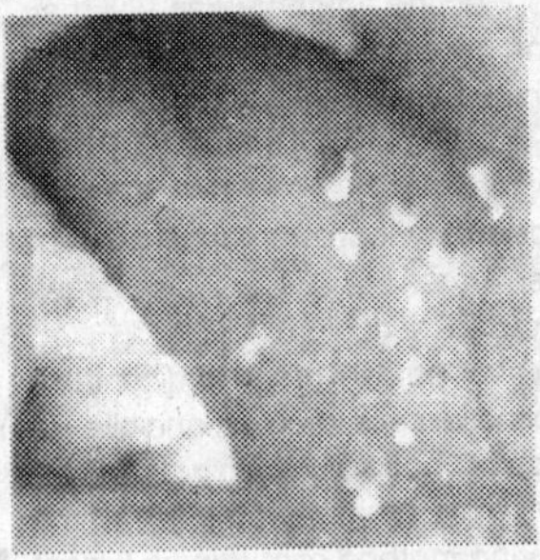

Koplick's spot in measles

Measurement of growth

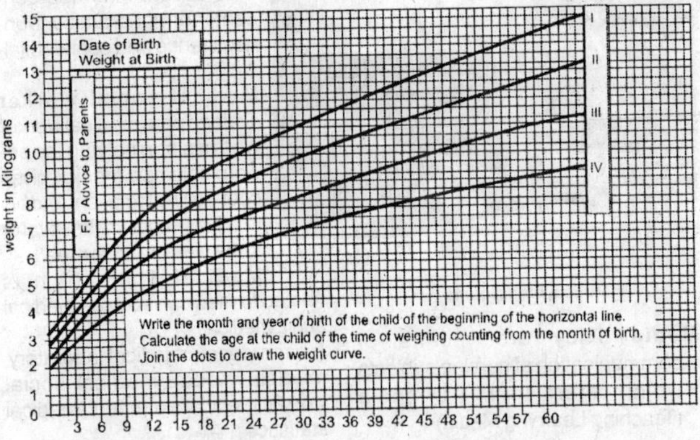

Growth chart for measuring growth

Meatus The opening into the ear channel is called external auditory meatus, The ear channel is called external auditory canal.

Meckel's diverticulum This is the connecting link between yolk sac and intestine in embryo stage which become remnant after birth, Is the remains of tube in the ileac region.

Meconium Soon after birth newborn discharges the intestinal discharges is called meconium,

This will be dark green and contains epithelial cells, mucous and bile.

Medela breast pump It is an automatic breast pump which is time saving method of obtaining breast milk on a longterm basis.

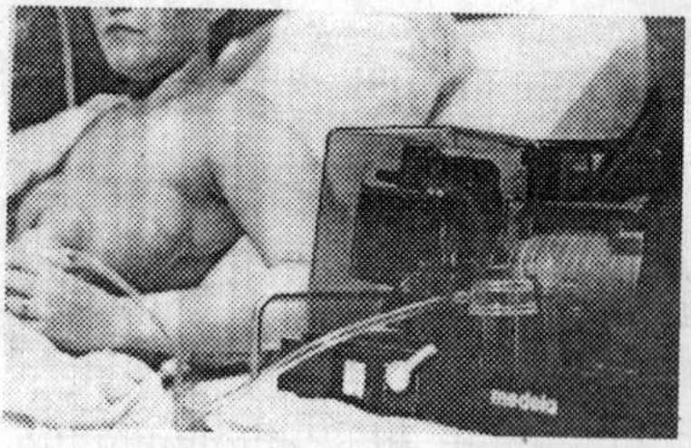

Medela breast pump

Media They are means of communication of nursing subjects which refers to T – L media (Teaching Learning Media)

Non projected	*Projected*
Black board	OHP
Display board	Slide projector
Charts	Epidiascope
Models	T V
Photos	Multimedia.

Table: T L media

Median When data is arranged in ascending order or descending order, the mid value taken forms an average called median, one which is placed in the centre of a distribution.

Mediastinum It is the place or space in the centre of the chest and between two pleurae.

Medical ethics That which deals with traditional and modern ethical values related to medical and health science for a social action to achieve desirable end

This covers informed consent, normal practice, non-negligence and confidentiality.

Medical social worker Trained para medical worker who assist in solving the social problems of the sick, gives counselling to patient and his relatives either in a hospital or in the field practice area.

Medical That which is related to medical, such as medical audit, medical

Jurisprudence, medical laboratory, medical model, medical social worker, medical statement, medical statistics.

Medicament All substance that are used for the relief of sickness and for treatment.

Medicated A substance is included in another substance which is of medicinal value such as Iodine is impregnated in salt.

Medication Patient treatment with drugs, a substance which is usually a chemical that is administered to patient for therapy.

Medication It is one of the forms of medical treatment where drugs are given orally, parentally or applied externally.

Medications Drugs that are used as therapeutic agents in clinical practice.

They are enumerated as under:

- Oral tablets.
- Oral capsules.
- Oral mixtures.
- Oral elixir.
- Tropical douche.
- Tropical eye, ear nose drops.
- Topical inhalant.
- Topical via nasogastric tube.
- Topical nitroglycerin
- Topical rectal
- Injectable I M
- Injectable I V
- Injectable S C
- Injectable I D
- Injectable insulin pumps.

Medicinal That which is related to medicine or that which has got therapeutic value.

Medicine A remedy for cure Science and art of disease diagnosis, disease investigation and disease treatment by medicaments.

Types of Medicine are :

- Emergency medicine
- Nuclear medicine
- Space medicine
- Sports medicine
- Forensic medicine
- Preventive medicine
- Community Medicine
- Family medicine.

Medico It refers to a medical student studying in medical college.

Medicolegal Medical matters related to law .

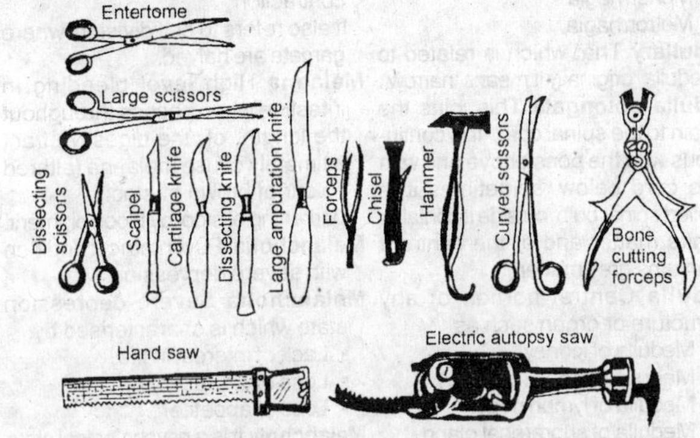

Medicolegal postmortem examination instrument

Medicosocial When both medical and social factors are involved in disease process.

Meditation transcendental An exercise by habit which can give a feeling of complete relaxation ,
It has shown low O_2 consumption, low cardiac output and changed electroencephalographic changes.

Medium Refers to culture medium which is used to allow growth of organisms,
A bacteriological term.

Medlars This is abbreviated as MEDLARS which is **Med**ical **L**iterature **A**nalysis and **R**etrieval Systems,
It is an on line data base system.

Medroxy progesterone Female sex hormone which is synthesised, It is used and indicated under following conditions:

- As contraceptive.
- Treating endometriosis.
- During treatment of endometrial cancer.
- DUB.
- Menorrhagia.
- Metrorrhagia.

Medullary That which is related to medulla, originally it means 'narrow'.

Medulla oblongata This joins the brain to the spinal cord. It is continuous with the pons above and with the cord below, sometimes it is called spinal bulb, outside it contains white matter and at the centre it contains grey matter.

Medulla Central portion of any structure or organ such as

- Medulla of kidney.
- Medulla of bone (marrow).
- Medulla of lymph node.
- Medulla of suprarenal gland.
- Medulla oblongata.

Megacolon Dilatation and hypertrophy of colon that can be acquired or congenital (Hirschsprung's disease).

Megakaryocyte This is present in bone marrow which is large in size and is responsible for production of blood platelets.

Megaloblast They are large nucleated cells which produce RBC.

Megalocephaly Condition where head is very large of an individual.

Megalomania One of the symptom of GPI (**G**eneral **P**aralysis of the **I**nsane) which manifests as delusions and self-esteem.

Mega ureter Clinical condition with enlarged ureter.

Meibomian cyst Other name for Chalazion, ducts of sebaceous gland gets obstrued to produce cyst first described by German anatomist.

Meibomian glands Small sebaceous glands beneath conjunctiva named after German anatomist Meibom.

Meiosis It refers to pupillary contraction
It also refers to cell division where gamete are halved.

Melaena High level bleeding in intestine when passes throughout the length of the digestive tract ultimately cause melaena (altered colour of brown of stool)
Darkening of stool by blood pigment.

Melancholia Psychiatric condition with severe depression.

Melancholia Severe depression state which is characterised by:

- Lack of interest in life.
- Loss of sleep.
- Loss of appetite.

Melancholy It is a psychological state of too much of sadness.

Melanin Melanin is a dark pigment, this is present in following organs:
- Skin.
- Hair.
- Choroid of the eye.
- Tumours (melanotic).

Melanin Dark pigment that is produced by natural means in the skin, in the eye and in the hair, It may be more, moderate or less in quantity which gives the colour to the area mentioned,
And tanning also produce melanin in the skin.

Melanocyte It refers to melanin tissue cells.

Melanoma Cancerous growth arising from pigmented tissue very commonly from a skin mole,
A malignant tumour.

Melena passing stool which is dark, blood stained or with altered blood

Mellitus This is a Latin word meaning 'honey', in clinical practice it is applied for sweet taste of urine in diabetes.

Membrane serous A connective tissue sheet lubricated with slippery serum.

Membrane This fibrous tissue layer which separates adjacent cavities or which surrounds a part or an organ
Mucous membrane and basement membrane are two common types available in description.

Memory It is the capacity of a person to retain, recall all experienced ideas, sensations and impressions, this comes from the process of learning As per physiologists the memory centre is situated in temporal lobe of the brain.

Menarche Attaining menarche is the start of menstrual cycle in girls at the age of 12 to 13 years.

Mendel's law It states–in the inheritance of certain traits or characters,the offspring are not intermediate in character between parents but inherit from one or other parent in this respect
Example:
TT tallness SS shortness ... parents TT, TS, ST, SS are possibilities in offspring.

Mendel's theory Similar to Mendel's law in nature.

Meniere's disease Otitis interna causing progressive deafness; clinically manifested with vertigo and tinnitus.

Meniere's disease Disease of inner ear which produce vertigo and hard of hearing.

Meninges The brain and spinal cord are covered by membranes called the meninges, outer dura mater, middle arachnoid mater and innerpia mater.

Meningioma Benign tumour of arachnoid mater and pia mater.

Meningism It is manifested with signs of cerebral oedema and there will be no evidence of pathogens.

Meningitis Infection and inflammation of covering of brain and spinal cord, meningococcal and tubercular meningitis are common.

Meningocele Cyst filled with CSF which is the protuberance of meninges through skull or spinal cord ,otherwise called spina bifida.

Meningococcus Common organism which cause meningitis and the genus is Neisseria meningitides, a diplococci.

Meningoencephalitis Infection and inflammation of brain and meninges.

Meningomyelocele A defect in the vertebral column causing protrusion of spinal cord and meninges Colloquially it is spina bifida.

Meniscus It is the semilunar cartilage of knee joint ,
If a lens has one side convexity and the other side concavity,
The upper surface of a liquid which is observed when the liquid is in a tubular container and which is seen as concave or as convex surface.

Menopause AT the age of 45 years and above women observe stop of menses and bodily changes which is quite normal to the aging process, After the age of 45 years in women, menstrual cycle wanes and stops indicating the stop of ovulation, This is associated with hormonal imbalance
Menopause is influenced by woman's heredity, her general health status and climate where she lives.

Menorrhagia Excessive flow of menstrual flow a gynaecological condition in women.

Menses Uterine bleeding at the time of menstruation in women.

Menstrual Related to or pertaining to menstruation.

Menstruation During the period of puberty and menopause women have monthly discharge of blood and endometrium from the uterus, Common gynaecological types of menstruation mentioned are:

- Ovular menstruation.
- Anovular menstruation.
- Vicarious menstruation.

Mental deficiency This refers to feeble mindedness, low I-Q of an individual.

Mental retardation It is one of the major conditions which affect human brain, some are born without the mental capacity to cope with the world which may be due to unfortunate accidents heredity or congenital defects or illness of the mother affecting the unborn child.

Mental Anything which is related to mind such as:

- Mental disorder.
- Mental handicap.
- Mental age.
- Mental health.
- Mental illness.
- Mental hygiene.
- Mental impairment.
- Mental acumen.

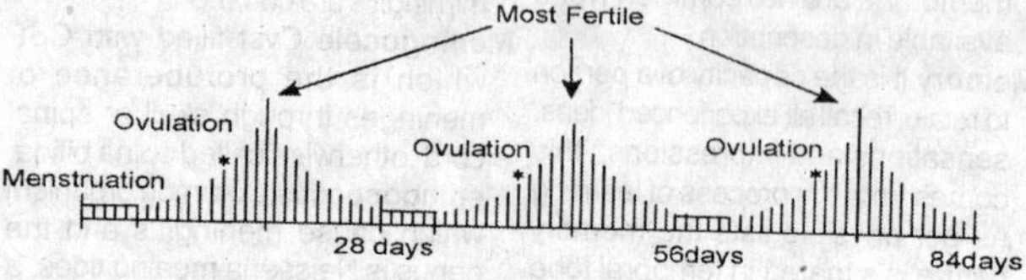

Menstrual cycle

Menthol It is derived from oil of peppermint and available as crystalline substance, Its uses are:
- Used in rhinitis.
- Used in neuralgia.
- Used as local anodyne.
- Used as local antiseptic.

Mentor One who gives advice or one who guides or one who facilitates,
Nursing tutor who helps in professional career development.

Mepacrine Chemotherapeutic agent used in malaria and giardiasis.

Meprobamate A therapeutic agent used in anxiety neurosis
A pharmacological agent which is used as a tranquilliser.

Mercaptopurine A chemotherapeutic agent in leukaemia,
It acts by preventing the synthesis of nucleic acid.

Mercury It is an element which is heavy and liquid in nature, in hospital practice we come across many thermometers and manometers set with mercury,
Occasionally in given dilution it is used as salt for antiseptic use.

Meridian Energy flowing lines in the body which is used in naturopathy like acupuncture.

Mescaline It is derived from an alkaloid which has the effect of hallucination and hence it is addiction producing drug.

Mesentery The small intestine is attached to the posterior wall of the abdomen by a relatively small double fold of peritoneum called mesentery.

Mesion It is the plane that divides the body into symmetric halves called right and left halves.

Meso Greek prefix meaning middle or intermediate.

Mesoderm In embryo, it is middle layer of 3 primary layers of cells which go to form connective tissue.

MesotheliomaThis highly cancerous growth seems to be associated with asbestos occupation,
It involve pleura, peritoneum or pericardium in the order of its occurrence,
It is one of the rapidly growing cancer where lifespan is in months.

Messenger RNA In chemical representation is is represented as mRNA, m RNA links amino acids to form protein in cellular level.

Meta-analysis In the year 1976-Professor Glass coined the word which denotes the combination of results of many clinical studies on the same subject to arrive at statistical conclusions,
This helps to take a decision on best clinical approach to a clinical problem.

Metabolic Any thing related to metabolism.

Metabolism For general function in the body, for growth of the body and for repair of the organs continuous *anabolism* and *catabolism* are going on (called metabolism) where food eaten gets transferred to tissue elements and then to energy,
In nursing care, two common terminologies used are:
- Basal metabolism.
- Inborn error of metabolism.

Metabolite Substance that take part in metabolism.

Metacarpal It is one of the five bones of the hand which joins wrist with fingers.

Metacarpus They are metacarpal bones mentioned under metacarpal.

Metacercaria Usually an infective stage of trematodes.

Metal splint splints made up of tin and aluminium are common in use. They are made in sections and are usually moulded as a gutter to fit the natural curvature of limb, metal splints are padded with felt and used.

Metal stretcher They are light and decontaminatable metal stretcher used in day to day first aid work., It has tubular poles and is provided with wire mesh bed and is comfortable for transporting patient with spine fracture.

Metamorphosis Transitional change from one shape to other in insects.

Metaphase In regular cell division called mitosis, metaphase is second phase.

Metaphysis It is the junction in a long bone where epiphysis and diaphysis come in to contact.

Metaplasia Metaplasia is an indication of malignancy where we notice abnormal changes in the structure of tissue.

Metastasis They are secondary deposits of cancer from primary cancer which is transferred by blood, by lymph or direct transfer.

Metastasis A cancerous growth when spreads by circulation to other parts of the body, secondary growth start growing in remote area of the body.

Metatarsal They are five bones which join toes to the tarsus.

Metatarsus They are metatarsal bones mentioned under metatarsal.

Metazoa They are multi-cellular organisms,

All animal kingdom except protozoa.

Metformin Oral hypoglycaemic agent used in diabetes,

Chemically it is biguanide derivative.

Methadone Pharmacologically it is an analgesic but not sedative and is used in the following conditions:

- Pain relief and palliative care.
- Terminal illness for symptomatic treatment.
- Treatment of drug addicts particularly in heroin addicts.

Methaemoglobin Drug action on RBC produces this altered form of Hb which cannot carry oxygen to tissues,

Aniline compound and phenacetin are known to produce methaemoglobin.

Methaemoglobinaemia High quantity of methaemoglobinaemia in the blood results in cyanosis and poor oxygen supply to tissue.

Methane Organic compound when gets decomposed, methane is produced, Methane is an inflammable explosive gas.

Methicillin One of the Penicillin group which is resistant to penicillinase, *Staphylococcus aureus* exhibits this phenomenon

MRSA is an abbreviation for **M**ethicillin **R**esistant ***S**taphylococcus* ***A**ureus.*

Methionine It is sulphur containing amino acid one of the essential amino acids.

Methotrexate Anticancerous drug which inhibit cell formation by antagonising folic acid.

Methyl orange It is an indicator used in chemistry which works in the pH range of 3.2 to 4.4 (yellow at pH 3.2 and pink at 4.4 pH).

Methyl red It is an indicator used in chemistry which works in the pH range of 4.4 to 6.0 (red at pH 4.4 and yellow at pH 6.0).

Methyl salicylate A liquid with characteristic odour produced from steam distillation of Gaultheria leaves or Betula lenta bark,

$OH.C_6H_4CO_2.CH_3.$

Methylated spirit It is called industrial spirit which can cause alcohol poisoning,

It contains 5% methyl alcohol and remaining will be ethyl alcohol.

Methylcellulose Indicated in constipation as a laxative since it forms bulk forming substance.

Methyldopa Drug used in hypertension, Its action is enhanced if used with thiazide diuretics.

Methylene blue It is an organic chemical compound which is used under following conditions:

- in cyanide poisoning.
- in methaemoglobinaemia.
- in staining techniques in pathology.
- in staining techniques in microbiology.
- as an antiseptic.

Metre It is a fundamental unit of length in metric system.

Metritis infection and inflammation of uterus.

Metronidazole Common chemotherapeutic agent used in

- Amoebic dysentery.
- Anaerobic bacterial infection.
- Giardiasis.
- T V infection.

Michel's clip They are surgical closure equipment and used along with suture or separately in surgery. For the removal of Michel's clip, dissecting forceps and clipremoving forceps are used.

Michel's suture clip Suture clips developed by French surgeon Dr.G.Michel, which are used for suturing wounds.

Miconazole Antifungal antibiotic used in clinical and nursing practice:

Common indications are:

Systemic fungal infections – I V infusion

Mouth and GI fungal infection - oral preparation

Athlete's foot, vulvovaginal Candidiasis – Topical.

Microaneurysm Dilatation of small arteries,

Common in diabetes and thrombocytopenic purpura

Diabetic retinopathy is typical example of microaneurysm.

Microbe Microorganism visible under microscope.

Microbiology Scientific study of microorganisms and their characteristics .

Microbion Related to microbe.

Microfilm Photographically to reproduce micro films of 16 mm or 35 mm sized films by high speed automatic machine.

Micrognathia Clinically receded chin due to failure of development of lower jaw.

Microgram One millionth of a gram which is represented as ìg.

Micron The other name for microgram.

Micro-organism It is a general term to denote bacteria, virus, rickettsia, parasites, some of the helminths which are microscopic in nature.

Microphage Phagocyte which is small in size.

Microscope Used in laboratory to view minute organisms which cannot be seen by naked eye.

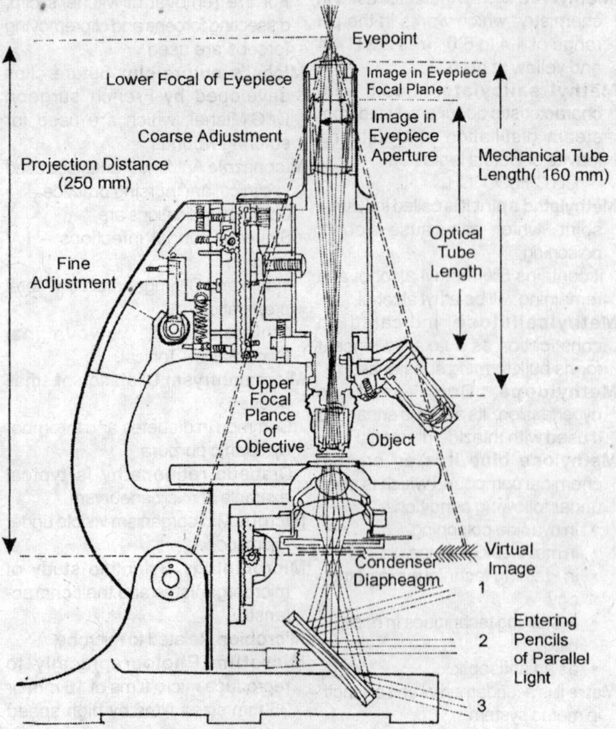

Path of Light through the Microscope

Microscope

Microscopic That which is visible only by microscope.

Microsurgery Minute detailed surgery done under microscope with the help of miniature surgical instruments.

Microvilli Finger like projection of cell membrane which gives greater surface area.

Microwave It refers to an electro-magnetic radiation with short wavelength , common sources are:

- Cathode tubes.
- Induction furnaces.
- Electrotherapy.
- Radar.

Usual descriptions of these waves are:

- Infrared wave upto 1 mm.
- Micro wave 1 mm to 30 cm.
- Radio wave above 30 cm.

Micturition The act of urination.

Mid deltoid injection site Injection given on lateral aspect of upper arm when 1 ml injectable is to be given and when injection is to be given occasionally mid deltoid injection site is selected for I M injection.

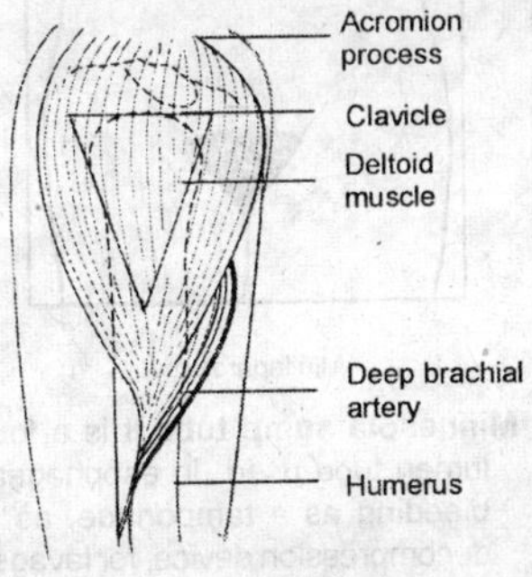

Mid deltoid injection site

Midbrain It is connecting part that connects brain and cerebellum and pons.

Midlife crisis Colloquially it is known as "empty nest syndrome",

In the stage of human cycle this stage is linked with dissociation when children move away from parents for their settlement,

Anxiety, depression and fear developed by elders when they are devoid of protection from their children.

Midwife This term has undergone many changes during the course of history of nursing,

Midwife ▸▸ Nurse ▸▸ Uni purpose worker female ▾▾

M.P.W. female.

Midwifery It is an art of attending to pregnant women in her pregnancy, in her delivery and in her post-delivery period.

Migraine Severe headache associated with nausea vomiting and visual disturbances in a person, paroxysmal attacks of severe headache

Headache which is very severe, which is associated with visual disturbances and often one sided.

Milestone It is the basis for the measurement of motor, social and psychological development of a child, developmental norms.

Miliary The term denotes to a generalised haematogenic spread of tuberculosis,

Usually refers to lung tuberculosis spread by blood.

Milk alkali syndrome It occurs in prolonged treatment of peptic ulcer, It is explained by the following findings:

- High level of calcium in the blood.
- Low calcium in the urine.
- Low phosphates in the urine.

Milk Nutritional fluid produced and made available to offspring by mother or mother animal through breast human milk is rich in carbohydrates where as cow's milk is rich in protein.

Human milk G.%	*Nutrients*	*Cow's milk G.%*
2.0	Protein	3.5
3.5	Fat	3.5
6.0	Carbohydrate	4.0
0.2	Mineral	0.7
88.0	water	88.0

T*able: Difference between cow's milk and human milk by composition*

Miller abbot tube It is an intestinal tube used to insert into the intestine for diagnostic and therapeutic purpose

Used in managing intestinal tubes in nursing care.

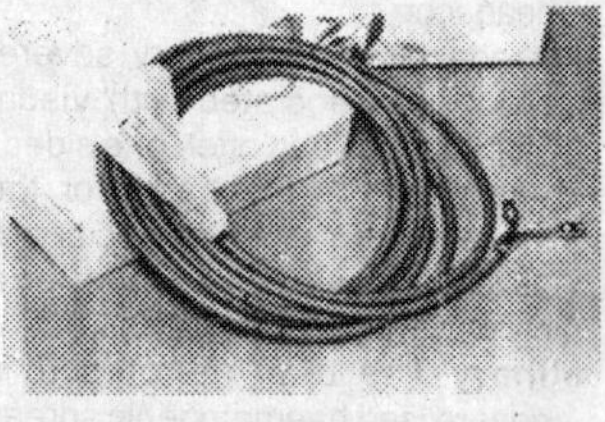

Miler Abbott tube

Millilitre One thousandth of a litre.

Millimetre One thousandth of a metre.

Milroy's disease It is one of the familial disease where accumulation of lymph leads to the swelling of limbs.

Mimicry A chance for the survival shown by animal kingdom which imitate others to improve survival chance.

Mineral Any metallic substance found in nature, Some of the minerals are essential nutrient to man and animals which are often trace elements, Latest terminology is micronutrients.

Mineralocorticoid It is produced by adrenal cortex which maintain the salt and water balance in the body.

Minilap operation With a small incision under local anaesthesia, tube is identified, ligated and sterilised. This is also called as pomeroy technique

Because of safety, efficiency and ease, it is used in tubectomy camps. It is suitable for post-partum tubal sterilisation.

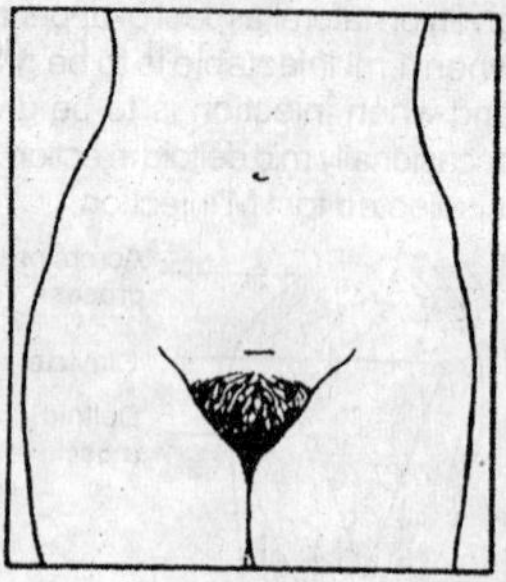

Minilaparotomy

Minnesota sump tube It is a four lumen tube used in esophageal bleeding as a tamponade, as a decompression device, for lavage, in general as a compression device.

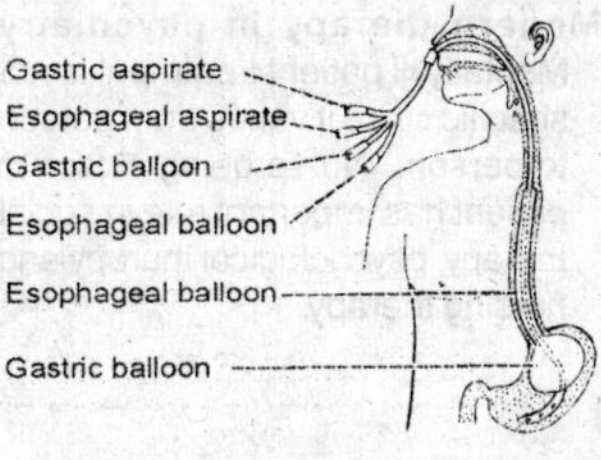

Minnesota sump

Miosis Pupillary contraction.

Miscarriage Labour occurring before the 28th week of pregnancy is called miscarriage (before 20th week it is abortion), violent exercise heavy lifting, sexual intercourse, long automobile trips, over work , excessive fatigue, painful dentistry and exposure to infections are found to be associated with miscarriage in women.

Mite They are spider like in their appearance. Medically importants are:

- Trombiculid mite, Itch mite
- Trombiculid mite transmits scrub typhus and itch mite causes scabies.

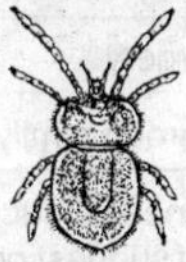

Adult Trombiculid mite

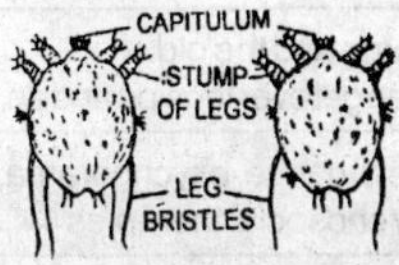

Adult itch mite

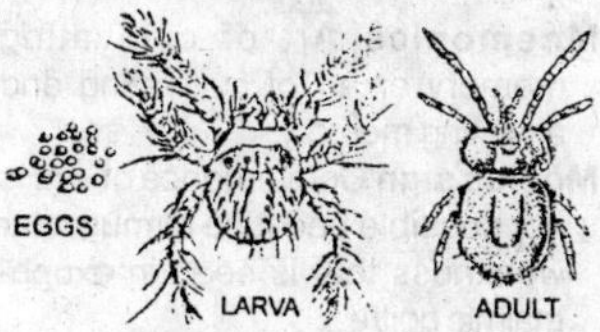

Life cycle of Mite

Mitochondrion Intracellular material which is responsible for production of energy and food oxidation.

Mitosis It is the process of cell division.

Mitral That which is connected with mitral valve of the heart such as:

- Mitral valve.
- Mitral stenosis.
- Mitral incompetence.
- Mitral vavlotomy.

Mixture Latin word meaning combination of different drugs or different ingredients, mixing fluids or fluid with solids for medica mentation.

MLD Abbreviation for **M**inimum **L**ethal **D**ose.

MMR Abbreviation for **M**aternal **M**ortality **R**ate.

The death of woman while pregnant or within 42 days of termination of pregnancy irrespective of duration and site of pregnancy from any cause related to or aggravated by the pregnancy or its management but not from accidental or incidental causes.

$$MMR = \frac{\text{Female death due to complications of pregnancy, childbirth or within 42 days of delivery from puerperal causes in an area during a year}}{\text{Total live births in that area for Yr}} \times 1000$$

Mnemonics Art of cultivating memory or art of cultivating and assisting memory.

Mobius sign Convergence of eye is not possible because of muscular weakness that is seen in exophthalmic goitre.

Modern sewage treatment plant Sewage is treated both by aerobic and anaerobic treatment to make sewage harmless and also useful.

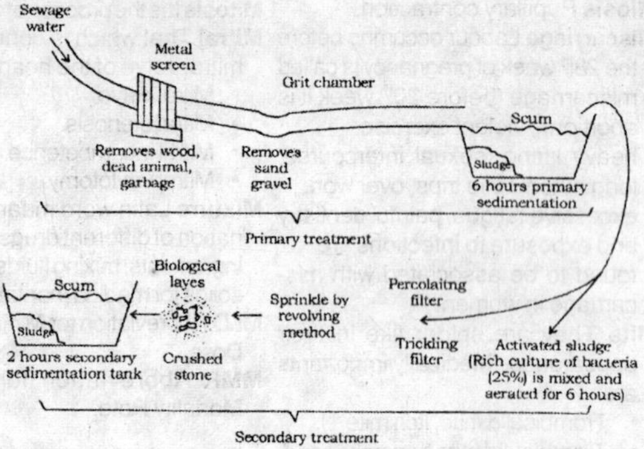

Modern sewage treatment

Modern therapy in psychiatry Mentally ill patient treatment is not specific since it varies from person to person. Nurse being closer to patient has important role in social therapy, psychological therapy and nursing therapy.

Physical therapy	Drug therapy, ECT, psychosurgery
Psychopharmacology	Psychotherapy of individual, group, family
Hypnosis	By altered state of consciousness induced by conditioning and skilled use of suggestions
Play therapy	Very helpful for young and the old. Diversion by play can get over tension and anxiety
Activity therapy	Occupational, music, dance, psychodrama, recreation and psy chosocial therapies

Table: Modern therapy in psychiatry

MOH Abbreviation for **M**edical **O**fficer of **H**ealth.

Moiety One portion of an another portion which are almost equal.

Molar It denotes molar tooth used for grinding at mastication,
Adult jaw contains total 12 molar teeth and child's jaw contains total 8 molar teeth.

Molds They are spore bearing fungi in nature, some of them cause allergy
They grow in decaying material
It also refers to a casting material for a shape.

Mole It refers to pigmented nevus
It refers also to uterine tumour
It also refers to molecular weight of a substance in G.

Molecular That which is connected with or made up of molecules.

Moles They can be ignored with safety unless located clothing tends to irritate them, any growth any bleeding, any soreness, any change in colour needs medical attention.

Malformation Any deformity of defect in a structure or in an organ.

Molluscum Skin manifestation with round tumours.

Moment of death Moment of death passes on to final death state in a series of pathological changes in the body
Somatic death, followed by cellular death through autolysis and decay occurs
Brain death or brainstem death is the requirement for legal, ethical and organ donation purpose
Moment of death may be noticed or unnoticed.

Noticed	*Unnoticed*
*passes through stage of pain, suffering, fear and giving up state	*Goes undescribed through the dying patient's mind
*Heart throbbing to family members	*Described by members of family according to their faith and feeling

Table: Noticed and unnoticed moment of death

Mongolism Old term for Down's syndrome or Trisomy 21.

Monilia It is the other name for fungus belonging to Candida.

Monoamine oxidase This is an enzyme which reacts and breaks down serotonin and noradrenaline in the body.

Monoclonal That which is derived from one single cell.

Monocular That which happens or occurs to one eye.

Mononucleosis Infectious mononucleosis colloquially called 'kissing disease' is a disease of young and adolescent groups in the society.

Monosaccharide They are simple sugars like glucose, fructose, galactose, etc.

Mons Any prominence or any mound such as Mons pubis.

Montgomery's tubercle They are sebaceous glands around nipple, Grow large in pregnancy to become tubercle
Named after Irish Obstetrician Dr.Montgomery around 1820.

Mood Depression and excitement are common moods which show off as emotional reaction in a person.

Moonface Clinical manifestation of Cushing's syndrome, steroid therapy adds the blown up picture.

Morbid it refers to illness, abnormality or disorder.

Morbidity It is the morbid state of a person or a group of people.

Moribund Terminal stage of a dying patient, one who is dying.

Morning sickness Layman's term for nausea of pregnancy in early pregnancy.

Moro reflex Moro reflex is also called Startle reflex where we notice sudden movement of a newborn for a loud noise.

Morphine It is an opium derivative which dulls the pain in patients, It produces addiction and is responsible for drug abuse Opium alkaloid which produce addiction in a person $C_{17}H_{19}NO_3 + H_2O$.

Morphologic It is related to the structure of an organism.

Mortality Death occurring due to illness, suffering or disease.

Mortification Necrosis of tissue.

Morula Early part of ovum development in the study of embryology.

Mosaic If a person has cells of varying genetic composition.

Mosquito Little flying insect which sucks blood and transmits many diseases,

Anopheles, culex, aedes and mansonia are common mosquitoes in public health consideration.

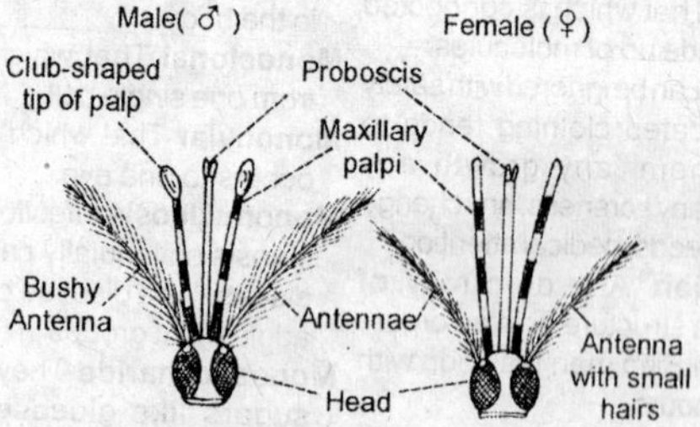

Head of anopheles

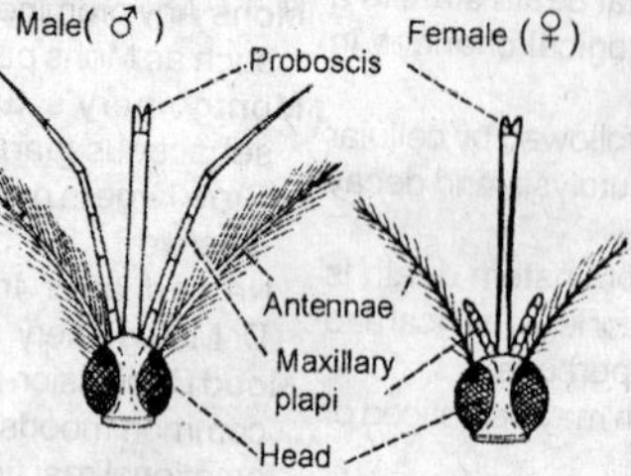

Head of anopheles and culex mosquitoes

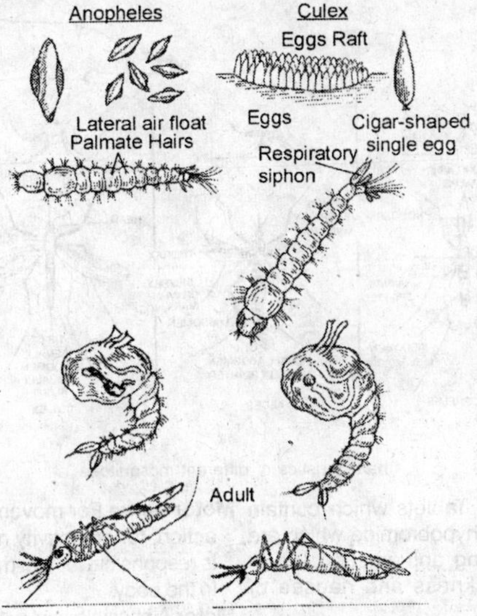

Life cycle of mosquito

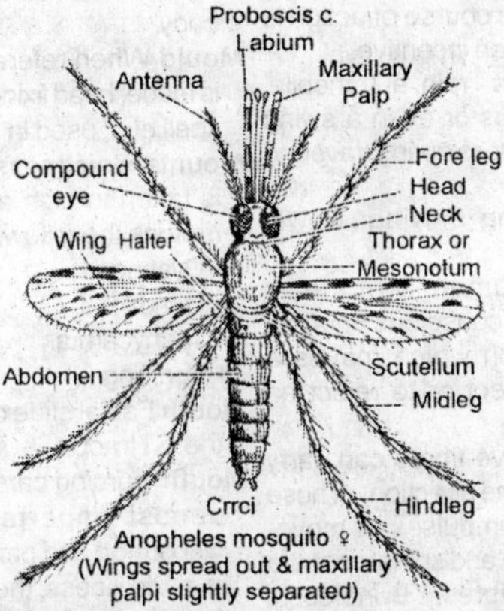

Anopheles mosquito ♀
(Wings spread out & maxillary palpi slightly separated)

Adult anopheles mosquito female

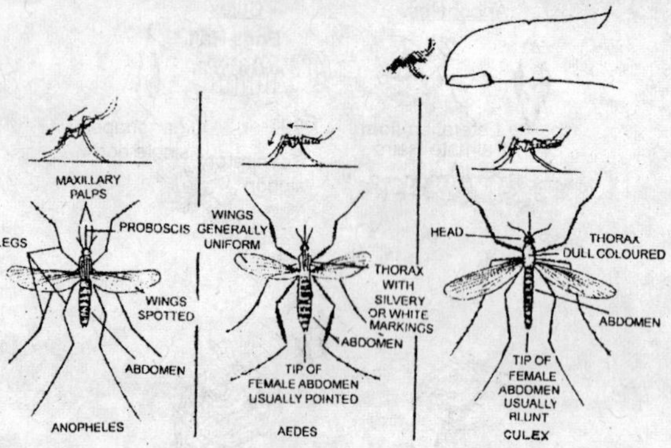

Characteristics of different mosquitoes

Mothersils Tablets which contain hyoscine hypobromide which are short-acting anti-emetic used in travel sickness and nausea of pregnancy.

Motile Any course of action or any direction of the course of action is determined by an incentive.

Motion sickness Train, automobile, ship, plane, bus or even a swing can produce illness during travelling or at motion.

Motion Anything moving, Bowel movement.

Motivation Human attitude is determined by conscious or unconscious reason which makes a person to accept or to reject an action.

Motor fibre Nerve fibres can carry messages in one direction . Those which convey impulses of movement from brain and spinal cord are called motor fibres. Bundles of motor fibres go to form motor nerve

Motor nerve For movement, for an action, for an activity nerve which is responsible for that motor activity in the body.

Motor A physiological action causing movement of parts, of organ or of a body.

Mould When reference to a fungus is made, head fixing shell, limb fixing shell etc., used in radiotherapy.

Mountain sickness When a person is taken to high altitude he experiences the following:

- Dyspnoea.
- Headache.
- Tachycardia.
- Vomiting.

Mouth Facial slide of the opening of the G I tract.

Mouth nursing care of the mouth is utmost important to prevent discomfort and parotitis.

In acute illness, the mouth requires frequent and careful attention

This is required in patients who are on a limited fluid diet and regular two hourly attention should be given.

In unconscious patient, danger of inhaling material into the air passage should be borne in mind.

Mouthstick When there is no functioning hand in a person or a patient, this device is used.

Mouthwash Mouth cleansing solution which is used to wash the mouth, but do not have any medicinal value or whatsoever.

Movable joint Movable joint is one in which the bones have smooth cartilage covered surfaces, which are lubricated by synovia and are bound together by more or less perfect capsules.

Movement Refers to movement of extremity, or of a part of the body, or of the bowel.

MPW Abbreviation for **M**ulti **P**urpose **W**orker,

One MPW (male) and one MPW (female) are posted to subcentres which cover a population of 5000. They are given the assistance of voluntary workers.

This scheme is as per the recommendation of Kartar Singh Committee Report 1973.

MRCP Abbreviation for **M**ember of **R**oyal **C**ollege of **P**hysicians.

Mucilage Artificial viscid paste used in pharmacy.

Mucinase Enzyme acting on mucin.

Mucin It is mucous membrane secretion that contains mucopolysaccharide.

Mucocele A tumour arising from mucous membrane such as from lacrimal mucocele or gallbladder mucocele.

Mucocutaneous Anything that is related to skin and mucous membrane.

Mucoid That which resembles mucous.

Mucolytic Drug which brings down the viscosity of bronchial secretion.

Mucopolysaccharide It is present in synovial fluid and mucous secretions,

It is also called as glycosaminoglycan.

Mucoprotein It is a complex substance containing mucopolysaccharide and protein.

Mucopurulent When both mucous and pus are present.

Mucosa It refers to mucous membrane.

Mucoviscidosis Other name for fibro cysti disease of the Pancreas.

Mudaliar committee This is called "Health Survey and Planning Committee". This studied the progress of Bhore committee report and made certain recommendations for health service expansion.

Multicellular Refers to multicellular organism other than protozoa.

Multidisciplinary approach When many disciplines are involved in addition to health sector all related sectors and aspects of National and community development in particular agriculture, animal husbandry, food industry, education, housing, public works and communication are to join and give health care through multidisciplinary approach.

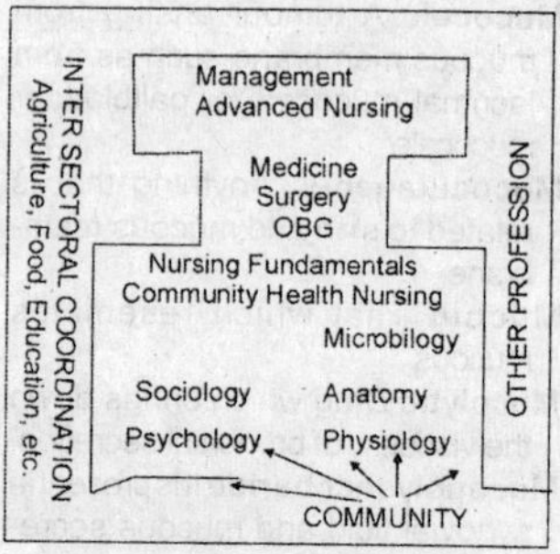

Multidisciplinary approach in health care

Multidisciplinary Who many disciplines are involved.

Multigravida Woman when has more than two pregnancy in her reproductive life.

Multilocular When a structure has many locules such as multilocular cyst of ovary.

Multiple When a thing occurs simultaneously in different parts of the body.

Multipara Woman who has had more than two children.

Multiple sclerosis Deterioration of brain and nervous tissue due to hardening of brain tissue or nerve, It is a nervous disorder.

Multivariate analysis All related variables are taken into consideration for analysis of data to find out their significant relation in the causation.

Multivitamin oral or parenteral preparation containing many vitamins for therapeutic use.

Mumps A viral infection of parotid gland which can affect testes, ovary, bone, brain, pancreas causing acute infection of mentioned organs and as a consequence of which function of such organs are lost such as sterility in case of testes or ovary.

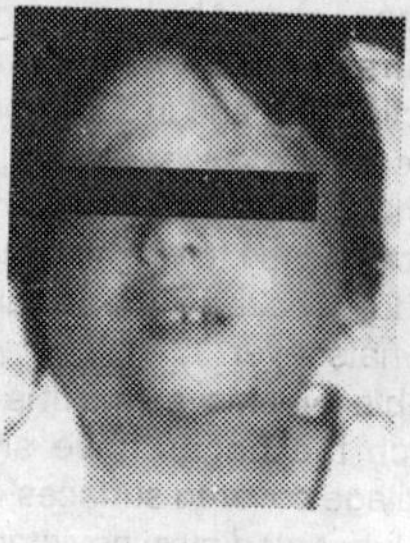

Unilateral mumps

Murmur Sound heard at auscultation of the heart which gives the clue to the defects of valve or damage of valve.

Murphy's sign Pressure on gallbladder causes 'catch breath' at the peak of respiration, this is the diagnostic of gallbladder inflammation American Surgeon Dr. Murphy first elicited this sign.

Musca domestica It is the zoological name for common house fly.

Muscarine Fungus alkaloid which is poisonous that cause muscle paralysis.

Muscle Fibrous tissue that has the power of contraction and that help in the movement of part of the body, They may be striated or unstriated in nature

Referable to both bone and muscle.

Musculoskeletal Related to muscle and bone, pertaining to the framework of the body which include muscle and skeleton.

Muscular dystrophy Gradual wasting of muscles of the body giving rise to dysfunction.

Museum They are health galleries in science which deal with human beings themselves, here people can inform themselves about themselves for better health.

Mustard bathe It is a medicated bath which is ordered for its general stimulating effect, or to treat colds and chills.

4 to 6 oz. of mustard may be placed in a muslin bag, which is squeezed in the water or it may mixed to a paste with sufficient tepid water and added to the bath. the average full bath is 30 gallons.

Mutant That which is produced by mutation,

A genetic terminology.

Mutation Genetic change which is chemical in nature that brings about either change in characteristics or disorders.

Mute One who cannot speak or who has lost speech.

Mutilation Body injury is caused by specific purpose or deliberately.

MutilationLoss of configuration of an organ, organ or tissue which looses its natural integrity, loss of portion of the body.

Mutism Person who cannot speak because of loss of hearing which cause not learning or because of disease such as stroke.

Myalgia pain experienced in muscle due to many clinical conditions.

Myasthenia gravis Severe muscle weakness of one specific group of muscles.

Myasthenia It refers to muscular weakness.

Mycetome It is referred to as madura foot, a chronic fungal infection of skin and internal organs.

Myco An abbreviation for Mycobacterium.

Mycobacterium Gram-positive acid-fast rod-shaped bacteria which include the following:

Mycobacterium tuberculosis

Mycobacterium leprae

Mycology Scientific study of fungi.

Mycosis Diseases caused by fungi.

Myeloblast It is bone marrow cell which is primitive and from which granular leucocytes are developed.

MyelinThe covering of nerve fibres which are medullated and looks fatty.

Myelitis It refers to both inflammation of spinal cord and bone and are used as myelitis and osteomyelitis respectively.

Myelocele Hernial protrusion of spinal cord substance through defect in bony canal.

Myelocyte This is produced from myeloblast and is the cell in bone marrow.

Myelogram X-ray of spinal canal after pushing radio-opaque chemical.

Myelography By L.P. radio-opaque substance is introduced to view spinal cord.

Myeloid Similar to bone marrow, Related to spinal cord.

Myeloma It is plasma cell tumour.

Myelomatosis Multiple myelomas are present in cancer of bone marrow.

Myiasis Myiasis is a clinical condition caused by the attack of larvae of common house fly. They attack tissues, intestine or bladder.

It is not "obligatory Myiasis" since development of housefly larva in

human tissue is not essential for their complete development. Housefly larva can be "facultative Myiasis"
Maggots or larvae of flies invade wounds which give the appearence of worms in the wounds.

Myocardial That which is related to myocardium such as myocardial infarction.

Myocarditis Inflammation of myocardium.

Myocardium This is the muscle tissue of the heart.

Myoclonus Severe spasmodic contraction of muscles or of a muscle.

Myofibrosis Muscle tissue is replaced by fibrous tissue which is a degenerative disorder.

Myohaemoglobin Hb like substance which is present in muscle tissue, Myoglobin is stored in the muscle.

Myokymia Harmless quivering of muscle, a clinical condition.

Myoma Benign tumour of muscle.

Myometrium The muscle tissue of uterus.

Myoneural That which is related to muscle and nerve.

Myopathy It refers to the diseases of muscles.

Myope It refers to a person who is suffering from myopia.

Myopia Short sight in a person,

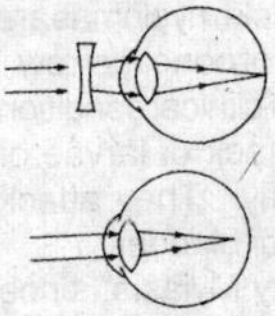

above picture under this is with correction by Concave lens for Myopia. Below picture this is before correction showing rays focussed in front of retina.

Myoplasty In rehabilitative surgery and reconstructive surgery, a muscle is detached and used for correction of movement of an organ or limb.

Myosarcoma Sarcoma of muscle tissue.

Myosin This is a muscle protein
It is a myoprotein or muscle protein that helps in muscle contract ion.

Myositis Inflammatory disease of muscle tissues
Infection and inflammation of muscle tissue.

Myotonia When there is no tone or reduced tone of a muscle.

Myringotome This is used to puncture the eardrum during middle ear infection associated with pus in the ear.

Myxoedema Hypothyroidism or lowered functioning of thyroid gland, Clinical presentations are:

1. Swelling of the face.
2. Swelling of the limbs.
3. Swelling of the hands.
4. Skin is dry and rough.
5. Loss of hair.
6. Pulse and temperature are below normal.
7. Lowered metabolism.
8. Mentally dull.

Myxoma Mucous tumour of connective tissue which is not cancerous.

Myxovirus Mucoid tissue is present in a sarcoma.

N

N95 mask In the case management of SARS, N95 Mask is suggested to attending doctors and nurses in the isolated ward to prevent the doctor and nurse in getting the infection.

Naegele rule It is a method of counting the expected date of delivery by subtracing 3 months from first day of (LMP) and add 7 days.

Naevus Flammeus It is capillary haemangioma which is diffuse poorly defined area varying from pink to dark blue involving otherwise normal skin.

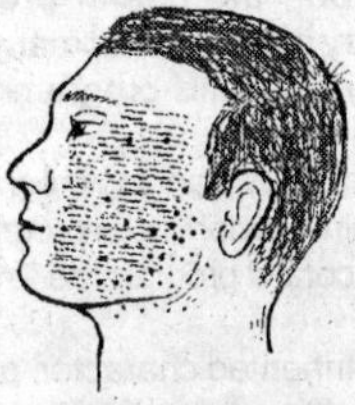

Naevus Flammeus

Naevus Birth mark which is an area of pigmentation of the skin.

Negative Absence of a person, of a substance, of an item, not positive.

Nail Keratinised portion of epidermis found in fingers and toes, *Spoon nail* and *in growing nail* are common occurrence, finger nail and toe nail are specialised form of skin.

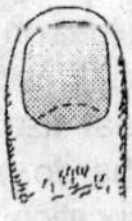

Nail

Naked Person without any cloth on the body, born free status, fully exposed for the view.

Nalidixic acid Chemotherapeutic agent used in urinary infections.

Named nurse Nurse posted to look after certain patients is accountable for the Nursing care and who effects good continuity or follow up.

Nandrolone Anabolic steroid used in health care.

Nanism Too short a stature, a dwarf.

Nano One in billion, 10^{-9}, 0.0000000001 describes smallness in comparison, nanogram.

Nape Area in the back of the neck.

Nap Sleep of small duration.

Naphthalene It is an anti-moth agent, derived from coal tar.

Naphthol Crystalline antiseptic substance, two types are alpha and beta

$C_{10}H_7.OH$.

Napkin rash Skin rash in infants in napkin area due to ammoniacal dermatitis, napkin wash by detergent can cause skin rash.

Narcissism Self admiration of one's own naked body, sexual pervert.

Narcolepsy Desire for sleep which is not controllable.

Narcosis Loss of consciousness by the use of narcotic drugs.

Narcotic Drug that produces unnatural sleep, induced sleep.

Narcotics Drugs which induce sleep or depress body functions.

Nares Other name for nostrils.

Nasolacrimal Word indicates the covered area by both nose and lacrimal apparatus.

Nasal cannula It is called low flow system in respiratory therapy, used in patient with MI and COPD for oxygen therapy.

Nasal duct It is the part of lacrimal apparatus, this carries the tear fluid down into the nose.

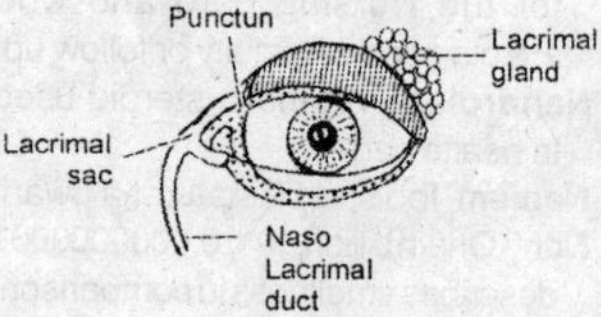

Nasal duct

Nasal feeding Feeding tube is passed through to the stomach and liquid are pushed, indicated in a case of not swallowing by mouth.

Nasal Referable to the nose.

Nascent Just liberated substance from a compound, person or animal just born.

Nasogastric tube Used in feeding and for medicine administration.

Nasogastric Referable to both nose and stomach.

Nasojejunal feeding Indicated in babies to prevent aspiration with nasogastric tube feeds, indicated in sick baby which is on ventilator for CIP (Continuous inflating pressure), a method of baby feeding when it is sick.

Nasopharyngo-scope An electrically lighted instrument for examining the throat and larynx.

Nasopharynx Referable to both nose and pharynx the upper part of the throat which is behind the nose.

Natal Pertaining to birth of a newborn.

Nates Colloquially it is called buttocks, anatomically it is called gluteal region.

National Formulary National level compilation of pharmacological formulations, Recipes and prescriptions which are standards for pharmaceutics.

National health problems There are 5 categories of health problems in India. They are:

- Population problem.
- Health care accessibility.
- Environmental sanitation problems.
- Nutritional problems.
- Communicable diseases problems.

National health programmes To act upon the health problems, country has launched many National health programmes, to mention a few

National F W planning programme
Vitamin A prophylaxis programme
AIDS control programme
UIP.

Native Inherited character, person if born with a disease or a defect.

Natraemia It indicates the presence of sodium in the blood.

Natriuresis High quantity of sodium is excreted in the urine.

Natural childbirth Active participation of woman and her husband for childbirth which can allow avoiding medical interference and pain killers.

Naturopath A practitioner of healing cult which relies on so called natural methods such as diet, air, sun and water to treat disease:

Naturopaths do not have formal medical education.

Naturopathy Natural way of allowing healing through diet, exercise, hydrotherapy, no artificial or allopathic treatment.

Nausea Vomiting sensation of the patient or of pregnancy.

Navel Navel region, umbilical region.

Navicular Tarsal bone of the feet which is boat-shaped it refers to boat-shaped item, Navicular bone.

NBIN emulsion It contains the following:

Benzyl benzoate	68 %
DDT	6%
Benzocaine	12%
Polysorbate	14%

It is a scabicidal agent.

NCD Non Communicable Diseases.

Nebuliser Apparatus used for aerosol therapy in clinical conditions like asthma, in therapeutic conditions like oxygen therapy.

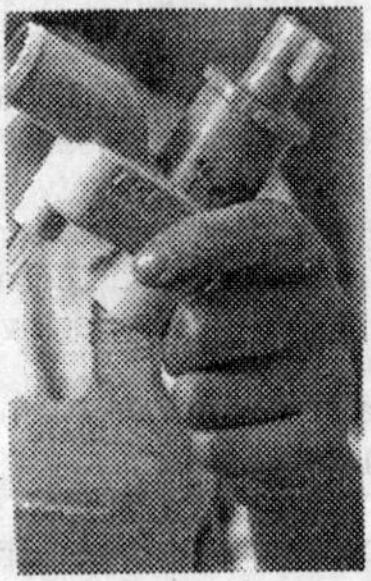

Nebuliser

Nephritis Proper word is glomerulonephritis, popular name is Bright's disease, associated with infection of the throat.

Nebula Corneal opacity caused by injury or ulcer.

Nebuliser It is an atomiser, instrument to make liquid to be sprayed as spray.

Necator Hookworm group of helminths, *Necator americanus*.

Neck Part of the body which connects head with thorax, words like anatomical neck and surgical neck are used by orthopaedicians.

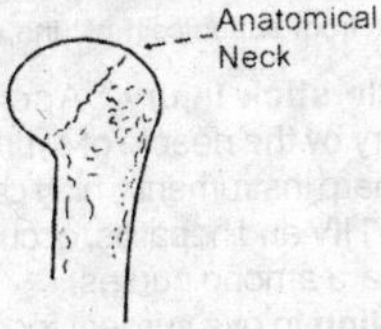

Anatomical neck of femur

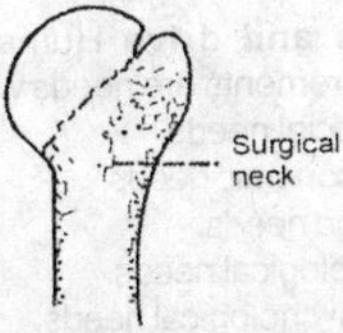

Surgical neck of femur

Necrobiosis Death of tissue due to degeneration.

Necrosis Death of tissue.

Necrotising enterocolitis An infective condition in preterm babies which cause diarrhoea and bleeding in intestine.

Needle Sharp instrument for puncture, common known needles are:

- Aspirating needle.
- Ligature needle.
- Hypodermic needle.
- Harelip needle.
- Hagedorn's needle.
- Exploring needle.

- Cataract needle.
- Aneurysm needle.

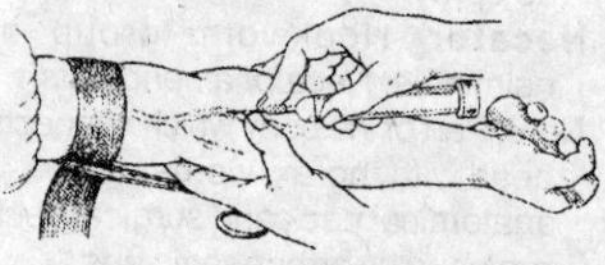

Needle in position for obtaining blood from superficein of the arm

Needle stick injury Accidental injury by the needle of syringe or of a sharp instrument which can infect with HIV and hepatitis, occupational hazard among nurses.

Needling In eye surgery for cataract lacerating and splitting of lens is done.

Needs and drive Human basic requirements are needs which are:
- Social needs.
- Economic needs.
- Ego needs.
- Biological needs.
- Psychological needs.
- To acquire the needs there are motives or drives in human beings.

Negligence Describe the legal duty of a nurse to provide health care which when absent results in bodily injury of the patient.

Neil Robertson stretcher Very useful first aid for removing casualties from confined spaces and is widely used in the navies.

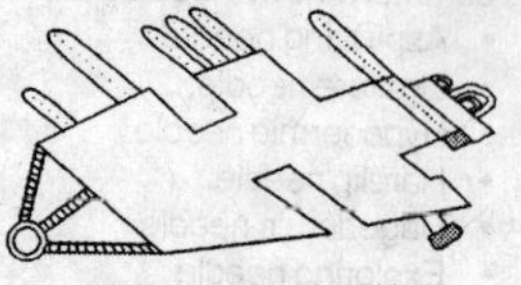

Neil Robertson stretcher

Neill Mooser reaction It is a laboratory test by doing animal experiment, animal inoculation with rickettsiae of murine typhus produces scrotal swelling which contains large mononuclear cells filled with rickettsiae which are intracytoplasmic in nature.

Neisseria *N.gonorrhoea* which is paired, spherical and gram-negative.

Nelson's inhaler Traditional method of treatment for inflammation of upper air passage, an earthenware inhaler is filled with boiling water to which medicine is added and inhaled in a closed space artificially provided with a cover by shawl or small blanket.

Nematoda It is a class of roundworms and threadworms, nemathelminthes.

Neo Marxism Updating the insights of Marx by a group.

Neoglycogenesis It is also called glyconeogenesis, liver glycogen formation from noncarbohydrate source.

Neomycin Wide range antibiotic used, indicated in eye and skin infection, given orally in pre-operative bowel preparation.

Neonatal nursing Procedure Birth weight, height and head circumference recording, APGAR scoring, check for birth defects, snap test for hip dislocation etc.

Neonatal Period of 28 weeks of life after birth of a child.

Neonate Newborn baby up to one month of age.

Neonatologist Paediatric specialist who deals with neonatal problems including intensive care of the new born.

Neonatology Study of paediatric medicine which deals with disorders of the newborn.

Neon It is inert gas in nature, which rarely available.

Neoplasm Usually refers to a tumour which may be or may not be malignant.

Neorealism This theory excludes theology and philosophy as source of knowledge and truth, which looks to science as its primary source.

Nephrectomy Surgical excision of kidney.

Nephrotic As caused by kidney infection or inflammation, by nephrosis.

Nephritis Inflammation of the kidney but loosely used to cover other kidney diseases.

Nephrogram Kidney radiograph with contrast medium in renal tubules, Excretion urogram.

Nephrolith Renal calculus.

Nephrolithotomy Removal of renal calculus by incision and opening the kidney.

Nephroma Refers to tumour of the kidney.

Nephron It is the functional unit of the kidney

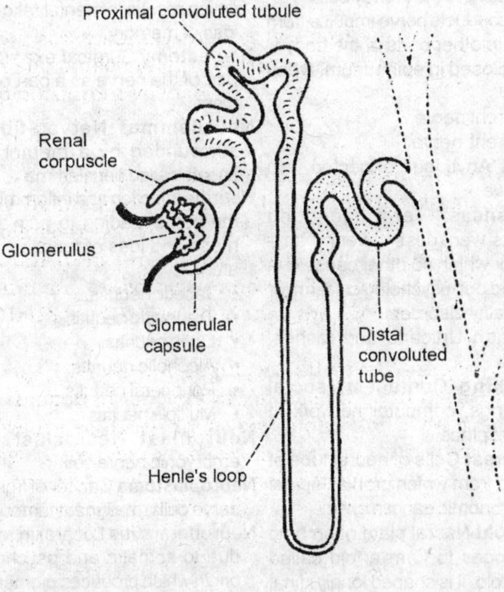

Nephron

Nephropexy surgical fixation of movable kidney to the nearby muscles

Nephrosclerosis In arteriosclerosis and in malignant hypertension conditions there is constriction of the arterioles of the kidney.

Nephrosis Any inflammatory and non-inflammatory disease of the kidney, It is characterised by oedema, albuminuria and low plasma albumin.

Nephrostomy Permanent opening is created in to the renal pelvis.

Nephrotomy Surgical incision of the kidney.

Nephrotoxic Substance which is destructive to the kidney cells.

Nerve It conducts nerve impulse from centre to other parts of the body. It is enclosed in epineurium, types are:

- Efferent nerve.
- Afferent nerve.

Nervous Anything connected with the nerve.

Nervousness Term denoting nervous weakness covering anything for which no other cause can be found out, psychological term for personality disorder.

Nettle rash Urticaria and rashes, urticaria.

Networking Contact by social gatherings, computer network in different place.

Neural crest Cells of neural tube of embryo from which cranial, spinal and autonomic ganglia arise.

Neural fold Neural plate of embryo which goes to form a fold called neural fold, it is shaped longitudinal elevation on the neural tube.

Neural plate Ectodermal band along the dorsal surface of the embryo, this is a thickened band of ectoderm

Neural Anything related to the nerve.

Neuralgia Neurological disturbance causing pain along the course of the nerve.

Neurapraxia Compression on the nerve causing temporary loss of function,
Nerve paralysis due to pressure effect.

Neurasthenia Chronic fatigue and weakness the cause of these symptoms is now sought in concealed disease conditions.

Neurasthenia A neurotic condition which results in mental fatigue and loss of memory.

Neurectomy Surgical excision of a part of the nerve as a part of treatment.

Neurilemma Nerve fibre is surrounded by a membranous sheath called neurilemma

Neuritis Infection and inflammation of the nerve leading to pain, tenderness and loss of function , types are:

- Tabetic neuritis.
- Traumatic neuritis.
- Optic neuritis.
- Alcoholic neuritis.
- Peripheral neuritis.
- Multiple neuritis.

Neuroblast Neuroblast is an embryonic nerve cell.

Neuroblastoma Cancer of immature nerve cells, malignant tumour.

Neurodermatitis Local skin reaction due to somatic and psychogenic origin which produces pigmentation and thickening of the skin.

Neurofibroma Tumour oı .ıerve and fibrous tissue which is benign in nature.

Neurofibromatosis Otherwise called Von Recklinghausen's disease, it is a hereditary disorder with amty number of fibromas of skin on whole body.

Neurogenic Neurogenic shock, a clinical condition caused by nerve stimulation.

Neuroglia It is a special connective tissue which support nervous tissue, tissues that support brain and nerves, other name for astrocytes

Schwann cells.

Neurohypophysis Other name for posterior lobe of pituitary gland which secretes

Vasopressin and oxytocin.

Neuroid That which resembles a nerve.

Neurolathyrism Neuroparalysis because of contamination of edible dhal with non-edible kesaridhal (lathyrus satibus).

Neuroleptic Drug which acts on nerves and connected tissue.

Neurology The study of nervous system and its disorders.

Neurology medical speciality concerned with physical diseases of the brain and nerves.

Neuroma It is a tumour which consists of nervous tissue.

Neuromuscular Related to nerve and muscle, referred to neuromuscular junction,

Motor end plate of muscle fibre which is supplied by nerves.

Neuromyelitis Infection and inflammation of nerve and myeline sheath,

Similar to multiple sclerosis, neuritis and myelitis.

Neuron It is a nerve cell.

Neuroparalysis Paralysis of parts due to nervous disorders.

Neuropathy Degeneration of nerve and subsequent loss of function, Common types are:

- Diabetes neuropathy.
- Alcoholic neuropathy.
- Pressure neuropathy(entrapment)
- Ischaemic neuropathy.

Neuropil Network of delicate nerve fibres permeating the nervous system.

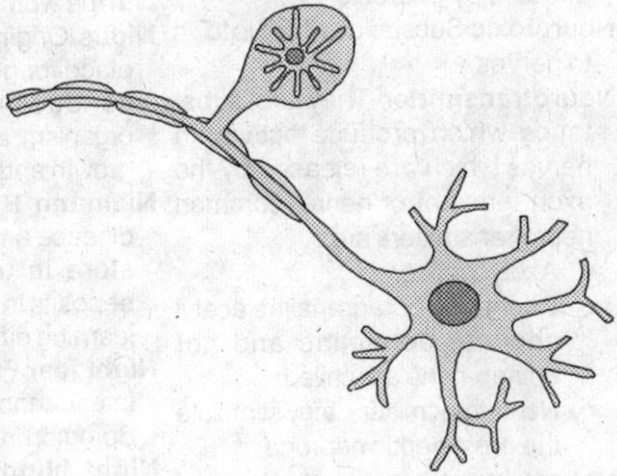

Neuropil

Neuroplasty Repair of damaged nerve by surgical intervention.

Neuropsychiatry Organic disorders causing damage to mind and behaviour.

Neurosis Mental illness partly involving personality and causing anxiety and nervous tension, Obsessive compulsive and anxiety are two common types of neurosis seen in clinical practice.

Neurosis Abnormal way of meeting a situation which is an emotional disorder.

Neurosurgery Discipline which deals with surgical intervention in neurological illness of brain, spinal cord and nerves.

Neurosyphilis Third stage of syphilis involving brain, types of neurosyphilis are:
- Tabes dorsalis.
- General paralysis of the insane.
- Meningovascular syphilis.

Neurotic Connected with and affected by neurosis.

Neurotoxic Substance which is toxic to nerves.

Neurotransmitter They are substance which produce activity in nerves which are released by the axon terminal of nerve, common neurotransmitters are:
- Acetycholine.
- Dopamine noradrenaline acetyl choline, dopamine and nor epinep-hrine are called.
- Neurotransmitters, they stimulate the presynaptic neurone.

Neurotripsy Surgical crushing of nerve for treatment of relief of pain Eg., trigeminal neuralgia.

Neurotropic Pathogens that attack nerve cells, one which has affinity to nerves.

Neutropenia Low count of neutro phils in the blood.

Neutrophil It is a polymorphonuclear leucocyte which do not react either with acid or with an alkali.

New social movement It is called NSM, interests and identities such as gender,ethnicity, sexuality, religious feeling, etc.

NFPP National Family Welfare planning Programme.

Niacin Other name for nicotinic acid, one of the B complex group.

Niche A depression on the usual smooth surface, ulcers produce niche.

Nicking Retinal vein compression at the site where artery crosses.

Nicotine Tobacco extract from plant which is an alkaloid.

Nicotinic acid Water soluble vitamin B complex, niacin.

Nidation Implantation of fertilised egg in the womb.

Nidus Originally it means a nest, a place for getting infection, a place conducive for the growth of organism, a favourable condition for growth and development.

Niemann Pick disease Inherited disease among jews, physically fat store in the body and lecithin deposits in organs associated with learning difficulties.

Night fear Frightening at sleep and later cannot recall the cause of it, Common in childhood period.

Night blindness Vision problem during night which is associated with deficiency of vitamin A , common in malnourished children in developing countries, nyctalopia.

Nightingale Pledge Well known pledge by the nursing profession from the days of
Florence Nightingale,

"I solemnly pledge before God and in the presence of this assembly to pass my life in purity and to practice my profession faithfully. I will abstain from whatever is deleterious and mischievous and will not take or knowingly administer any harmful drug. I will do in all my power to maintain and elevate the standard of my profession and will hold in confidence all personal matters committed to my keeping and all my family affairs coming to my knowledge the practice of my calling. With loyalty I will endeavour to aid the physician in his work, and devote myself to the welfare of those committed to my care".

Nikethamide It is a respiratory stimulant given IV in respiratory failure.

Nimesulide Anti-inflammatory agent which also acts as an analgesic.

Nipple Tip of the breast, structure available for feeding the newborn by the mother, abnormalities are:
- Inverted nipple.
- Retracted nipple.
- Accessory nipple.

Nissal granules It is responsible for protein synthesis, described as RNA unit.

Nit Egg stage of the head louse, body louse, and pubic louse.

Nitrazine tape Used to find out the rupture of amniotic membrane, determination of pH of leaked fluid over garment of patient, since amniotic fluid pH is alkaline and is at 7.2, and if the test tape is darker then it is likely that membrane has ruptured.

Nitrogen balance Balance between protein intake and its utilisation.

Nitroglycerin disk To apply nitroglycerin ointment to the skin of patient with angina pectoris and cardiac ischemia, the disc is advantageous because of its neatness, dose accuracy and known duration of action, continuous release is present, it is adhered to that side of skin which is dry and hairless and remaining protective strip paper is removed.

Nitroglycerin It is a vasodilator used in coronary insufficiency or heart attack, one of the drug which reduces spasm in arteries.

Nitrous oxide Anaesthetic gas commonly called laughing gas.

NMR Nuclear magnetic resonance, signals by magnetic influence are used in chemical analysis in magnetic spectroscopy and in magnetic resonance imaging, radiological diagnostic tool.

NNT Neonatal tetanus.

No scalpel vasectomy Vasectomy done by using a small puncture in the scrotum and by one needle puncture anaesthesia, which has many advantages.

Nobel Prize Alfred Bernard Nobel who lived during 1833 to 1896 established the prize to be given annually for the encouragement of work for the sake of humanity, they are awarded every year for the most important work of the year in physics, chemistry, medicine and physiology, literature and world peace.

Nocardia Micro-organism belonging to actinomyceae.

Nocturia Urine production in excess during night.

Nocturnal Tumescence Erection of male genital organ during sleep described as a physiological phenomenon.

Nocturnal Connected with night such as nocturnal enuresis or bed wetting.

Node It means a protuberance:
- S A node.
- A V node.
- Ranvier node.

Nodule It means a small protuberance.

Noma It refers to gangrene of an organ, other name for cancrum oris, Specifically refers to abnormal conditions of mouth.

Nominal When we categorise the object, event or people, we assign a A number or a letter viz., A B C D or 0 1 2 3 etc.,

Sex of the nurse	0 =	female
	1 =	male
Qualification of nurse		
	1 =	certificate course
	2 =	basic nursing course
	3 =	diploma in nursing
	4 =	degree in nursing
	5 =	PG in nursing
	6 =	PhD in nursing
Hygiene of patient	0 =	worst
	1 =	bad
	2 =	good.

Non-compliance Patient when not following the instructions given by the nurse.

Non-maleficence Used in medical ethics, avoid harm to other in your professional Duty.

Non-retention Enema Enema medication used in nursing practice. Equipment required are:
- A container.
- Tubing with a clamp.
- Bed saver pad.
- Water soluble lubricant.
- Toilet paper.
- Disposable glove.
- 4 × 4 gauze pads.
- Bedpan.
- IV pole or bedside stand.
- Normally rectal enema is given by warming enema solution to 40.5^0 C.

Non-specific urithritis Commonly it is gonococcal infection of the urethra, grouped under STD caused by Chlamydia trachomatis.

Non-specific Cause not known in the occurrence of the disease.

Non-striated muscle Involuntary muscles controlling actions of the internal organs.

Non-union Orthopaedic term to denote failed union of fractured bones.

Noradrenaline Hormone from suprarenal gland which cause vasoconstriction.

Norethisterone Progesterone like substance, it is an anabolic steroid, is an Ingredient of oral contraceptive.

Normal Usual thing, it is equal to a standard thing.

Norm sociological term denoting normal, social regulations.

Normoblast Precursor of RBC in the bone morrow.

Normochromic normocyte Normal in colour and in size, refers to RBC.

Norms Social rules which define what is expected of individuals in certain situations.

Norton score It is geriatric term, a score of less than 14 require hourly change of posture to overcome pressure sore.

Norwalk agent Name of a virus which induces G.E.

Nose Natural airway for respiration and organ of smell (special sense).

Nosocomial Hospital acquired infection.

Nosology Criteria based classification of diseases.

Nostril Singular, refers to anterior orifice of nose.

Nostrum One's own medication, it also means quack, it also means secret medicine kept with somebody.

Notifiable disease Under Municipal Act diseases that are to be notified either to District surgeon, District H & F W officer or to city health officer.

Notifiable Refers to a disease which has to be notified to health authorities e.g., diphtheria, cholera, etc.

NPCB National Programme for the Control of Blindness.

NREM One of the types of sleep called Non-rapid Eye Movement sleep.

NSAID Non Steroidal Anti Inflammatory drug.

NTP National Tuberculosis Control programme.

Nuclear explosion It causes blinding flash of light, intense heat and radiation,
A health hazard situation.

Nuclear family Consists of adult male, adult female and children.

Nuclear medicine Discipline of medicine which deals with the use of radioactive isotopes and radioactive nuclides for the purpose of investigation, diagnosis and treatment of diseases.

Nuclear When radionuclide is used in the diagnosis and treatment.

Nuclease Enzyme which breaks the nucleic acid.

Nucleolus Dense body in the nucleus which contain RNA.

Nucleoprotein Compound which contain nucleic acid and protein.

Nucleotide Chemical compound which is made of pentose sugar, phosphoric acid and purine.

Nucleus Main component of a cell,

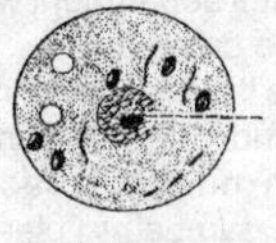

Cell showing the nucleus

Null hypothesis This word is used in tests of significance in statistics, we assume that there is no difference existed between study group observation and control group observation, $H_1 = H_2 = 0$.

Nullipara No birth has taken place by a woman, no viable child is produced by a woman.

Numb No sense at all, denotes dead, dying.

Numbness It is the disturbance of sensation called *limb going to sleep*.

Nuremberg code Code was enunciated in 1947, Nazi physicians were fined for cruel experiments on the prisoners and those held up in concentration.
The code has given an outlook to sociological, penological and Constitutional values and norms.

Nurse's aide Trained woman employed in hospital to perform nonmedical services such as bed making, meal serving, wound dressing.

Nurse Professional and qualified health personnel who is trained in nursing skills and nursing care a trained person capable of performing nursing services under doctor's supervision, she is referred to as practicing nurse, a hospital graduate is often called as registered nurse who is graduated and registered with Nursing Council.

Nursery Hospital department where newborns are cared for.

Nursing ethics It is the code of moral behaviour and rules of conduct related with nursing practice, compassion, sympathy pleasant manner are dealt with in nursing ethics which is based on major principles of nursing ethics like

Do good	Impartial
Respect patient	No harm.

Nursing home A place to live and get well, Nursing in terms of physical therapy, occupational therapry, psychiatric therapy, recreational programme and healthful diet are given care.

Nursing Nursing profession which performs the function of nursing care of the patient.

Nutmeg East India plant item which is used as a flavouring agent.

Nutrient The food that nourishes the body , they are grouped under Proximate principles (fat, carbohydrate and protein), vitamins, minerals and trace elements.

Nutrition value of food Availability of calorie, proximate principles and nutrients in 100 grams of food stuffs.

FOOD STUFF	*PROTEIN*	*FAT*	*CARBOHYDRATE*	*CALORIES*
Cereal	9.9	2.3	71.0	344
Bread	7.8	0.7	51.9	245
Salt biscuit	6.6	32.4	54.6	534
Sweet biscuit	6.4	15.2	71.9	450
Pulses	22.6	2.0	58.4	342
Green leafy Veg.	3.8	0.6	6.0	45
Roots, Tubers	1.2	0.2	16.0	70
Other vegetables	2.2	0.3	6.3	36
Nuts, Oilseed	15.2	46.6	20.4	578
Condiment, spice	9.8	6.6	40.6	261
Fruit	1.1	0.4	7.6	79
Meat	21.0	4.9	0.8	131
Egg	13.3	13.3	0.0	173
Milk	3.6	5.8	4.7	85
Curd	3.1	4.0	3.0	60
Butter	0.0	81.0	0.0	729
Ghee	0.0	100.0	0.0	900
Oil	0.0	100.0	0.0	900
Sugar	0.1	0.0	99.4	398
Honey	0.3	0.0	79.5	319
Jaggery	0.4	0.1	95.0	383
Sago	0.2	0.2	87.1	351

Nutritive value of foods

Nutritional surveillance Keeping a watch over nutrition of a community to take decision on required improvement for better nutrition.

Nutritional programmes This is to tackle the problem of malnutrition in the country, the aim is to provide additional nutrients to target groups to fill the gap between intake and requirement

Main programmes are:

- Applied nutrition programme.
- Special nutrition programme.
- Balwadi nutrition programme.
- Mid day meal programme of the centre and of the state.
- Vitamin A prophylaxis.
- programme.
- Prophylaxis against nutritional anaemia.
- Control of iodine deficiency disorders.
- ICDS and IPP.

Nutrition Food consumption, food assimilation and its utilisation in the body.

Nutrition of the old age Therapeutic diet advised for the old age, geriatric therapy.

Foodstuff	*Requirement (Grams)*	
	Male	*Female*
Cereals	350	225
Pulses	50	40
Vegetables	200	150
Leafy vegetables	50	50
Roots, Tubers	100	100
Fruits	200	200
Milk and Milk products	300	300
Sugar	20	20
Fats and Oils	25	25

Balanced diet for the geriatric age

Foodstuff	*Requirement (Grams)*	
	Male	*Female*
Calorie	2200.00	1700.00
Protein	65.00 G	50.00 G
Fat	50.00 G	40.00 G
Calium	1.00 G	0.90 G
Iron	38.00 mg	30.00 mg
Vitamin A (retionl)	1030.00 μg	930.00 μg
Thiamin	1.96 mg	1.45 mg
Riboflavin	1.78 mg	1.51 mg

Nutrient required for the old age

Nuts Oil yielding food stuff like groundnut, peanut, coconut, etc.

Nux vomica A plant seed containing strychnine which is a poison.

Nyctalopia Other name for night blindness, common causes are vitamin deficiency and occasionally retinitis pigmentosa.

Nylon Synthetic polymerised plastic which in fiber form is used as suture material.

Nymph Usually third stage in the development of insect

Egg → Larva → Nymph → Adult

Nymphomania Over desire of sex in woman excessive sexual desire which is abnormal in women.

Nystagmus It is involuntary rapid movement of the eyeball due to nervous or muscular diseases.

Nystatin Antifungal antibiotic used in clinical practice.

Nysten's rigor mortis Rigor mortis after death starts from muscles of mastication and progresses downwards.

O

O P Out Patient meaning patient can take consultation and treatment without staying in a hospital.

Oat It is a cereal and a staple diet in some community.

Obesity Overweight of a person which is more than 15% above normal weight that has come up by fat and not by bone and muscle, or BMI of over 30 kg per square meter of the body.
Excessive development of fat in the body.

Objective sign and symptom At clinical examination by the medical doctor, eliciting a sign on the examining patient which is seen, heard or felt or elicited is called objective signs,
At clinical history, patient comes out with certain manifestations which give clue to the diagnosis of an illness and are called objective symptoms.

Objective Desired end result or a purpose in an act of life,
It also denote the lens which is nearer to object in a microscope.

Oblique That which has got a slant or a slanting objects.

Oblongata That which is oblong such as medulla oblongata.

Obscenity An act which is offensive or outrageous to accepted standards of decency or modesty.

Obscure Not distinct or hidden manifestations of a patient.

Obsession A compulsive thought which is regarded as senseless.

Obsessive compulsion It is persistent and uncontrolled thoughts and irrational beliefs that cause an individual to perform compulsive rituals that interferes with his daily life;
Categories of OCD are:
- Dirt and contamination.
- Aggression.
- Orderliness of inanimate objects.
- Sex.
- Religion.

OCD is believed to be due to deficiency of serotonin, a neurotransmitter which play an important role in causing OCD.

Obstetrician Medical doctor who is trained in obstetrics.

Obstetrics The discipline that deals with pregnancy, labour and puerperium which is a branch in Medicine.
Discipline that deals with care of women in her pregnancy and in her childbirth.

Obstipation Very severe constipation.

Obstruction Blocking occurring in intestine or clogging occurring in a vessel.

Obstructive lung disease When air passage is obstructed in the lung due to certain clinical entities like bronchial asthma or chronic bronchitis with emphysema.

Obturator That which closes an opening such as obturator foramen.

Obtuse Dull in case of living, Blunt in case of non-living.

Obtusion In some diseases normal sensation is lost.

Occipitobasilar Pertaining to occiput and the base of the skull.

Occipital lobe Lobe of the brain situated toward back of cerebrum.

Occipital That which is related to the occiput.

Occipitoatloid Pertaining to the occipital bone and the atlas bone.

Occipitoaxoid Pertaining to the occipital bone and the axis.

Occipitoanterior This is the position of foetus in womb where foetus' occiput lying front of maternal pelvis.

Occipitobregmatic Pertaining to occiput and bregma.

Occipitoposterior This is the position of foetus in womb where foetus' occiput lying back of maternal pelvis.

Occiput Area of the back of the head.

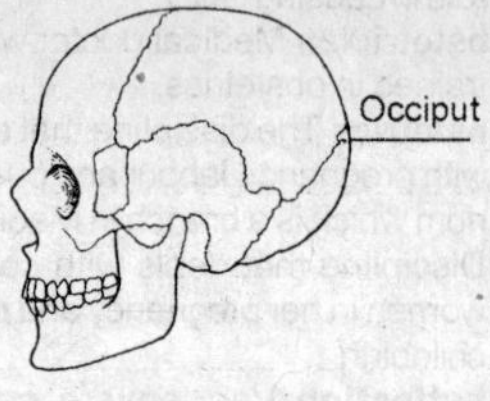

Skull showing occiput

Occlusion Meaning closure of an item such as:

- Teeth alignment in jaw.
- Occlusion of coronary artery.
- Occlusion of the pupil.

Occult blood This is testing stool for hidden blood in patients who loose blood in stool.

Patient should not eat red meat for 24 hours.

Stool is smeared on to filter paper which is kept on a glass plate and reagent is added. Colour change is observed. In many tests, the filter paper will turn blue if the faeces contain blood.

Occult That which is not revealed such as microbleeding in intestine which can be detected by sensitive tests,

Concealed by observation.

Occlusion It indicates closure of a blood vessel or of a lumen of intestine.

Occupational cancer Cancer occurrence is seen associated with certain occupation, such as.

Occupations	*related cancer*
X-ray technicians, workers in Isotopes, benzol	Blood cancer
Nickle, chromium, arsenic, uranium, asbestos, tob	Lung cancer
X-ray, oil,dyes, gas workers,tar distillery, chimney sweeping	Skin cancer
Rubber, aromatic amines,dyeing industry, electric cable,magenta and aniline	Urinarybladder cancer

Table: Occupational cancers

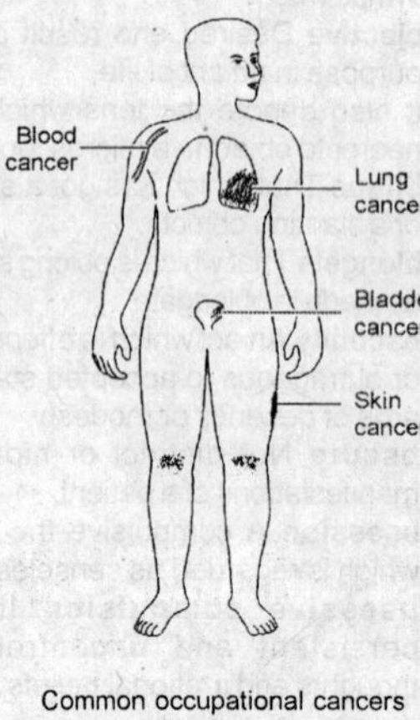

Common occupational cancers

Occupational Anything related to work and working condition common terminologies are:
- Occupational health.
- Occupational hazard.
- Occupational health nurse.
- Occupational medicine.
- Occupational therapy.

Octogenarian 80th year of age in a person or one who is in eighties,

Ocular That which is related to the eye such as:
- Ocular myositis.
- Ocular myopathy.

Oculist Physician who takes care of eyes who is called as ophthalmologist.

Oculocardiac reflex Pressure on the eyeball produces bradycardia.

Oculogyric Movement of eyeball is done by oculogyric nerves and muscles
Which cause movement of eyeball.

Oculomotor nerve It is the name of III cranial nerve, arises from midbrain, supplies extrinsic muscles of eye but not superior oblique and lateral rectus muscles.

Odontoid When a structure resembles a tooth such as odontoid process.

Odontoma Tumour of tooth or tooth structure.

Odorant It is a sense stimulator, Sense that stimulates or irritates the nose.

Odoriferous Heavily used perfumes to attract others.

Odorous That which has fragrance.

Oedema Fluid collection as a result of inflammatory process,
Visible and demonstrable swelling due to collection of fluid.
Common terms in nursing practice are:
- Pitting oedema.
- Pulmonary oedema.
- Dependent oedema.
- Cardiac oedema.
- Cerebral oedema.
- Angioneurotic oedema.

Oedipus complex Oedipus was Greek hero who developed fixed arrogance after series of conflicts is the root of this word,
Affection towards mother and aversion towards father in child hood by conflicts in childhood , if not solved, lead to Oedipus complex 'the suppressed sexual desire of son to his mother'.

Omentum The peritoneal fold that connects stomach and other abdominal organs, there are two omentum called greater omentum from greater curvature and lesser omentum from lesser curvature of stomach.

Oesophageal feeding It is called tube feeding to describe the administration of fluid food through a tube passed into the stomach either through mouth or through nose, they are done under doctors' order, this procedure requires assistance of another nurse in nursing care

Oral oesophageal feeding:-
Requirements:
- An oesophageal catheter (14 – 22 size).
- Glass funnel.
- Rubber tubing to fit glass funnel.
- Glass connection from tubing to oesophageal tube.
- Sterile water.
- Feed to be fed which is liquid.

- Bowl for the apparatus.
- Mackintosh and feeding cloth.
- Mouth tray.
- Mouth wash.
- Linen for wiping mouth.
- Gag for unconscious patient.

Nursing procedure:
If artificial denture remove them, mouth is cleaned, tube is passed taking care not to touch posterior pharyngeal wall, feed is poured slowly, little water is poured slowly, tube is pinched tightly and removed in one quick movement. Mouth wash is given

Nasal oesophageal feeding:
Requirement:

- Glass syringe, glass funnel.
- Fine catheter.
  - * Size 4 for infant.
  - * Size 6 for children.
  - * Oesophageal small size for adult.
  - * Ryle's duodenal tube may also be used.
- Glass connection.
- Wool swabs.
- Mackintosh bib and feeding cloth.
- Bowel.
- Sterile water.
- The liquid feed.

Nursing procedure:
One nostril is cleaned, tube is passed along the floor of nose backwards and downwards, Tested for the tube passed down the oesophagus and is in stomach, Any difficulty doctor is asked to verify that all is well before the nurse proceeds with the feeding.

Oesophageal That which is related to oesophagus such as oesophageal varices, oesophageal atresia.

Oesophagitis Infection and inflammation of oesophagus.

Oesophagoscope The instrument called endoscope to visualise inside of oesophagus.

Oesophagus GI tract from pharynx to stomach which is 23 cm. in length, colloquially it is called 'gullet'.

Oestradiol Ovarian hormone, Synthetic preparations are used in amenorrhoea and menopausal syndrome.

Oestrogen One of the steroidal hormones produced from ovary, Also are extracted from adrenal cortex, placenta and testis.

Official Recognised by Government, Recognised by the organisation which meets the accepted standard.

Ogive It is the terminology of Biometry, It refers to ς shaped curve.

Ohm's law It is an expression of electric current in amperes,

$$\text{Current (amperes)} = \frac{\text{EMF (volts)}}{\text{Resistance}}$$

Ohm It is the unit of electric resistance, An electric resistance of a column of mercury for the following dimentions:

Cross section = 1 Sq. mm
Length = 106 cm.

OHP It is a common projected media in nursing education, this is useful in teaching with eye to eye contact and there is no need to darken the class

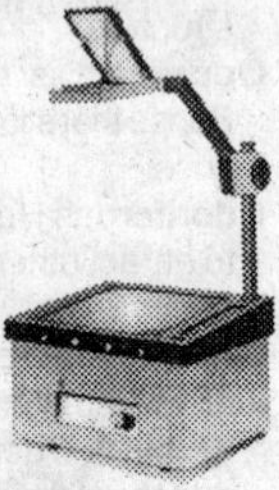
Over head projector

Oil Liquid combustible substance which may be fixed or volatile, which can be animal mineral or vegetable in origin,
Insoluble in water but soluble in ether,
Common oil used in nursing practice is:
- Almond oil.

Ointment Remedy for external application is mixed with greasy base and is used as ointment.

Old age problem The change in old age is called senescence which is natural process
Common effects of old age are:
- Senile cataract.
- Nerve deafness.
- Osteoporotic changes.
- Bronchitis with emphysema.
- Changes in mental outlook.

Old age In developing countries 64 years of age and above is referred to as old age,
The age when senescence has occurred.

Olecranon The ulna bone lies on the inner side of the forearm; its upper extremity helps to form the elbow-joint. At this point is a large projection called *olecranon process* which can be felt at the back of the elbow.
- Bony knob at the back of the elbow which is actually upper end of the ulna is common site for fracture.
- Fractured olecranon needs applying a splint along the front of the limb, extending from the upper third of the arm to the palm of the hand, to prevent bending of the elbow.

Oleum Pharmacy term for an oil.

Olfactory That which related to smell sensation such as olfactory nerves.

Olfactory organs Sense of smell is contained in the olfactory organ located in the top of the nasal cavity, They are like a chemical detector, odour when dissolved in the mucous secreted by the nasal mucous membrane then one can smell the odour.

Oligaemia When cellular component is less in the blood.

Oligodendroglioma CNS tumour of glial tissue.

Oligohydramnious Low quantity of amniotic fluid.

Oligomenorrhoea Gynaecological conditions with less flow and infrequent menses
Scanty and infrequent menses.

Oligospermia Low sperm count in semen, infertile person.

Oliguria Urinary secretion is reduced in urinary organ dysfunctions.

Olivary Organ that is olive-shaped such as olivary body (mass of grey matter in medulla oblongata).

Olive Refers to an elevated round structure such as olivary body in the pyramid of the medulla oblongata,
The oil which contains olein and palmitin used as food, laxative and for external application to bruises,
It is plant origin.

Omnivorous Animal or man who eat mixed diet (vegetarian and non-vegetarian).

Omphalitis Infection and inflammation of umbilicus.

Omphalocele It refers to umbilical hernia.

Onchocerca A genus from filarial worm which cause skin and sub cutaneous lesions in tropical areas.

Onchocerciasis Clinical condition produced by infestation of onchocerca.

Oncogenesis Development and occurrence of tumours.

Oncogenic That which produce tumour or tumour like growth in the body.

Onco Greek word meaning mass of tissue usually refers to cancerous mass.

Oncology Scientific study of the discipline which deals with nature, occurrence and management of cancerous growth

It is the branch of medicine that deals with science, diagnosis, investigation and management of cancer.

Onlay This refers to a graft which is grafted to the surface of an organ, Examples are:

- Skin graft on the skin.
- Nerve graft on the nerve.
- Bone graft on the bone.

Onychia Nail has fallen due to inflammation of nail matrix with suppuration.

Oöcyte Immature cell in the ovary.

Oögenesis Development and production of ovum in the ovary.

Ookinete Zygote of parasite Plasmodia which is motile in nature.

Oöphorectomy Surgical removal of the ovary for the treatment.

Oöphoritis infection and inflammation of ovary.

Oöphoron Medical term for the ovary.

Oösperm Ovum which is recently fertilised by sperm.

Opacity Opacities in vitreous humour and in the lens of the eye.

Opaque enema An aperient is given 36 hours before and a colon washout 4hrs before the examination is given.

Barium sulphate emulsion contains the following:

Barium sulphate	40 oz.
Tragacanth powder	60 grains
Water	to 80 fluid oz.

The enema is allowed to run in slowly through a rectal tube while radiologist examines patient under fluoroscopic screen

Patient is required for 24 hours in X-ray department. On the morning of examination a cup of tea is given and usual diet afterwards.

Open reduction It is also called internal reduction by surgical opening and bringing the fractured ends together,

Orthopaedic surgical intervention of a fracture.

Open-heart surgery Surgery done on heart along with usage of cardio-pulmonary heart lung machine,

Any surgery which require opening of heart, any surgery which needs opening of blood vessel that needs Heart lung machine,

Close heart surgery.

Operation Surgical operation as surgical treatment by using surgical instruments.

Operculum Latin word meaning a covering structure,

Common operculums heard in nursing practice are:

- Orbital operculum.
- Trophoblastic operculum.
- Occipital operculum.

Ophthalmia neonatorum Severe purulent conjunctivitis of newborn by gonococcal infection.

Ophthalmia Severe infection and inflammation of the eye structures such as

Ophthalmia neonatorum.

Ophthalmitis Infection and inflammation of the eyeball.

Ophthalmologist A consultant surgeon specialised in eye disorders and who treats eye conditions by treatment and by surgery.

Ophthalmology Discipline that deals with diseases and disorders of the eye and which takes care of conservation of vision

Study which deals with eye structure, eye function and eye disorders including their management.

Ophthalmoplegia Condition with paralysis of muscles of the eyeball.

Ophthalmoscope Instrument which help to illuminate the interior of the eye for clinical examination, fundoscope.

Opiates As such word means 'sedatives',but it denotes drugs derived from opium

Any medicine that contains opium.

Opisthotonos This posture is seen clinically in case of tetanus, meningitis and strychnine poisoning,

The head is seen retracted and whole body is seen arched like a bow,

This is due to muscle spasm and muscular rigidity

Body bending backwards seen in *Dhanurvayu* or Tetanus

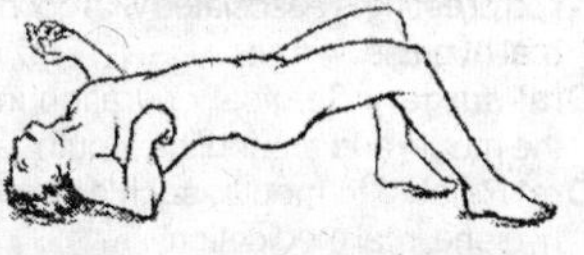

Opisthotonos

Opium It is a narcotic extracted from dried poppy juice and is an addictive drug.

Opponens They are muscles controlling the movements of the fingers,

Act of opposing the thumb with little finger by adduction of thumb

This opposing action is brought out by Opponens pollicis.

Opportunistic Pathogens which becomes pathogenic under certain circumstances and they ordinarily do not cause illness.

Op-site It is a transparent polyurethane self-adhering dressing. It prevents the escape of fluid, provides moist environment which will enhance granulation and epithelization during wound healing.

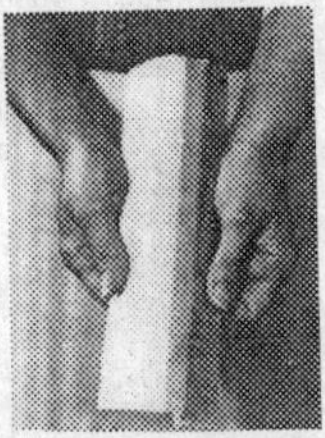

A: Self-adhering dressing by Op-site (before application)

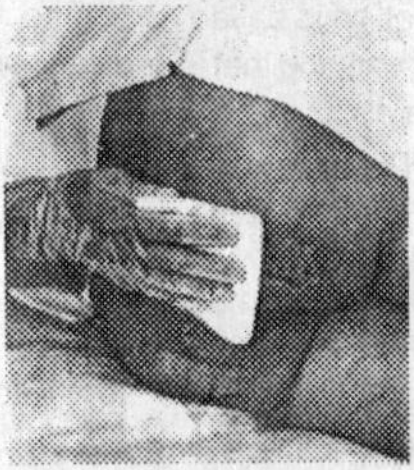

B: Self-adhering dressing by Op-site (process of dressing)

Self-adhering dressing by Op-site

Opsonic index This index measures the power of bactericidal activity of phagocytes in the blood.

Opsonin Opsonin is present in bacteria which are specific to given bacteria.
Opsonin in the blood renders bacilli destroyed by its action.

Optic atrophy Atrophy of optic nerve head with the appearance of chalky white optic disc.

Optic chiasma It is the junction where optic nerve fibres decussation occurs.

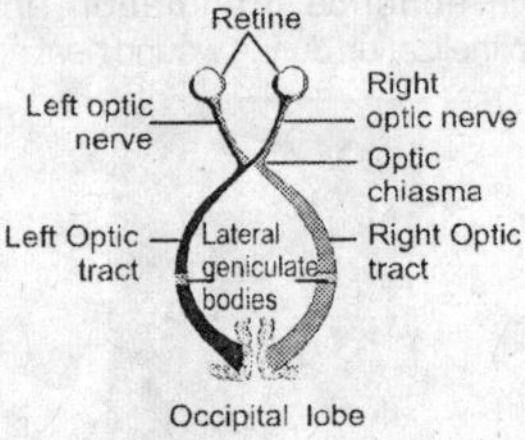

Optic chiasma

Optic disc Ganglion cells go to form optic nerve at the posterior pole of the retina is called optic disc.

Optic Anything that is related to vision, such as:
- Optic nerve.
- Optic foramen.
- Optic disc.
- Optic chiasma.
- Optic atrophy.

Optical Pertaining to sight such as Optical density.

Optician Person who produces lens and optical instruments to help eye specialist to treat patient with eye problem.
He is professionally trained to detect refractive error by testing and is capable of prescribing spectacles for correction of such errors.

Optimum The most desirable state of affairs which can be for any physiological variables, also suggests a thing to be best and favourable.

Optometrist He is paramedical person helping eye doctor by examining refractive error, by fitting glasses for short sight and long sight.

Optometry Method of putting correction for visual acuity and fitting glasses for its correction.

OPV Abbreviation for **O**ral **P**olio **V**accine.

Ora serrata This is the retinal portion behind the ciliary body.

Ora Latin word meaning that it is edge or margin such as ora serrata.

Oral contraceptive Tablets taken by mouth to see that ovulation do not occur and there by conception do not take place with consumation.

Oral hygiene It implies good teeth, good gum and good healthy buccal cavity.
Mastication produces and promotes saliva and gastric secretion which help in digestion. Emotional satisfaction of eating is associated with good oral hygiene.

Oral surgery Surgical operation in the mouth and around the mouth

Oral Related to mouth, such as oral hygiene, oral medication,
It also suggests the oral side of a tooth.

Orbicularis oris It is the muscle of the mouth around the lips which help in pursing of the mouth.

Orbit Bones of the face form the framework of the face and help to make the sockets of eyes called orbit,
Eyeball lies in the orbit which is held in place by muscles which can turn it in any direction.
It also depicts the path where an object moves around another object (earth moves in the orbit).

Orchidectomy Surgical removal of testis, It is called *castration* if both the testes are removed.

Orchidopexy Surgical correction and placement of undescended testis.

Orchiepididymitis Infection and inflammation of testis and epididymis.

Orchitis Infection and inflammation of testis.

Orderlies Appointed workers in the hospitals who does heavy manual work and who does all maintenance work of the hospital.

Ordinal When characteristics are put into categories which give meaning, but distance between the categories are not properly known it is ordinal scale. For example in final B.Sc., Nursing – Asha, Rita and Zinat secured I,II and III ranks respectively. This does not tell us by how many marks they differ,
Examples:

Socioeconomic class	*I.Q.*
1 = Low	0 = Idiot
2 = Middle	1 = Moron
3 = High	2 = Normal
	3 = Genius

Orf Boils seen among meat handlers which is due to virus infection from sheep

Organ donation Organ donation is imminent part of treatment for damaged organs among patients. It involves use of organ to the sick. It is not possible without formal procedures. Values and norms are dreawn and ethical issue has a great significance in organ donation and organ transplantation.

Organ Organ refers to one part of human body which can perform a known biological function.

Organelle Minute portions of living cell which perform specific function, Nucleus, nucleolus, mitochondria are called organelle.

Organic Disease due to bodily pathological status, One can demonstrate the bodily changes when disease occurs
Diseases due to organic mean that structural changes of an organ has brought out the illness,
Chemicals containing carbon atoms go to form organic compound
That which is related with living organisms,
Chemical compound containing carbon,
Lesion or illness due to body change or physical changes
Related with organ.

Organism Living being unit which can be plant, animal or man.

Orgasm This is the climax stage of sexual excitement,
Intense pleasure of sexual intercourse at climax,
This is manifested by the following characters:
- Pelvic throbbing
- Contraction of levator ani muscle.

- Contraction of anal sphincters.
- Mucous secretion or wetting of vagina in female.
- Seminal ejaculation in male.

Orientation Person who has the sense of place, time and persons, Imparting a course for understanding.

Orifice Openings in the body such as anal orifice, vaginal orifice, oral orifice, etc.

Origin It refers to the 'origin' of a muscle which denote from where a muscle begins,
It can mean the origin of a nerve when starts the course with branching,
It can also mean the origin of a vessel when starts the course with branching.

Ornithodoros It is an orgasid tick which tranmits spirochetal infections and relapsing fever,
Common vector is ornithodoros moubata.

Ornithosis Colloquially called 'parrot fever' acquired through birds caused by virus,
A form of bronchopneumonia by virus transmitted by pigeons or parrots.

Orogastric tube If the nasal intubation is contraindicated, orogastric tube is inserted through mouth.
First distance between tragus of ear to mouth and to the tip of xiphoid process is determined which is the distance up to stomach, tube is guided toward the back of throat,
Patient flexes head forward and begins swallowing,
At stomach placement, tube is taped to patient's cheek.

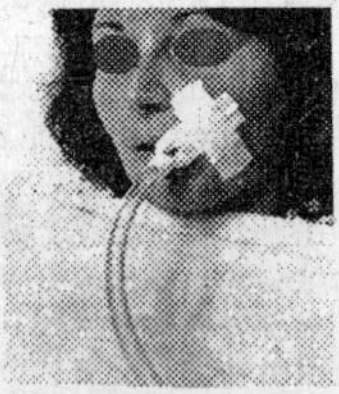

A : Assessment by measurement for orogastric tube

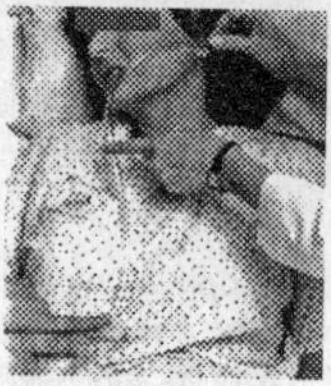

B: Orogastric tube is positioned by taping

Orogenital Anything that is related to mouth and genital organs.

Oropharyngeal tube S-shaped plastic device that fits over tongue and extends into pharynx is indicated to assist airway after anaesthesia, in semiconscious patient who gets obstructed airway by tongue.

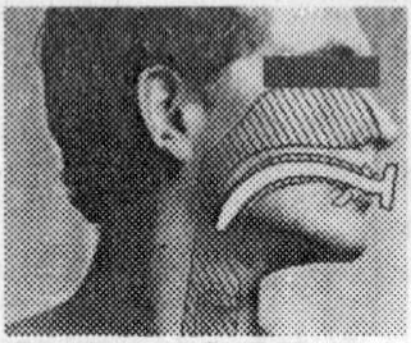

A: Diagram to show how Oropharyngeal tube fits

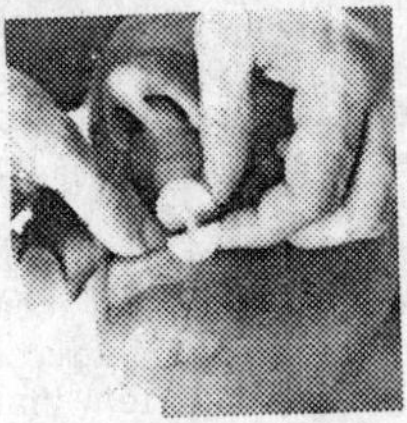

B: Oropharyngeal tube in position

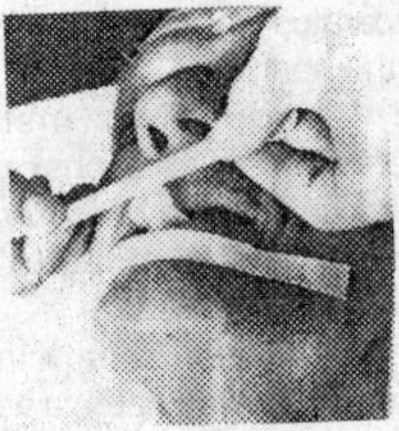

C: Orogastric tube, taping to patient's cheek

Oropharynx Pharyngeal portion which is behind mouth and above the level of oesophagus and larynx.

Oroya fever It is the other name of Bartonellosis.

Orphans Children who, for one reason or another are deprived of both natural parents where the child looses family care.

Orphenadrine A chemotherapeutic agent used in the treatment of Parkinsonism and associated depression.

ORS Abbreviation for **O**ral **R**ehydration **S**olution.

Orthodontics Speciality which does the job of corrective dental work other than filling of cavities and teeth extraction. Speciality that deals with malocclusion correction and correcting irregularities of teeth.

Orthodontist Dentist who corrects malocclusion and defective bites, Correction of irregularities of teeth and poor bite correction by dentist who is specialised in that area.

Orthodontry Malocclusion leading to facial deformity, when space maintainer is required, when deciduous teeth are too long, dentist gives orthodontic treatment which is called orthodontry.

Orthopnoea Difficulty in breathing in lying down position but feel comfortable in upright position Breathing is very difficult without upright position of patient.

Orthopaedics Speciality that deals with injury and diseases of bone, joints and muscles, specialist in bone and joint diseases,
It takes care of injury, deformities and diseases of bone and joints.

Orthopercussion Purcussion on the chest by using distal phalanx of the pleximeter finger which is held perpendicular to chest wall.

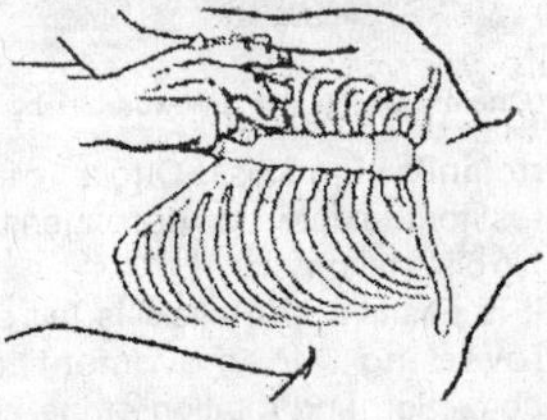

Orthopercussion

Orthoptics Non-surgical methods of treatment practiced in case of abnormalities of vision such as squint.

Orthostatic Anything that occurs in patient when he stands upright, examples are:

- Orthostatic hypotension.
- Orthostatic albuminuria.

Orthotic Treatment by supportive appliance to a physically handicapped to improve the function of the part.

Orthotist Person practicing Orthotic supportive treatment of handicapped.

Ortolani click test It is done to assess for congenital hip dislocation, Middle finger is positioned over greater trochanters and thumbs on medial side of thighs, Then flex the hips and knees

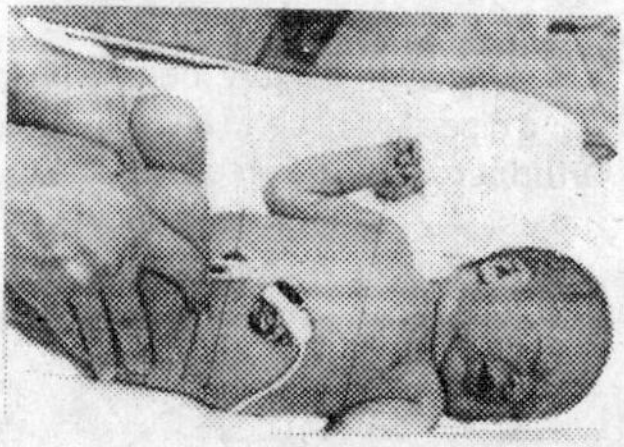

Ortolani click test in a newborn baby

Ortolani's sign This is Ortolani click test for the detection of congenital hip dislocation
It is positive if a "click" is felt on reversing the movement of abduction and rotation of the hip while the child is lying with its knee flexed.

Os "Os" is Latin word singular meaning 'any opening'
In singular it also means 'mouth'
In singular it also means 'bony'.

Osazone They are compounds obtained by heating sugar with phenylhydrazine and acetic acid, common compound is glucosazone.

Oscillation Any item that show forward and backward motion,
In living body if there is vibration.

Oscilloscope Cathode ray used apparatus to visualise performance of the heart.

Oscilloscope This instrument monitors the oscillations of EMF,
It is a cathode ray vacuum tube to measure EMF (**E**lectro **M**otive **F**orce).

Osler's disease This is the other name for polycythaemia vera.

Osler's node Subcutaneous painful swelling in limbs following sub acute bacterial endocarditis described by Canadian Physician around 1900, It is one of the classical subjective manifestations of a clinical disease entity.

Osmoreceptor They are specialised nerve cells to monitor osmotic pressure of blood and body fluids. Path from these areas to the hypothalamus is well established.

Osmosis It is a chemical process of permeation of fluid from lower concentration to higher concentration through a semipermeable membrane.

Osmotic That which is related to osmosis, such as osmotic pressure.

Osseous The word meaning "bony".

Ossicle It refers to a small bone, example is auditory ossicle containing 3 small bones namely incus,
Malleus and stapes
In the middle ear, within tympanic membrane there are 3 tiny bones which are called ossicles, they are referred to as under:

- Hammer.
- Anvil.
- Stirrup.

- Malleus.
- Incus.
- Stapes.

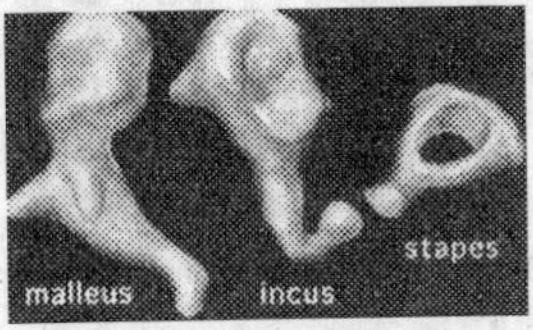

Ossicles of middle ear

Ossification Bone development process or osteogenesis in the body.

Osteitis Infection and inflammation of bone.

Osteoarthritis Non-crippling form of arthritis in elderly people,
Inflammation of a joint or many joints along with inflammatory changes in bones.

Osteoblast Osteoblast develops into osteocyte to form a bone tissue
Bone cells that are concerned with forming new bone and also concerned with repair of bone tissue.

Osteochondritis Inflammatory conditions of both bone and cartilage causing pain and deformity, Common sites in clinical practice are:

- Hip.
- Tibia.
- Scaphoid.

Osteochondroma Tumour of bone and cartilage.

Osteoclasis It refers to orthopaedic correction of fracture and restructuring of osseous tissue in repair of bone damage.

Osteoclast An orthopaedic instrument used in orthopaedic surgery, Large osteoclast cells breaks down and absorbs to form into callus
Bone cells that are concerned with eliminating bone tissue that are not needed for skeletal strength as after fracture or after injury.

Osteocyte Bone cells that are concerned with continuous maintenance activity in the bone.

Osteodystrophy One of the metabolic disorders of the bone.

Osteogenesis It is called bone formation.

Osteoma A benign tumour of the bone.

Osteomalacia Softening of the bone due to vitamin D and calcium deficiency,
Failure of ossification which is related with low serum calcium level.

Osteomyelitis Infection and inflammation of the bone due to pyogenic organism.

Osteopath Traditional healer who treats bone displacement by his theory of putting them to alignment, They are not many after it is taken over by orthopaedicians
One who practices osteopathy.

Osteopathy It is a method of treatment of bone fracture and bone disorders by manipulations.

Osteoperiostitis Infection and inflammation of periosteum and bone.

Osteopetrosis It is also called as "Albers-Schönberg disease which is a congenital disorder of bone in which the bone becomes very dense.

Osteophyte It is an outgrowth that occurs after the damage of bone in a joint due to osteoarthritis.

Osteoporosis Reduced precipitation of lime salt leads to thinning of bones that can lead to pathological fractures, common causes are:

- Aging.
- Nutritional deficiency.
- Hormonal imbalance.
- Excessive bone resorption.
- Inadequate calcium absorption.

Osteosarcoma It is a malignant bone tumour.

Osteosclerosis Density and hardness of bone is high that lead to pathological states

There are two common variants:

- Congenital: Achondroplasia which is called osteosclerosis congenita.
- Acquired: Osteopetrosis which is called osteosclerosis fragilis.

Osteotome Surgical instrument to cut bone, A chisel for cutting bone.

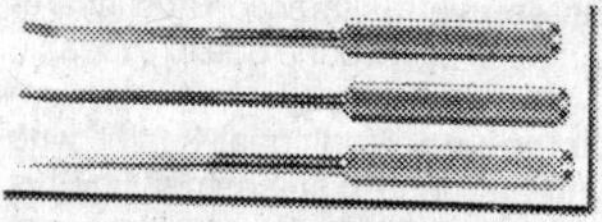

Osteotome

Osteotomy Surgical cutting of a bone for its repair in certain deformity.

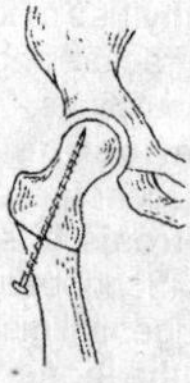

Osteotomy with faxator (hip)

Ostium The opening at the end of a tube such as fallopian tube opening into the peritoneal cavity.

Ostomy belt Under managing stomal care in G I surgical management, at applying a drainable pouch, if patient is obese and has a stoma that is flush with the peristomal area, ostomy belt is advisable.

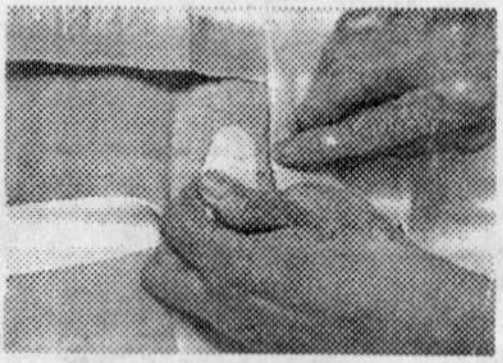

A: Ostomy belt positioning to a patient

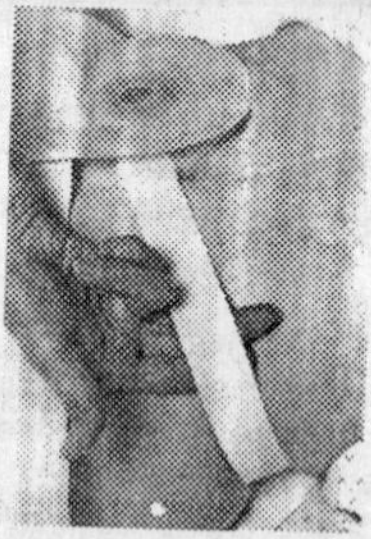

B: Ostomy belt in position to a patient

OT disinfection An important hospital practice to prevent hospital acquired infection. Following are usual procedures:

- Soap water clean, aeration, sunlight.
- Wash with chlorinated lime (25 PPM).
- Wash with 1% formaldehyde solution.
- Wash with 2.5% cresol

- 500 ml. formalin in I litre per 30 cub.mtr as fumigation.
- 200 grams Potassium permanganate in 500 ml formalin in 1 litre water for 30 cub.mtr.

Otic That which is related to the ear.

Otitis Infection and inflammation of the ear, Common clinical conditions are:
- Otitis externa.
- Otitis media.
- Otitis interna.
- Otitis labyrinthica.
- Otitis mastoidea.

Otolith Minute calculus in inner ear at the base of the semicircular canal.

Otologic One which is referable to the ear.

Otomycosis Fungal infection of auditory canal.

Otorrhoea Ear discharge due to infection by pyogenic organisms.

Otosclerosis Hard of hearing following ringing in the ear which may be due to hereditary predisposition,
Spongy bone is formed in labyrinth of the ear leading to deafness
Hardening of small bones of middle ear leading to deafness.

Otoscope ENT instrument used for the examination of the ear, an auriscope.

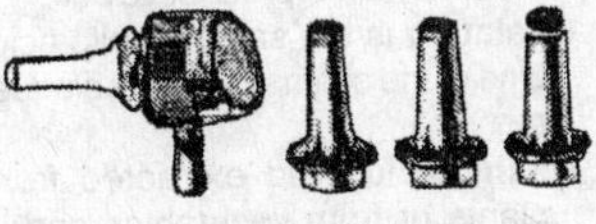

Siegle's otoscope

Ototoxic An agent which is toxic to organ of hearing.

Out patient service Care of patients in the hospital done without getting them admitted.

Ovarian That which is related to the ovary such as ovarian cyst.

Ovariotomy Surgical removal of ovary in certain disorders of ovary including ovarian tumour.

Ovariectomy Surgical excision of the ovary.

Ovary One of the reproductive organ, one pair in females which produce ova.

Over investigation This is condemned by the code of ethics from time to time.
Over investigation includes the following:
- More frequent lab investigations in the name of periodic health check up.
- For want of nothing repetition of routine investigation done.
- unwanted investigations are ordered.
- During inappropriate time interval follow-up, investigation is or dered which is of no use.
- Doing repeated screening test on a person or on a patient for the sake of doing survey or social or welfare activities.

Over the needle catheter Insertion of catheter for(angiocath) vascular catheterisation,
Skin is prepared,
Catheter is advanced to vein,
Backflow confirms correct position,
After removing needle, the distal end of the primed infusion tubing is attached to needle,
To double check pressure is applied to the vein just proximal to insertion site,

If the dripping stops in the drip chamber we are sure that vein is patent and needle has is in correct position.

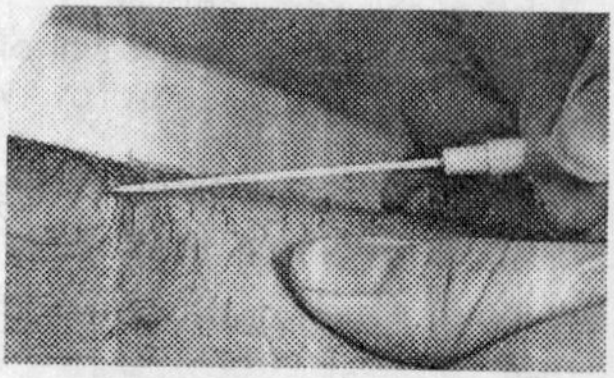

A: Positioning the tip of the over-the-needle catheter

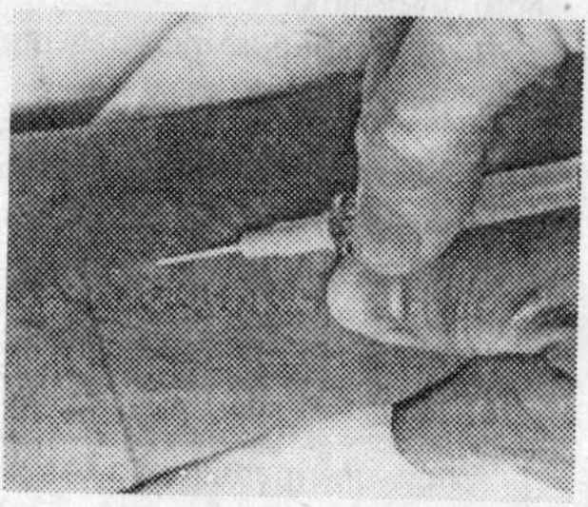

B: Advancing the catheter into the vein

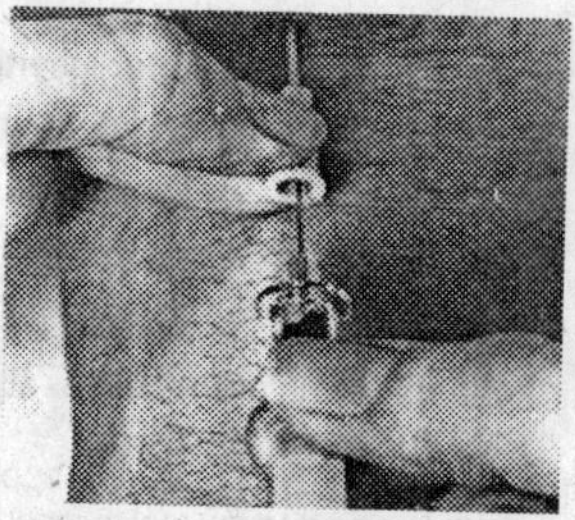

C: Backflow of blood tested for proper position of catheter

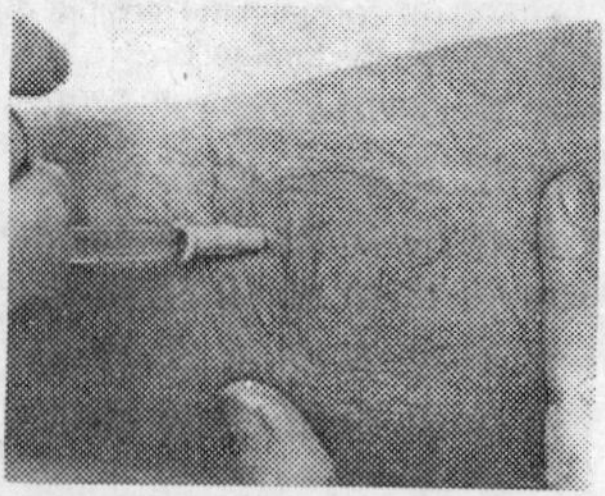

D: Fixing the catheter to distal end of infusion tubing

Over urbanisation The conditions of insecurity which affect many of the inhabitants of cities in the third world.

Overcorrection In the correction of defective vision, too powerful lens is used.

Overweight If the weight of the body is above 10 percent of permissible weight for the given age and for the given sex.

Oviduct It is the fallopian tube.

Oviparous Animal that produce eggs.

Ovulation It is the process of rupture of Graafian follicle and liberation of ovum.

Ovulation When the ovum is matured it is discharged from the ovum and this process is called ovulation.

Ovum Latin word meaning 'the egg', is the female reproductive cell.

Oxalate It is the salt of oxalic acid, One of the common urinary bladder stone.

Oxalic acid Acid extracted from plants or from vegetables and is used as a reagent.

Oxaloacetic acid This is one of the major by product in citric acid cycle and in metabolic cycle.

Oxford respirator It is used for resuscitation over a short period, The principle is that the lungs are inflated by forcing air into the air passages,
Positive pressure through the airway is the mechanisim.

Oxidation Chemical process of uniting with oxygen, burning of calories occurring in the body is normally by oxidation.

Oxidising agent They are a group of chemical disinfectants such as $KMNO_4$.

Oxime Also called Oxim which is obtained by the chemical reaction of hydroxylamine on an aldehyde or on a ketone.

Oximeter Photo-electric instrument used to determine the oxygen saturation of blood.

Oxycephalia This happens by symmetrical premature closure of the coronal sutures with parietal and occipital bones which becomes turret shaped.

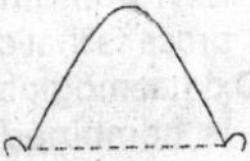

Oxycephalia

Oxygen analyser It analyses the receipt of oxygen in a tent, in a hood or in incubator
The unit measures the patient's oxygen concentration when delivered to incubators.

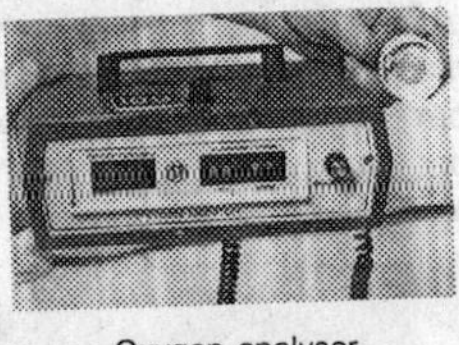

Oxygen analyser

Oxygen hood It is used in cribs, incubators or for radiant warmers where controlled concentration of oxygen, temperature and humidity are desired.

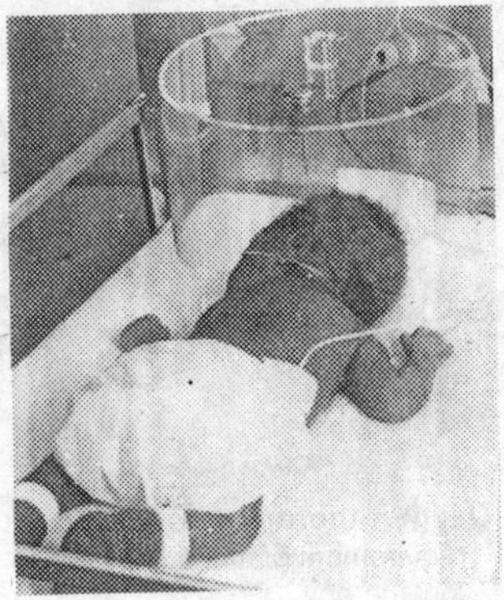

Oxygen hood

Oxygen mask Controlled oxygen, temperature and humidity are required,
At nursing care, nurse should see that tubing is free from condensation.

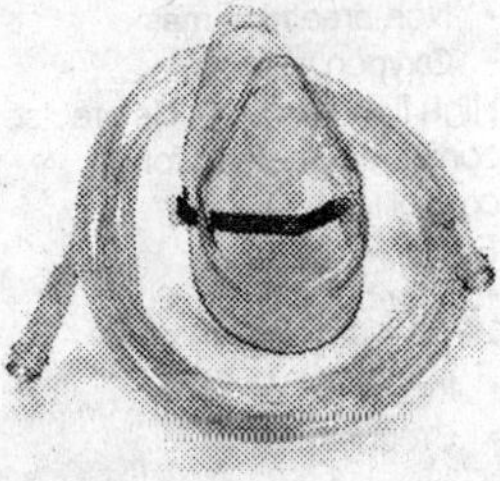

Facemask (Polymask) Oxygen mask

Oxygen tent In this tent, about 60% of oxygen is made available for oxygen therapy. It is made of transparent plastic material attached to a frame.

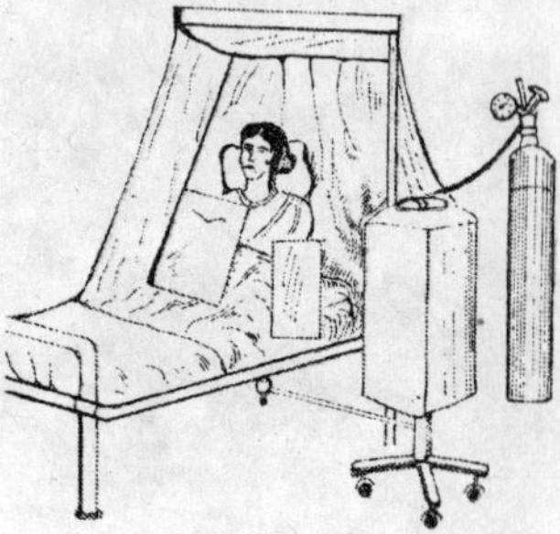

Oxygen tent

Oxygen therapy It is an utmost requirement of managing respiratory therapy.

There are two types of therapy;

Low flow system: Room air is inhaled with oxygen, fraction of inspired oxygen is adjusted (FiO_2)

Examples are:

- Facemask.
- Nasal cannula.
- Partial re-breathing mask.
- Non-breathing mask.
- Oxygen hood.

High flow system: It is precise and consistent method for controlling FiO_2

Examples are:

- Non-breathing mask.
- Ventury mask.
- Incubator.
- Croupette.

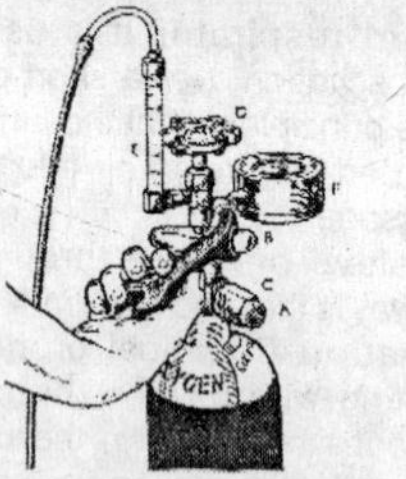

Oxygen cylinder with valve

Oxygen Natural gas present in atmosphere which colourless and odourless and is very much required for the body,

In medical therapy, we come across the following during oxygen therapy:

- Oxygen tent.
- Oxygen therapy.
- Oxygen saturation.

Oxygenation Haemoglobin is saturated with oxygen to form oxyhaemoglobin a biological process that occur in the lung.

Oxyhaemoglobin Haemoglobin that is combined with oxygen that circulates in the artery.

Oxytocin It is secreted by the pituitary gland which stimulates uterine contraction, the preparation is used in induction of labour in PPH.

Ozone Oxygen containing 3 molecule of oxygen which is represented as "O_3"

Ozone is an oxidising agent and an antiseptic, it is seen discharging from electrical machines and X-ray apparatus.

Ozonide Ozone which is bactericidal by producing nascent oxygen.

P

P U O It is an Abbreviation for **P**yrexia of **U**nknown **O**rigin.

Paracetamol Antipyretic and analgesic commonly used,
Chemically it is Para Acetyl Amino Phenol.

PABA Para Amino Benzoic Acid which is vitamin B group, used in lotions creams for external application.

Pacemaker Natural and artificial pacemakers are known in maintaining heart rate in case of arrhythmias,
Sinoatrial node is the natural pacemaker,
Electronic pacemaker is used which can stimulate myocardium at frequent interval to maintain equivocal rate of heart,
The word is common terminology in Biological Chemistry which denote " a substance, a tissue, an organ, an instrument whose rate of reaction sets the pace for a series of linked reactions,
Electronic pacemakers are of two types:

- External source pacemaker which run on battery for stimulation
  with frequent change of battery whenever pulse rate slows down by 5-6 beats per minute.
- Permanent source pace maker which are implanted in the subcutaneous tissue.
- Demand pacemaker is electronic pacemaker which is programmed to produce rhythm when heart do not produce regular contraction and relaxation.
- Fixed pacemaker is electronic pacemaker which are programmed for delivering pulse at regular interval irrespective of heart con traction or relaxation.

Pachydactyly Hugh size of toes and fingers in a person.

Pachydermia Hypertrophy of skin leading to abnormal thickening which gives the sense of thick toad skin or elephant skin.

Pachymeningitis Infection and inflammation of dura mater of the brain
Types of pachymeningitis in clinical use are:

- External pachymeningitis.
- Internal pachymeningitis.
- Purulent pachymeningitis.
- Syphilitic pachymeningitis.
- Serous pachymeningitis.

Pacing code It is letter code which describe the type and function of pacemaker
Three letter code is commonly used which denote as under:

- First letter denotes the heart chamber paced.
- Second letter denotes from where electrical activity is sensed.
- Third letter denotes the response to sensed electrical activity.

Bipolar limb leads (standard)

Right arm	– left arm	Lead I
Right arm	– left leg	Lead II
Left arm	– left leg	Lead III

Unipolar limb leads

a VR	- the exploring electrode placed on the right arm
a VL	- the exploring electrode placed on the left arm
a VF	- the exploring electrode placed on the left leg.

Unipolar chest leads

V_1 electrode position is 4th intercostals space just to the right of sternum		
V_2	"	4th intercostals space just to the left of sternum
V_3	"	lies midway between V_2 and V_4
V_4	"	5th intercostals space in midclavicular line
$V_{5,6,7}$	"	lie on the same horizontal line as V_4 in anterior, mid and posterior axillary lines respectively

Table: Pacing code in ECG

Pacinian corpuscles They are present in skin innervations of hand and foot and is helpful in sensation of deep pressure stimuli.

Pacinian corpuscles are elliptical semitransparent bodies along nerve supply of certain area of skin.

Packed cell Blood without plasma containing only cells.

Packs hot Used in acute poliomyelitis, This reduces pain and spasm and allow movements at an early stage, Blood circulation is increased, Earlier ordering to promote sweating in case of renal disease is not advocated nowadays.

Pads They are pressure relief pads to give relief of pressure around bony prominences and reduces skin breakdown,

Sheep skin pad is commonly used

Flotation pad contain gel-like inner substance to overcome pressure

Air mattresses are pads that minimise pressure over bony prominences

Lapidus airfloat system is a mattress pad used.

Paediatrician Specialist or consultant who deals with diagnosis, examination, treatment and management of illnesses of children,

He is doctor of medicine.

Paediatrics This the branch of medicine which deals with care, treatment and management of sick children and maintenance of health among healthy children.

Paedophilia This is one of sexual offence seen in the community, Sexual exploitation of young children.

Paget's disease This is named after British Surgeon Sir J Paget who lived during 1814 to 1899 who made detailed picture of Osteitis deformans, Bone with dense thickening and Ares of rarefaction,

Paget's disease also refers to nipple inflammation secondary to cancer of lactiferous ducts (mammary gland).

Pain receptors They are bare nerve endings in skin tissues which produce pain sensation from that area.

Pain It describes agony, intolerance, suffering and distress feeling,

It is one of the sign of infection or/and inflammation,

Different types of pain are encountered in nursing care. They are:

- Labour pain.
- False pain of pregnancy.
- Gas pain (distension).
- Bearing down pain of delivery.
- Lancinating pain.

- Phantom pain.
- Referred pain.
- Rest pain of leg ischemia.
- Menstrual pain.
- Hunger pain (physiological).

Paired organs Two organs present in our body such as:

- Eyes.
- Kidneys.
- Ovaries.
- Testes.
- Fallopian tube.
- Lungs.
- Adrenal glands.
- Ears.

Palatine bone One pair palatine bone form part of hard palate and nasal cavity.

Palatoglossus It is a constrictor of faucial isthmus and this muscle arises from sides and under surface of tongue and is inserted to palate.

Palliation By this patient's feelings gets improved and there is no cure of the disease.

Palliative It is relief treatment and curative treatment.

Pallium It is the area of cortex of the cerebrum in which white substance contains olfactory and non-olfactory part,
Colloquial terms used are **mantle** and **brain mantle** for this area.

Pallor Paleness of skin due to anaemia, paleness of conjunctiva due to anaemia, paleness of nailbed due to anaemia.

Palmar That which is related to the palm such as palmar arch, palmar fascia.

Palm Flexor surface of the hand which is hollow in nature,
It also is the name of a tree belonging to palmaceae.

Palpation Hand is put over a part and by touch and pressure organ examination is done,
It is second in the list of clinical examination which can be seen by list:
1) Inspection 2) Palpation
3) Percussion 4) Auscultation.

Palpating arterial pulses Common is radial pulse count. By going to known anatomic landmark other arterial points are also can be used for palpating and counting the arterial pulses
Criteria:

Infants	80 – 180 beats per minute
At 4 year	80 –120 beats per minute
At 10 years	70 – 110 beats per minute
From 14 years	50 – 100 beats per minutes
Adult	72 beats per minutes (average)

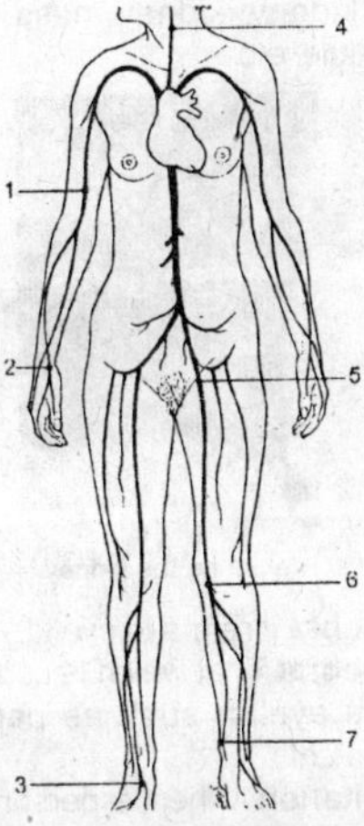

Common sites for palpating arterial pulses

1. Brachial artery.
2. Radial artery.
3. Dorsalis pedis artery.
4. Carotid artery.
5. Femoral artery.
6. Popliteal artery.
7. Posterior tibial artery.

Palpating the kidneys Nursing examination should include palpation of kidneys under assessment of renal urinary system,
Hands are positioned on both sides of patient's flank at the area between iliac crest and lower costal margin, At each breathing of patient, nurse shall increase the pressure between hands till one gets maximum depth entry by palpation. At the end, nurse can feel lower edge of kidney between her hands.
Done to assess for size, absence of kidney, kidney mass, kidney nodule, etc.

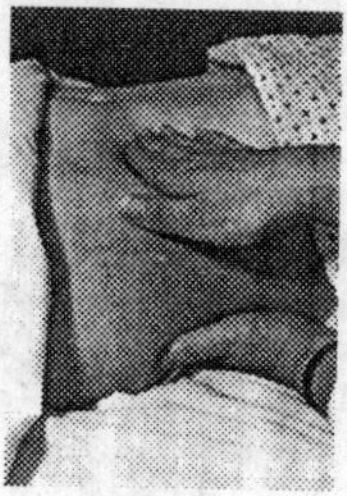

Palpating the kidney

Palpebra It refers to eyelid.

Palpebral That which is connected with eyelid, such as palpebral ligament.

Palpitation When a person starts feeling his heart beat, which otherwise is not perceivable.
When patient is conscious of forceful and rapid heart contraction he complaints ' palpitation is heard and experienced.

Palsy The term denotes paralysis which is associated with trembling and shaking,
Common clinical paralyses in nursing practice are:
a) Cerebral palsy (stroke palsy).
b) Bell's palsy (Facial nerve palsy).
c) Crutch palsy (by crutch).
d) Palsy agitans (Parkinsonism).
e) Palsy polio.
f) Palsy traumatic.

Panacea It is a mythological remedy for all illnesses in the world.

Panchayat Raj system It is a 3 tier health system at 3 levels . They are:
- Panchyat village level.
- Panchayat samiti at Block level.
- Zilla parishad at district level.

Pancoast's syndrome Cancer of the ling which has eroded to brachial plexus,
Horner's syndrome.

Pancoast's tumour In Ca. lung which is located in the apex of lung produces neurological involvement which produce the following triad:
1. Pain.
2. Wasting.
3. Weakness of arm.

This type of Bronchogenic carcinoma was described by American Radiologist Dr.Pancoast around 1910.

Pancreas It is one of the digestive gland situated behind the stomach, islets of Langerhans is located in pancreas which secretes insulin by virtue of which body can utilise sugars and starches,

It is an elongated recemose gland, retrogastric and head in the duodenal curve.

Pancreatectomy Surgical removal of part of pancreas or whole of pancreas.

Pancreatin It is secreted by pancreas which helps in digestion.

Pancreatitis Infection and inflammation of the pancreas,
Clinically acute pancreatitis and chronic pancreatitis are known.

Pancuronium It is a muscle relaxant used in surgery/anaesthesia.

Pancytopenia Lowered blood cell count due to bone marrow depression.

Pandemic A disease occurring simultaneously in many countries.

Panel It is a 'large group' method of teaching – learning process with one moderator (a senior nursing professor) and 4-6 nursing teachers and hold an orderly and logical conversation on one topic.
This allows exploring a problem from all angles.

Panic Abnormal fear for which no reason can be sought out ,
Usually it is present in schizophrenics and in patients who suffer from anxiety neurosis.

Panniculitis It is subcutaneous fat inflammation causing painful nodes, Common sites are thigh, thorax and abdomen.

Pannus It is sequelae of trachoma and corneal ulcers,
Pannus produce granulation of cornea and leads to impaired vision Latin word meaning 'cloth'.

Panophthalmia Infection and inflammation of all layers of eyeball.

Panting It is shallow rapid breathing.

Pantothenic acid It is one of vitamin B complex and is water soluble.

Pap test Short form for Papaniculao test named after its discoverer, it involves the examination of smear specimen of body secretions for early diagnosis of cancer,
Common screening test for Ca.cervix.

Papain It is extracted from papaya fruit which is a proteolytic enzyme.

Papilla Any projection which is shaped like a nipple, common types are:

- At the back of the tongue-Circumvallate papilla.
- In optic disc - Optic papilla.
- Skin projection with nerves–Tactile papilla.
- In main tongue – Filiform papilla.

Papillary That which is having projections shaped like nipple.

Papilloedema Colloquially called 'choked disc' due to hyperaemia of optic disc one of the sign of increased intracranial pressure.

Papilloma Other name for wart which is a benign epithelial tumour.

Papovavirus Warts producing viruses which are DNA viruses.

Pappus This is the first tiny hair which appear during puberty.

Papule Skin lesion which is raised above the surface of the skin such as pimple or papule of chickenpox.

Paracentesis To drain fluid from a cavity a puncture is made.

Paradigm When a theoretical postulation is made, some of earlier examples are taken before proceeding to action.

Paradox It means incredible self contradictory word from Greek root paradoxos

Examples of paradox are:

- Weber's paradox (Very much stretched muscle cannot contract depicting that it stretched too much).
- Kretz's paradox (Vaccine prevent illness by immunisation , but reacts violently on person who is previously immunised with that).
- Opie's paradox (Local anaphylaxis leading to necrosis show protective action).

Paradoxical That which occurs not in the natural way or abnormally.

Paraesthesia Abnormality in sensation in neurological pathology, colloquially it is called 'pins and needles' tingling sensation.

Paraffin Petroleum product which is hydrocarbon (saturated) ,

Derivatives of paraffin are:

- Liquid paraffin (laxative).
- Wax paraffin (wax treatment in arthritis).
- Soft paraffin (skin protection).

Paragonimus They are lung flukes belong to trematodes helminths, Paragonimus westermani is common lung fluke in tropical countries.

Paraguard rescue stretcher It is made of light metal closely fitting stretcher with plastic cushioning. It is convenient to use in a confined space. One more advantage is that it can be made flexible in the middle for negotiaing narrow corners, can be folded for compact storage and for carriage.

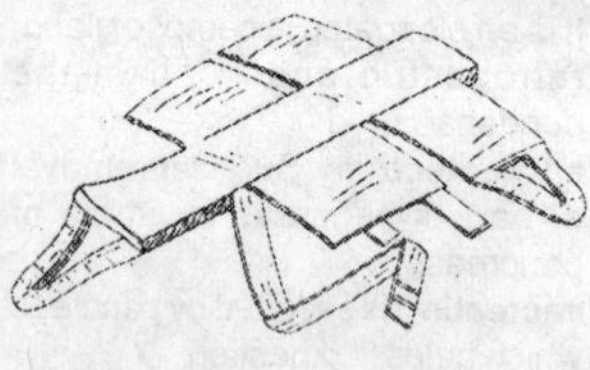

Paraguard rescue stretcher

Paraguay tea Decoction from South American herb mate. It has social value and no medicinal value.

Paraldehyde Nowadays its use is restricted, It is anticonvulsant, sedative and hypnotic.

Paralysis When there is loss of nervous function leading to loss of motion

Loss of motor function by neurological lesion,

Types of paralysis in nursing practice are:

- Infantile Polio paralysis.
- Flaccid paralysis.
- Spastic paralysis.
- Facial paralysis.
- Bulbar polio paralysis.
- General paralysis of the Insane.
- Paralysis agitans of Parkinsonism.

Paralytic ileus In emergencies when patient comes with late obstructive process in peritonitis, nurse should auscultate the abdomen to find out bowel sounds which are typically absent.

Paralytic That which is related with paralysis such as paralytic ilelus.

Paramedian Lying parallel to the midline such as paraspinal muscles.

Paramedical In integrated health services, associated health workers who are trained in their skilled profession, help the doctor in giving health care services, paramedical include:

- Nurses.
- Laboratory technicians.
- Medical record officers.
- X-ray technicians.
- Dialysis technicians.
- O T technicians.
- Health inspectors.
- Public health nurse.
- Lady health visitors.
- MPW male.
- MPW female.
- Physiotherapist.
- Medical social workers.
- Speech pathologists.
- Speech therapists.
- Trained first aid and ambulance workers.
- Occupational therapists.
- Councillors for marriage, sex, genetics.

Medical service related items are done by skilled and trained people, Technically trained persons in medical service such as Technician, health worker, medical social worker, medical record officer, health inspector, etc.

Parametritis Infection and inflammation of tissues surrounding uterus,
Pelvic infection.

Parametrium Connective tissues surrounding the uterus.

Paraamino salicylic acid It is a chemotherapeutic agent used in the treatment of tuberculosis
Commonly called as PAS.

Paramnesia It is a psychological condition where patient has defect in memory,
Always patient recollects false events and events that which did not happened.

Paranoia Delusion filled mental disorder and patient maintains good personality.

Paranoid It is one of the mental illnesses manifested mainly by suspicion
Delusions of persecution are marked and resemble paranoia.

Paraparesis Lower limb paralysis which is not complete paralysis.

Paraphimosis Painful constriction which occurs when prepuce gets retracted behind glans penis.

Paraphrenia Schizophrenia without personality defect which is seen in adult type of schizophrenia.

Paraplegia Acute or chronic paraplegia which occurs due to injury or disease of spinal cord,
Lower trunk paralysis and lower limb paralysis below the lesion.

Paraprofessional Paramedical is a paraprofessional who assists a medical profession, see list under paramedical.

Parapsychology Any psychological disorders which fall outside the scope of physical law of the nature
Effects and experience of psychological illness which the modern science cannot previews.

Parasite It can be plant or an animal which live on another animal or plant to fetch nourishment and thrive.

Parasiticide Drugs used in parasitic infestations.

Parasympathetic nerves One of the component of autonomous nervous system,

Parasympathetic nerves reverse the action of the sympathetic nerves.

Parasympathetic Part of autonomic nervous system which lies in craniosacral region.

Parasympatholytic Nervous system that oppose the effects of parasympathetic nervous system.

Parathormone Parathyroid gland secretions.

Parathyroid Small endocrine glands associated with each lobe of thyroid gland,

Parathyroid hormone control calcium metabolism.

Paratyphoid Milder and short duration form of typhoid caused by *Salmonella* other than s.typhi.

Parecentesis Puncture of the wall of a cavity to draw fluid for diagnosis or to release tension.

Parenchyma Active connective tissues of an organ which is differentiated by its high vascularity.

Parenteral All injectable including intravenous administration of drugs.

Paracentesis It is tapping the abdomen to draw fluid from peritoneal cavity (ascites) seen liver disorder, malignancy

Requirements:

- Local anaesthetic.
- Syringe and needle.
- Spirit.
- Swabs.
- Adhesive plaster.
- Pail.
- Mackintosh.
- Receptacles.
- Forceps.
- Hypodermic tray.
- Ascites trocar and cannula.

Procedure: Patient must empty bladder. Patient sits upright,

He is supported by the pillows; Binder is placed in position so that it can be applied soon after trocar and cannula are inserted.

When introduced the fluid drains and nurse should tighten the binder.

Parenthood Responsibilities that are to be discharged by father and mother to their offspring(s),

It is a dramatic experience in the life of a young husband and wife which changes their whole outlook on life and living.

Paresis Paralysis which is incomplete in nature.

Parietal That which is related to the wall of a cavity such as:

- Parietal bone.
- Parietal cells.
- Parietal pleura.

Paris green It is copper acetoarsenate, a green powder. It is used at 2% dust spray for killing larvae of mosquitoes.

Parity This depicts live births to a woman, para one means that the woman has one live born child in her maternal life.

Parkinson's disease In extrapyramidal system, nuclear masses seen degeneration giving rise to the following clinical manifestations:

- Characteristic tremor of resting muscles.
- Slowed down of voluntary movements.
- Gait which is festinating in nature.
- Posture which is peculiar.

- Weakness of muscles.
- Mask like facies.

Paralysis agitans described by Dr.Parkinson a British Physician A nervous disorder affecting nerves and muscles which cause muscle stiffness and muscle trembling.

Parks For the safety of children in play and playground, parks are provided in residential area which are visible to parents and who can have a vigilance on their kids at play Park also a safety area to sit and relax (park) by the elderly.

Paronychia Fingernail abscess called whitlow.

Parotid Salivary gland which is situated in front of the ear on both side.

Parotitis Infection and inflammation of parotid gland.

Parous Derived from para meaning woman having one or more children

Paroxysm Recurrence of an attack which is sudden and acute in nature Refers to asthmatic attack, a convulsive attack.

Paroxysmal That which is related to paroxysm such as paroxysmal tachycardia, paroxysmal dyspnoea

Parrot disease Refers to Psittacosis, viral infection spread by birds (parrots).

Parrot fever It is caused by a virus and is transmitted by birds either parrot or parrot related birds.

Partial rebreathing mask It is mask for low flow system oxygen therapy in the management of respiratory therapy.

In cardiac conditions and in pulmonary diseases it is useful for short-term treatment when patient is having increased FiO_2 demand

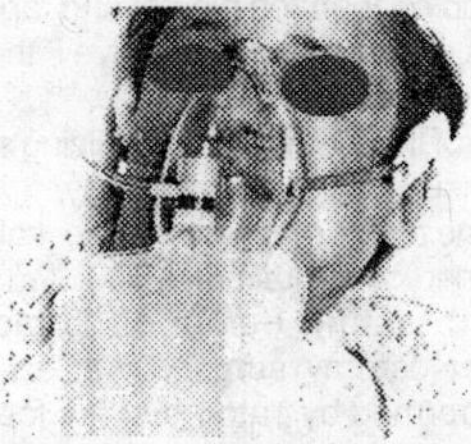

Partial rebreathing mask (Low flow system)

Particle Small unit of a substance or minute substance.

Parturition The process of birth of the child in delivery.

Parturient That which related to the childbirth.

PAS Abbreviation for **P**ara **A**mino **S**alicylic acid.

Passive smoking Inhalation of nicotine when other smoke in the society.

Passive That which is not active, common terminology in nursing practice are:

- Passive immunity.
- Passive movement.
- Passive smoking.
- Passive surveillance.

Pasteurella Gramnegative bacilli which cause plague.

Pasteurisation It was discovered by Louis Pasteur who showed that heating of milk to a certain degree can kill pathogens,

Milk pasteurisation is common item in dairy development

Heating milk to 72^{0}C for 15 to 20 minutes and then rapidly cooling.

Patch test This is testing sensitivity of a substance on the person by keeping them on plaster and taping to skin which show positive if there is inflammation

One of the method of determining skin sensitivity or general allergy,

Done for the diagnosis and for safety of medicamentation.

Patch testing Before using tapes after ostomy surgery skin test is performed by patch test for foam, silk and paper tapes ,

They are kept on to abdomen skin and tested for 24 hours,

Documentation is done if patient is allergic to patch and one should use non-sensitive patch for stomal patch Patch test should not be done on hairy skin.

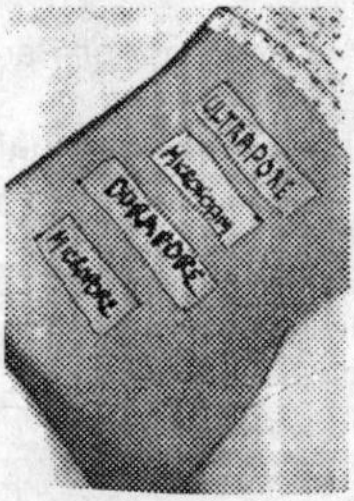

Prior to ostomy surgery patch test done

Patella Sesamoid bone which form knee cap.

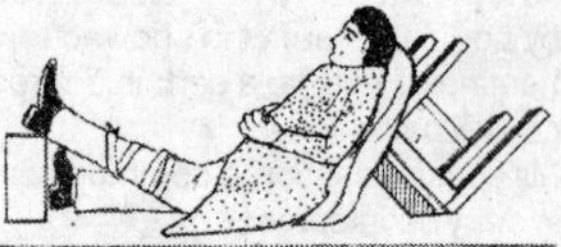
Patella fracture (treatment completed)

Patellar reflex Done for L2, L3 and L4 innervations by percussing the patellar tendon just distal to the patella. In normal process, the knee should extend and the quadriceps muscle should contract.

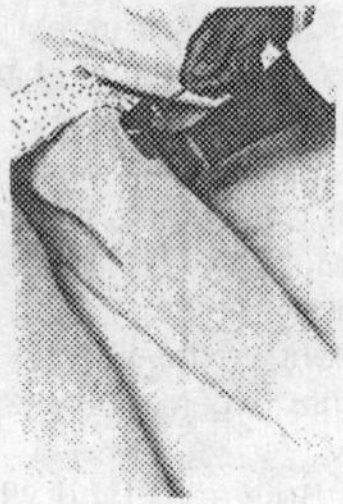
Patellar reflex

Patent medicine Commercially promoted drug preparation of secret composition,

Patenting require disclosure of its composition.

Patent That which is open such as patent ductus arteriosus.

Patent ductus arteriosus When ductus arteriosus is not closed, it causes shunt of blood from aorta into the pulmonary artery and produce heart murmur.

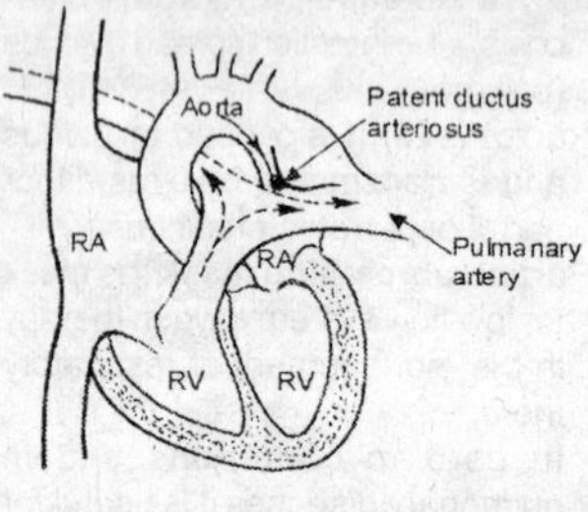

Patent ductus arteriosus

Paternity test Tests like blood grouping, HLA are done to find out the real father of a child in case of legal dispute.

Pathogen It is referred to germs which cause diseases in man and in animals.

Pathogenicity This refers to the ability of germs to cause diseases.

Pathognomonic A subjective or objective manifestation of a disease which help to identify a disease.

Pathological It is the description of morbid and microchanges of tissues in a disease

That which is related to pathology.

Pathology Discipline that deals with identification of abnormality of tissues abnormal processes and abnormal reactions,

Structural and functional changes in tissues and organs of the body which cause illness.

Pathophysiology The science which throw light on the physiological changes in diseases.

Patient related ethics They are guiding principles for nursing profession such as compassion, confidentiality, element of informed consent, obligation to treat, respect for person, solidarity and well being or beneficience.

Patient self-determination Act The Patient Self Determination Act USA (1990) is self-explanatory

The patient can direct health profession. He can reject the treatment.

Patient's right Rights of patient in hospital treatment are: (1) moral and (2) legal in nature

Moral rights are:

1. Right to know about illness and its course.
2. Right to privacy about illness and its course.

Legal rights is:

1. Right to treatment for illness and its sequelae.

Patient Person who is under the care of doctor and nurse for his treatment over an illness.

Paul Bunnell test It is an agglutination test (antigen and antibody reaction) which is diagnostic for glandular fever.

Dr.Paul and Dr.Bunnell the American Physicians discovered this test, which is an immunological test.

Pavlov reflex The reflex is named after Russian Physiologist which is popularly called as conditioned reflex.

In his dog experiment, ringing the bell produced the condition of an anticipation of food to eat and dogs started salivary and gastric secretions.

Payer's patch Oval elevated areas of lymphoid tissue on the mucosa of the small intestine.

Pearson correlation It is a statistical technique to study relationships by mathematical methods.

Pearson correlation is repre-sented as "r".

Relationship ranges from +1.00 through 0.0 to – 1.00 (perfect +ve no relation and perfect negative relationship respectively)

Peau d'orange Resemblance of orange skin due to blockage of the skin lymphatic which is common in breast cancer.

Pecten Named to the crest of pubic crest to which inguinal ligament is attached.

Pectoral That which is related to the chest such as pectoral muscles.

Pectus Chest is named as 'pectus'.

Percussion It is the clinical examination by tapping with fingers to observe any changes in underlying organs.

Pedagogy The science of teaching.

Paediatric Medical speciality that deals with the diseases of children, Diseases of children up to the age of 16 years according to Planning Commission of India Diseases of children upto the age of 12 years according to existing treatment modalities in hospital services.

Paediatrician Medical specialist who is trained and is a consultant in dealing with diagnosis, treatment and management of illnesses in children.

Pedicle It refers to neck or stem of a tissue or organ.

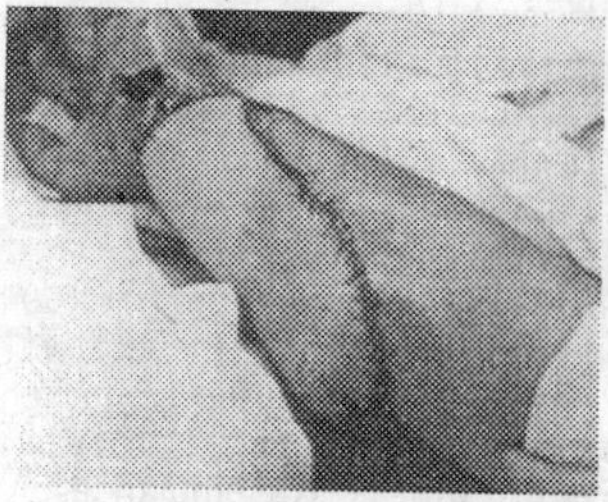

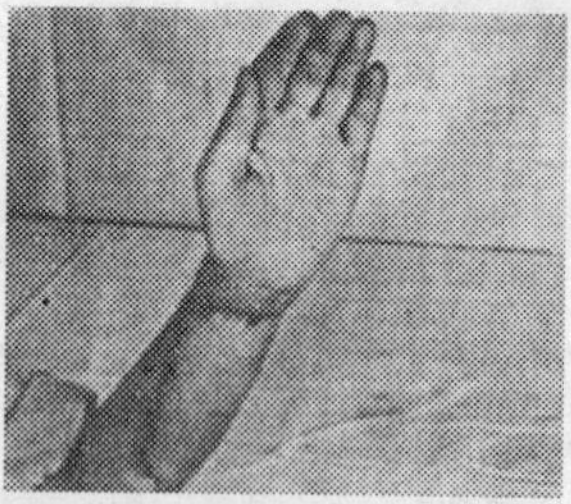

Pedicle graft

Pedicular Related with the infection of lice.

PediculosisLouse infestation of a person, may be head louse or body louse.

Pediculus Name of genus of louse such as:

1) Pediculus capitis hominis.
2) Pediculus corporis hominis.
3) Phthirus pubis.

Paedodontics Speciality that deals with diagnosis, treatment and management of teeth problems of children.

Peduncle Narrow supporting part of a tissue or organ such as cerebellar peduncle.

Peer review It is a quality assurance programme wherein nursing care service is reviewed by the peer group of nurses.

Peer Associate of equal age or contemporary.

Pellagra Condition caused by niacin deficiency which is common among alcoholic and drug addicts.

Pelvic inlet It is formed by two hip bones, the sacrum and coccyx.

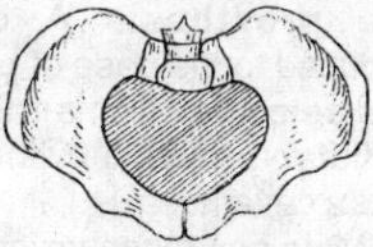

Normal pelvis

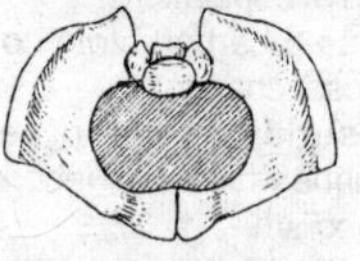

Flat pelvis

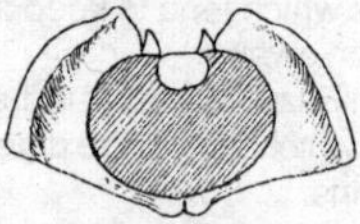

Rachitic pelvis

Pelvic inlets

Pelvic belt It is applied for patients with sciatica, low back pain and muscle spasm in lower back, It should encircle the pelvis than waistline.

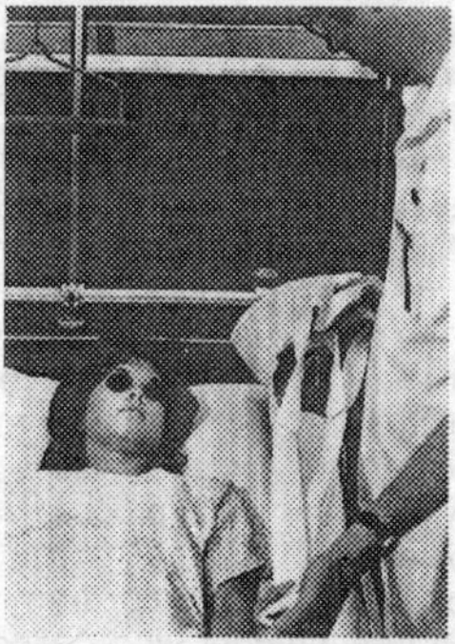

Pelvic belt (assessing before putting the belt)

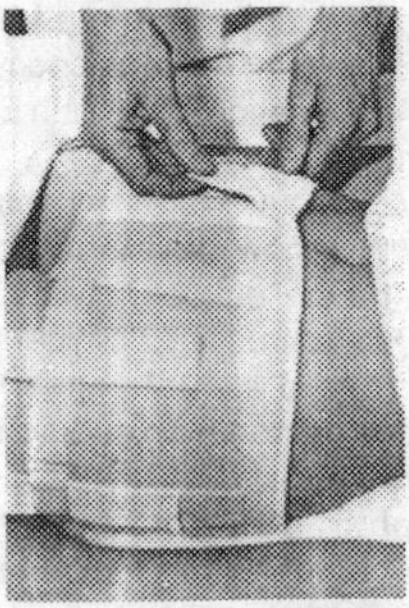

Pelvic belt put in position

Pelvic girdle Ring formed by bones which form the hip and lower abdominal area.

Pelvic traction Pelvic belt is applied and is fixed to traction tapes and are connected to 8 to 10 pounds weight for traction to pelvis, as indicated in pelvic belt.

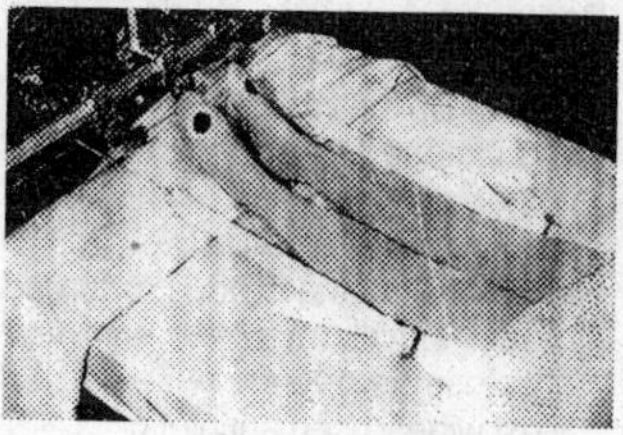

Pelvic traction through straps of pelvic belt

Pelvic That which is related with pelvis such as pelvic girdle, pelvic inflammatory disease.

Pelvimetry One of the gynaecological examination to measure pelvic brim to assess the possibility of normal vaginal delivery or to assess CPD.

Pelvis Pelvic girdle formed by two hip bones, sacrum and coccyx.

PEM Abbreviation for Protein Energy Malnutrition,
PEM affects infants by retarded growth, show development and poor mental outlook, Kwashiorkor and Marasmus are 2 clinical types.

Pemphigoid skin changes where blisters beneath the epidermis is seen or resembling pemphigus.

Pemphigus Blister causing skin disease which has the capacity to alter general health
Greek word pemphix meaning blister, considered to be an autoimmune disease.

Pendulous That which is seen hanging such as hanging abdomen.

Penicillamine Pharmacologically it is a chelating agent, its uses are:
- Used in metal poisoning.
- Wilson's disease.
- Rheumatoid arthritis.

Penicillin Antibiotic obtained from Penicillium was discovered by Fleming in the year 1929.

Penicillinase This enzyme is present in staphylococci which inactivates the antibiotic Penicillin.

Penicillin It is the product of bread mold penicillium which was first antibiotic discovered,
Most widely used antibiotic.

Penicillium Genus belonging to fungi, Penicillin is obtained from Penicillium.

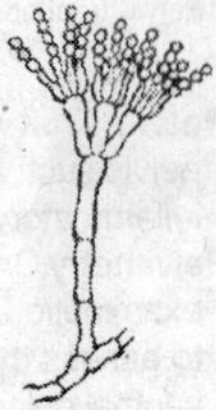
Penicillium

Penile prosthesis A device introduced to the base of penis to achieve erection which is in the form of inflatable plastic cylinder (to corpora cavernosa).

Penis Male sex organ which is the organ of copulation.

Pentose 5 carbon atom containing monosaccharide.

Pentosuria Presence of pentose in the urine which is an inborn error of metabolism.

Pep pills They are habit forming drugs which tend to keep a sleepy person awake.

Pepsin Enzyme present in the gastric juice which help in the digestion of proteins.

Pepsinogen Pepsinogen is the precursor of pepsin, Pepsinogen is activated by HCl.

Peptic ulcers It refers to ulcer in stomach or in the duodenum.

Peptic That which is related with pepsin or gastric juice such as pepticulcer.

Peptide On hydrolysis peptide yield amino acids.

Peptone Peptone is produced by the action of pepsin on protein.

Percentile It describes the level of existence of a characteristic,
When a characteristic is arranged from lower to higher in a group of 100, 50th value is 50th percentile or median, 70th value is 70th percentile, 90th value is 90th percentile, etc.

Perception Man perceives a thing which is a mental process called perception.

Percussion According to Dr.Auenbrugger who described Percussion in 1761,

"It is the Act of striking a part with short, sharp blows as an aid in diagnosing the condition of the parts beneath by the sound obtained".
Common clinical types of percussion are:

- Finger percussion.
- Coin percussion.
- Deep percussion.
- Topographic percussion.

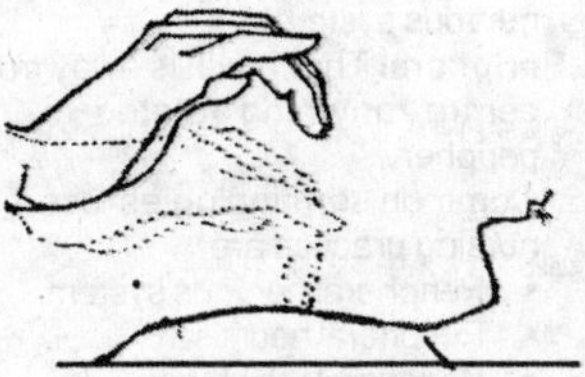

A: Immediate percussion

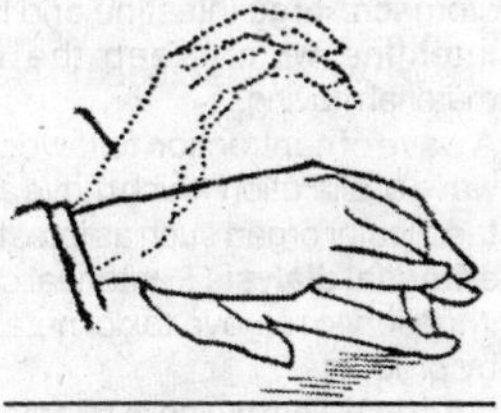

B: Strong percussion

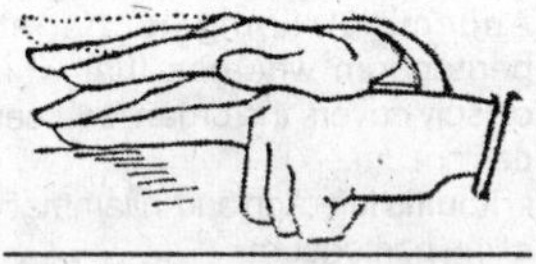

C: Weak percussion

Percutaneous Refers to external applications like ointment, emulsion, etc.

Perfuse To pour over another liquid

Perfusion Isolating the circulation in a limited portion of the body or the for cancer treatment of that area with antimetabolites

Passage of blood through lung which is meant for oxygenation.

Perianal That which is located around the anus such as perianal abscess.

Periarthritis Infection and inflammation of surrounding tissues of a joint.

Pericarditis Infection and inflammation of pericardium, Types of pericarditis are:

- Bacterial pericarditis.
- Viral pericarditis.
- Rheumatic pericarditis.
- Adhesive pericarditis.
- Chronic constrictive pericarditis.

Pericardium Outer layer covering the sac of heart which contains both fibrous and serous coats along with serous fluid.

Periodontics Treatment of gum diseases (tissues around teeth) .

Perifolliculitis Infection and inflammation around hair follicle.

Perimetry Eye examination to measure the field of vision and visual acuity throughout the whole field.

Perinatal This is the period around the childbirth which starts shortly before birth to 7th day after birth of the child.

Perinatology It is the branch of medical science which includes obstetrics and paediatrics which deals with the health of perinatal period.

Perineal That which is related to the perineum.

Perineum bandage Specific bandage used over the perineum as first aid or for treatment.

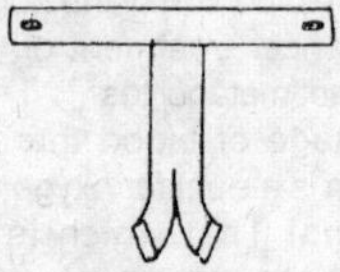

Perineum bandage

Perineorrhaphy The laceration occurred during labour is repair by suturing the lacerations at birth.

Periodic That which occurs in regular interval.

Periodicity That which recurs at regular intervals of time.
Common terminologies in clinical use are:
- Periodicity of malaria paroxysm.
- Periodicity of microfilaria in blood.

Periodontitis Inflammation of tissues and gum around teeth which cause loosening of teeth
Infection and inflammation of the Periodontium.

Periodontium It refers to the connective tissue between teeth and their sockets.

Periodontosis Wasting away of the bone surrounding the teeth, with consequent loosening of the teeth.

Periosteal That which is related with periosteum.

Periosteum It is the membrane that covers bone surface, they are absent where ligaments are attached, they are also absent where bone becomes cartilaginous, The fibrous tissue covering the surface of a bone.

Periostitis Infection and inflammation of the periosteum.

Peripheral nervous system They include the following:
- Nerves running to the sense organs.
- Nerves running to heart.
- Nerves running to internal organs.
- Nerves running to skeletal muscles.

Continuing on from the central nervous system.

Peripheral That which is away from centre, anything related to the periphery,
Common terminologies used in nursing practice are:
- Peripheral nervous system.
- Peripheral neuritis.
- Peripheral resistance.
- Peripheral iridectomy.

Peristalsis Wave like motion of stomach, large intestine and large intestine which keep the food material moving,
A wave of contraction followed by a wave of dilatation which move along the tubular organ such as intestine.

Peritoneal dialysis Peritoneal cavity irrigation to remove toxic metabolic by products.

Peritoneal That which is related with peritoneum such as peritoneal dialysis, peritoneal cavity, etc.

Peritoneum The serous membrane that covers the abdominal organs, Abdominal lining is parietal peritoneum whereas that which closely covers the organ is visceral peritoneum.

Peritonitis Infection and inflammation of the peritoneum.

Peritonsillar Depicts that which is around the tonsil such as quinsy.

Perineal care This is routine gynaecological technique done and or supervised by the nurse.

Method 1: Squeeze bottle filed with tap water warmed to 100°F for cleaning perineum after every voiding

Method 2: A sitz bath is prepared for patients with vulvar pain and swelling and who require warmth to heal the perineal area. Indicated after vaginal hysterectomy, Vulvectomy childbirth, haemorrhoidectomy

Method 3: For any perineal discomfort nurse can teach the patient how to use surgigator perineal care system for cleansing and providing warmth to the perineum.

Permeability It is the status of fluid flow through any semipermeable membrane.

Pernicious That which is dangerous.

Person years in good health The philosophy of life from time immemorial is prolongation of life, which has a philosophical basis in blessings, for a century of life (Shatamanam Bhavati).

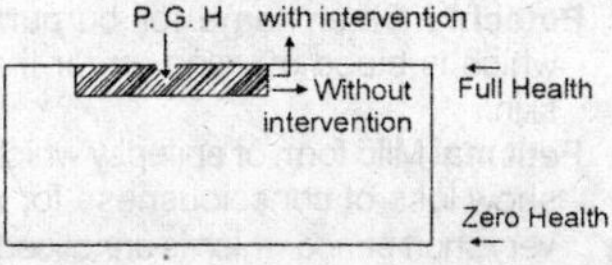

P G H (Person years in good health)

Personal hygiene It deals with practices of an individual which help in maintaining and promoting his health physically, mentally, socially and spiritually to get maximum health benefit.

Components of personal hygiene are:

- Skin care.
- Importance for clothing.
- Care of the hand.
- Care of the hair.
- Hygiene of toilet.
- Bowel habit.
- Menstrual hygiene.
- Care of special sensory organs
  - * Eye
  - * Ear
  - * Nose
  - * skin
  - * Oral cavity
- Balanced diet.
- Exercise.
- Posture.
- Sleeping habit.

Personality This is mental make up and attitude of a person which is built up by heredity, environment and literacy,

In nursing psychology, following personalities are observed:

- Good personality.
- Balanced personality.
- Imbalanced personality.
- Antisocial personality.
- Cyclothymic personality.
- Dual personality.
- Split personality.
- Double personality.
- Schizoid personality.
- Psychopathic personality.

Human behaviour is moulded by personality, personality of health professional influences prognosis of sick and the hospitalised.

It is defined as body pattern which are influenced externally by status role and internally by thinking, desire, goals and motivation

Types: Extrovert, introvert and mixed.

Perspiration The process of sweating which is controlled by nervous system and balanced by physical environment.

Perthes' disease Named after German Surgeon for "Osteochondritis of the head of the femur".

PERT Abbreviation for **P**rogramme **E**valuation and **R**eview **T**echnique, This is helpful in detailed planning and in comprehensive supervision. It is made by sequence arranged logically with arrow marks for steps and timings.

PERT helps in planning, scheduling monitoring, communication, problem identification, gives progress report and thus is a good evaluating method in nursing service administration.

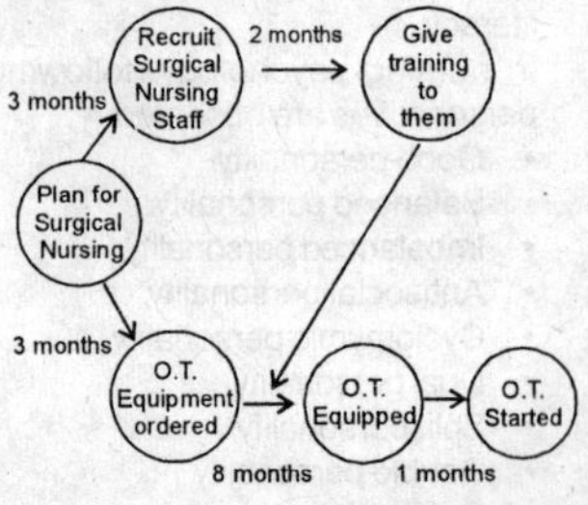

Network analysis of surgical nursing for O T functioning in a hospital

Pertussis The name of whooping coughs a bacterial disease of young children.

Perversion Visible deviation from normal social norms such as sexual perversion, here we observe behaviour changes.

Pessaries It is an instrument for introducing into the vagina for giving support in cases of prolapsed uterus. They are made of coils of watch spring covered with rubber, Perspex or vulcanite.

Though surgery is permanent cure, sometimes nurse has to introduce ring pessary,

Pessary is also used for antiseptic purpose

Requirement:

- Clip forceps, sterilised.
- Pessary sterilised.
- Swabs.
- Lotion of Bradsol 1:2000Gloves.
- Mackintosh.
- Receptacle.
- Hand lamp.

Nursing procedure: In left lateral position Mackintosh is arranged, swab the vulva, put on sterilised gloves, ring pessary is dipped in lubricant, It is inserted into the vagina with the posterior rim along the length of the orifice gradually turning it over directing upwards and backwards till one side of the rim is in posterior fornix and cervix is felt in ring.

Pessimistic One who is always show negative attitude for everything,

Dejected mind.

Petechia Other name for purpura which is blood effusion under the skin.

Petit mal Mild form of epilepsy which show loss of consciousness for a very short period which is unnoticed.

Petrous That which is stone like such as petrous bone.

Pets Veterinary Association has shown that dog, cat, cattle, hogs, sheep, goats, horses, mules are common pets of man,
Pets are disease carriers and their care is essential
Pets at home allow vermin which are health hazardous
Rabies is well known diseases from pets which show 100% mortality.

Peyote It is a mescal weed preparation from India,
Indians use this for religious ceremonials,
It is a stimulating drug often misused for kicks.

pH It is called buffer or hydrogen ion concentration of a liquid
pH 1 to 6 is acid, pH 7 is neutral, pH 8 to 14 is alkaline.

Phaeochromo cytoma Tumour of adrenal medulla which leads to hypertension in a person.

Phage typing It is a bacteriological examination to detect strain that cause disease,
One of the tool in epidemic of food poisoning.

Phage It refers to bacteriophage.

Phagocyte WBC which destroy bacteria and tissue debris.

Phagocytosis Process of engulfing pathogens or foreign bodies by the phagocyte.

Phakoma Tumour of retina.

Phalanges It refers to bones of toes or to bones of fingers.

Phallus Name for the male sex organ penis.

Phantom Originally pseudo or false impression or false image obtained by an image,
Model of an organ or part of the body created for demonstration
When radiation interaction is produced in the human body,
Similar terminologies in nursing practice are:
- Seudocyesis called phantom pregnancy.
- Tumour like swelling called phantom tumour.
- Pain in an amputated limb called phantom pain.

Pharmaceutical It is related to drugs and pharmacy Preparation formulation and distribution of a drug by company.

Pharmacist He is a trained person in pharmacy who is licensed to compounding and licensed to sale prescribed drugs.

Pharmacogenetics Drug response of an individual which is prefixed by genetically induced variations.

Pharmacology The science that deals with property, nature, preparation, body reaction and complications on human body,
Drug effects on human body is studies in this discipline.

Pharmacopoeia Standard preparation, standard preparation and standard doses are published by authorities in a country, such as:
- British Pharmacopoeia.
- American Pharmacopoeia.
- Indian Pharmacopoeia.

Prenatal sex determination Human society is 'boy child' dominated societies. 'Girl child' is abanded and has many ethical issues involved in prenatal sex deter mination or detection. This is associated with allowing abortion, asking for MTP and no care in in fancy.

Pharmacy Medical store where drugs are stored and distributed for use,
This is the science of and Art of formulation, preparation and compounding of medicamentation.

Pharyngeal That which is related to pharynx such as pharyngeal pouch.

Pharyngitis Infection and inflammation of pharynx.

Pharynx The part at the back of the mouth which has mucous lining and which is a muscular tube useful for deglutition
Space at the back of the mouth called throat which connects nasal cavities, oesophagus and larynx.

Pheneybutazone A chemotherapeutic agent which is used in the treatment of gout, arthritis and rheumatic conditions.

Phenobarbitone It is Phenyl Ethyl Barbituric Acid,
Chemically it is 'Phenylethylamlonylurea' used as hypnotic and sedative in epilepsy,
$C_6H_5(C_2H_5).C(CO.NH)_2CO$.

Phenol It is a coal tar derivative which is used as disinfectant,
Carbolic acid.

Phenolphthalein It is a laxative or cathartic,
It has limited used because of some of the complications such as rashes, albuminuria and haemoglobinuria.

Phenomenon An event or an occurrence which is noteworthy in clinical history
It can also be one of the objective manifestations of a patient.

Phenotype Characteristic of a person which is developed and is due to both environmental influence and genetic influence.

Phenylalanine It is one of the essential amino acid,
In phenylketonuria this amino acid cannot be synthesised in the body.

Phenylketonuria P.K.U. or Phenyl Keton Uria is a defect in metabolism of phynylala nine which is a congenital disorder,

Lack of enzyme phenylalanine hydroxylase

▼

Conversion of phenylalanine to tyrosine does not take place

▼

Accumulation of phenylalanine in blood take place

▼

Phenylpyruvic acid in urine is seen.

Metabolic error in phenylketonuria

Phenylketonuria A defect in the body chemistry that prevents the body's assimilation of an amino acid found in most protein foods which cause mental retardation.

Phenylpyruvic acid This is an abnormal constituent of urine in the clinical condition of phenylketonuria.

Phimosis Prepuce cannot be drawn back over glans penis because of constriction of the prepuce,
This is corrected by surgical intervention (Circumcision).

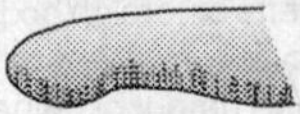

Phimosis

Phlebectomy It is surgical excision of a vein or part of a vein.

Phlebitis Infection and inflammation of vein which is characterised by the presence of pain swelling and redness along the vein,
Phlebitis is common in leg veins.

Phlebogram Tracing of venous pulse by sphygmograph.

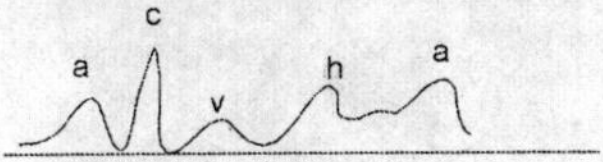

Phlebogram

a = Right atrial contraction
c = Right ventricle contraction
v = Blood filling ventricle
h = Abnormal wave.

Phlebolith A stone present in a vein (concretion in a vein).

Phlebotomus Sand fly genus which transmits sand fly fever.

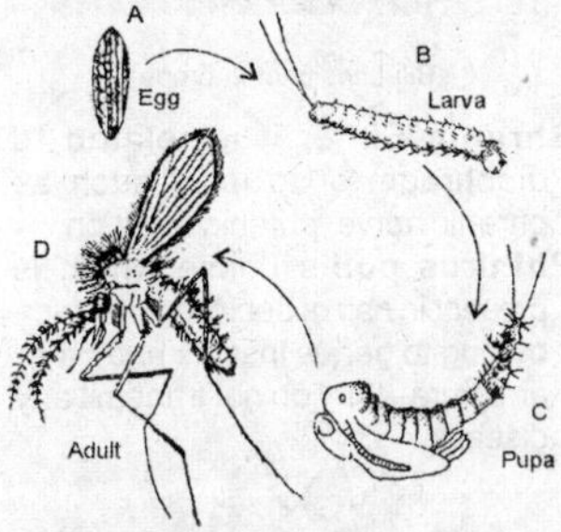

Life cycle of Sandfly (Phlebotomus)

Phlegm Phlegm is mucous secretion of air passage.

Phlegmatic Anything that which is dull and not active.

Phlyctenula It refers to a small or tiny pustule.

Phobia It is morbid fear with or without foundation in certain diseases such as hydrophobia, cancer phobia, AIDS phobia, etc.

Phocomelia It is a developmental anomaly where proximal portion of limbs found attached to the trunk through a single attachment.

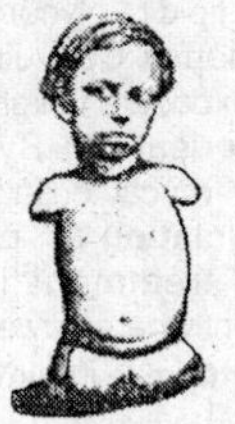

Phocomelia

Phonocardiogram Phonocardiographic recording of heart sounds and heart murmurs.

Phosphate crystals Deposits of salt of phosphoric acid found in urine producing symptoms.

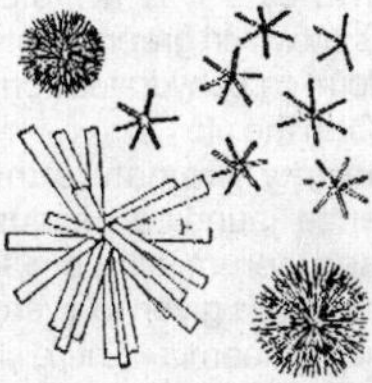

A : Stellar phosphates

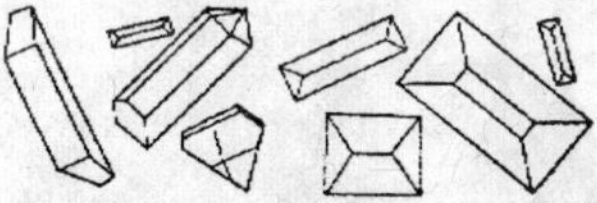

B: Triple phosphate crystals

Phosphatase This is required in phosphate metabolism. One of the common and major enzyme in this group is alkaline phosphatase.

Phospholipid Mainly seen in nervous system at cellular level which is a lipid of glycerol fat.

Photic epilepsy Convulsion following the exposure to light.

Photocauterisation By using radium or X-ray cauterisation is done.

Photocoagulation An ophthalmic mode of treatment in retinal detachment where powerful light is used to produce inflammation of retina.

Photophobia One who cannot tolerate light and has abnormal intolerance to it.

Photophthalmia Eye inflammation due to U.V light.

Photosensitivity Person showing severe reaction to sun light exposure.

Photosynthesis It is a biological process by which green plants use light to form carbohydrates from CO_2 and H_2O in the air.

Phototherapy Premature infants experience jaundice because of increased serum bilirubin level. Phototherapy is given to overcome hyperbilirubinaemia. Entire skin of infant is exposed to light for given period of time.

Bili Lites are used for phototherapy.

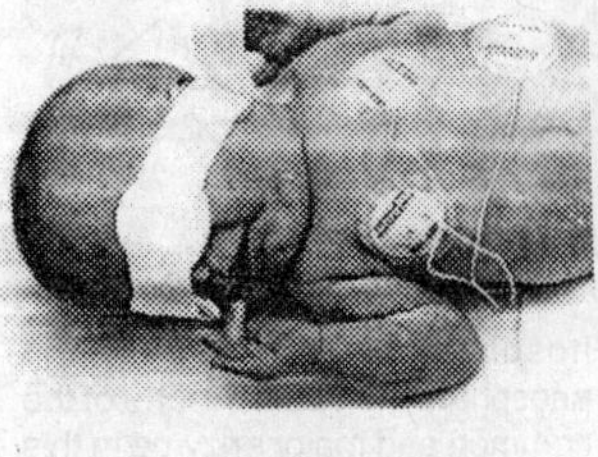

A: Phototherapy of newborn

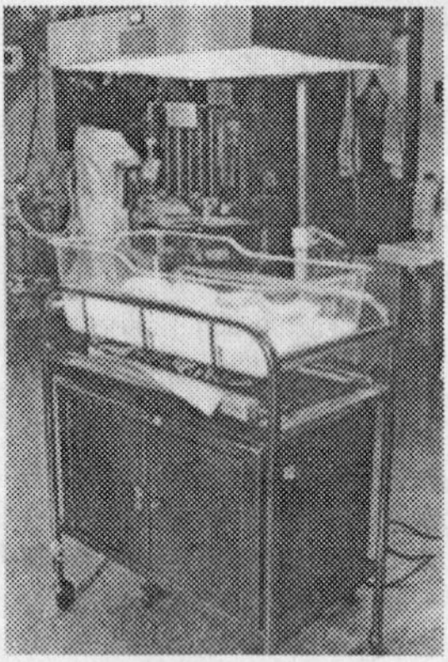

Bili-Lites phototherapy

Phrenic Either it is related to diaphragm or to mind such as phrenic nerve, phrenic avulsion.

Phthirus pubis Louse which is present in hair of pubic region which belong to genus insects and order anoplura, they do not transmit any disease.

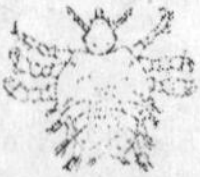

Phthirus pubis

Phthisis Literally mean shrinking of an organ or body,

It refers to pulmonary tuberculosis,

Shrinking of eyeball is called phthisis bulbi.

Phylum It is the primary division of animal kingdom or plant kingdom.

Physical medicine In the treatment of illness when physical agents like heat, water, light, massage and or exercise are used.

Physical Anything that is related with human body such as physical medicine, physically handicap, physical examination.

Physician Qualified doctor who practices general medicine after obtaining M D degree,
Those who have obtained superspeciality training are called consultant physicians.

Physiological Anything which is normal in nature such as physiological jaundice
Physiological solution.

Physiology The science that deals with the function of human body, this is a discipline in medical science in preclinical sciences.

Physiotherapy Treatment with physical agents such as heat, light, electricity,massage, vibration, water and or exercises; also called physical treatment
treatment by using natural force.

Physique This explains the structure of human body such as good physique.

Physostigmine An alkaloid which miotic in its property, It also has the property of antispasmodic and motor depressant,
Its preparations are used in the following conditions:

- Intraocular tension (glaucoma)
- Trismus
- Asthma
- Tetanus
- Emphysema.

Phytobezoar It is an accumulated vegetable matter in the stomach which give rise to stomach upset, Commonly hair accumulation is seen in clinical practice.

Phytosis It refers to illness that are caused by parasites seen on vegetables.

Pia mater The innermost covering of the brain and spinal cord.

Pica Colloquially it is 'dirt eating' is a bad habit sometimes encountered in good habits
It is a bad habit in a good child
It is from Latin which refers to a bird that eats everything unfit for food (magpie)
Commonly seen in pregnancy and among children with learning disability.

Pick-a-back For the transport of the sick and injured this pick-a-back method is used when patient is conscious and is able to support himself on the first aider's back.

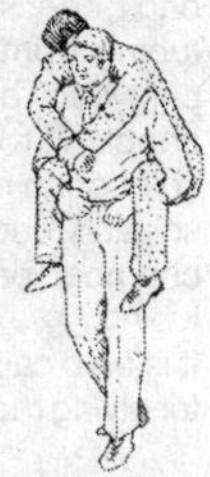

Pick-a-back

Pick's disease Dementia due to loss of brain cell cortex in elderly which was described by Dr.Pick a Czechoslovakian physician.

Picornavirus RNA group of viruses which contain echovirus and rhinovirus.

PID Abbreviation for **P**elvic **I**nflammatory **D**iseases.

Pie chart Data is represented in the form of circle where variables are put to proportions.

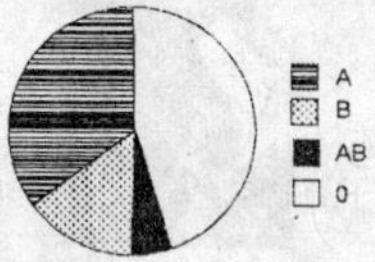

Pie diagram (Distribution of blood groups)

Pigeon chest Unduly prominent sternum among children suffering from rickets.

Pigeon's`breast Projected sternum in children due to rickets.

Piggyback medication Through an established I V set, medication is given by a secondary bottle called Piggyback bottle

Piggyback bottle is attached to the upper injection port on the primary line. The primary line must have a back check valve to prevent the tubing from running dry after the piggyback bottle empties.The back check valve allows the primary solution to run after the piggyback solution reaches the level of the drip chamber on the primary infusion tubing.

It is also called partial fill container for giving medication.

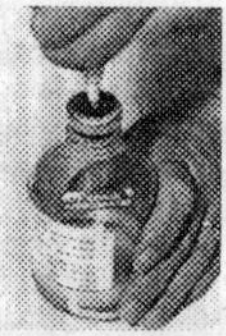

A: Piggy back infusion bottle ready for attachment

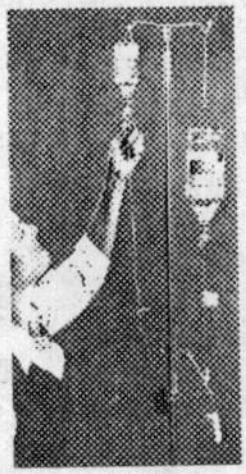

B: Piggyback bottle is fixed to the established IV set

Pigment Colouring matter of an organ or tissue such as blood pigment, bile pigment

This is the colouring matter present in the skin, hair, eyes.

Pigmentation Abnormal deposit of melanin pigment in a tissue or an organ.

Pile This is colloquial word for haemorrhoid.

Pill An oral preparation of medicament in illness treatment.

Round circular medicinal disc given orally in medical treatment.

Pilobezoar Accumulation of hair in the stomach giving rise to abdominal upset which may need surgical intervention.

Pilocarpine Drug used in the treatment of glaucoma which is an alkaloid from jaborandi leaves, Pupillary constructor.

Pilonidal An area where growth of hair is seen, having growth of hair.

Pilot study Planned preparatory study to finalise the study material in research,

This helps to overcome problems and bottlenecks in a study undertaken in a large scale.

Pimple Papule or pustule on the face, attributed to hormonal disturbances.

Pin care This is one of the major item of nursing care to be given to patients who are having skeletal traction to reduce fracture, particularly in case of distal femur, proximal tibia and the proximal ulna.

Pin or wire put should be inspected once every 4 hours to assess migration, infection, erythema, oedema, foul smelling, purulent discharge or gross bleeding.

No iodine preparation should be used since they corrode pins,in case of indications the area of pinning is cleaned with hydrogenperoxide leaving intact any superficial crust followed by an application of an antibiotic ointment,

If pin becomes loose intimate doctor in rounds and ask the patient to be immobile till doctor visits

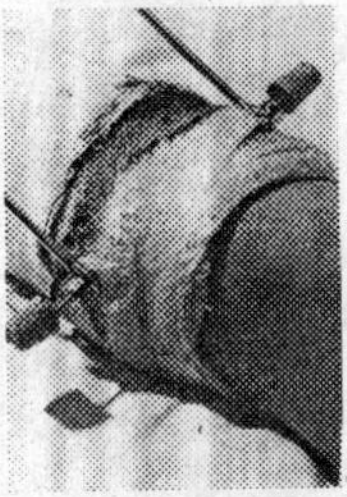

Pin skeletal traction to distal femur

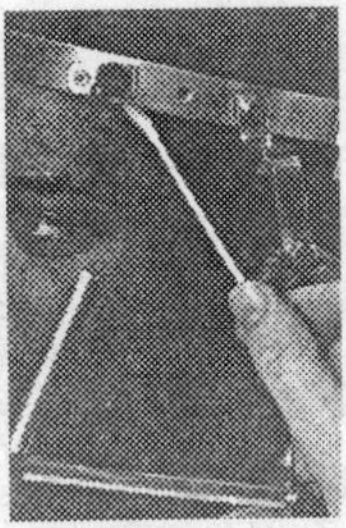

Pin care in case of Halo vest

Pineal Any structure shaped like a pin cone such as pineal body in the brain.

Pinguecula Harmless yellow spot on conjunctiva common elderly, due to degeneration of elastic tissues.

Pink eye Colloquial word for eye inflammation by local infections of conjunctiva or cornea or both General illness like measles, influenza, streptococcal infection of throat ARI, and pneumonia.

PinnaThis is ear flap sometimes called the auricle. In the centre of the pinna opening of ear channel lies, Pinna directs sound wave into ear channel.

Pons varolli The Pons Varolli is a bridge of white matter or nerve fibres which join together all the various parts of the brain, linking the two cerebellar hemispheres and joining the cerebrum above to the medulla below.

Piñta A non-STD caused by *Treponema carateum* which can be well differentiated from syphilis, Infection by a spirochete.

Pinworm Other name for thread-worm *'E.vermicularis'*.

Piperazine Antihelminthic drug used in the treatment of threadworm and roundworm.

Pitchman Always he is a promoter posing as a health lecturer for food fads or other forms of quackery.

Pituitary An endocrine gland at the base of the skull which is bilobed This is located in the middle of the lower surface of the brain,

It is the principal gland of internal secretion.

Pityriasis Scaly desquamation of skin a known skin disorder,

Types of Pityriasis are:

- Pityriasis capitis (dandruff)
- Pityriasis rosea (skin inflammation)
- Pityriasis alba (White scaly patches [children]).

Pityriasis Brany scales on the skin , Following clinical entities are seen:
- Superficial fungal infection (Pityriasis versicolor).
- Macular patch in children (Pityriasis alba).
- Exfoliative dermatitis (Pityriasis rubia pilaris.
- Acute pink macule (Pityriasis rosea).

PKU Abbreviation for **P**henyl **K**eton **U**ria.

Plagiocephaly Head looks twisted and suture union is not symmetrical which gives rise to a look of bent head and uneven head.

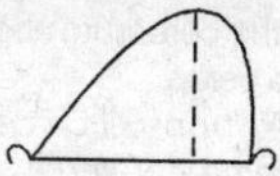

Plagiocephaly

Placebo Drug given to a patient which do not contain pharmacological ingredient and which is given to satisfy the patient,
Placebo are used in clinical trial which can be:
a) single blind method.
b) double blind method or.
c) treble blind method.

Placenta This is a special organ which nourishes the unborn baby (foetus), Colloquially called afterbirth,

Plague A bacterial disease caused by Yersinia pestis and transmitted by rat fleas,
Common type is Bubonic plague, Other acute types are:
a) Pneumonic plague.
b) Septicaemic plague.

Planes of trunk It is a determined flat surface for the description of anatomy.

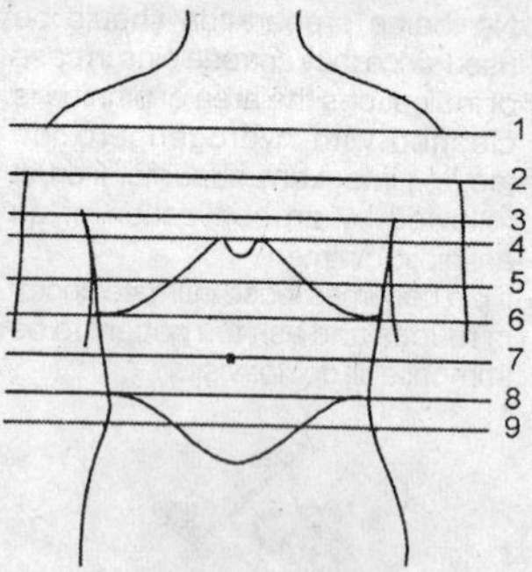

Different planes of trunk

1. - Suprasternal
2. - Ludwig's
3. - Thoracic
4. - Sternoxiphoid
5. - Transpyloric
6. - Subcostal
7. - Umbilical
8. - Intertubercular
9. - Spinous.

Plantar arch This refers to the arch of the foot.

Plantar reflex This is done to elicit Babinski reflex. A positive Babinski reflex is normal in infants under 1 year of age or even upto 1 ½ years. But it is a sign of motor nerve dysfunction in adult if positive.
How to test plantar reflex?
Stroke along the lateral surface of the sole of foot as shown in photograph.
Inference: If toes curl downward = it is normal
If smaller toes fan apart and large toe dorsiflexes toward patient's

head = Positive Babinski = Motor nerve dysfunction.

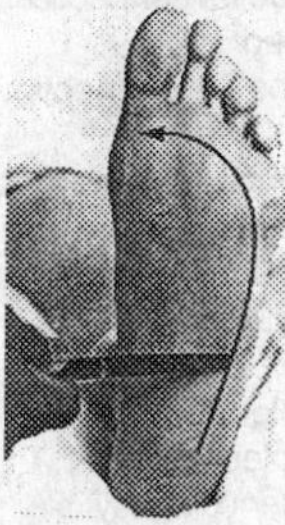

Eliciting plantar reflex (Babinski reflex)

Plantar That which is related to sole of the foot such as plantar arch, plantar wart, plantar extension, plantar flexion.

Plaque Hardened food particle on teeth

And also refers to flat patch on the skin.

Plasma It is the liquid portion of the blood, if fibrinogen is removed from plasma it is called serum.

Plasmin It is present in plasma which fibrinolytic which can dissolve fibrin clot.

Plasmodium They are protozoal parasites in RBC which produce Malaria,

Four major diseases producing Plasmodium are:

- *Plasmodium vivax.*
- *Plasmodium malariae.*
- *Plasmodium ovale.*
- *Plasmodium falciparum.*

Plaster of Paris bandage Given length of butter muslin or book muslin is foundation of plaster of Paris bandage. Dry plaster is rubbed into material, red thread identity helps to find out end on soakage, Quick setting plaster is used, Finished bandages are stored in airtight tins.

Plaster Certain material when mixed becomes hardening which are used to immobilise parts in fracture,

Also refers to adhesive plaster which is used in wound dressings,

Common types of plaster in nursing practice are:

- Plaster of Paris (for casting).
- Corn plaster (for corn).
- Frog plaster (for hip dislocation).
- Bohler's plaster (for Pott's fracture)..

Plastic surgery Surgery aimed at restoration of appearance and function.

Reconstructive surgery and skin transplant are included in this discipline.

Plastic That which is pliable, any substance that can be adoptable to many purposes,

Synthetic substance adaptable to many purposes

Common pliable materials seen in the market are vinyl, orlon and nylon.

Plateau This refers to persistent phase of high fever in an illness.

Platelet Platelet is the blood component which is involved in the clotting,

A thrombocyte.

Platysma This neck muscle which produces wrinkling on neck and depression of jaw.

Plethora If the tissue is reddened or an organ found bright red,

Anything that is red coloured.

Pleura Lining of the thorax which also

envelops lungs, which is serous membrane.

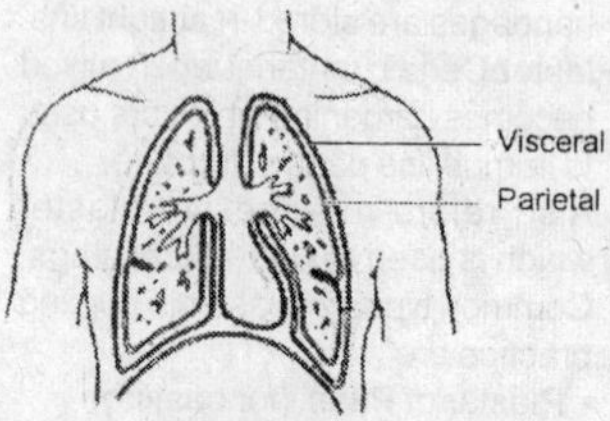

Pleura

Pleural effusion This is associated with restriction of upper chest movement,

This needs teaching apical expansion exercise to patient at nursing care,

Following exercise is advices and taught to patient by the nurse;

Fingers are positioned before clavicles, moderate pressure is applied, Patient is asked to inhale while pushing his chest upward and forward expanding his chet upward and expanding against nurse's finger pressure. Patient is encouraged to retain the expansion for a few minutes, and then asked to exhale quietly and passively,

These help in lung expansion and minimize flattening of upper chest.

Pleurevac system It is a disposable chest drainage system that is attached to a chest tube to relieve pressure from a build up of air or fluid in pleural space. (in thoracic trauma, pleural tears, spontaneous pneumothorax, haemothorax, etc.)

This system has 3 chambers:

- Suction control chamber.
- Water seal chamber.
- Collection chamber.

Two tubes are attached to this are;

Short tube for connection to suction if it is used

Long tube for connection to chest tube.

Pleuritis Infection and inflammation of the pleura,

Inflammation of pleura secondary to injury or tumour,

Types of pleuritis are :

- Dry pleurisy.
- Wet pleurisy.
- Purulent pleurisy.
- Fibrinous pleurisy.
- Pleurisy with effusion.

Pleurodynia Rheumatic pain in intercostals muscles.

Plexus It can be nervous plexus or venous plexus, Plexus denotes network, Common anatomical plexus are:

- Brachial plexus.
- Coeliac plexus.
- Choroid plexus.

Plication Plication in surgical procedure is that unfolding or tucking is done to shorten any structure.

Plumbism Common occupational hazard by lead intoxication.

Pneumococcus Gram-positive diplococcus that cause pneumonia.

Pneumoconiosis Because of the inhalation of dust chronic fibrous reaction in the lung is seen ,

Common types of pneumoconiosis are:

1) Bagassosis (cane sugar).
2) Byssinosis (cotton).
3) Tobacosis (nicotine).
4) Anthracosis (coal).
5) Silicosis (silica).
6) Asbestosis (asbestos).

Pneumocystis pneumonia One of the common respiratory complication of HIV/AIDS,

Pneumonia and pneumothorax are usual in such patients,

In an HIV positive patient following manifestations helps in the diagnosis of PCP (Pneumo Cystis Pneumonia):

I. Hypoxemia found out by arterial blood gas analysis
II. Presence of PCP in sputum obtained by nebulised saline
III. X-ray showing nodular reticular shadows, extensive infiltration, cavitation and sometimes pneumonitis.

Pneumoperitoneum When air is present in the peritoneal cavity, Types are:

- Pathological pneumoperitoneum.
- Diagnostic pneumoperitoneum.
- Therapeutic pneumoperitoneum.

Pneumothorax Air in the pleural cavity which can be:

- Spontaneous pneumothorax.
- Tension pneumothorax.
- Artificial pneumothorax.

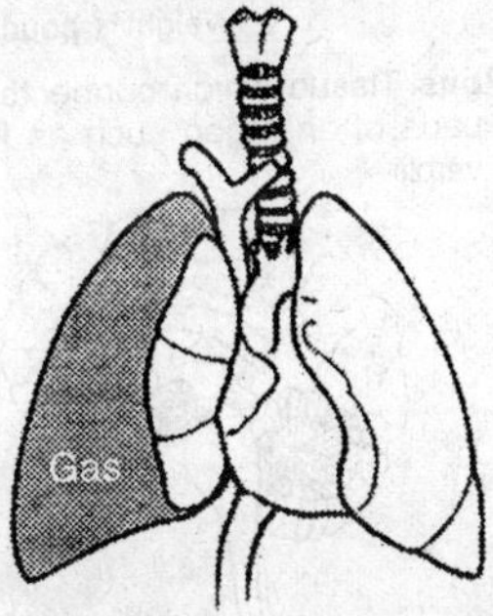

Artificial pneumothorax

Podiatry Art and science that deals with treatment and care of feet disorders.

Poikilocyte Abnormal shaped RBC.

Poison ivy It is a wild plant which secret toxic oil that can cause skin irritation.

Poison oak It is a wild poison plant which secret toxic oil that can cause skin irritation.

Poison Substance that produces injury or death of an organ of the body.

Polarisation Referring to light, a condition in which the vibrations take place in one plane,

Polarisation reduces glare in glasses and mirrors.

Poliomyelitis Acute viral infection that cause lameness, paralysis or death,

Infantile paralysis.

Poliosis Full discolouration of hair giving rise to white royal hair style.

Polyposis Presence of multiple polyp in intestine.

Political socialisation Individuals are initiated into the dominant values and traditions of a society.

Politzer bag Rubber bag used in ENT to inflate middle ear.

Pollen Andresium or male cell of plants which are disbursed to air for pollination through air,

Pollen grains are sometimes are allergic and produce allergy in person who comes in contact with this.

Pollution Spoiling of natural resources by noxious or dangerous contaminants, Common types of pollutions are:

- Air pollution

- Water pollution.
- Noise pollution.
- Soil pollution.
- Atmosphere pollution.

Polyandry Woman having many husbands or married to many men

Polyarteritis nodosa Smallvessels inflammation showing segmental necrosis

Polyarthritis Inflammation of many joints at the same time, Rheumatoid arthritis

Polyclinic Clinic run by physician or doctor of medicine which manages all variety of illness

Polycystic kidney Some people are born with kidneys in which there are little lakes of fluid called cysts. These cysts take up space that should be occupied by normal kidney tissue. If cysts are infected they further reduce healthy kidney tissue

Polycystic An organ that contains many cysts such as polycystic kidney

Polycythaemia Increased number of RBC in the blood which is called Erythrocythaemia

High RBC count in certain pathological conditions

Polydactylism More than 5 fingers or 5 toes in an individual

Polydipsia Common symptom of diabetes - excess thirst

Polygamy a Tribal culture which allow many wives

Polymer A synthetic material which is made up of many molecules

Polymorphous Attributed to many forms of a condition,

Occurring in many forms by lower animals

Polyopia Multiple vision in an individual

Polyp Abnormal growth from a mucous membrane, usually not malignant

Mucous membrane tumour of mucous membrane which has a peduncle

Polysaccharide Carbohydrate containing more than 4 molecules of simple carbohydrates combined with each other,

Examples are:

a. Dextrin b. Starch
c. Glycogen d. Cellulose
e. Gum f. Inulin
g. Pectose

Polyserositis Inflammation of all serous cavities like Pleura, abdomen and pericardium

Polymorphonuclear A cell which has many nuclei of different shapes such as polymorphonuclear leucocytes

Polyneuritis Many nerves show inflammation at a given point of time

Ponderal index It is the tool for measuring obesity and also a good anthropometric measurement,

$$\text{Ponderal index} = \frac{\text{Height (inches)}}{\text{Weight}^3 \text{ (pounds)}}$$

Pons Tissue which connects two parts of an organ such as Pons varolii

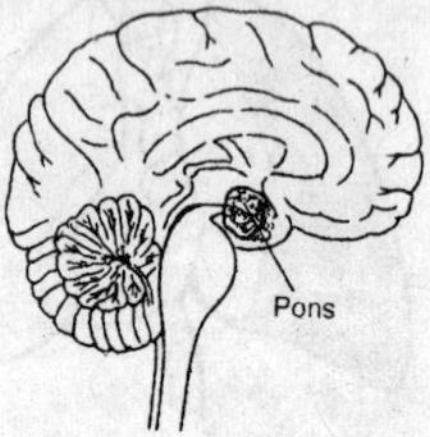

Brain section to show Pons

POP Abbreviation for Progestogen Only Pill,
Women who use progestogen only pill swallow a pill everyday to prevent pregnancy. POP contain very small amounts of only progestin (1/10th of dose of combined pill), they are best for breastfeeding women. They do not reduce milk production

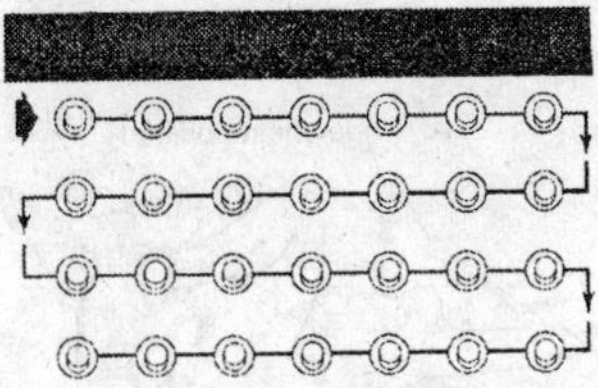

P O P Pill

Popliteal Posterior part of knee.

Popular culture The mass features of the media in postmodern societies.

Population dynamics Population dynamics is the study of mode of change of population and the factors responsible for such changes.

Population explosion It is meaning over population and its effect in human living condition, Major effects are poor national development, unemployment illiteracy, poor housing, non-availability of health care facility poor environment sanitation, fast growth of slums and shanty town
Fast doubling of population in the world occurring as under:

- In 130 years II billion population added in the world (1930).
- In 30 years III billion population added in the world (1960).
- In 15 years IV billion population added in the world ((1974).
- In 12 years V billion population added in the world (1987).
- In 12 years VI billion population added in the world (1999).

Since then every year 92,543,000 population added to the world.

Population Number of people in a country, State or District or village, This can be a group from which a sample is drawn for the study Specific trait holding group.

Pores enlarged This represents the opening of a special type of hair follicle, the sebaceous follicle which has fine and invisible hair.

Pornography Sex stimulating literature of photos.

Porphyria It is an inborn error of metabolism,
Porphyrin metabolism is deranged resulting porphyrinuria,
Types (1) Hepatic
(2) Erythropoietic.

Porphyrin Is a pigment which help in the production of the haem portion of haemoglobin.

Portable wound drainage system Nursing care is a requisite in case of patient who has postsurgical indwelling drain that connects to a portable vacuum container.
Inspection of the tubing, emptying at every shift and vacuum container to be pinned to the bed are underlined.

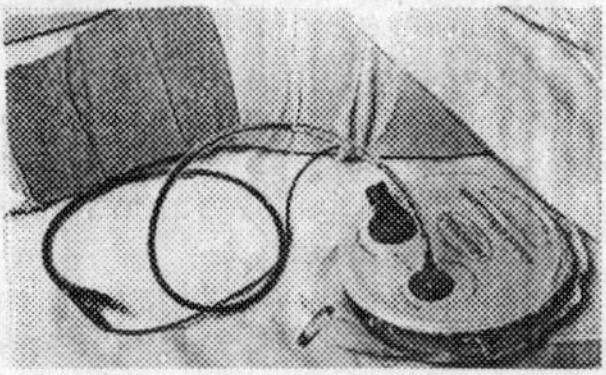

Portable wound drainage system

Portal system It refers to portal vein and its branches which drain to inferior vena cava.

Portal vein This vein is formed from superior mesenteric vein, inferior mesenteric vein, splenic vein, gastric vein, cystic veins.

Portfolio Described achievement relevant to professional practice, Description of professional development.

POSDCORB Gulick has indicated the component function or activities involved in administration through an acronym "POSDCORB"

Meaning of POSDCORB is as under:

Planning the things that need to be done.

Organising the formal structure of the agency.

Staffing the agency.

Directing the work of the agency and making decisions relating there to.

Coordinating all staff activities.

Reporting to the executive and through him to those to whom he is responsible.

Budgeting and all other aspects of fiscal management and control.

Position Usually refers to posture of a man or a woman,

Common positions in nursing practice are:

- Knee chest: Body weight is put on knee and chest and the head is rested on hands.
- Lithotomy: Weight of the body on the back, legs flexed on to the thigh, thighs flexed on to the belly but abducted.
- Sim's: Body weight is on to the left side of the body, right knee and thigh drawn up, left arm is along the back.
- Trendelenburg : Body weight is on the back but inclined at 45 degrees, legs and feet hanging over the end of thetable.

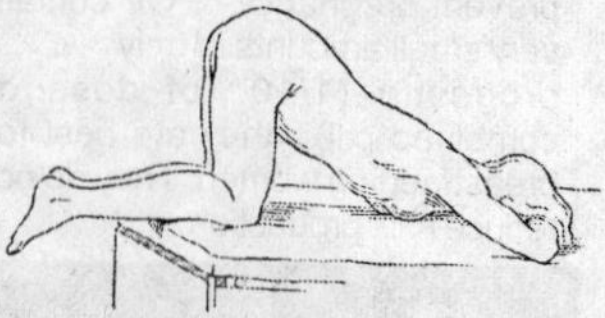

A: Knee chest position

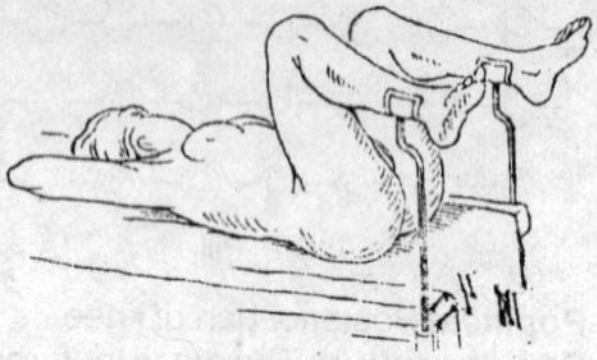

B: Lithotome position

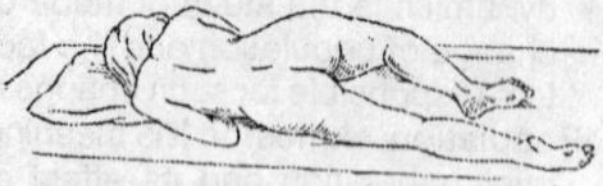

C: Sim's position

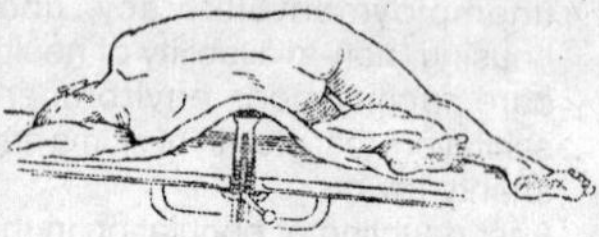

D: Trendelenburg position

Positioning Careful planned positioning is important to prevent the complications of prolonged bed rest. Advantages of positioning are:

- Pressure on bony prominences are reduced.
- Correct body alignment is maintained.
- Stress and strain to joint is reduced.
- Helps in proper breathing with lung expansion.
- Prevents contractures.

Common positioning that are mainly attended by the duty nurse are:

- Supine positioning for lower body.
- Supine positioning for upper body.
- Simi-Fowler's position with 30^0 head elevation.
- Side lying positioning.
- Prone positioning.

Positioning aids To prevent abnormal movements of parts of the body positioning aids are given, they are:

- Trochanter rolls.
- Sand bags.
- Foot supports.
- Hand rolls.

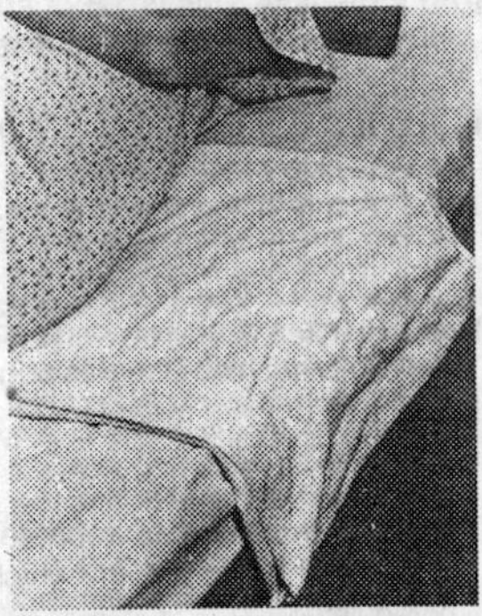

Trochanter roll is being started at bed

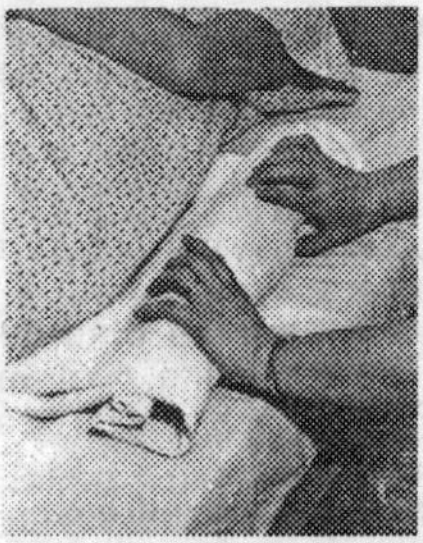

Trochanter roll ready to tuck against patients hip

Positive That which exists,
Value move than zero,
A test showing the evidence of presence of disease.

Posseting Infant's regurgitation after breastfeed.

Postcoital contraceptive They are recommended within 48 hours of unprotected intercourse.
Common ones are:

- IUD Copper T is inserted if acceptable.
- Double the dose of standard combined pill namely 2 tablets of oral contraceptives immediately followed by another 2 pill 12 hours later.
- As emergency contraception 4 tablets of pills containing 30 mg.oestrogen, at one time itself – is given.

Postexposure prophylaxis Preventive steps taken for a person who is exposed to an infection,
Vaccine, chemotherapeutic agent, antibiotics given after exposure to an infection,
Action in HIV infection or Rabies exposure by a man.

Postganglionic Which is distal to a ganglion, refers to autonomic nervous system.

Posttransfusion syndrome Some of the clinical manifestations that follow blood transfusion,
They are:
- Fever.
- Splenomegaly.
- Lymphocytosis which not typical in nature.

Posttraumatic stress disorder Person experiencing disorder following injury, rape, natural disaster or an accident.

Postconsussional syndrome Postinjury insomnia in a patient.

Posterior Behind or dorsal in an anatomical position.

Posthumous Event occurring after the death of a person such as posthumous birth, posthumous honouring.

Postmature Refers to the period that comes after the expected date of confinement,
Prolonged labour.

Postmortem Refers to the condition of time after death of a person such as Postmortem examination.

Postnatal This is the period after child birth,
Common terminologies in nursing practice are:
- Postnatal advice.
- Postnatal care.
- Postnatal clinic.
- Postnatal mortality.

Postpartum technique Mother is assessed for the following:
- Palpating the fundus for location and tone.
- Palpating the bladder.
- Evaluation for Lochia for amount. character and odour.
- Examination of the perineum in Sim's position for healing stage, presence of oedema, bruising, dehiscence, infection, haemorrhoids.
- Inspection of breast.
- Palpation of breast (areolae, nippies, engorgement).

Mother is assisted for baby feeding;
- Positioning the infant by cradle hold method by football hold method.
  by side lying method.
- Help to burp the infant after feeding.
- If needed manual expression of breast milk .
- If needed how to use breast pumps.

Postpartum That which occurs after delivery.

Postprandial After the food, after the meal such as PPBS test.

Postural Related with posture such as postural drainage.

Potable Refers to water which is fit for human consumption.

Potency Male sexual strength for effective intercourse
Usefulness of vaccine to produce immunity.

Pott's disease This is TB of spine described by Dr.Pott a British Surgeon during 1750.

Potts fracture It is fracture dislocation of ankle which include
- Fracture of lower end of tibia.
- Displacement of talus.
- Fracture of medial malleolus.

Pouch It refers to a cavity or a pocket like cavity such as Douglas pouch.

Pouches They are meant for
a) faecal collection.
b) urine collection.
Drainage pouch is appropriate for patients who has ostomy which is unregulated
Postoperative disposable pouches are available.

Poultice Traditional method of applying heat which has limited value in treatment, some of the traditional poultice are:

- Ragi flour in oil heated.
- Lard heated mixed with cereal.
- Mullein leaves boiled in vinegar in flour.
- Catnip in oil and cereal flour.
- Ground worms simmered in lard and flour.

Latin origin meaning a soft, moist, pultaceous mass applied hot to the surface of a part for the purpose of supplying heat and moisture.

Poupart's ligament This is the Inguinal ligament described by Dr.Poupart French Anatomist, Lower border of the external oblique muscle of the abdominal wall from anterior iliac spine to os pubis.

Poverty cycle Explanation of how poverty is transmitted from generation to generation.

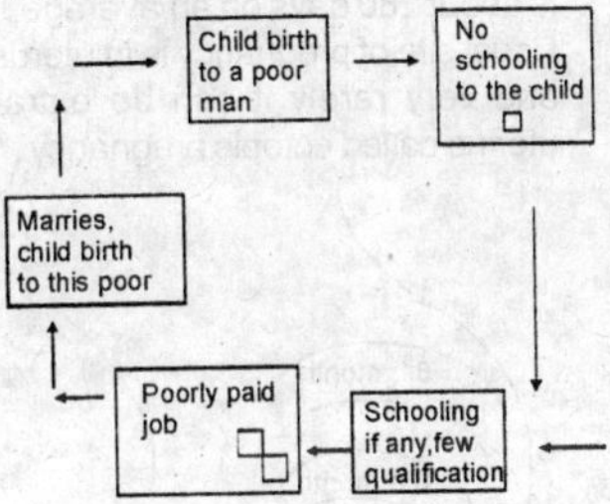

Poverty cycle

Pox Name given eruptive diseases such as:

- Smallpox.
- Chickenpox.
- Monkeypox.
- Greatpox (syphilis).

PPBS Abbreviation for Planning – Programming – Budgeting System This technique helps nursing service administrators to take decision to allocate resources so that the resources are used in an effective way.

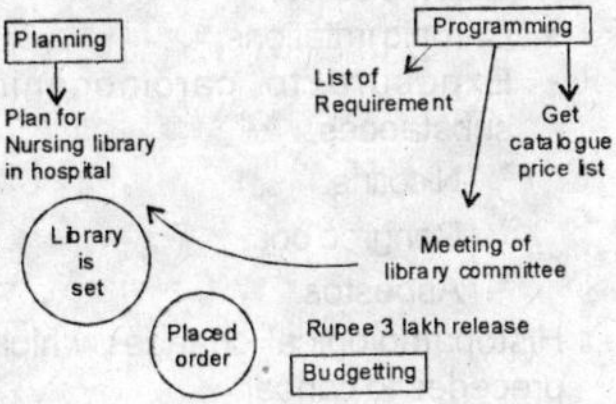

PPBS for a nursing library

PPC Abbreviation for Post Partum Programme.
It is a maternity centered FP approach started in the year 1969 It is coordinated in OBG department of a Medical college and in the District Hospitals.

PPH Abbreviation for Post Partal Haemorrhage.

Practioner A person who practices a profession such as a nurse practice the Nursing profession.

Pre-eclampsia Clinical condition peculiar to pregnancy which occur during II trimester and manifest with following clinical manifestations:

- Albuminuria.
- Hypertension.
- Paedal oedema.

Premarital examination It is now called 'marriage counselling' a method of excluding some of the diseases that are known to run in families by heritance, Others are metabolic diseases, HIV, VD, etc.

Precancerous Certain conditions that are found developing to malignant stage

They are:

- Chronic sores.
- Chronic irritations.
- Exposure to carcinogenic substances.
  - * Nicotine.
  - * Congroo pot.
  - * Asbestos.

Histopathological changes which precedes to cancer.

Preceptor One who works under a senior person to become matured professional person by undergoing training.

Precipitate Solid matter appearance in the liquid by a chemical reaction.

Precipitate labour Sudden expulsion of baby by quick delivery which is rapid than expectation, This is related with child trauma and perineal lacerations.

Precocious Physical or mental development developed well in advance in a child such as precocious puberty.

Precordium Anatomical area in front of heart on the chest

Predisposition One who is disposed to illness, susceptible to illness.

Prednisolone Synthetic corticosteroid, its common uses are:

1. Asthma.
2. Allergic disorders.
3. Dermatitis of allergic in origin.
4. Inflammations of acute nature.
5. Rheumatic condition which is acute in nature.

Pre-exposure prophylaxis 3 doses of ARV vaccine given on 0, 7, and 28 days to prevent rabies exposure of a risk person, each 1.0 ml through IM .

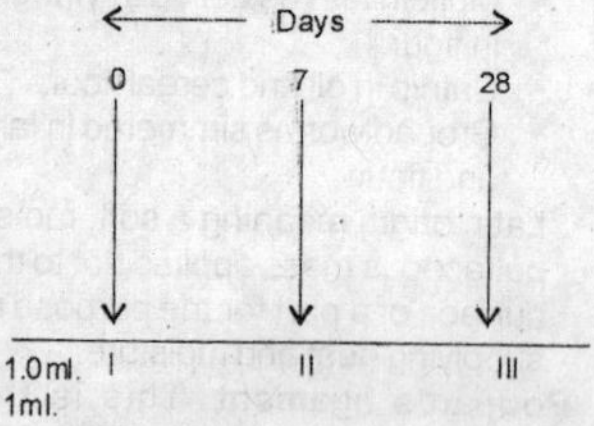

Pre-exposure prophylaxis (Rabies)

Pregnancy test By assessing the urine of pregnant woman for chorionic gonadotrophin one can diagnose pregnancy.

Pregnancy It starts with conception and implantation of fertilised ovum to normal or assisted delivery, This is about 280 days on an average, Usual site of pregnancy is in uterus and very rarely it can be extra-uterine called ectopic pregnancy.

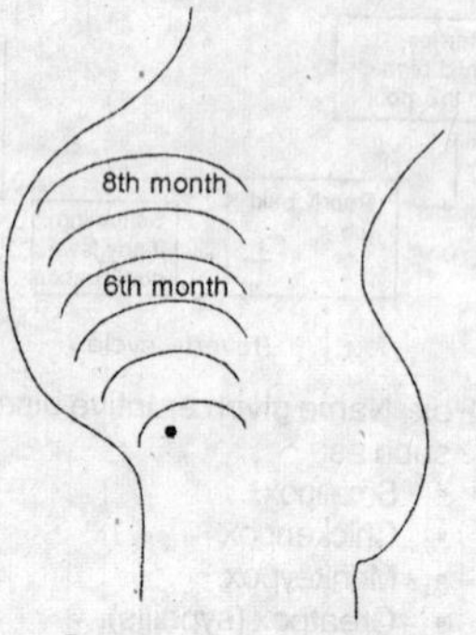

Pregnancy – uterus level

Pregnancy weight gain

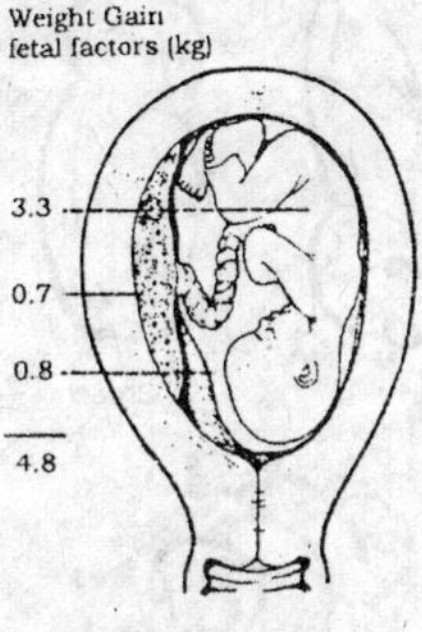

A: Weight gain (Foetal)

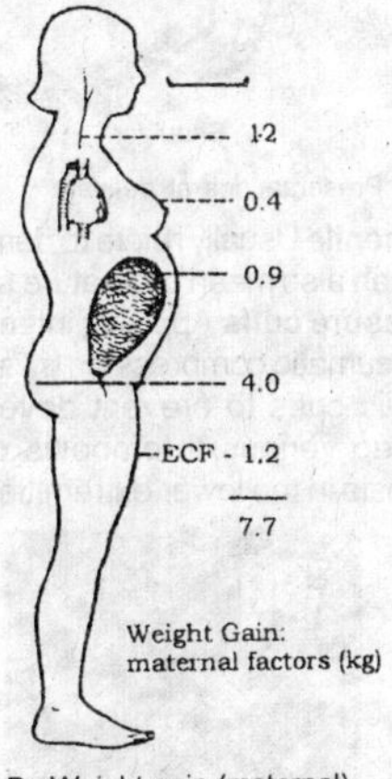

B: Weight gain (maternal)

Premature ejaculation Seminal ejaculation occurring in very early part of sex act and well before climax.

Premature infant Newborn with birth weight of less than 2.5 Kg or born before the completion of 37 weeks of gestation

Premature Occurrence of a biological event well before the expected time,

Common nursing terminologies used are:

I. Premature baby.
II. Premature ejaculation.
III. Premature contraction of heart.
IV. Premature delivery.

Premedication Drug administered well before surgery to alleviate anxiety and to facilitate induction of anaesthesia.

Premenstrual Anything before menses such as premenstrual tension.

Premolar Teeth in front of molar which are bicuspid in nature.

Premonition When a person gets the feeling of future impending event

Prenatal technique Following assessments are done during ANC; (by duty nurse)

- Fundal height is measures to calculate gestational age by using McDonald's Rule (refer McDonald's rule).
- Perform Leopold's maneuvers (refer Leopold's Maneuvers) to palpate foetal parts.
- Auscultate foetal heart sound by foetoscope.
- Auscultate foetal heart if ultrasonic (Doppler) is available.
- If there is leg cramps, apply counter pressure by pressing upper planter upwards.
- If there is back pain, apply pressure from central line of midline on the back at lumbar area
- If there is suspicion of rupture of membrane, nurse can do Nitrazine tape test to test for amniotic fluid.

Amniotic fluid is alkaline at a 7.2 pH and the darker the test strip, the more likely it is that the membranes have ruptured

Prenatal Period before birth of the child which is called antenatal period.

Prepuce Loose skin which covers the glans penis.

Presbycusis Old age deafness which progresses to bilateral deafness.

Presbyopia Farsightedness in old age which is called chalisha which is due to loss of elasticity and reduced accommodation of the lens.

Presbyopic Reference to presbyopic.

Prescription Doctor's slip containing the drug advised for therapy, dose,duration, also indicating the mode of administration,

Nurse's slip containing the required medicamentation for therapy,

Prescription for drug is given by a registered medical practitioner or by registered nurse.

Presentation This describes the part of foetus that appears in the centre of the neck of uterus at delivery or before delivery.

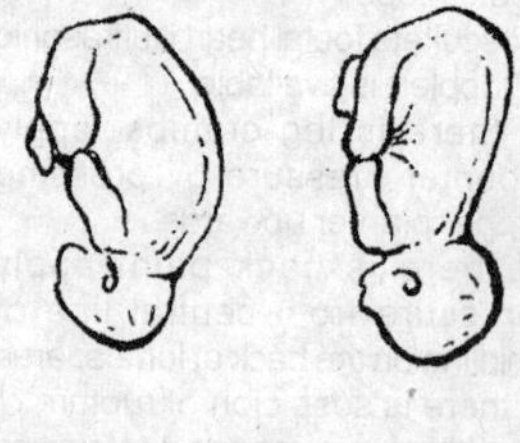

Vertex Brow

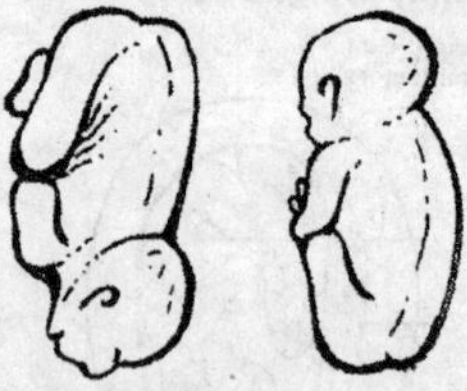

Face Breech

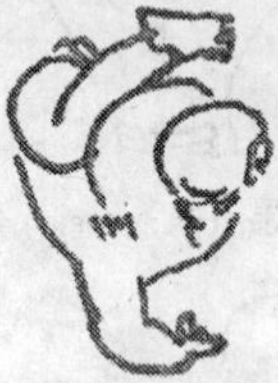

Shoulder

Presentations at delivery

Presenile Usually refers to dementia, It can also mean premature senility.

Pressure cuffs Applying intermittent pneumatic compression by antiembolic cuffs to prevent developing deep venous thrombosis due to stasis in the lower extremities.

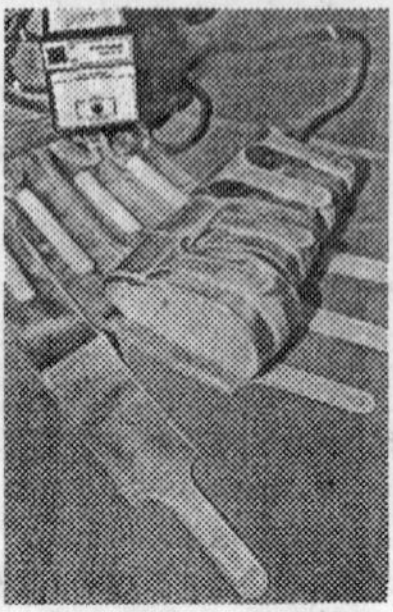

Pressure cuffs

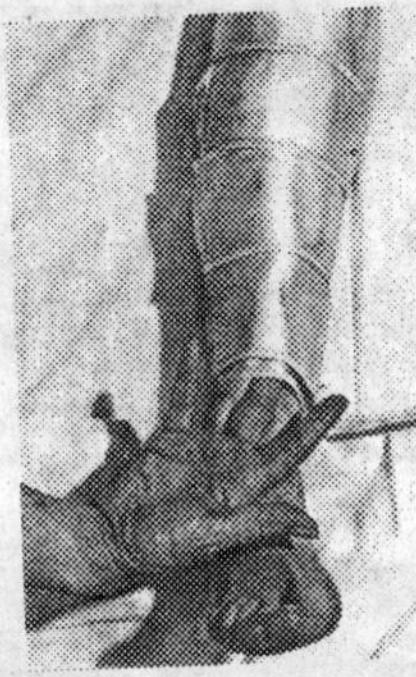

Pressure cuffs with attached straps

Pressure points Points which are susceptible for bedsore in a chronic patient,
Point at which pressure arrests the bleeding.

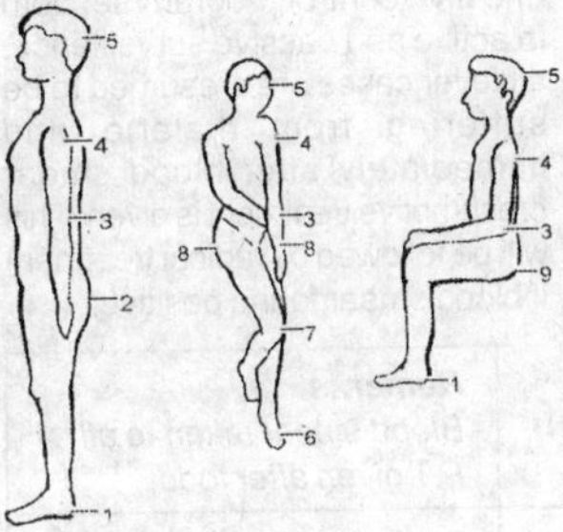

Pressure points

1. Heel
2. Buttock
3. Elbow
4. Shoulder
5. Head
6. Feet
7. Knee
8. Hip
9. Sacrum

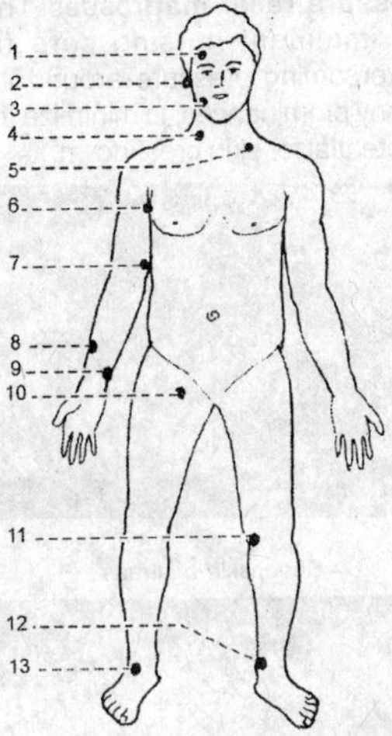

Arterial pressure points

1. Temporal
2. Occipital
3. Facial
4. Carotid
5. Subclavian
6. Axillary
7. Brachial
8. Radial
9. Ulnar
10. Femoral
11. Popliteal
12. Dorsalis pedis
13. Posterior tibial

Pressure point In the treatment of haemorrhage, pressure points are found in sites where artery is superficial and lies over a bone such as:

- Brachial artery.
- Ulnar artery.
- Radial artery.
- Femoral artery.
- Subclavian artery.
- Carotid artery.
- Temporal artery.
- Popliteal artery.

Pressure relief mattresses This is imminent nursing care for overcoming pressure around the bony prominences, to minimize the potential for skin breakdown.

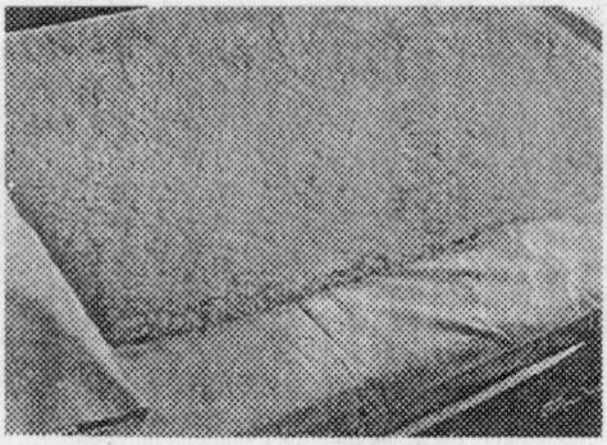

Sheepskin mattress

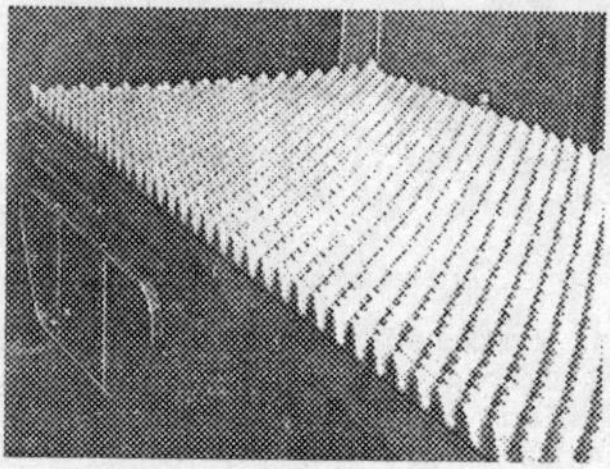

Egg crate mattress

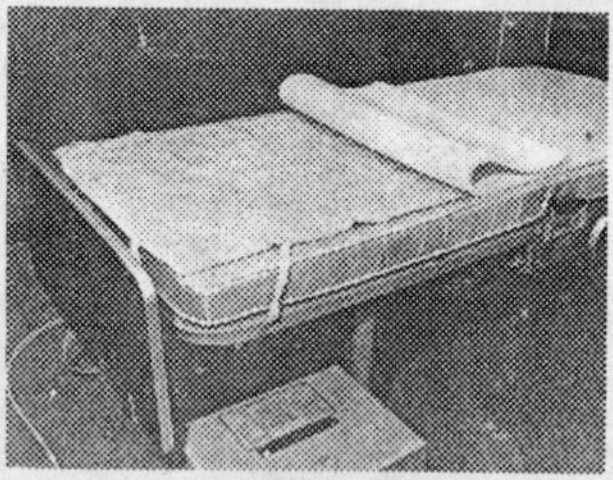

Air locked mattress

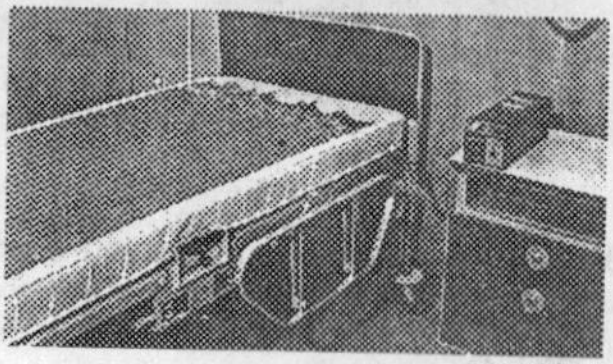

Air float system adopted mattress

Presumptive treatment In malaria effective control programme, both in active and passive surveillance, all fever cases are presumed to be suffering from malaria and immediately after blood smear presumptive treatment is given. This will be followed by radical treatment if blood smear found positive.

Age	***Chloroquine***	***Remarks***
Below 1 year	*75 mg. (half tablet)*	*Blood smear taken to all P T given after food*
1 – 4 years	150 mg. (1 tablet)	- do -
4 – 8 years	300 mg. (2 tablets)	- do -
8 – 14 years	450 mg. (3 tablets)	- do -
Above 14 years	600 mg. (4 tablets)	- do -

Table: Presumptive treatment of malaria with chloroquine in low risk area

Age	Chloroquine (mg) Day I	Day II	Day III	Primaquine (mg) Day I	Remarks
Below 1 year	75	75	37.5	-	Blood smear taken PTgiven after food No primaquine for Pregnant and infant
1-4 years	150	150	75	7.5	- do -
4-8 years	300	300	150	15	- do -
8-14 years	450	450	225	30	- do -
Above 14 years	600	600	300	45	- do -

Table: Presumptive treatment with chloroquine and primaquine in high risk area

In case of chloroquine resistant cases (adult dose)

Amodiaquine	600 mg
OR	
Sulphaline	1000 mg
Pyrimethamine	50 mg

Presystole This is the period just before systole in a cardiac cycle.

Preterm Age of the growing foetus in uterus which is less than 37 weeks of pregnancy.

Prevalence This is for available cases or available events at a given point of time,
Prevailing status of illness in the community.

Preventive medicine Discipline that deals with steps that are taken to see that diseases do not occur medicine applied before the occurrence of illnesses.

Priapism Erection of penis which is always present irrespective of sex stimuli which could be due to spinal cord injury.

Prickly heat Other wise called heat rash in the form of skin eruption or red spots on the body which is exposed to hot sun.

Primaquine This drug is used along with chloroquine for the treatment of benign malaria.

Primary care First contact care given by health workers at sub centre and PHC,
Initial care or first contact care given by health workers outside health institutions.

Primary health care It is " Essential health care based on practical, scientifically sound and socially acceptable methods and technology made universally accessible to individuals and families in the community through their full participation and at a cost that the community can afford to maintain at every stage of their development in the spirit of self-determination"

Primary health centre P.H.C is an outcome of Bhore Committee Report. PHC provides integrated health services. We have about 23000 PHC in the country, it covers a population of about 30000 and has about 6 **S**ub **C**entres under it

Following is the staff pattern:

- MOH.
- Pharmacist.
- Nurse midwife.
- Health worker female.
- Health worker male.
- BEE.
- Health assistant male.
- Health assistant female.
- UDC.
- LDC.
- Lab technician.
- Driver.
- Class IV employees

Following are functions of PHC:

- Medical care.
- RCH services.
- Family welfare planning.
- Water supply and Sanitation.
- CCD.
- Collection of vital statistics.
- Health education.
- Carry out National Health Programmes.
- Referral service.
- Training of health assistants, health workers, health guides and local dais.
- Basic lab services.

PHC is equipped with the following services:

- Tubectomy.
- Vasectomy.
- MTP.
- Minor O T procedures.

Prime movers This is one of the task performed by the muscle. Prime Movers are muscles which play the major part in moving the joint. Other types of muscles which help prime movers are muscles of fixation and synergists.

Example:

In golf play :

- Powerful swing is by prime movers.
- Stance is by muscles of fixation.
- Guiding the direction is by synergists.

Primigravida First pregnancy of a woman in her married life.

Primipara First delivery with live birth by a woman in her life.

Probability This describes the chance of occurrence of an event or of a character, this is expressed as 'P' which can be 1 in 20; 1 in 100 ; 1 in 1000 etc., (in other words P=0.05; P=0.01; P=0.001).

Probenecid Drug used for excretion of uric acid in gout.

Procaine Is a local anaesthetic, commonly used with Penicillin.

Process Outgrowth of a part is called process,

Systematic nursing care is called Nursing process.

Procidentia This refers to prolapse of uterus,

Proctalgia Pain in the rectum, One of the symptom of haemorrhoids.

Proctitis Infection and inflammation of rectum.

Proctoscope An electrically lighted instrument by which the larger bowel can be examined and treatment can be performed, Instrument to examine rectum.

Prodromal Related with Prodrome

Prodrome Premonitory symptom or early manifestations before the true symptoms of an illness appear.

Profession People who have procured skills and higher knowledge to function autonomously and are committed to higher standards of conduct and service to the community.

Profile Outline of an organ, side view of head, representation of characters through tests, records of achievement of a person.

Progeny Succeeding generation or offspring of parents, Discendants.

ProgesteroneThe hormone that regulates menses and pregnancy, It is secreted by corpus luteum.

Progestogen Steroid hormone similar to progesterone.

Prognathism Protruded and enlarged jaws.

Prognosis Forecasting the probable future course of a disease or of an operation,

It is expressed either as good or bad Survival rate after surgery of treatment for 5 years or 10 years prediction is also done under prognosis.

Proguanil Antimalarial drug used as chemoprophylaxis.

Prolactin Hormone of the anterior pituitary gland which stimulates mammary gland.

Prolapse Downward displacement of a part or of an organ such as prolapse of uterus, prolapse of rectum.

Proliferation Rapid multiplication of cells seen in primary union or in cancer.

Prolongation of life It is increasing life expectation and is the hall mark of professional ethics. One of the goal of medical treatment is prolongation of life.

Prominence It refers to a projection on a bone.

Pronation Opposite of supination where the hand is turned downwards.

Prophylactic That which is related with prophylaxis, an agent or a drug used in prevention of illness.

Proprioceptor They are present in the following organs; Movements are perceived by these sensory end organs:

- Labyrinth.
- Joint capsule.
- Tendon.
- Muscle.

Proprioceptive neuromuscular facilitation exercises This is an alternative to ROM exercises. This has advantage that they combine movements at several joints simultaneously thereby reducing the amount of time necessary to complete the series.

This in positioning and mobilisation.

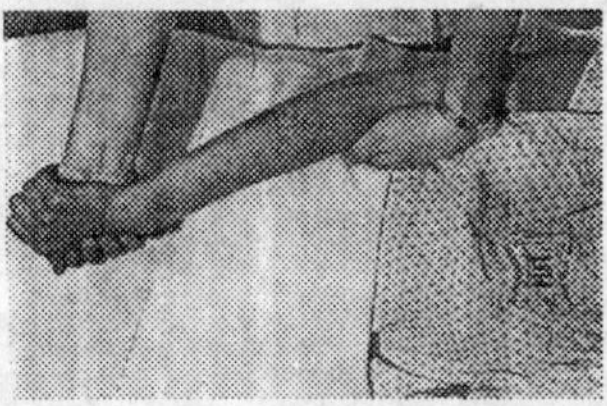

Diagonal movement of upper limb for proprioceptive neuromuscular facilitation exercise

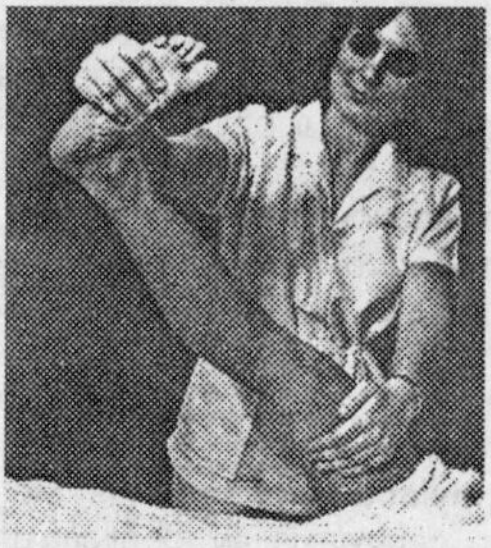
Diagonal movement of lower limb for Proprioceptive neuromuscular facilitation exercise

Proptosis Projected eyeball which gives a fierce look, exophthalmus.

Prostaglandin They are fatty acids present in semen, brain, lung, uterus and can produce cardiac, gastric and respiratory effects,
They are metabolites of arachidonic acid and are unsaturated fatty acids, Four types of prostaglandin known are: (preparation of the prostate glands of bullocks)
- Prostaglandin D_2
- Prostaglandin E_2
- Prostaglandin F_2
- Prostaglandin I_2

Prostate It is a gland surrounding urethra , prostatic secretion is mixed with semen during ejaculation:

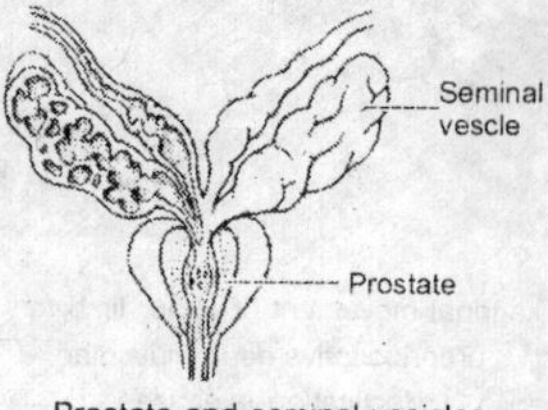

Prostate and seminal vesicles

Prostate Gland which surrounds the bladder opening in the male, Commonly it is mispronounced and miscalled as prostate.

Prosthodontics The discipline in dentistry which applies science to find the mode for special appliances to compensate for oral malformations.

Prostitution It is one of the oldest known social evils very much commonly seen in broken homes, illegitimate love making, easy money as sex worker and poverty.

Prostration It is a state of severe exhaustion.

Protease This helps in metabolism of protein and it is a proteolytic enzyme.

Protein One of the major proximate principle, made up of complex organic nitrogenous compounds from amino acids,
In nursing practice, following terminologies are seen:
- Reference protein.
- Bence Jones protein.
- First class protein.
- Second class protein.

Proteinase Enzyme which helps in the breakdown of protein in digestive process.

Protein Main item under proximate principles in food,
Contains nitrogen essential for body growth and maintenance
Sources are:
- Pulses.
- Meat.
- Fish.
- Egg.
- Poultry.
- Cheese.
- Leguminous vegetables.

Proteinuria Presence of high quantity of proteins in the urine.

Proteolytic That which promote proteolysis, refers to proteolytic enzyme.

Proteus Genus of Gram-negative bacteria commonly found in infected wound and urinary tract infections.

Prothrombin It is the precursor of thrombin present in plasma.

Proton It is an atom which is positively charged particle.

Protoplasm It is living matter of cells and tissues which is an essential chemical compound.

Protozoa Unicellular organism which itself is a Phylum,

Entamoeba and Plasmodium are common protozoal parasites of man.

Protuberance A round projecting part of an organ such as occipital protuberance.

Provitamin They are precursors of vitamins such as:

- Provitamin A is carotene.
- Provitamin D is ergosterol.

Proximal Opposite of distal, nearest to central point anatomically.

Prudent diet This is the diet developed by National Nutrition and Food Policy to achieve high level health. It is called prudent diet if the following criteria are adopted in a diet:

a) Fat intake below 20 to 30% of total calories.
b) Saturated fat below 10% of total calories.
c) Carbohydrate should contain high fibre.
d) Fats, alcohol restricted.
e) Salt below 5 grams per day.
f) Protein below 15 to 20 % of daily intake.
g) Junk foods avoided (ketchup, cola).

Prurigo Skin lesions with popular eruptions, A chronic skin condition.

Pruritus Localised or generalised itching which is intolerable.

Prussic acid Among less common poisons in clinical practice, Prussic acid is also one that is consumed which produces excitability, confusion and convulsion,

Emetic, artificial respiration and early transportation to the hospital saves the patient.

Pseudocrisis Symptoms of acute exacerbation occurs during the course of a disease which mimic true crisis.

Pseudocyesis Presence of all symptoms of pregnancy without pregnancy in a woman, psychological origin in nature.

Pseudogynaecomastia Fat tissue deposit in male giving appearance of enlarged breast.

Pseudohypertrophic The enlargement perceived is only false and not true.

Pseudomonas Gramnegative bacilli which is found in pus and in UTI.

Psittacosis 'Parrot fever', a disease caused by virus, transmitted by parrots or related birds

Paratyphoid like disease caused by *Chlamydia psittaci* in parrots that spreads to human beings.

Psoas It is the flexor of the hip joint which arises from spine (lumbar) and gets inserted to lesser trochanters of the femur.

psoralen They are prepared from plants which are used in psoriasis and vitiligo, It is obtained also from see weed.

Psoriasis A chronic skin disease which disfigures the person,
Reddish marginated patch with silvery scaling on extensor surfaces,
Seems to be familial skin disease which is chronic and recurrent in nature.

Psyche This refers to both conscious and unconscious mind.

Psychiatrist A consultant in psychiatry who treats mental illnesses
Doctor of medicine who has an advanced training in the diagnosis treatment and management of mental disturbances and emotional disturbances such as:

- Psychosis.
- Neurosis.
- Psychoneurosis.
- Paranoid syndromes.
- Personality disorders.

Psychiatry A discipline which covers the area of advanced tool to treat and manage diseases of mind and problems of emotional character
Medical science which studies the diagnosis, treatment and prevention of mental illnesses.

Psychoanalysis It is a branch of psychiatry which involves prolonged exploration of the patient's personality,
A study of free association, interpretation and dream analysis developed by Dr.Sigmund Freud.

Psychoanalyst A specialist who does psychoanalysis.

Psychogenic Diseases that are psychogenic in origin.

Psychologist A trained person who is not a medical doctor but has studied Human behaviour in depth and Psychology,
One who studies normal and abnormal mental processes, mental development and mental behaviour.

Psychology It is a science in medical field as medicine allied subject that deals with the study of mind and mental process.

Psychomotor That which affects motor activity or muscular activity in the body.

Psychoneurosis One of the type of psychiatric illness where mental response is abnormal to a normal stimulus as in the cases of hysteria, Obsessive compulsive neurosis.

Psychopath Mentally disturbed antisocial personality.

Psychopathology It deals with cause of mental illness and the processes of mental illness.

Psycho pharmacology Study of drugs which has effect on mind and how it acts.

Psychosis It is one of the specific mental illness,
A major mental disorder of emotional origin and show the following features:

- Personality disorders.
- Delusion.
- Hallucination.
- Illusion.

Psychosomatic Psycho = emotional, Soma = physical or bodily disease in which mental or emotional aspect influences the physical changes in the body (either produce or aggravate),
Examples are:

- Asthma.
- Anorexia nervosa.
- Peptic ulcer.

Psychotherapy Treatment of mental illness by drug and behaviour change.

Treatment aimed at helping the patient to solve his psychic problems and his emotional problems.

Psychotrophic Refers to the drugs that has an effect on the mind such as:

- Nervous stimulants.
- Antidepressants.
- Sedatives.
- Tranquillisers.

Pterygium Patch of thickened conjunctiva which extends even to cornea,

It is usually fan-shaped with apex toward the pupil and the base towards the inner canthus,

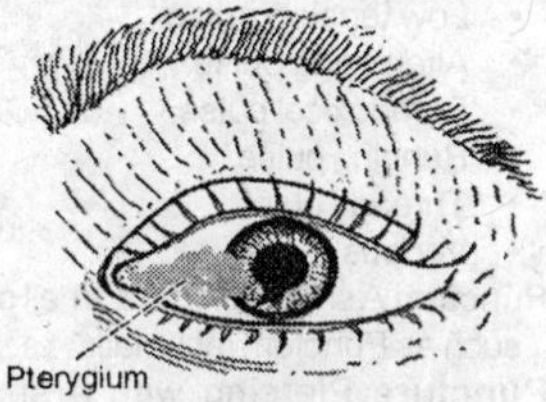

Pterygium

Pterygoid process It is a bony projection of sphenoid bone at the junction of body of sphenoid and greater wing of sphenoid bone.

Ptosis Drooping of eyelid.

Ptyalin It is salivary enzyme, It helps in starch metabolism.

$$\text{Starch} \xrightarrow{\text{Ptyalin}} \text{Maltose}$$

$$\text{Glycogen} \xrightarrow{\text{Ptyalin}} \text{Glucose.}$$

Puberty Time of maturation of sex organs, Development of secondary Sex characteristics in boys and girls (usually 12 to 17 years).

Pubes It refers to public hair growing area.

Pubic That which is related to pubes.

Public health This is the branch of medicine which takes care of physical, mental and social well-being of the community at large. Earlier version of preventive and social medicine is being told as community health for this discipline.

Pubis Anterior part of hip bone called pubic symphysis.

Pudendal block Pudendal nerve block by 1% lignocaine for episiotomy and also for forceps delivery.

Pudendum This refers to the external genitalia of woman.

Puerperal That is related with child birth such as puerperal sepsis.

Puerperium After delivery up to 42 days physiological changes to bring back normal in women is called puerperium.

Pulex It is called human flea, with full name as pulex irritans.

Pulmonary That which is related to lung such as pulmonary infection, pulmonary vain, pulmonary circulation.

Pulp capping Pulp chamber of the tooth is capped to prevent the pulp infection.

Pulp dental It is the inner substance of a tooth including the nerve

Pulp Vegetable tissue or animal tissue which is juicy and liquid in nature, Common nursing terminology that are used are:

- Splenic pulp.
- Digital pulp.
- Pulp cavity of tooth.

Pulsation Anything tissue or organ that throbs or its beating is heard, Such as cardiac pulsation, arterial pulsation.

Pulse deficit When a nurse examines radial pulse and apical pulse simultaneously there may be difference in pulse rate which is called pulse deficit.Peripheral pulse deficit occurs when the cardiac systole is not strong enough to produce a palpable arterial pulse as in case of atrial fibrillation.

Nurse, if finds pulse deficit, she should ask associate nurse to count radial pulse and she shall count apical pulse to confirm the pulse deficit which should be reported to duty doctor.

Pulse immunisation Oral Polio Vaccine is given to all 0 to 5 years children in a country on a single day regardless of previous immunisation. This is maintained as an annual event. Hence the name Pulse.

Pulse pressure It is the difference between systolic blood pressure and diastolic blood pressure, Normal range is between 30 to 50.

Pulse It is the heart beat which can give normalcy or pathological state when properly examined;

Physiological range is:

i. 72 per minute in adults (50 to 90).

ii. Infants 120 to 140.

iii. old age it tends to slow down.

It is local rhythmical expansion of an artery which are palpable,

Pathological alteration in the pulse:

Tachycardia:

a) Fever.

b) Thyroid over function.

c) Haemorrhage.

d) Anaemia.

e) Nervous disorder.

f) Failing heart muscle

g) Drugs like atropine, amyl nitrite.

Bradycardia:

a) Tumour, haemorrhage or injury of cerebrum.

b) Opium.

c) Myxoedema.

d) Convalescence period.

e) Heart block.

f) Jaundice.

Different types of pulse in clinical practice are:

- High tension pulse.
- Low tension pulse.
- Alternating pulse.
- Paradoxical pulse.
- Running pulse.
- Thready pulse.
- Venous pulse.

Punctum A small point or a small spot such as Punctum lacrimalis.

Puncture Piercing with a sharp instrument in surgical procedure, This is commonly done to collect body fluids for laboratory examination

Common such investigations done are:

- Lumbar puncture.
- Sternal puncture.
- Ventricular puncture.
- Cisternal puncture.
- Vene puncture.

Pupil check It means size and shape of pupil are examined. Pupil gauge is used for documenting size.

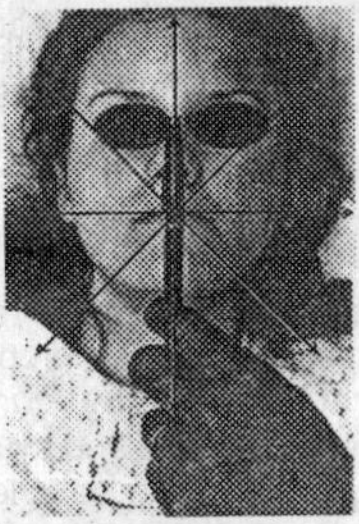

Pupil check

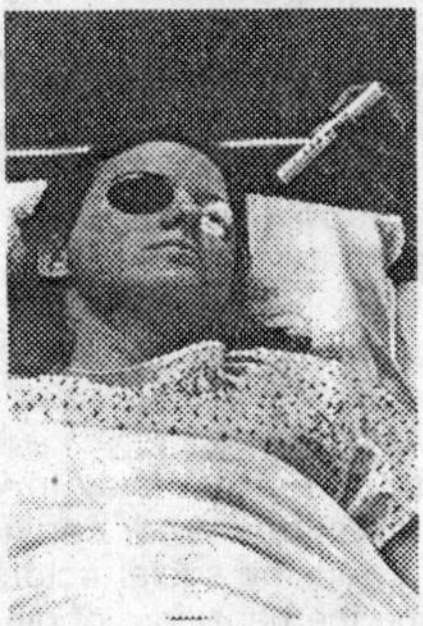

Pupil gauge

Pupil In the black or brown coloured portion of the eye there is an opening called pupil which allows light to enter the eye to produce image, Circular aperture in the centre of the iris through which light passes on to the retina,

Different kinds of pupil in nursing practice are:

- Fixed pupil.
- Artificial pupil.
- Multiple pupil.
- Tonic or slow reacting pupil.
- Argyll Robertson pupil (syphilitic pupil).

Purgative A drug to help passing motion or used as laxative, It is also called aperient drug.

Common purgatives are:

- Bulk purgative or mechanical purgatives eg., Agar, Bran.
- Lubricant purgative eg., Liquid paraffin.
- Irritant purgative eg., cascara, Rhubarb, Castor oil, Senna.

Purin bodies It is protein constituent and the source are red meat and internal glandular organs,

It is known to produce goat.

Purine It is the base for Adenine and Guanine in DNA and RNA.

Purkinje Anatomist and physiologist who described the following and are after his name in anatomy:

- Purkinje fibre (Muscle fibre).
- Purkinje cell (Large neuron).
- Purkinje phenomenon (Pupillary movement).
- Purkinje network (Fibrous network)

Purpura Disease of the blood which causes bleeding under the skin and bleeding in tissues including joints, Extravasations of blood in skin and mucous membranes producing purple spots which may be:

1) Idiopathic or

2) Thrombocytopenic in origin.

Common clinical purpuras seen are:

- Senile purpura.
- Steroid purpura.
- Thrombocytopenic purpura.
- Idiopathic purpura.
- Allergic purpura.
- Anaphylactic purpura.
- Non-thrombocytopenic purpura of Schönlein-Henoch.

Purulent That which contains pus in it such as infected wound, pustule.

Pus This is produced by the infection and inflammation in the tissue,
This contains:
1) Dead WBC 2) Cell debris
3) Tissue fluid, Blue pus is due to Pseudomonas infectin and Yellow pus is due to Staphylococci or Streptococci infection.

Pusher Person who sells illegal narcotic drugs which is punishable by Act.

Pustule Skin eruption which is elevated above the surface of the skin and which contains pus in it, One of the stages in eruptive fevers Commonly it refers to 'pimple' Anthrax pustule is called Malignant pustule.

Putrefaction Animal tissue or plant tissue when gets decomposed by certain micro-organisms it is called putrefaction.

P wave The deflections or waves of the ECG are designated by the letters P, Q, R, S, and T;
Here P wave is associated with atrial excitation.

Pyaemia Pyogenic micro-organisms from a site of infection get into circulation and produce Pyaemia, high fever, rigors and multiple abscesses are characteristics of Pyaemia.

Pyelitis Infection and inflammation of renal pelvis among children, Characterised by urgency, frequency, dysuria and pyuria.

Pyelography Water soluble iodine opaque substance is injected and radiological examination of urinary tract is done as diagnostic purpose.

Pyelolithotomy Surgical operation for excising a renal calculus from the pelvis of the kidney.

Pyelonephritis Infection and inflammation of the body of the kidney.

Pyeloplasty Plastic surgery or reconstructive surgery of renal pelvis.

Pygmalion effect Way in which expectations and consistent behaviour by social actors can shape the behaviour of others in society.

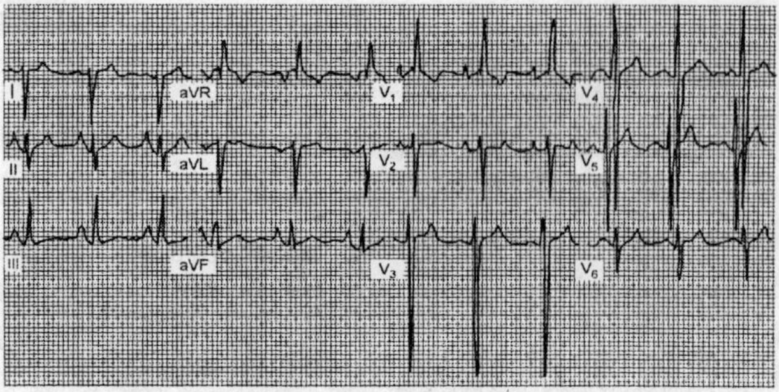

Tall 'P' wave (Right atrial enlargement)

Pygmy It refers to dwarf or to a small person,
Short living being.

Pyloric Pertaining to pylorus such as pyloric stenosis.

Pylorospasm Contraction of the pylorus which delays food movement from stomach.

Pyloroplasty Surgery for pyloric stenosis

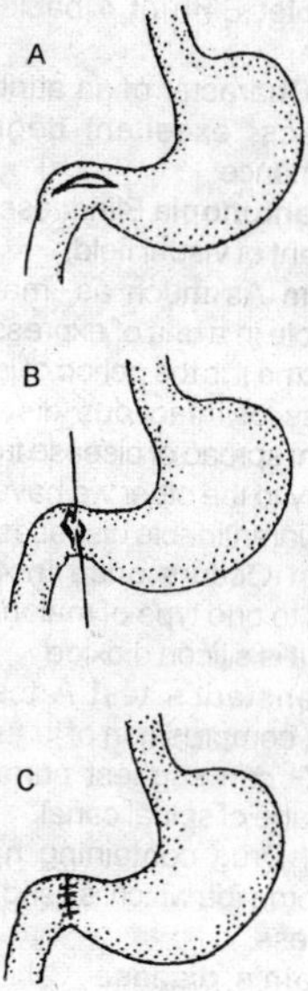

Pyloroplasty

A. Longitudinal incision
B. Pulled pransversely
C. Resutured.

Pylorus This is an opening at the lower end of the stomach which opens to duodenum.

Pyloric sphincter Muscle surrounding the opening at the lower end of the stomach.

Pyoderma Skin disease with pus discharge.

Pyogenic That which produces pus.

Pyorrhoea This refers to the discharge of pus secondary to severe infection.

Pyramidal That which is pyramidal in shape, such as pyramidal cells, pyramidal tract.

Pyrexia Fever or febrile condition from Greek word pyressein meaning to be feverish.

Pyrogen A substance that produce fever in man or in animal.

Pyrrole A chemical substance in the blood which is heterocyclic in nature and is a requirement for haemoglobin synthesis.

Pyrethrum It is from chrysanthemum flower used as space spray insecticide.

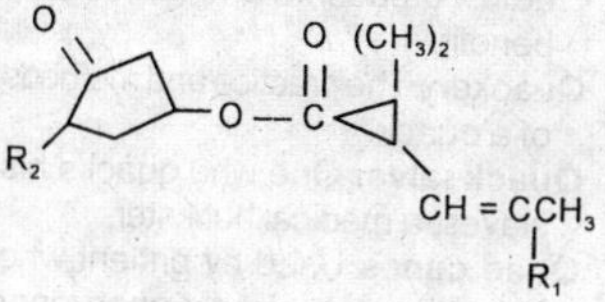

Pyrethrum

Pyruvic acid This is the intermediate product of carbohydrate metabolism and also of fat metabolism, Thiamine regulates the level of pyruvic acid in the blood.

Pyuria Clinical condition where urine contains pus cells, As per definition Pyuria is said if 3 WBC per high power field is present.

Q

Q fever A rickettisal infection caused by *Coxiella burnetti, Rickettsial pneumonia* like infection of cattle.

Q wave of ECG In ECG ' Q 'wave is downward projection, It is prominent in M I.

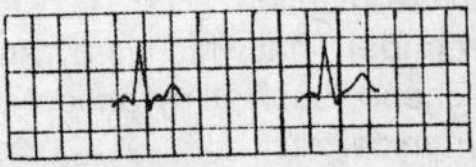

Q wave in ECG

QRS complex Prominent R wave and weak Q and S is routinely seen in ECG, cardiac impulse when passes through ventricle it produces QRS wave.

QT Segment the period of ECG from Q to T in ECG graph.

Quack A person, usually not a physician who pretends to have medical knowledge and experience which he does not possess to defraud patients and for his own benefit.

Quackery The practice and methods of a quack.

Quacksalver One who quacks his slaves, a medical huckster.

Quad canes Used by patient who have the use of only one upper extremity.

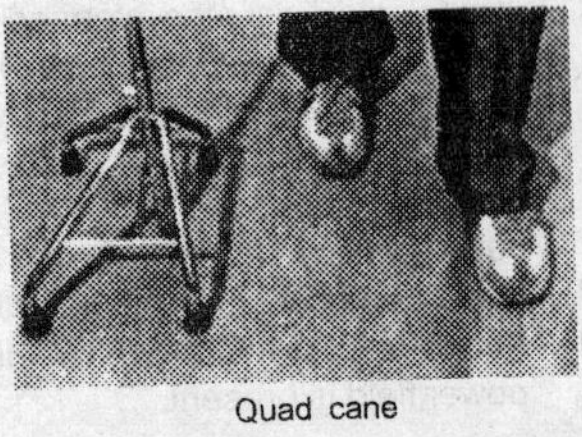

Quad cane

Quadrate lobe Liver lobe on the visceral surface of the liver, lobe of liver towards duodenum.

Quadratus Four-sided muscle of the thigh.

Quadriceps Extensor muscle of the thigh with four heads.

Quadriplegia Paralysis of all four limbs due to various known diseases

Quadruplet Birth of 4 babies to a woman.

Quality Character of an attribute in statistics, excellent degree of performance.

Quandrantonopia Blindness in one quadrant of visual field.

Quantum As much as, maximum available in a unit of expression.

Quarantine It is the period of isolation in case of infectious disease to prevent spread of disease from one country to the other we have specified quarantinable diseases.

Quartan Occurs once in 4 days, refers to one type of malaria.

Quartz It is silicon dioxide.

Queckenstedt's test A test done at L P, compression of jugular vein at L P can suggest normalcy or blockage of spinal canal.

Quells Drug containing hyoscine hypobromide which is used in travel sickness.

Quervain's disease Clinical condi-tion of chronic tenosynovitis of extremities.

Question bank In nursing education, we have an opportunity to develop question back with stored questions for an unbiased set, OSCE, OSPE.

Quick lime Calcium oxide used for white wash and with betel leaves.

Quick's test LFT to measure hippuric acid.

Quickening Feeling of foetal movement by the mother for the first time, movement in womb in 4th or 5th month.

Quince A plant fruit which is used as demulcent, mucilage from a plant.

Quinine Important alkaloid of cinchona bark used in malaria treatment.

Quinsy Peritonsillar abscess an acute infection of tonsil.

Quintuplet Woman giving birth to 5 babies in her single confinement.

Quotidian To occur every day, daily

Quotient Ratio obtaining by dividing one number by another, such as I Q, Respiratory Quotient.

R

R E system Reticulo Endothelial system, They are present in liver, spleen, bone marrow and lymph glands that produce macrophages which are having the capacity to produce antibodies.

Rabbit fever It is another name for Tularaemia.

Rabid Animal or a person who is infected with rabies viruses.

Rabies Common zoonotic disease caused by rabies virus and transmitted through infected saliva of dogs when they bite the man, Wild animals and bats are also known to transmit the disease, Hydrophobia.

Racemose That which has grape like appearance such as salivary gland.

Rachial That which is concerned with spine.

Rachischisis Congenital fissure of the spinal column.

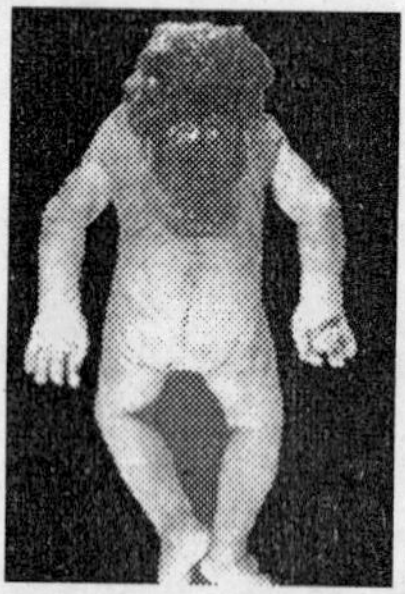

Rachischisis

Rachitis This is the other name for rickets.

Racquets Used in physical fitness under sports medicine, Racquets are used in 4 wall court games, Squash racquets are popular in these games.

Radial nerve Radial nerve examination include evaluation of sensation by pin prick of web area between thumb and index finger. Next evaluation of motion is by asking patient to hyperextend his thumb and then to extend all four fingers.

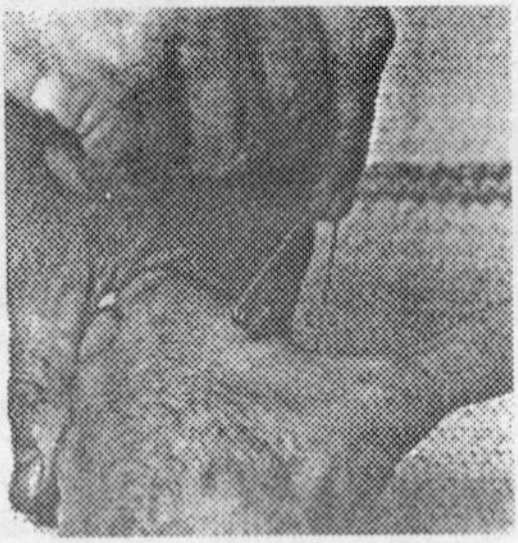

Testing for sensation by pricking the web between patient's thumb and index finger for radial nerve.

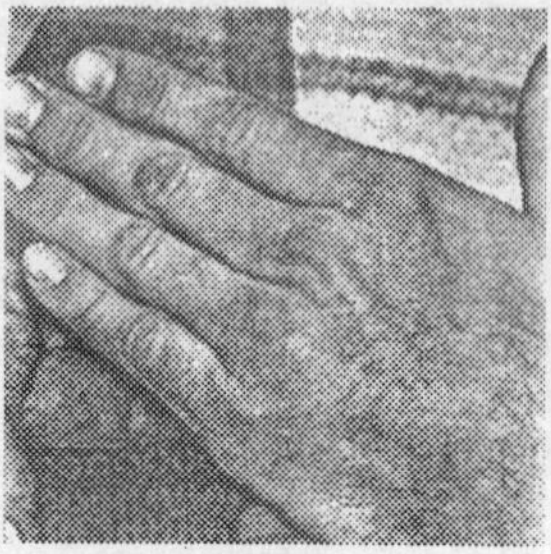

Testing for movement by asking him to hyperextend his thumb and then to extend all four fingers for radial nerve

Radiant That which emits rays.

Radiation implant For endometrial cancer radiation implants inserted through vagina into cervix, Warning signs should be looked into by the duty nurse,

Pregnant nurse should not be posted in this type of duties.

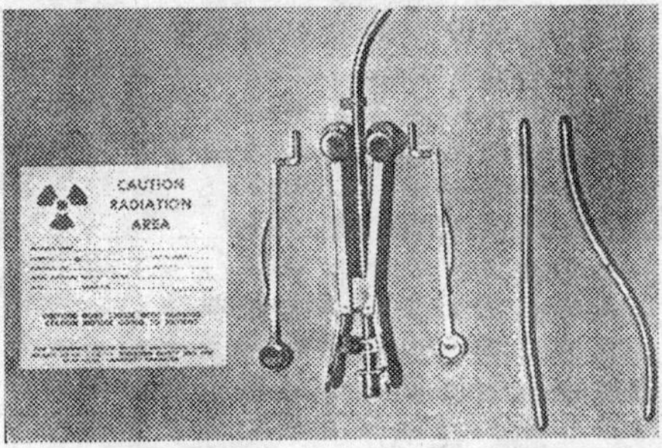

Radiation implants for cervicouterine cancer

Radiation sickness Acute manifestation in the form of nausea and vomiting in a person who is exposed to radiation either natural or artificial.

Radiation Invisible energy rays by X-rays by Radium and other chemicals when exposed to radioactive sources, Energy in the form of electromagnetic waves such as X-rays, Gamma rays, infrared rays and ultraviolet rays.

Radical treatment Under National Malaria effective control programme, active and passive surveillance is under way to find out all cases of fever. Blood smear is taken and soon presumptive treatment is given. If found smear positive , then radical treatment for total cure is done.

Age	*Chloroquine (mg)*	*Primaquine (mg)*	*Remarks*
Below 1 year	75	-	No Primaquine for pregnant and infant
1-4 years	150	2.5	
4-8 years	300	5	
8-14 years	450	10	
Above 14 years	600	15	

Table: Radical treatment for vivax, malariae, ovale

Age	*Chloroquine (mg) Day I*	*Day II*	*Day III*	*Primaquine (mg) I Day*	*Remarks*
Below 1 year	75	75	37.5	-	No Primaquine for Pregnant & infant
1-4 years	150	150	75	7.5	
4-8 years	300	300	150	15	
8-14 years	450	450	225	30	
Above 14 years	600	600	300	45	

Table: Radical treatment for falciparum and malariae

Chloroquine resistant cases (adult dose)

Sulphaline	1000 mg.	Single dose
Pyrimethamine	50 mg.	
Primaquine	45 mg.	

Radical treatment in chloroquine resistant cases

Radical Rerouting the illness or take away the cause of illness, Dealing with the cause of a disease.

Radioactive isotope Isotopes are variations of an element which have identical chemical properties but different atomic weight. Radioactive isotopes are produced by the bombardment of the nuclei of the atoms in an atomic piles. (By-products of the atomic research stations)

Common Isotopes are:

- Radioactive iodine for Ca. thyroid (oral).
- Radioactive phosphorus in polycythaemia (oral or intra venous).
- Radioactive cobalt for cobalt therapy in cancer treatment (beamunit treatment).
- Radioactive gold (local) in cancer pleura or peritonium.

Radioactivity When elements disintegrates to element of lower atomic weight, it emits alpha and beta particles and gamma rays.

Radiograph Picture taken on special film by passing X-ray through the body.

Radiography Making of radiographs of internal organs of the body by exposing film which is sensitized to X-rays or gamma rays

Radioimmuno-electrophoresis Labelled radioisotopes are used in electrophoresis.

Radioimmunoassay determination of presence of protein bound hormones in picogram

An immunological method of determining the concentration of a substance in the blood or in body fluids.

Radioisotope Elements when bombarded with neutrons isotopes are formed which emits radioactivity

Radiologist Qualified doctor who is specialised in radiodiagnosis or in radiotherapy.

Radiology Science that deals with radiation which is used in diagnosis and in treatment of diseases
One of the medicine and allied subject which deals with use of radiation in the diagnosis and treatment of illness, it also include radiotherapy discipline at present.

Radiolucent Substances that permit the x-ray to pass through them.

Radiosensitive Tissues or organs that responds to radiotherapy.

Radiotherapy Treatment of illness by radiation or by radioactive isotopes.

Radium needle Radium is impregnated in needle that are needled to tissues in the treatment of cancers (Radiothe-rapy by radium needle).

Radium An element from Uranium which has great radioactive power that is found useful in cancer treatment
One of the sources of radiation useful in treatment of disease.

Radius It is the line radiating from a centre,
The distance from the centre of a circle to the limit defined by the circle which is half the measure of diameter of that circle.

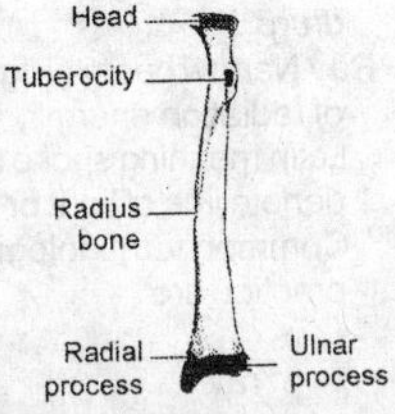

Radius bone

Radix Latin word meaning 'root'.

Radon When radium is disintegrated this gas is liberated,
Radon is known to cause lung cancer.

Radon Gaseous radioactive element which is obtained by breaking up of Radium.

Rage It is the stage of outburst of motor activity, this is described in decorticated animals,
Fear and rage is seen in insulin hypoglycaemia and in carbon monoxide poisoning.

Ragweed Ragweed are tiny weeds which are wind blown pollen that cause autumn hay fever.

Rale Rattling sound diagnostic of fluid in bronchi,
It is an auscultation of chest findings with stethoscope.

Ramstedt's operation Surgical correction of congenital stricture of the pylorus described by Dr. Ramstedt, German surgeon.

Ramus It can be the branch of artery, nerve, vein in anatomical description.

Rancid Usually fatty acid decomposition gives rise to very bad smell.

Random-controlled trial In a drug trial, study group or control group are selected at random which is an experimental study by nature with control.

Random sample A small sample is selected from a population without bias,
Sample selected by giving equal chance to all will have the same characteristics of population.

Randomisation It is blinding in clinical trial where subjects are selected by unbiased methods like lottery, by tossing, by numbers.

Range It is the value between minimum and maximum.

Ranula Blockage of sublingual duct produce a retension cyst under the tongue.

Rape Sexual intercourse without consent, A sexual offence.

Raphe Tissue which indicate junction of two parts of an organ.

Rapid eye movement (REM) It is paradoxical sleep where sleep is associated with dreaming with rapid eye movement in that sleep.

Rapport Good relationship between two individuals or between two groups

A good nurse patient relationship in nursing practice.

Rarefaction Tissue or bone becoming less dense.

Rash Refers to skin eruption due to infections or allergy.

Rashkind catheter It is a balloon catheter used in cardiac surgery developed by Dr. Rashkind, an American paediatric cardiologist.

Rat Domestic rodent commonly seen in human habitations.

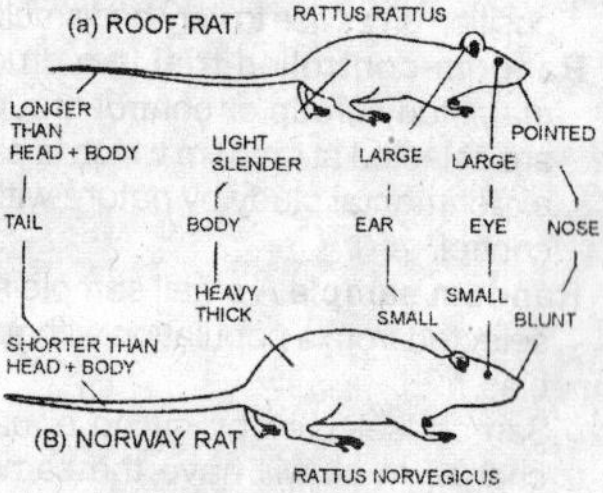

Black rat and Norvey rat

Rat bite fever Fever produced by the bite of rat which introduces either a (spirilium minus or b) streptobacillus moniliformis.

Rate It is an expression of event per unit of population or per unit of time, Common terminologies in nursing practice are:

- Birth rate.
- Death rate.
- Infant mortality rate.
- Maternal mortality rate.
- Neonatal mortality rate.
- Postneonatal mortality rate.
- Marriage rate.
- Fertility rate.
- Pregnancy rate.
- Basal metabolic rate.
- Glomerular filtration rate.
- Pulse rate.
- Respiratory rate.

Rathke's patch It is an embryonic depression that gives rise to anterior lobe of pituitary gland.

Ratio It expresses one entity in relation to other entity which is called a quotient by quotient, Common examples are:

- Sex ratio.
- Albumin globulin ratio.
- Doctor population ratio.
- Nurse population ratio.

Rationalisation Conscious or unconscious act of giving reasons for human behaviour,

It is a mental process in psychology.

Rattle It refers to gurgling sound.

Rauwolfia It is a tropical plant and its root is useful as antihypertensive drug.

Ray Narrow beam of light, or Radiant of radiation energy,

Latin meaning spoke like which can denote line of light or heat,

Common terminologies in nursing practice are:

- α ray.
- β ray.
- γ ray.

- U V ray.
- Cosmic ray.
- Cathode ray.
- Infrared ray.
- Supersonic ray.

Raynaud's disease Cyanosis or pallor of fingers or toes on exposure to cold,

It is an abnormal response of vessels.

Raynaud's phenomenon Cold, drug, hormone, trauma and emotion induced digital ischaemia.

RBC They are minute circular discs floating in blood which carry oxygen to tissues and CO_2 away from tissues.

Red Blood Corpuscles

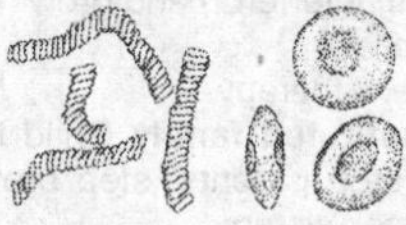

R B C

RCA latrine RCA stands for Research Cum Action

It is a water seal sanitary latrine recommended in developing country.

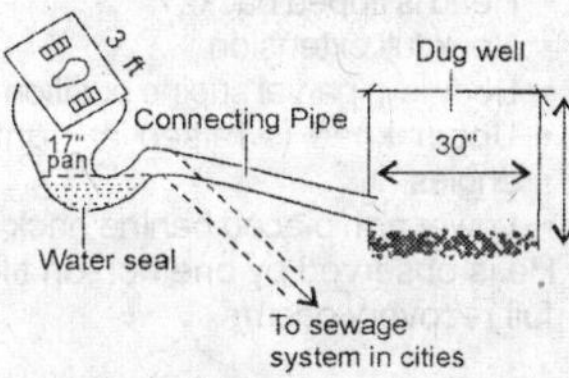

RCA latrine

RCH indicators Growth and development of child indicates the care given to a mother during her reproductive age. Similarly illness of mothers and children reflex RCH status. Of late, mortality rates are indicating the extent of RCH care in the community. These are:

- MMR.
- Foetal deaths.
- Stillbirth rate.
- Perinatal mortality rate.
- Neonatal mortality Rate.
- Post neonatal mortality rate.
- IMR.
- Child death rate.
- Child mortality rate.
- Child survival index.

RCH problems Reproductive and child health problems are:

I. Malnutrition II. Infection

III. Uncontrolled reproduction.

Reorientation of medical education (ROME) This was introduced in India in 1976 to fulfil the need of the country, By adopting rural and urban field practice areas teaching and training are imparted to students and interns in family background, Specialists are exposed to rural areas to look into the need of the society and to teach and help the treatment of patients within available resources,

Instead of training in bigger hospital, it is done in Primary Health Centres in society background or community background.

Re orientation of nursing education (RONE)

Training and teaching of nurses will be done in the health centres apart from hospital; which emphasis home nursing, nurse patient relationship and required counselling.

Reaction time It is time taken for a response from the time of stimulus, Stimulation to response time.

Reaction It is the response to a stimuli which is a counteraction
Term denotes untoward effect of a drug or of an operation.

Read only memory It is one of the part of computer memory which is usually a permanent memory.

Reagent A chemical substance used to demonstrate a chemical reaction.

Reality Occurrence of a thing, perception and behaviour are actual and not imaginary in nature.

Reason for respecting human life By respecting human life man gets joy and happiness through social organisation, family pattern and human dignity.

Reasoning It is highest stage of human thinking where he tries to solve problems in life which may be simple or complicated.
Thinking and allowing the use of intelligence brings about reasoning. Careful reasoning disallow fallacies.

Recall Coming back to conscious status or coming to recollection.

Receptor cells They are specialised cells that collect information for the organism, for the animal or for the man.

Receptors They are present in peripheral nerve endings in the skin and special sense organs of animals, that help in detecting the stimuli,
Molecular level effect producers,
Sensory nerve endings that receives stimuli.

Recessive That which is not dominant, that which recedes in its characters.

Recipe It is the prescription in doctor's formulations for treatment,
It is represented by R in doctor's prescription.

Recipient This refers to a person who receives blood, tissue or an organ from other donor.

Reclination An ophthalmic terminology used when the cataract lens is turned over into the vitreous, which is not practiced.

Recombinant DNA technology It is one of the major technique in genetic engineering.
Its use has been seen in:

- Diagnosis of inherited diseases
- Vaccine development
- Production of insulin, tPA, factor VIII, interferon and growth hormone
- Gene therapy.

Reconstituted family Child living with step parents, step brothers and step sisters.

Recovery position In case of asphyxia resuscitation is given by artificial respiration and when natural breathing rhythm is established the patient is to recovery position,
Recovery position includes:

- Head is tipped back.
- Neck full extension.
- Body is in partial supine position.
- Upper knee is raised at right angles.
- Lower arm placed behind back

He is observed by one person till full recovery occurs.

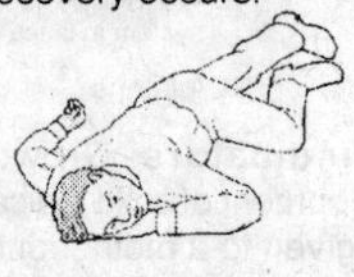

Recovery position

Recrudescence Reappearance of symptoms in severe form after a lapse of certain period.

Rectal crisis It is a neurological disorder which is manifested with severe rectal pain and tenesmus.

Rectal examination Before P R examination, privacy is provided, procedure is explained, patient is put in Sim's position, inspected for piles, skin change, cysts and fissures,

Procedure:

I. Put glove.
II. Lubricate index finger.
III. Ask patient to breathe deeply and to bear down.
IV. Slowly insert finger 2 – 4 inches into rectum.
V. Palpate along circumference of rectal wall.
VI. After removal of finger, check for presence of any stool, blood or mucous.

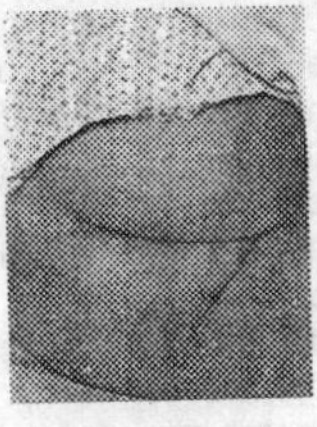

Position for P R

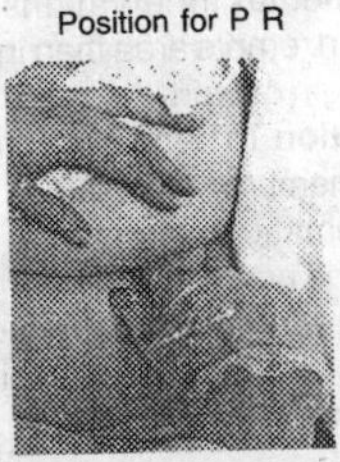

P R being done

Rectal That which is related with rectum such as rectal examination.

Rectal tube It is inserted to relieve gastric distension when it is caused by flatus.

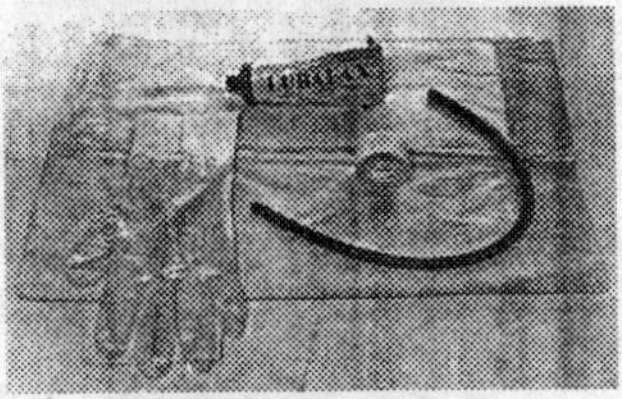

Rectal tube with lubricant

Rectified It refers to refined particularly for spirit,
Also refers when a structure is made straight.

Rectocele Hernial protrusion of portion of rectum into vagina

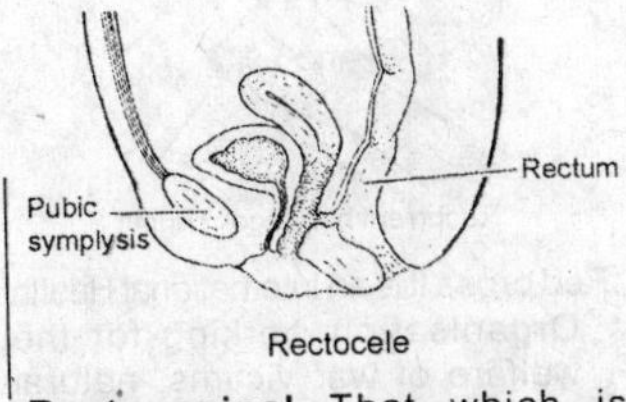

Rectocele

Rectovaginal That which is connected with rectum and vagina such as rectovaginal fistula.

Rectovesical That which is connected with rectum and urinary bladder.

Rectum This is the portion of large intestine from sigmoid flexure to anus.

Recumbent Refers to dorsal position or lying on back
This refers to the posture of lying down position

Recuperation The stage of recovery after an illness and gaining strength.

Recurrent That which recurs again and again such as recurrent fever.

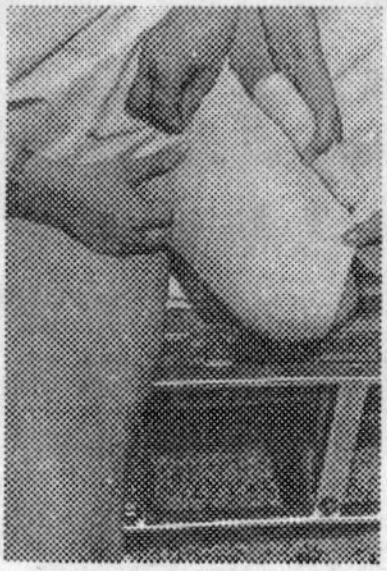

Recurrent bandage : Stump

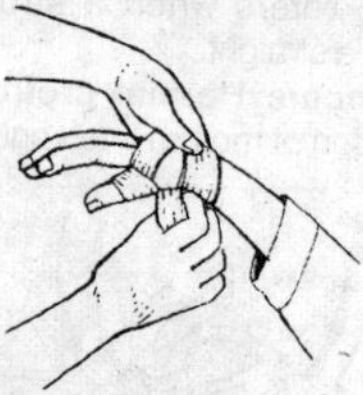

Recurrent bandage: Thumb

Red cross It is an International Health Organisation working for the welfare of war victims, natural calamities, disasters and in civilian distress.

Red marrow They are structure in the interstices of cancellous bones.

Red nucleus An area in the midbrain where gray matter is present.

Redivac drainage tube Post-operative drainage in abdominal surgical wounds,

Postoperative close drainage tube

Reduction Bringing to normal in case of hernia, in case of dislocation or in case of fracture,

Opposite oxidation where addition of Hydrogen is done in a chemical reaction.

Reference man He is between 20-39 years age weight 60 kg, is free from disease and physically fit for active work. On each working day he is employed for 8 hours in occupation that usually involves moderate activity. While not at work he spends 8 hours in bed, 4-6 hours sitting and moving about, and 2 hours walking and in active recreation or household duties.

Reference woman She is between 20-39 years age healthy, weight 50 kg. She may be engaged for 8 hours in general household work, in light industry or in any other moderately active work. Apart from 8 hours in bed, she spends 4-6 hours sitting or moving around in light activity and 2 hours walking or active recreation or household chores.

Referred pain Pain in different region due to sensory nerves of the same level

For example :

- In heart attack, pain in left shoulder.
- In diaphragmatic abscess, pain in shoulder etc.,

Segmental innervations causes pain in remote area than in the area of origin of pain

Reflection To bend back, reflection of a membrane,

Systematic thinking of a nurse in nursing practice.

Reflex arc It is a physiological mechanism necessary for a reflex action.

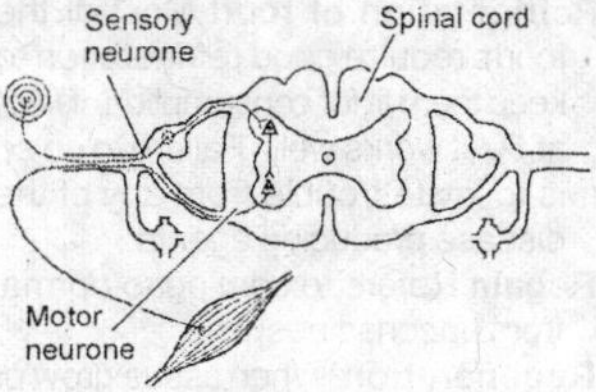

Reflex arc

Reflex They are present in all people. When absent or when heightened it could be due to some pathology It is an involuntary response in which a stimulus is received by a nerve and is transmitted, gets translated into muscie action, all in just a fraction of a second
Criteria for reflex scaling:

Non-reflexive	0
Hyporeflexia	1
Normal	2
Brisk	3
Hyperreflexia	4

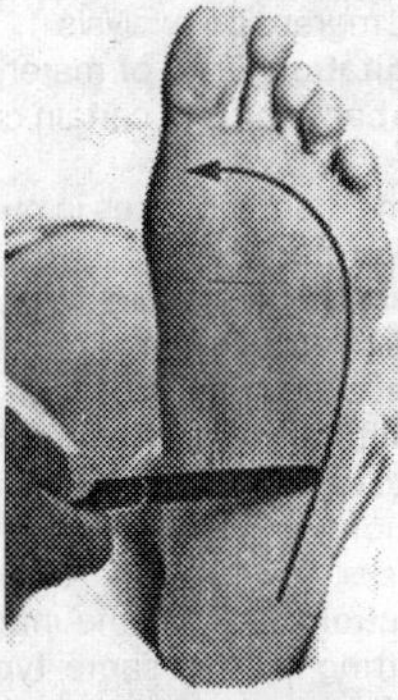

Plantar reflex

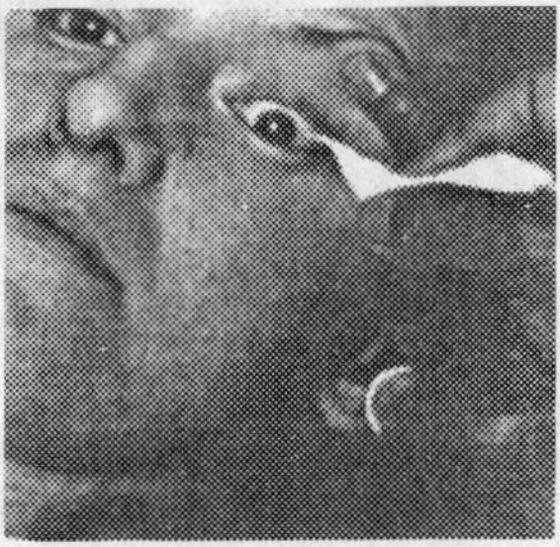

Corneal reflex

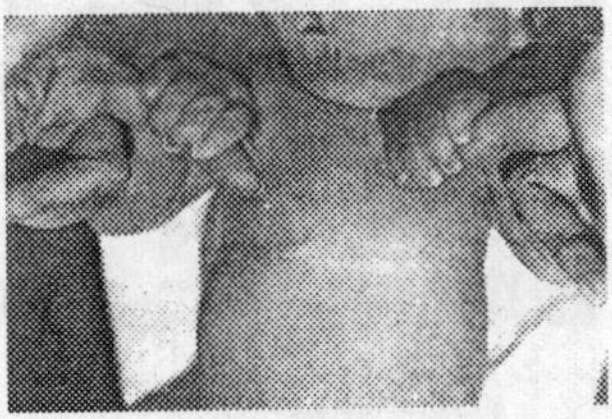

Grasp reflex

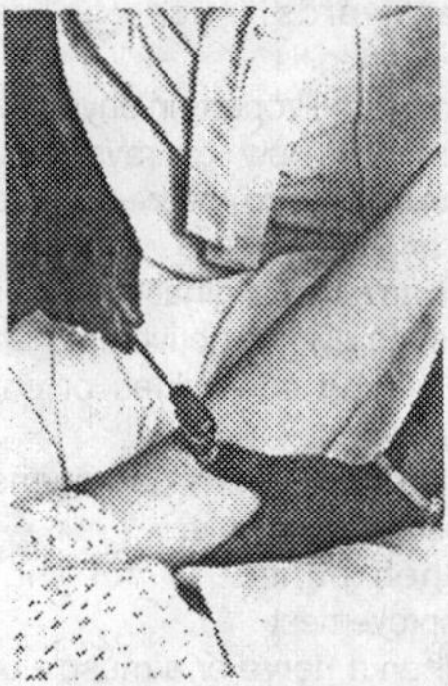

Biceps reflex

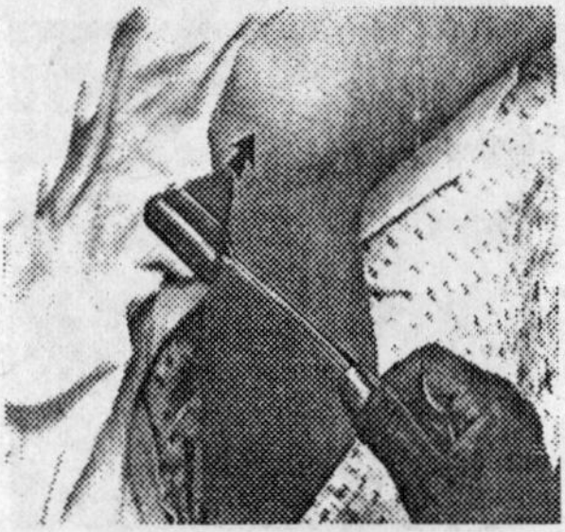

Triceps reflex

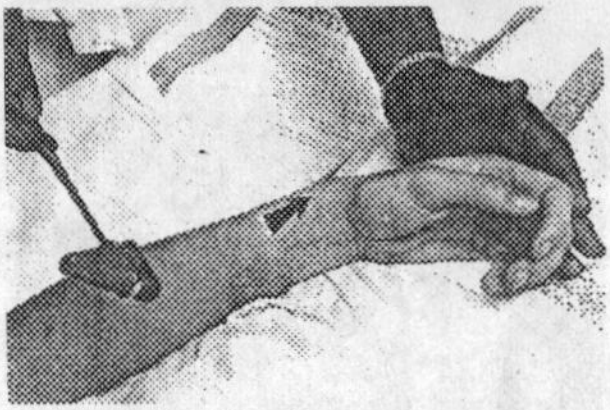

Brachioradialis reflex

Reflux Regurgitation or flow backwards such as reflux oesophagitis.

Refraction Property in physics which describes how light rays pass from one medium to another (one density to another)
It is an eye examination process for testing eye refractive error and for fitting spectacles or contact glasses.

Refractory When pathogens are resistant to drugs,
When patient is not showing improvement
When a nerve or a muscle do not show action after certain time.

Refrigeration of food Most of the foods require good refrigeration to keep them fit for consumption, if kept at 50^0 it works well. Failure to do so is to invite trouble from any of the disease producing agents.

Regain Refers to coming to normal from unconsciousness.

Regeneration When tissue grow or develop to grow after injury.

Regimen Regimen is a programme in medical treatment , also it can be a regimen for healthy living,
It is the systematic plan done for a treatment.

Register Entry of data done over a disease in the community or in a hospital.

Registrar One who keeps the register of cases, illnesses or vents.

Registration Entry of data done of vital events.

Regression To come back to previous state,
To come back to childish behaviour,
Also refers to statistical analysis called regression analysis.

Regurgitation Flow of material or liquid backwards in certain conditions,
Common terminologies in nursing practice are:
- Oesophageal regurgitation.
- Mitral regurgitation.
- Aortic regurgitation.

Rehabilitation It is third level of health care to restore to the best possible functioning state after serious illness or injury.

Reinfection Second time infection occurring by the same type of organism.

Reinforcement Force of strength is used in an action.

Action taken to strengthen a behavioural response,
It also means conditioning in biological science.

Reiter's syndrome Combination of arthritis, conjunctivitis and urithritis described by Dr.Reiter a German Bacteriologist.

Rejection phenomenon When a tissue or an organ is transplanted , there will be a tendency in the body to destroy that transplanted tissue which is called rejection phenomenon.

Rejection Reaction of the body on transplanted tissue or organ,
In psychology, it is a non-acceptance phenomenon.

Rejuvenators They are worthless methods since returning to youth is not possible in scientific concept,
Any preparation or any method supposedly capable of returning lost youth.

Relapse Reappearance of illness after the brief period of recovery.

Relapsing fever Also called recurring fever caused by Borrelia group of spirochaetes which are transmitted through ticks.

Relative poverty State of being poor with reference to a real, or perceived standard of living in a society.

Relative risk It is a ratio used in the epidemiological description,

$$R.R. = \frac{\text{Incidence rate among exposed}}{\text{Incidence rate among unexposed}}$$

Relaxant Drug that brings about relaxation of muscles.

Relaxation After the period of contraction, muscle gets relaxed over a period Mental calmness produced by various means.

Relief Free from pain, getting free from distress, removal of pain.

Religion Nurse to understand the faith in health, it is important in times of serious ill health and at tragedy, Religion covers this aspect.

Remarriage Divorced individual enters a marriage contract for a second time or more times.

Remedy It refers to the cure of a disease.

Remission No symptoms seen for a long period in certain diseases like TB.

Remittent When partial fall of body temperature occurs daily,
When frequency of vomiting gets partially reduced over a period of time.

Removal of urine from flaccid bladder

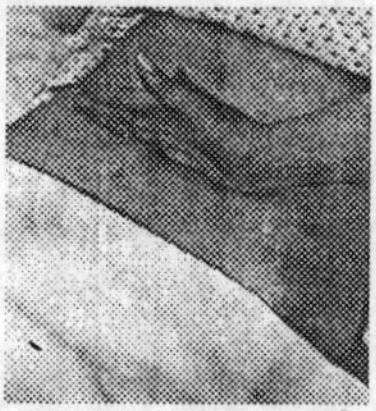

A: Assess the bladder distension

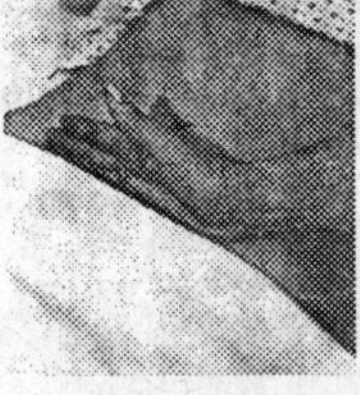

B: Press downward to initiate urination

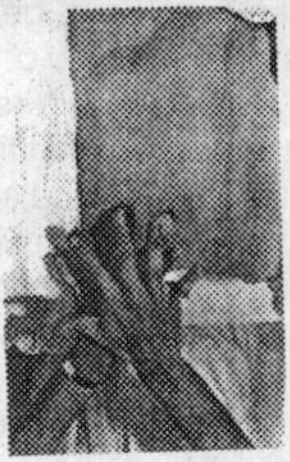

C: Percuss patient's bladder to ensure empty

Renal system The sys.em connected with excretion of waste products.

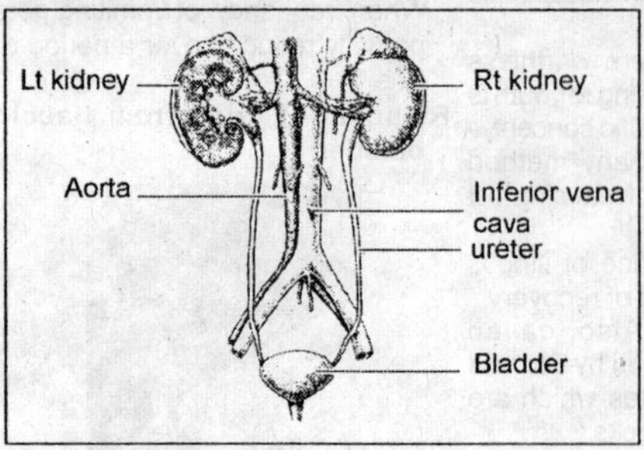

Renal system

Renal transplant Normal kidney from a healthy donor is taken out and is transplanted into the person who has diseased and non-functioning-kidney.

Renal That which is related with kidney such as:

- Renal failure.
- Renal dialysis.
- Renal tubule.
- Renal threshold.

Renal urinary disorder Nursing care commands application of external urinary device in cases of urinary retension,

Inserting a Robinson (straight) catheter into female and inserting a Robinson (straight) catheter into a male are asserted

Performing the Crede maneuver is another requisite in nursing care which is employed to facilitate the removal of urine for patients whose bladders are irreversibly flaccid.

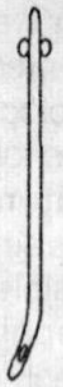

A: Female catheter

B: Male catheter

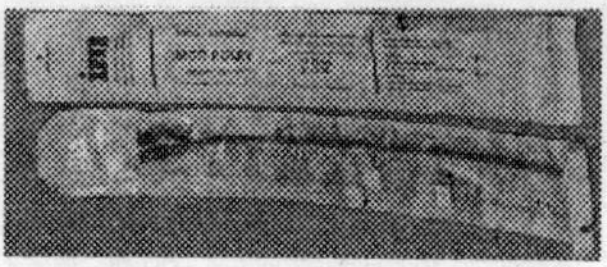

C: Foley catheter

Renin They are secreted by the kidneys during ischaemic conditions, Renin is a hypertensive and vasoconstrictor.

Reorganisation Referred to tissue healing by new tissue formation.

Reovirus RNA virus present in respiratory tract, intestinal tract, Commonly cause sickness in children.

Replication Refers to the dupli-cation of DNA.

Replogle tube An aspirator attached to a suction apparatus It is a double lumen aspiration apparatus.

Repository That which is responsible for restoration of an organ to its normal position.

Reproduction Reproduction by fusion of female germ cell with male germ cell which always refers to sexual reproduction.

Reproductive system Parts that represent male and female genital organs which are functioning to conceive, to up bring and to deliver an offspring.

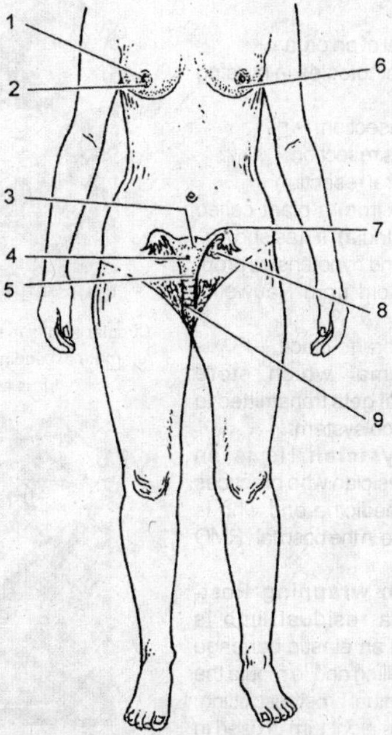

Female reproductive system

1. nipple
2. Areola
3. Uterine fundus
4. Uterus
5. Cervix
6. Breast
7. Fallopian tube
8. Ovary
9. Vagina

Research ethics This is the area of faithfully discrimination of doing right or doing wrong in professional activities. It includes animal experiments and clinical trial in human beings.

Research A scientific study which help us to prove the postulation of a hypothesis.

Resection Surgical removal of an organ,
Partial removal of an organ
Common terminologies in nursing practice are:
- Intestinal resection.
- Submucous resection.
- Transurethral resection.

Reserpine It is from a plant called snakeroot (in India), it has shown tranquilising and hypotensive property, An alkaloid from Rauwolfia plant.

Reservoir A storage place,
Man or animal which store pathogens that gets transmitted to other in the eco system.

Resident physician He is an employed physician who practices emergency medicine and who is readily available in the hospital, RMO of a hospital.

Residual limb wrapping Post-operatively a residual limb is wrapped with an elastic bandage to reduce swelling and to mould the stump for eventual prosthetic fitting. Modified figure eight turn is used in wrapping.

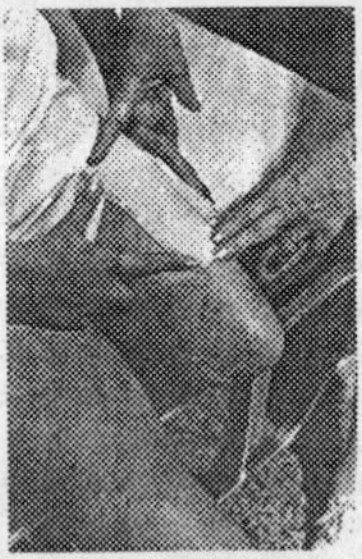

Positioning the end of elastic bandage

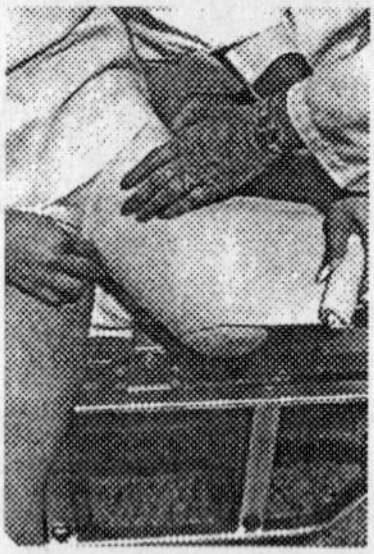

Circular turn is made for an anchor
Alternate ascending and descending turns are made

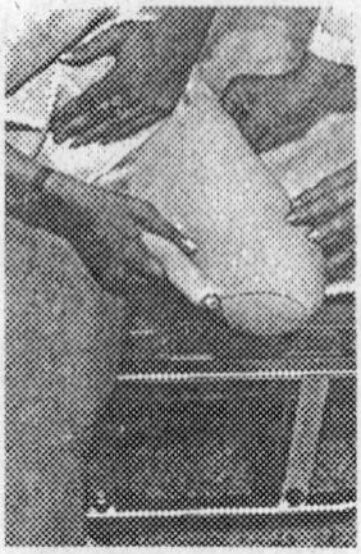

Residual limb wrapping

Residual That which is remaining such as residual Air, residual urine, residual volume

Refers to residual disability after an injury or after the full cycle of disease.

Residue What it remains after medical or surgical treatment with respect to illness,

Some thing that remains after removal of an anatomical structure.

Resilience When you undo the stretch the item comes back to its original state.

Resistance Degree of reaction to a action,

Degree of opposition to a force,

Resistance offered to the flowing current.

Resolution That which comes to normal such as resolution of the lung.

Resonance It is the reverberating sound by percussion on cavity or hollow organ,

The musical quality on percussing the air containing cavity.

Resources in health care It is important for equitable distribution of health care.

Considered resources are:

- Manpower.
- Money.
- Material.
- Technique.
- Skill.
- Knowledge.
- Duration.

Respect for persons Each person has the capacity and right to make a choice and decision about their body, their personal hygiene and the treatment.

Everything or all acts in nursing and medical profession must be free from unjustified interference by others.

Respiration Gaseous interchanges between tissues and atmosphere which include 1) Inspiration and 2) Expiration

Following are physiological and pathological respirations:

- External respiration.
- Internal respiration.
- Natural respiration.
- Artificial respiration.
- Laboured respiration .
- Stertorous respiration.
- Tissue respiration.
- Intermittent positive pressure respiration.

(A)

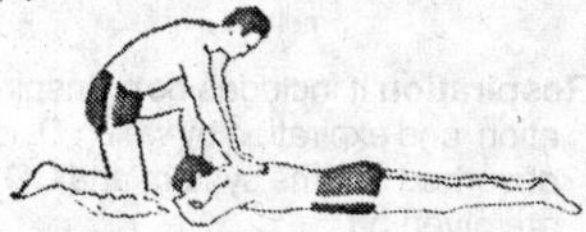

(B)

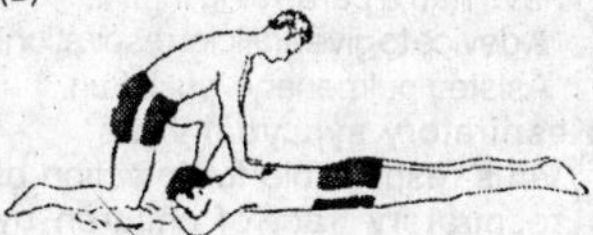

(C)

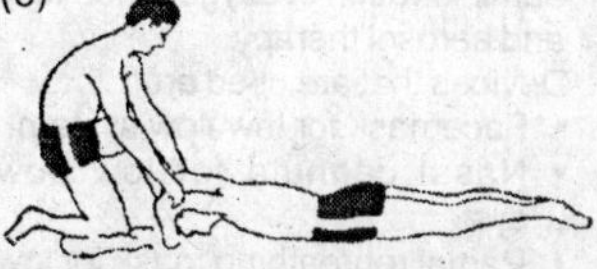

Artificial respiration The Holger-Nielsen

(A)

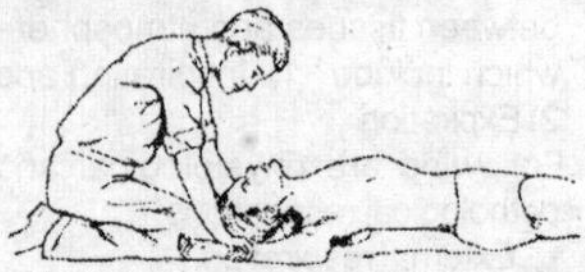

(B)

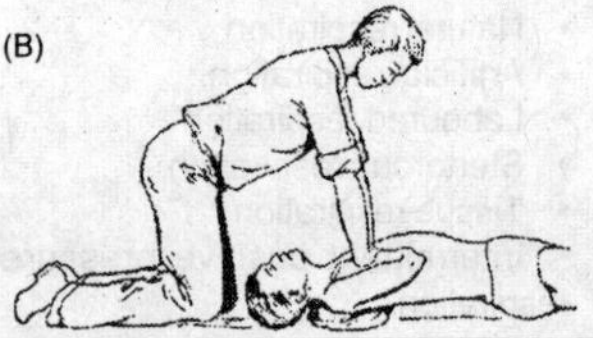

Artificial respiration by Silvester Broche method

Respiration It includes both inspiration and expiration by which O_2 is absorbed into the system and CO_2 are given off.

Respirator It is a device using alternate pressure and vacuum to help patients breathe when they have had a paralysing injury.,

A device to give artificial respiration, Asisted pulmonary ventilation.

Respiratory syncytial virus Virus responsible for infection of respiratory tract of children by inducing the formation of syncytial masses.

Respiratory therapy This includes administration of oxygen, humidity and aerosol therapy.

Devices that are used are:

- Facemask for low flow system.
- Nasal cannula for low flow system.
- Partial rebreathing mask for low flow system.
- Nonrebreathing mask for low and high flow system.
- Venturi mask for high flow system.
- Oxygen hood for infants.
- Incubator for infants.
- Croupette for children.

Respiratory That which is related with respiratory organs or process.

Restraints This is ordered by the physician to patient who are disoriented or combative and who dislodge the needle or catheter.

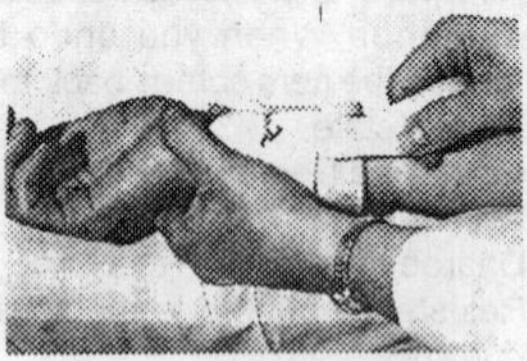

Wrist restrains (putting)

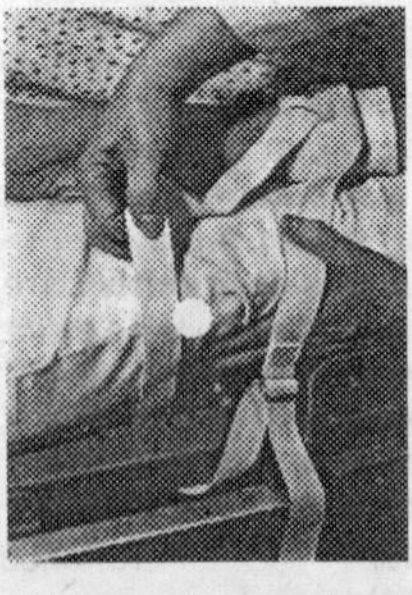

Wrist restrain to bed frame

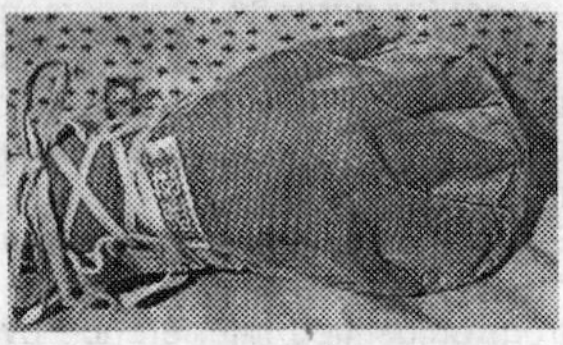

C: Mitt restrains to restrict hand movement

Resuscitation Restoration to normalcy of a person, who has ceased respiration,

Since heart and lung are to be maintained the common type of resuscitation is known as 'Cardio Pulmonary Resuscitation'.

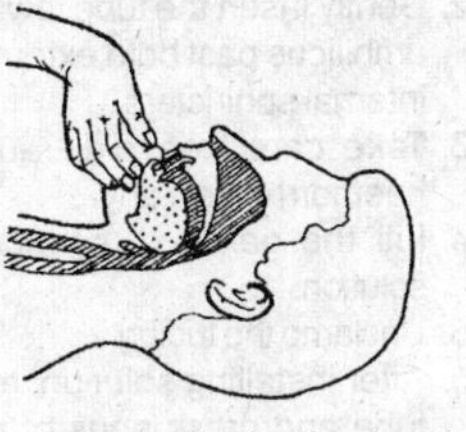

Resuscitation (pulling jaw for airway)

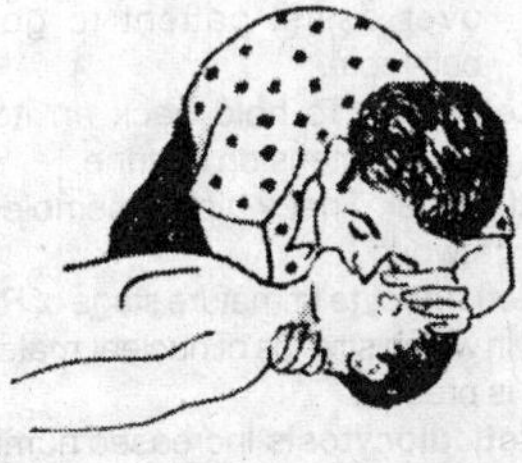

Resuscitation (Mouth to mouth breathing)

A

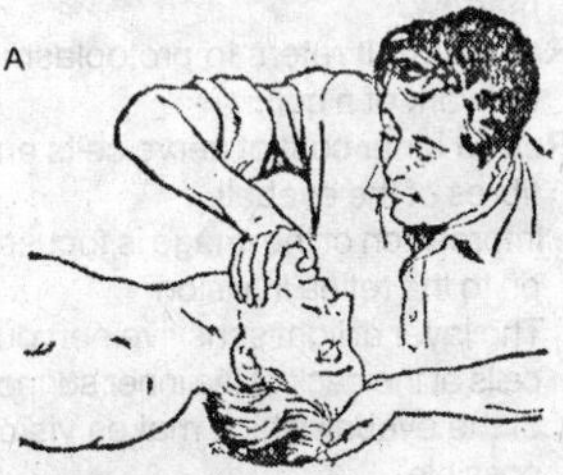

Extend head

B

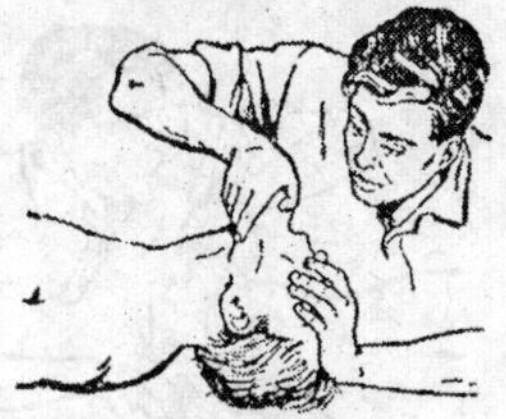

Lift jow + close nose

C

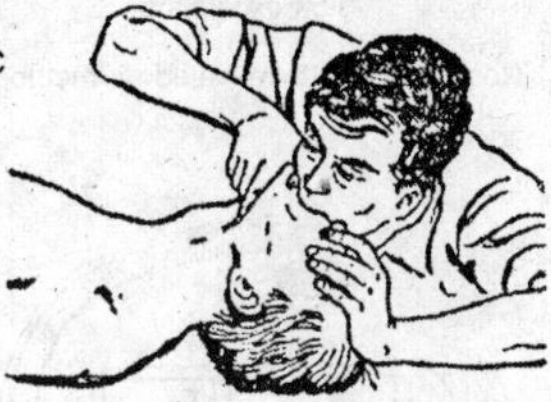

Mouth to mouth respiration

D

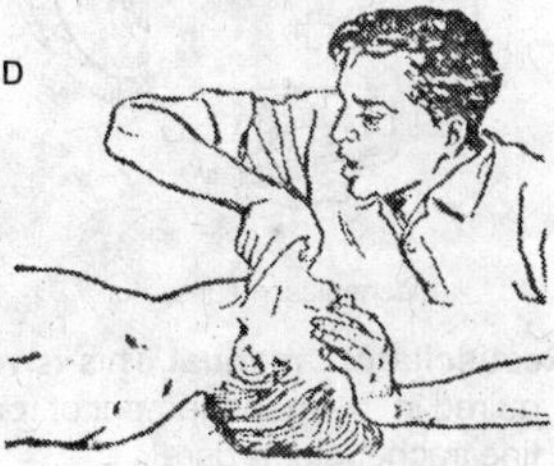

Allow exhalation

E

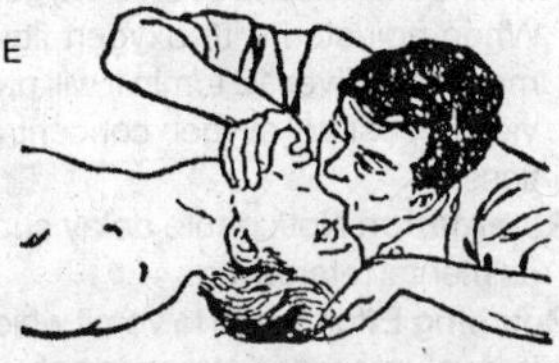

Mouth to nose respiration

F

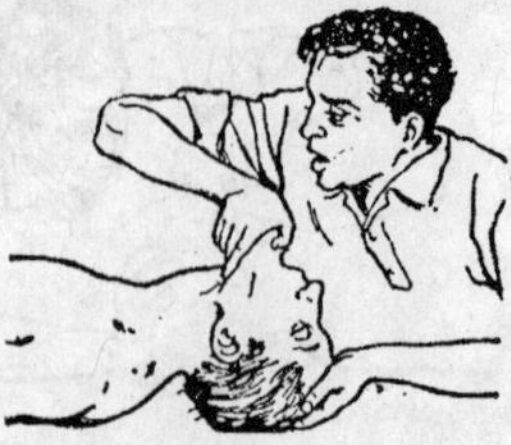

Allow exhalation

Resuscitation (by exhaled air method)

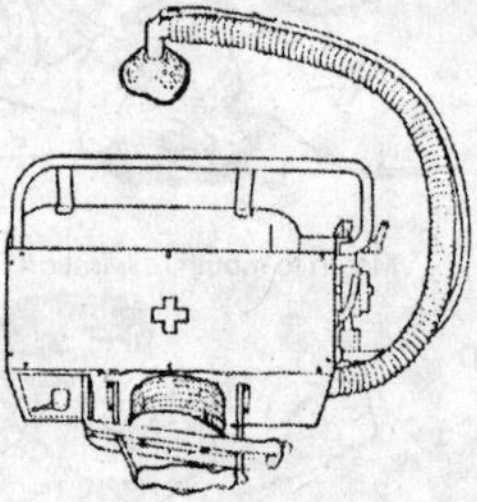

Mechanical resuscitator

Resuscitator manual This is required in the management of routine tracheostomy care,
Ambu or Laerdal manual resuscitator is attached to source oxygen, When adjusted with oxygen flowmeter to deliver 12 L/min it will provide necessary oxygen concentrations.

Retardation Noticeable delay such as mental retardation.

Retching Effort made to vomit which is involuntary and strong in nature.

Retension enema Enema given and retained in colon to provide the patient either nutrition or medicamentation.
Following steps are used in retention enema in nursing care:

1. Separate patient's buttocks.
2. Gently insert the tube toward the umbilicus past both external and internal sphincters.
3. Take care to avoid trauma to haemorrhoids if any.
4. Fill the barrel of syringe with solution.
5. Unclamp the tubing.
6. After installing solution, remove tube and press anus of patient for a few moments with gauze pad.
7. After prescribed retention time is over assist patient to go to bathroom.

Retention To hold back an item, such as retension of urine.

Reticular That which resembles a network.

Reticulocyte Immature stage of RBC in which strands of nuclear material is present.

Reticulocytosis Increased number of immature cells in the blood which is the sign of over activity of bone marrow.

Reticulum It refers to protoplasmic network of a cell.

Retina Inner coat of nerve cells and fibres of the eyeball,
Impression of the image is focused on to the retina in vision
The layer of light sensitive nervous cells at the back of the inner surface of the eyeball which makes vision possible.

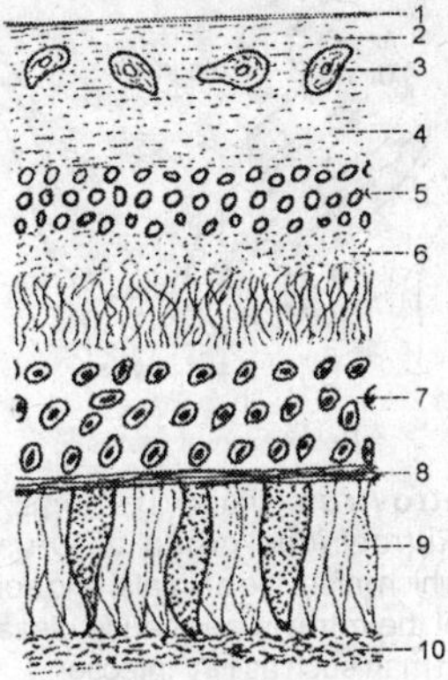

Retina (histology)

1. Internal limiting membrane
2. Nerve fibre
3. Ganglion cell
4. Inner molecular layer
5. Inner molecular layers
6. Outer molecular layer
7. Outer nuclear layer
8. External limiting membrane
9. Rods and cones
10. Pigment layer.

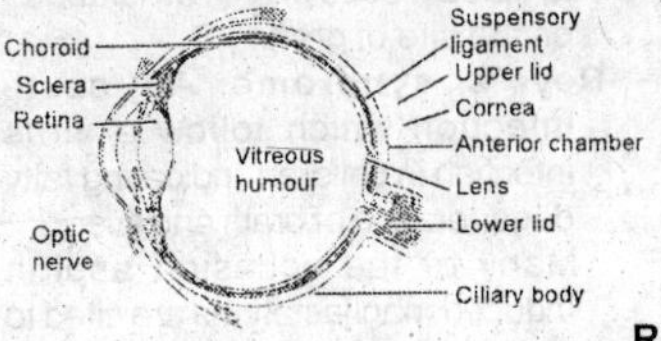

Retina (structure)

Retinaculum It refers to a structure that retains an organ or a tissue in its place.

Retinitis Infection and inflammation of retina.

Retinoblastoma Cancer tumour from retinal cells which calls for Enucleation.

Retinol It is one of the form of vitamin A.

Retinopathy Non-inflammatory diseases of the retina, common types in clinical practice are:

- Diabetic retinopathy.
- Hypertensive retinopathy.

Retinsocope An ophthalmic instrument to illuminate retina, helpful in the measurement of refractive errors.

Retractile Meaning that it is susceptible of being drawn back.

RetrobulbarRelated with the back of eyeball.

Retrocession of uterus Background displacement of uterus, It also mean's cancer spread to the interior organ from surface.

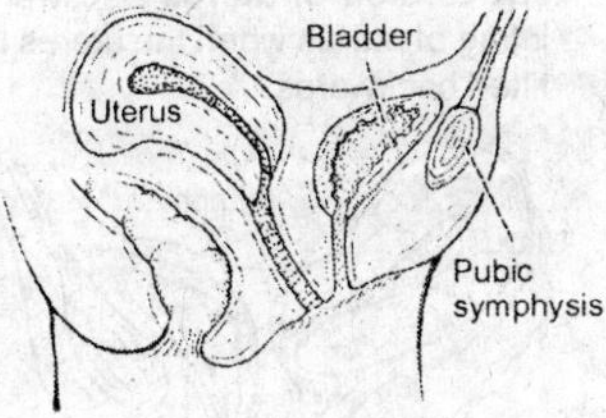

Retrocession of uterus

Retroflexed That which is bent backward such as retroflexed uterus.

Retrograde pyelography Cystoscope is introduced into the bladder, ureteric catheter opaque to X-ray is passed along the ureter into the pelvis of the kidney to be examined. Injection of opaque fluid is made through ureteric catheter (Sterile solution of sodium iodide 10%) (Water soluble preparation iodoxyl), X-ray is taken when pelvis of kidney is filled with solution.

Retrograde Going backwards against natural course such as retrograde urography.

Retrolental fibroplasias When premature baby is exposed to high content of oxygen, which produce fibrous condition of the vitreous body.

Retroperitoneal That which is behind the peritoneum.

Retropharyngeal That which is behind the pharynx.

Retropubic That which is behind pubic bone.

Retrosternal That which is behind the sternum.

Retroversion of uterus Backward lifting of uterus when the uterus is tilted backwards.

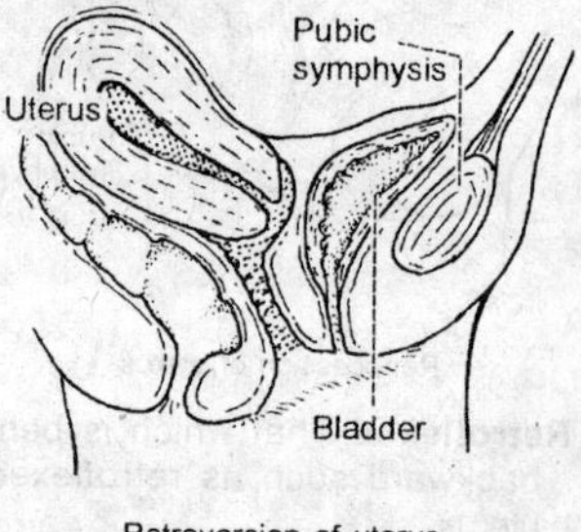

Retroversion of uterus

Retroflexon of uterus Uterus bent back at an acute angle but cervix will be in normal position.

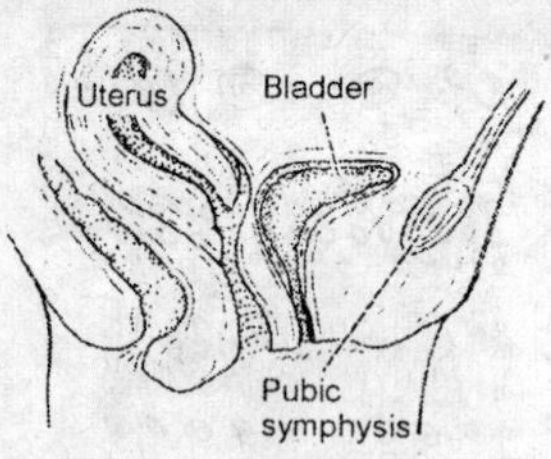

Retroflexon of uterus

Retrovirus This belongs to *Retroviridae* group of viruses which infect the animals, and some of the retroviruses cause disease in man such as HIV infection, Retroviruses contain reverse transcriptase.

Animal diseases by retrovirus	*Human disease by retrovirus*
Lymphoma Leukaemia	HIV AIDS

Reverdin's graft It is one of the types of skin graft developed by Dr.Reverdin

A Swiss Surgeon who described to place pieces of skin as islands on the site of graft.

Reye's syndrome An acute infection which follow a virus infection in children indicating fatty degeneration of brain and liver,

Many of the occasion aspirin induced manifestations are cited to be Reye's syndrome,

A syndrome named after Reye an Australian Pathologist.

Rh factor Blood grouping done by Rhesus factor which has important link with Rh incompatibility in pregnancy.

Rhabdo That which is rod-shaped such as Rhabdocyte.

Rhabdomyosarcoma Cancer of striated muscle which show rapid growth and rapid secondaries.

Rhazes Rhazes is an Arabian Physician who lived in 850 to 932 A.D. who has contributed in medical writings.

Rhesus factor It is called Rh factor, Genetically determined antigen if present it is Rh+,
Genetically determined antigen if absent it is Rh- ,
If mother is Rh- and newborn is Rh+ anaemia and jaundice occurs in the newborn due to Rh incompatibility ,
The condition is also called isoimmunisation.

Rheumatic fever An acute infection with severe manifestation in the form of sore throat,
Not the same as rheumatism
Rheumatic fever follows streptococcal sore throat,
Common manifestations are:

- Polyarthritis.
- Carditis.
- Chorea.
- Erythema marginatum.
- Subcutaneous nodule.

Rheumatism Disorders showing inflammation of joints and related tissues.

Rheumatoid arthritis Bilateral symmetrical polyarthritis of fingers and toes which show bone erosion and deformity of bones.

Rheumatoid That which resembles rheumatism such as rheumatoid arthritis
Severe and crippling form of arthritis.

Rheumatology Science that deals with the study of diseases of joints, muscles, tendons and ligaments.

Rhinitis Infection and inflammation of the mucous membrane of the nose
Common types of rhinitis are:

- Catarrhal rhinitis.
- Allergic rhinitis.
- Membranous rhinitis.
- Syphilitic rhinitis.
- Tubercular rhinitis.
- Vasomotor rhinitis.

Rhinophyma It is a clinical disorder manifested with nodular swelling and congestion of the nose,
It is a form of rosacea.

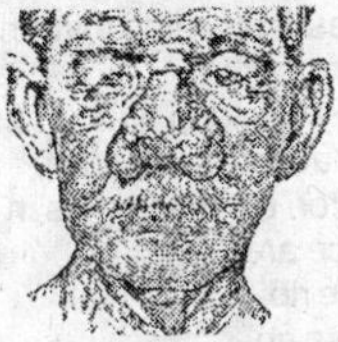

Rhinophyma

Rhinoplasty Plastic surgery of the nose where correction of distracted nose is undertaken.

Rhinorrhoea Running in the nose which is not normal and pathological.

Rhinovirus They are RNA viruses that cause respiratory infections including common cold.

Rhodopsin This is visual purple of the retina which is formed from vitamin A.

Rhomboid It is an oblique parallelogram.

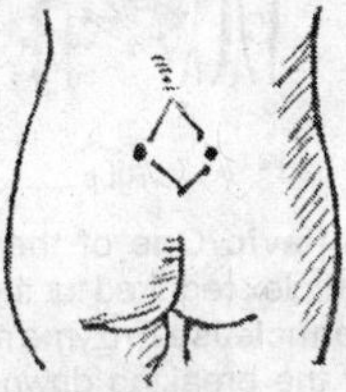

Michaelis' rhomboid

Rhonchus Wheeze in the bronchial area which is due to allergen that produces spasm,
Spasmodic bronchitis of allergy.

Rhubarb It is derived from the root of plant called rhubarb which has the purgative and astringent action.

Rhythm A method of (natural) family planning where sexual intercourse is restricted to infertile phase of menstrual cycle,
rhythm method of F P ,
A regular recurring occurrence such as a) cardiac rhythm b) Respiratory rhythm.

Rib They are long flat curved bones of thoracic cage of man,
Common terminologies in nursing practice are:
- True rib.
- False rib.
- Cervical rib.
- Floating rib.

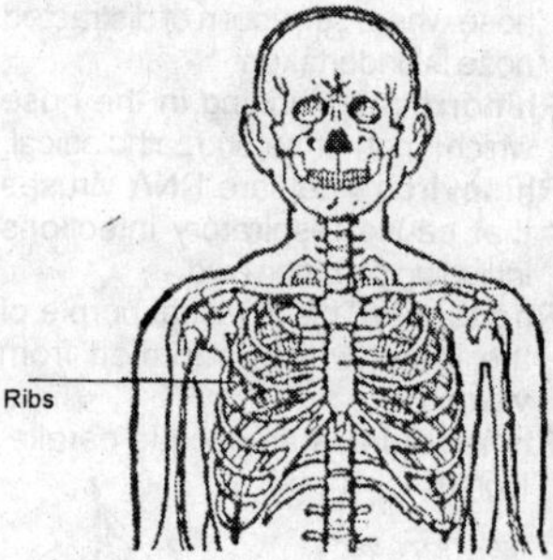

Ribs

Riboflavin One of the vitamin B complex required for the body.

Ribonuclease Enzyme responsible for the breaking down of nucleic acid.

Ribosome This is the site where protein is synthesised in the cell.

Rickets Deficiency of vitamin D among children,
Adult rickets is called Osteomalacia.

Rickettsia Group of micro organisms that produce typhus group of fevers.

Ridge It refers to a projection of an organ such as:
- Deltoid ridge.
- Genital ridge.
- Mammary ridge.
- Superciliary ridge.
- Supraorbital ridge.

Right to die with dignity Patients' Bill of Right Justified the Rights to die with dignity.
Patient can refuse treatment, surgery or even life supporting system
This has a relevance in cancer and any terminal illness of a patient.
'Mercy Killing' in the context is by no means available to patient.

Right to health It is the proclamation of social activists. We come across people with disease but fit enough to lead a healthy life. Also we see healthy person leading a miserable life.
Present concept is that 'right to health' is doing good for economic environmental and political conditions that will maximise good health.

Rigidity Muscles are stiff and not flexible due to neuropathology, injury or due to stress.

Rigor It is an attack of shivering occurs in acute infections, rigors may replaced by convulsions in infants and in adults.

Rigor mortis Within 6 hours after death, muscles become stiff and we call it rigor mortis.

Ring immunisation Under National Polio Eradication Programme, it is a mopping up operation in cities where door to door OPV to below 5 year children is done covering an area with a radium of 3 Kms.

Ringer's solution It is used in place of IV fluid to rehydrate a person This is mixture of NaCl , Ca , and K , Developed by Dr.Ringer a British Physiologist.

Ring A circular area or an organ in the body or a structure like:
- Benzene ring
- Amnion ring
- Ciliary ring
- Femoral ring
- Inguinal ring
- Tracheal ring.

Ringworm It is the name given to fungal infection of skin, hair and nails, By appearance it is circular, pinkish and has desquamating surface.

Rinne test This test is done to test hearing impairment in a patient. First vibrate tuning fork by striking the prongs against the palmar surface of hand, Patient is asked to cover one ear, Tuning fork is positioned on mastoid process of uncovered ear. Patient tells when she could not hear the vibration, Immediately move the prongs of tuning fork in front of the uncovered ear, patient should be able to hear sound twice as long in this position, Reverse is true in conductive deafness

Inference is:
- Positive if patient has normal hearing.
- Negative if the results are reversed.

Risk society Modern world with sense of danger and challenges.

Risk In nursing science it is the chance of developing a disease or a complication, meaning hazard to which a person is exposed, Epidemiologically relative risk and absolute risk are used.

Risus The word means 'laughter' and this facial expression is seen in tetanus because of facial musculature spasm.

RNA Abbreviation for **R**ibo **N**ucleic **A**cid.

RNTCP Abbreviation for **R**evised **N**ational **T**uberculosis **C**ontrol Programme RNTCP Case detection:
- 3 sputum examination of patients with cough of 3 weeks, (1) Spot (2) Early Morning and (3) Spot.
- Health awareness by health education on respiratory symptoms.
- Contact examination of AFB +ve children.
- Evaluation of chest X- ray.

RNTCP TREATMENT REGIMENS

TB Treatment	*TB Patients*	*Intensive Phase*	*Continuation Phase*
Category I	New smear-positive New smearnegative (Seriously ill) Extrapulmonary**	2(HRZE)3*	4(HR)

Category II	Sputum smear-Positive –Relapse*** – Failure*** – Treatment After Defaults	2(SHRZE)3 1(HRZE)3	5(HRE)3
Category III	New smear-negative (Not seriously ill) Extrapulmonary (Not seriously ill)	2(HRZ)3	4(HR)3

* The number before the letters refers to the number of months of treatment. The subscription after the letters refers to the number of doses per week. H: Isoniazid (600 mg), R: Rifampicin (450 mg), Z: Pyrazinamide (1500 mg), E: Ethambutol (1200 mg), S: Streptomycin (750 mg). Patients more than 50 years old receive streptomycin 500 mg. Patients in categories I and II who have a positive sputum smear at the end of the initial intensive phase receive an additional month of intensive phase of treatment.

** Examples of seriously ill extrapulmonary TB cases are meningitis, disseminated TB, tuberculous pericarditis, peritonitis, bilateral or extensive pleurisy, spinal TB with neurological complications and intestinal and genitourinary TB.

*** Very rarely, patients relapse with extrapulmonary or smear-negative pulmonary tuberculosis; such patients are considered as "Other" and treated with the category II regimen.

RNTCP Regimen

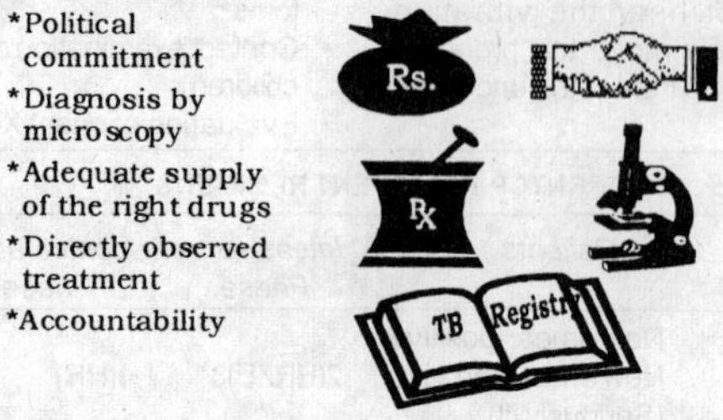

The DOTS' strategy

Robinson catheter It is a straight catheter inserted into female when indicated, It is indicated in urinary retention.

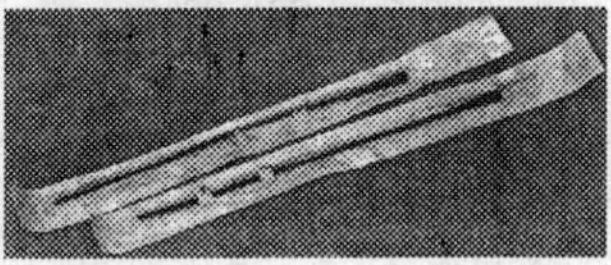

Robinson catheter (female catheter)

Rocky Mountain spotted fever It is a Rickettsial infection transmitted by the tick.

Rod Anything that is straight and thin in its structure such as retinal rod.

Rodent ulcer It is basal cell carcinoma which show destruction of tissue and bone and is commonly seen in face.

Rodents Rodents (rat, mice) are associated with plague, typhus which can be eliminated by environmental measures. Poor living condition and garbage menace allow rodents to populate and thrive.

R.rats	*R. norvegicus*
Slender body	Heavy body
Long nose	Blunt nose
Long tail	Short tail
Large eye and ear	Small eye and ear

Table: Character differences of R. rattus and R.norvegicus

Rods They are specialised cells of retina of the eye that are sensitive to fine degrees of light and dark.

Roentgen ray Roentgen was German Physicist who lived during 1845 to 1923, He discovered X-ray which is named after him as 'Roentgen ray' X-ray was discovered in 1895 which helped medical world in final diagnosis of many illness and many health problem.

Role The expected pattern of behaviour associated with a social status behaviour developed in response to the expectation of the society

Role play as father, mother, brother, sister, son, daughter, friend, teacher, student, are inherited and involuntary.

Roller bandage Its use is common in nursing care. Their common uses are:

1) To secure dressings to wounds.
2) To exert pressure in bleeding.
3) To exert pressure in varicose veins.
4) To give support to cases of sprains.
5) To reduce swelling in sprains.
6) To hold splints in fracture treatment.
7) To help correcting deformity.
8) To build up warmth.

Material used in roller bandage are:

1) Cotton.
2) Calico.
3) Domette.
4) Muslin.
5) Crepe velpeau.
6) Elastoplast.
7) Rubber.

Patterns of roller bandaging are:

1) By circular turn.
2) By spiral turn.
3) By reverse spiral turn.
4) By figure of eight turn.

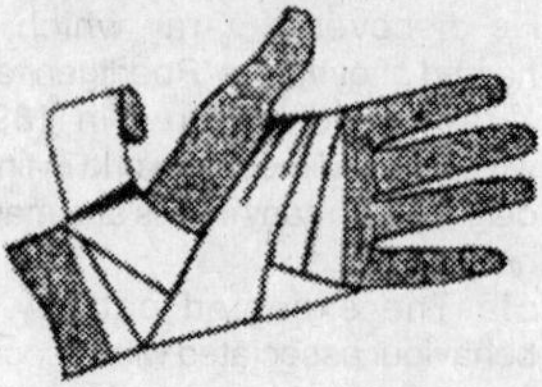

Roller bandage

Roller skating Roller skating has maintained a steady popularity in continent as required sports for physical fitness.

ROM evaluation This is under nursing assessment guideline when she assesses a patient for musculo-skeletal system by taking interview for subjective data, take vital signs and then evaluates the **R**ange **O**f **M**otion under the following heads:

1) Personal history.
2) Family history.
3) Occupation.
4) Activities of daily living.
5) exercises done.
6) Any assistive device used.
7) Any injury.
8) Any surgery.
9) Any medication.
10) Gait disorders.
11) Skeletal disorder.
12) Joint disorders.

ROM exercise ROM i.e. performing passive range of motion exercises are done to prevent contractures and ankylosis, is done in all cases of immobilisations

ROM is initiated by following motions:

a) Passive movement of all joints.
b) Active movement of all joints.
c) What is assisted range of motion is detected.
d) Abduction is done.
e) Adduction is done.
f) Extension is done.
g) Flexion is done.
h) Hyperextension is done.
i) Opposition is done.
j) Radial deviation is done.
k) Ulnar deviation is done.
l) Rotation is done.

Romberg sign It is done to test cerebellar function, Patient should stand still with his arms at his sides and his feet together when eyes are shut and also when eyes are opened.

Inference:

- When he has problem when eyes closed it is sensory ataxia.
- When he has problem when eyes closed and when eyes are opened it is cerebellar ataxia.
- Excessive swaying with eyes shot or opened is positive.
- Romberg's sign.

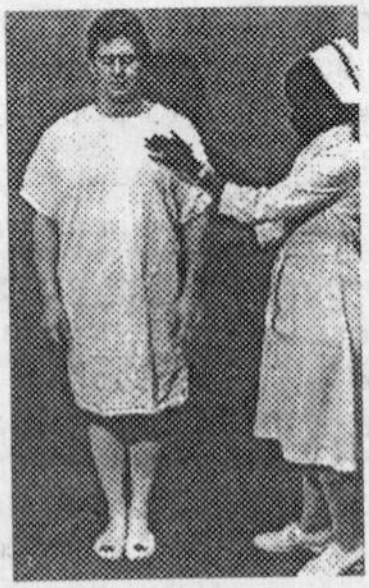

Romberg sign

- In tabes dorsalis, patient cannot stand erect without swaying if the eyes are closed.
- First described by Dr. Romberg a German physician.

Rooming in For mental stability, self-confidence and for early breast-feeding the baby is kept by the side of mother's bed. This is called 'Rooming-in'.

Root canal It is the pulp cavity in the root of teeth.

Rooting reflex Infant turns towards the finger to suck when cheek is stimulated by striking with finger.

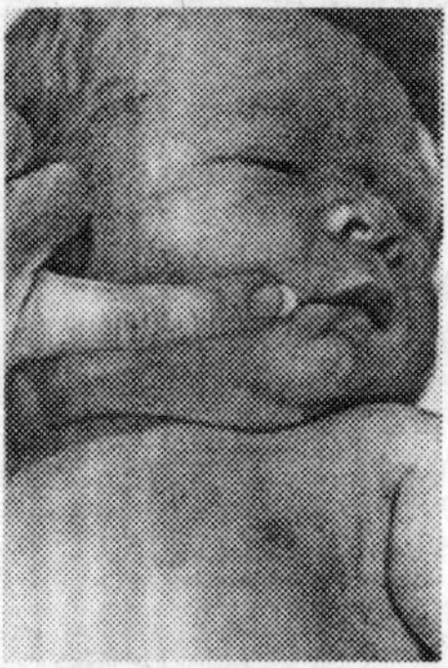

Rooting reflex

Rosacea Pimples on the face or acne rosacea,

Papules and pustules of sebaceous glands of the face which are often show hyperplasia of sebaceous glands.

Rose hips Rose seed or rose fruit is called rose hips,

They are used in pharmacy in their formulation,

They are promoted by food faddists.

Rosette A structure which resembles a rose or a small rose.

ROSLA **R**aising **O**f **S**chool **L**eaving **A**ge, Accepted normal programmes of study and examinations to allow to leave school early.

Rostellum Anterior end of scolex of tapeworm with hooks.

Rostrum Anatomical structure which resembles a beak,

An appendage or part of a structure which has beaklike shape.

Roth's spot One of the sign in subacute bacterial endocarditis where white spots which are minute in nature are seen in the retina,

Described by a Swiss physician.

Roto rest kinetic treatment table To produce continuous lateral rotation this table is used which helps in enhancing pulmonary blood flow, It is an automatic turning table that rotates every 3 minutes to achieve 60^0 lateral angle.

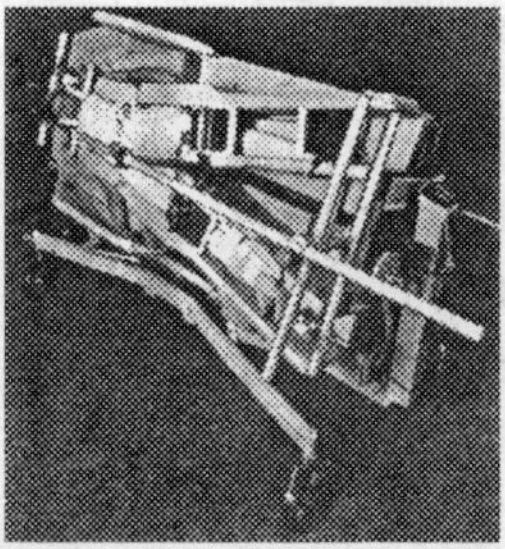

Roto rest kinetic treatment table

Roughage Dietary bulk by fibres and cellulose.

Rouleau When RBC pile on each other a rounded formation is seen in blood.

Round ligament Cord like anatomical structure from uterus into the broad ligament which run through inguinal canal to end in labia majora as soft tissue.

Roundworm Common nematode in developing countries which is colloquially called as *roundworm.*

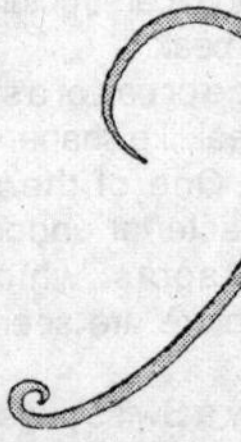

Roundworm male

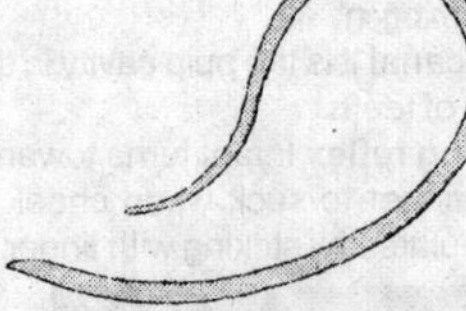

Roundworm female

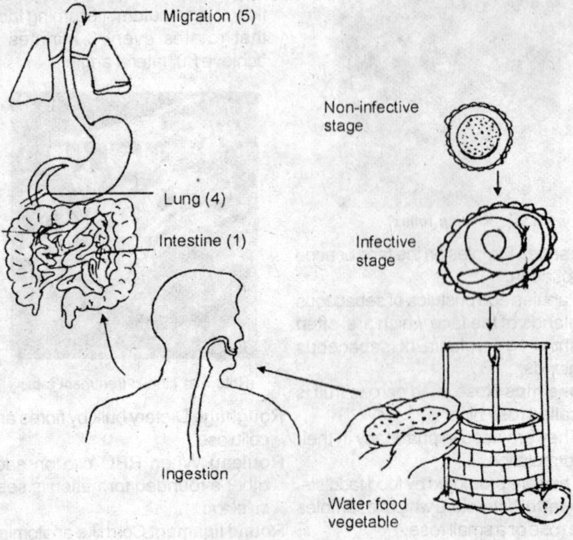

Life cycle of roundworm

Roundworm One of the common nematode which infest mostly children and also adults transmitted by the ingestion of contaminated food.

Rovsing's test This sign is positive if patient gets pain in right iliac fossa when surgeon presses in left iliac fossa.

Rowing Rowing with or without canoeing, sailing provide vigorous outdoor exercise.

Rubefacient Agent or drug which causes redness of skin, Turpentine liniment is a rubefacient.

Rubella It is German measles, colloquially called one day measles.

Rubeola Red measles, colloquially called 5 day measles.

Rugae It means folds or rugae (plural form of ruga).

Ruga Singular form of Rugae which means fold.

Rule of half World Health Organisation has noted that proportion of adequately treated for hypertension is only 10-12%. It is depicted by *rule of half*.

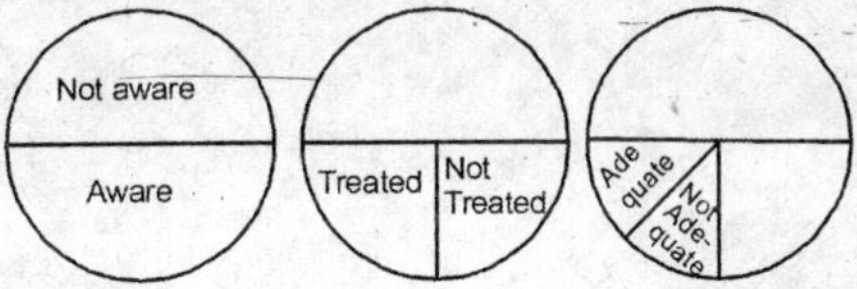

Rule of half

Rule of nine In the management of burns body surface area is calculated with the help of formula as under:

Head	9%
Front of the trunk	18%
Back of the trunk	18%
Left leg	9%
Right leg	9%
Left hand	9%
Right hand	9%
Perineum	1%

Rules of bandaging Following are the rules for bandaging in nursing care:

A. Nurse should stand in front of patient on the side of bandaging
B. Part to be bandaged should be in a long static position such as elbow in flexed position etc.,
C. Both hands are used for interchanging at bandaging
D. Outer side of roller bandage should be placed against the part
E. Oblique turn should be downwards for good secure
F. bandage must be fully and firmly rolled before unrolling
G. One should work within outwards on the limbs
H. Turns must be parallel to each other
I. To remove the bandage one has to roll it at removal
J. Skin surface needs putting cotton wool before bandaging
K. Wool dressing is used in axilla and groin before bandaging
L. Wet bandaging is avoided in nursing bandaging

M Recommended width are as under:

• Thumb	2.5 cm.
• Fingers	2.5 cm.
• Hand	5 cm.
• Head	5 cm.
• Foot	5 cm.
• Forearm	5 cm.
• Leg	10 cm.
• Thigh	10 cm.
• Upper arm	10 cm.
• Breast	10 cm.
• Spica of shoulder	10 cm.
• Axilla	15 cm.
• Trunk	15 cm.

Rum convulsion Convulsion occurring among drunkards as withdrawal symptom.

Rumination Cows regurgitate gross. eaten, chews again and then swallows again,

It also refers to recurring thoughts.

Rump Colloquial name for buttocks.

Rupia Bullae or vesicles of syphilis which looks like filth,

Gangrenous skin changes.

Rupture Refers to rupture of an organ by injury, of amniotic membrane at labour.

Ruptured ear drum Loud explosion and severe blow on external ear causes rupture of ear drum, Symptoms are bleeding from ear and sudden deafness,

Nurse should be careful to observe history of head injury where fracture of base of skull may be there and should look for watery discharge from ear after a head injury (which also has rupture of ear drum).

Russel body They are spherical hyaline bodies seen in tissue growth such as inflammatory growth, cancerous growth.

Rye It is a cereal used in beverages.

Ryle's tube Used for th withdrawal of gastric contents and used for administ ration of fluids,

Stomach tube developed by Dr.Ryle a British Physician.

S

Sabatier's suture A surgical method in which approximation of the intestinal wound is effected by means of a piece of cardboard saturated with turpentine oil.

Sabin vaccine Live oral attenuated polio vaccine discovered by Dr. Sabin.

Saccharide Sugars under carbohydrate carbohydrate series items, Types are mono, di, tri and polysaccharides $C_6H_{10}O_5$ do compose saccharides.

Saccharin Substitute for sucrose in obesity and diabetes, chemically it is o-toluene sulphonamide, used in circulation time detection, $C_6H_4.CO.NH.SO_2$.

Saccharine One which has sugary taste.

Saccular That which resembles a sac

Saccule A minute sac small sac or small bag like structure.

Sac Small bag or a pouch like dural sac, abdominal sac.

Sacral related to sacrum.

Sacralisation Transverse process of 5th lumbar vertebra is seen as part of sacrum.

Sacroiliac Related to both sacrum and ileum.

Sacrovertebral angle Fifth lumbar vertebra and base of sacrum produce this angle.

Sacrum Made of 5 united sacral vertebras, back of pelvis.

Saddle nose Leprosy nose, syphilitic nose where cartilage is absent.

Saddle It is an artificial denture base structure specifically one section.

Sadism Sexual perversion where pleasure by inflicting physical and mental pain.

Sagittal Mean arrow shape, refer to Sagittal suture between parietal bones.

Sago starch derived from plant belonging to genus sagus.

Sahli's test Test done to find out digestive power of stomach, determination of stomach acidity after one hour of medicinal soup (made from water, flour, butter and salt).

Saint Vitus' Dance Chorea popularly known after Sydenham, Sydenham's chorea, Neurological lesion with purposeless involuntary movements.

Salicylate Salt of salicylic acid, antipyretic, analgesic, antirheumatic

Salicylic acid Bacteriostatic in skin infection helps in wart and corn removal.

Saline Sodium chloride and water solution, types are normal, hypertonic and hypotonic.

Saliva secretion of salivary gland clear alkaline viscid secretion of salivary glands for initial digestion.

Salivary glands They are six in number and are located three on each side of the mouth, they secrete the saliva which moistens the food during chewing and begins the digestive process.

Salivary Related to saliva of mouth.

Salk vaccine Killed viral polio vaccine given by injection, discovered by Dr. Salk.

Salmonella Organism responsible for causing typhoid and Paratyphoid, Typhoid fever causing bacteria.

Salpingitis Fallopian tube infection and inflammation.

Salpingo-oophorectomy Surgical removal of fallopian tube and ovary.

Salpinx Fallopian tube, Eustachian tube.

Salt Common salt, NaCl, any compound of a base as acid.

Salve Salve is a thick ointment.

Sample size In research we restrict to a sample from that of a population which is representation of whole population and which is the size of the sample for the study.

Sample Selected small group in the study which can give idea of a large group or a universe.

Sampling Method of selection of the sample for the study like simple, stratified, multistage.

Sanatorium Special hospital which is in isolated place for the treatment of tuberculosis patients.

Sanitarium Old name for instituion for the promotion of health, different from mental and TB hospital (coined by the seventh day Adventists at Battle Creek, Michigan).

Sand fly fever An arboviral infection transmitted by sand fly.

Sand fly Insect which transmits sand fly fever, phlebotomus insect.

Sane Person who is mentally sound.

Sanguine Related with blood and blood substances.

Sanguineous That which contains blood.

Sanitary napkin Perineal pad used by women during menstruation to avoid soiling their cloth or robes.

Sanitary well A well dig or bore for water source must have certain criteria like distance from stable, good wall, a parapet, a platform, a drain covered from above and a pump set.

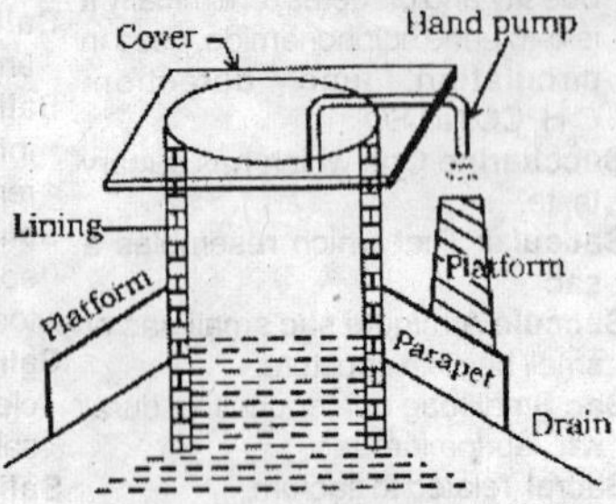

Sanitary well

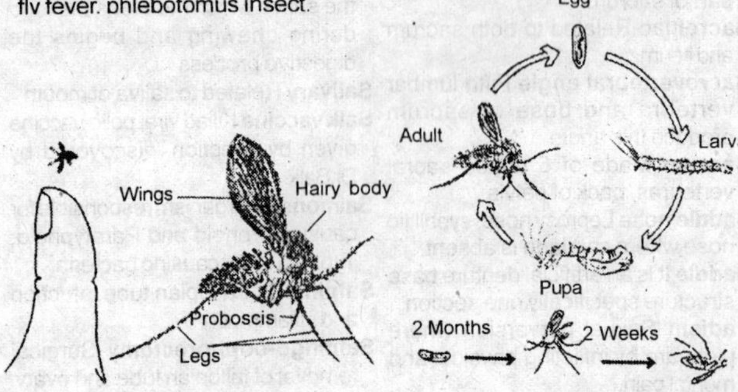

Sand fly

Sanitation Refer to sanitary disposal of solid waste, liquid waste and human excreta, include both personal and environment hygiene.

SAPEL **S**pecial **A**ction **P**rojects for **E**limination of **L**eprosy.

Saphenous Related with saphenous vein.

Saponification Soap formation, chemical action called hydrolysis of fat by alkali, Saponification produces glycerol and salts of fatty acid or soap, Ester is hydrolysed into an alcohol and an acid.

Sapremia It means rotten blood, septic intoxication by saprophytic bacteria.

Sarcocystis Animal disease caused by a parasite with lesion like bladder in internal organs, according to veterinary people sarcocystis of Cow's heart is common.

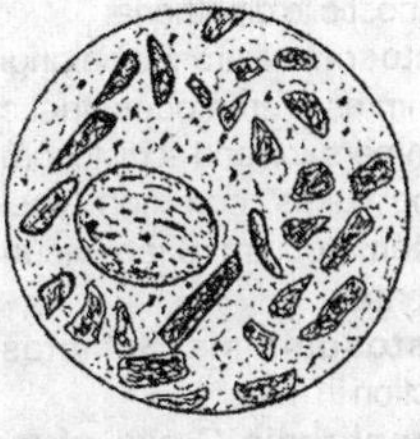

Sarcocystis in heart muscle

Sarcoid Non-caseating lesion, sarcoidosis.

Sarcoidosis Chronic progressive disease like tuberculosis affecting any organs.

Sarcoma Connective tissue cancer malignant tumour from bone, muscle or other organs of the body.

Sarcoptes scabiei Itch mite which cause scabiei or scabies.

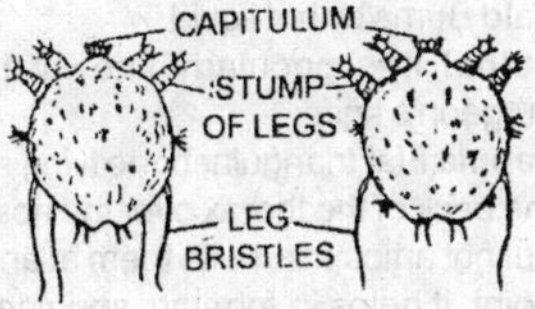

Itch mite

SAR Number of exposed persons developing the disease within the range of the incubation period following exposure to the primary case.

Sarsaparilla Plant from Mexico, its glycoside parillin is diuretic.

SARS **S**evere **A**cute **R**espiratory **S**yndrome.

Sartorius Long muscle of thigh.

Saturation Total dissolving of a substance in a liquid, after this any further addition will not increase the chemical concentration.

Saturday night palsy Radial nerve paralysis in alcoholics by nerve compression in their chair lying after drinks.

Saucerisation It is a surgical treatment of wound, tissue excavation to lay open the wound which allow shelving depression.

Scab Crust left after skin eruptive disorders, post-chickenpox scab.

Scabies Skin condition produced by the itch mite, indicative of poor personal hygiene.

Scalp Hairy skin that covers skull.

Scale An instrument used to measure.

Scalene Three sided structure, usually referred to scalenus muscle

Scalenus Muscle that move neck sideward, muscle that raise first two ribs during inspiration.

Scald Burns by hot liquid.

Scalpel It is popularly known as surgeon's knife.

Scapula Flat triangular bone lying at the back of the thorax over the ribs, but not articulating with them at any point, it helps in forming shoulder joint with arm bone, shoulder blade which help in the formation of shoulder girdle.

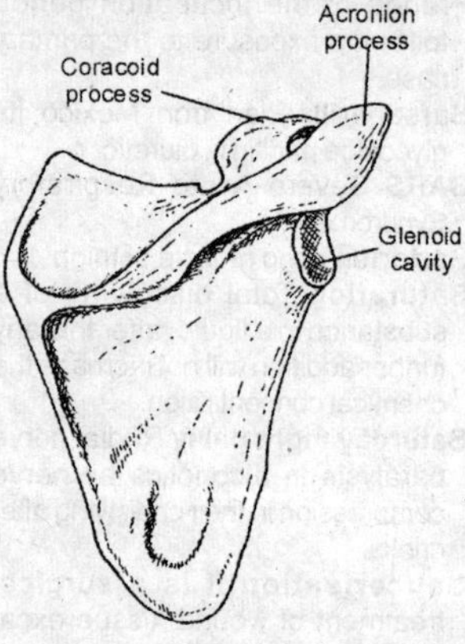

Scapula bone

Scan Moving detector produced image, sweep of radiation beam, Ultra-sonography, computed tomography.

Scanning Visual examination of anatomical area by a scan.

Scaphoid Boat-shaped wrist bone

Scar Mark followed by a wound or injury, repaired tissue.

Scarlet fever Group A beta haemolytic streptococcal infection of children.

Schafer's artificial respiration One method of artificial respiration, patient is placed prone on the ground with the head on one side and a pillow of folded coat under the upper part of the abdomen nurse kneels at the side of the patient, placing her hands with the fingers lying together on the patient's back over the lower ribs and the thumbs parallel to the vertebral column. Swinging forwards, the chest is compressed; swinging back the weight is taken off the hands allowing the chest to expand. This is repeated 16 times per minute.

Schick test Skin test done as diagnostic to diphtheria.

Schistosome Parasite belonging to helminths (trematodes) that cause swimmers itch and schistosomiasis, Blood flukes, common types are S.haematobium, S.japanicum and S.mansoni.

Schistosomiasis Schistosoma infection in man.

Schizophrenia Group of mental disorder with lowered mental function level, delusion, social withdrawal by the patient, speech defect and hallucinations, paranoid, catatonia.

Schuffner's dot Malaria infection causes minute granulation in RBC, vivax malaria infection manifestation.

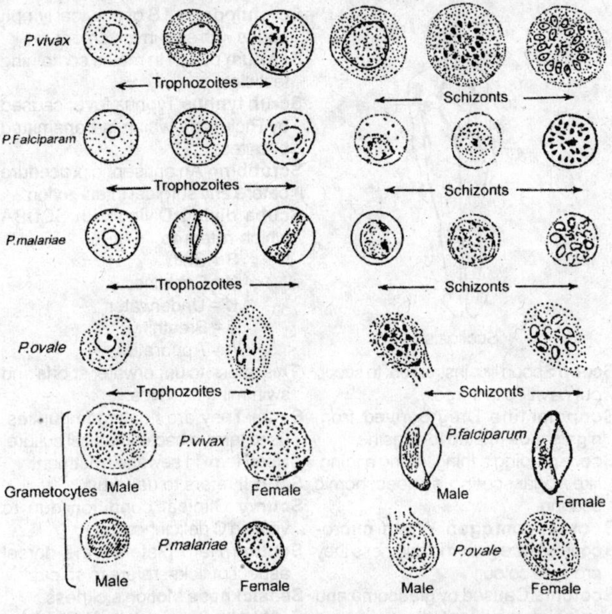

Schuffner's dot

Schwann cell Precursor of neurilemma, these precursor cells are derived from ectoderm.

Sciatica Pressure on sciatic nerve causing run down pain of leg which are supplied by sciatic nerve.

Scissors Cutting instrument in surgery with two blades.

Sclera White of the eye which joins cornea in front.

Scleroderma Clinical condition with progressive hardening of the skin, Chronic condition called Raynaud's phenomenon.

Sclerosis Connective tissue and fibrous tissue are overgrown giving the condition of hardening of tissue or organ of part of body. Types are:

- Disseminated sclerosis.
- Multiple sclerosis.
- Amyotrophic lateral sclerosis.
- Systemic sclerosis.
- Hardening of tissue, a scar.

Sclerotic Part which is affected by sclerosis.

Scolio One which has twisted look, a crooked look.

Scoliosis Lateral deviation of spinal column lateral curvature of the spine which does not resolve as patient bends forward, structural changes in spinal column.

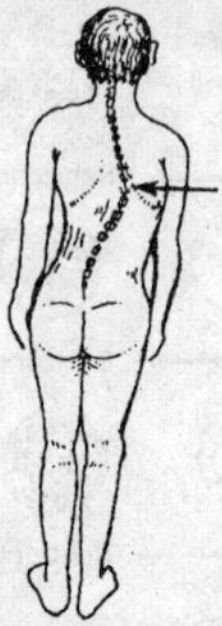

Scoliosis

Scoop Spoon like instrument to scoop out cavities in surgery.

Scopolamine Drug derived from nightshade related to atropine.

Score grading a thing, rating a thing, like Apgar scoring, socioeconomic scoring.

Scotochromogen When micro-oganism are grown in darkness they produce colour.

Scotoma Caused by glaucoma and retinal detachment, there will be a blind area of vision.

Scratch test It is the test for allergen in allergy patients, the substance in question is placed on a scratch made and observed for change, Development of wheal within 15 minutes indicate allergy.

Screening Not a diagnostic test, a community based large scale test for finding out prevalence of a condition, a procedure for health check up camps rapid superficial clinical and lab examination to find out the ill and further to allow specific diagnostic tests for confirmation, Help to find out sensitivity and specificity of a test.

Scrofuloderm TB of cervical lymph nodes with skin involvement.

Scrotum pouch In males containing testicles.

Scrub typhus Typhus fever caused by Rickettsia which is transmitted by mites.

Scrubbing An antiseptic procedure before any surgical intervention.

Scuba diving Diving with SCUBA which refers to:

S = Self.
C = Contained.
U = Underwater.
B = Breathing.
A = Apparatus.

This refers to underwater sports and swimming activities.

Scum They are floating impurities, used term in bacteriological culture, Used term in sewage treatment.

Scurf It refers to dandruff.

Scurvy Clinical condition due to vitamin C deficiency.

Scutum Hard plate on the dorsal aspect of ticks, refers to shield.

Seasickness Motion sickness.

Seat belts Belts installed in the front seat of cars, it will reduce the number of fatalities and severity of injury in road accidents.

Sebaceous Related with sebum, sebaceous cyst, sebaceous gland.

Seborrhoea Hypersecretion of sebaceous glands which leave greasy plugs on body which cause itching and burning.

Sebum Oily secretion of sebaceous glands.

Secondary Having second importance, secondary level, secondary prevention.

Secretin Which stimulates the secretion of pancreatic juice, secreted in duodenum.

Secretions Products of glands or glandular organs, of both exocrine and endocrine glands.

Sedation Help in sleep by drugs by allying the irritability.

Sedative Drug which produce calmness and sleep inducing drug that cause lowered excitement of a person, sleep inducing.

Sedentary Low profile of physical activity of a person, indicate insufficient physical activity.

Sedimentation The act of settlement of deposits in a liquid, centrifuge machine helps in sedimentation.

Seed Mature ovum, mature sperm, platinum shell in radiation therapy.

SE Variability measure to detect the standard error of the difference between two means.

$$\text{S.E.} = \sqrt{\frac{SD^2}{n}} \; or \; \sqrt{\frac{pq}{n}}$$

S.E. of the difference between 2 means

$$= \sqrt{\frac{SD_1^2}{n_1} + \frac{SD_2^2}{n_2}}$$

S.E. of the difference between 2 proportions

$$= \sqrt{\frac{p_1 q_1}{n_1} + \frac{p_2 q_2}{n_2}}$$

Segmental transfer technique Technique to move the patient from the stretcher to the bed, assisting the transfer of patient by asking patient to move onto the bed from stretcher by employing segmental transfer technique.

Seizures Epilepsy or fits, nursing protective device inclues padded tongue blade and soft seizure helmet.

Selene Moon-shaped structure, lunula of the nail.

Self-care performed act by the patient like taking bath, attending to toilet, having personal independence in his or her care at hospital.

Self-examination A procedure for early detection of cases where patient or a person does his body organ examination in a systematic way as told by a doctor or nurse, self-examination of breast, self examination of testes.

Self Antigenic constituent of a person, complete well being in terms of personality.

Sella turcica Anatomical position of pituitary body in sphenoid bone depression.

Semeiography Graphics which describe the signs and symptoms of a disease.

Semeiotic Refers to pathognomonic.

Semeiotics In medicine it refers to symptomatology.

Semen seminal fluid ejaculated during intercourse.

Semenuria Presence of semen in the urine.

Semicircular Anatomical structure formed with half arch, semicircular canal of internal ear.

Semicomatose Arousal of patient is possible in this stage.

Semilunar Half moon-shaped structure, semilunar cartilage, semilunar valve.

Seminoma Cancer of testes which respond to cobalt therapy.

Semiotics Signs in society for media and myths.

Semipermeable A permeable membrane which permits some selected substances.

Semiprone Lying face down with knees turning to one side.

Senescence It is natural process of becoming old.

Sengstaken Blakemore compression tube Used in the treatment of varicosity of varicose veins of oesophagus.

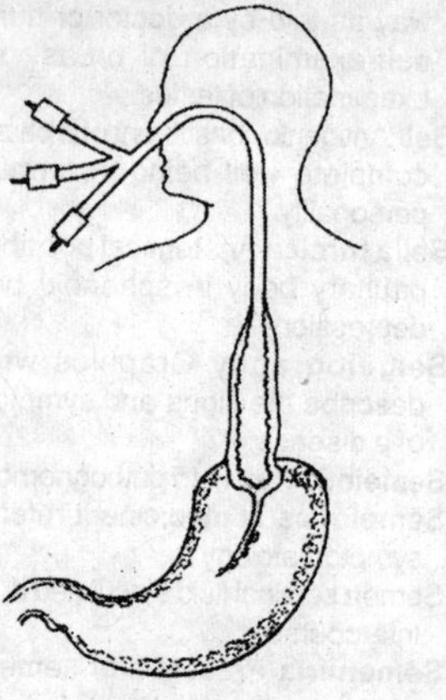

Sengstaken Blackmore compression tube

Senile dementia Loss of mental and emotional capacity through physical changes in the brain as a result of hardening of the arteries in the brain, or by its degeneration with age.

Senile Involuntary changes because of old age, senile dementia.

Senile Refers to old age.

Senior citizen Person who has attained the age of 65 years, categorised for the purpose of welfare activities.

Senna Cassia plant leaves that have cathartic effect, laxative.

Sensation Feeling felt by sensory nerve impulses.

Sense Physiological conditions which are perceivable in nature, pain sense, hunger sense, touch sense, pressure sense.

Sensitisation Increased susceptible to the exposure of certain foreign body exposure to foreign body produce body changes which when subsequently get exposed produce violent reaction in the body, commonly seen with protein, drug, chemicals.

Sensitivity One who respond to sensation, used term in screening test

Disease.

Test	+	–	
+ **a**	b	=	a + b
_ c	d	=	c + d
a + c	b + d	=	a + b + c + d

Sensitivity = a/ac × 100 which is True positive

Sensitivity formula

Sensory ataxia Trouble with maintaining balance only when his eyes are shut, patient has a loss of position sense referred to as sensory ataxia.

Sensory nerve Nerve which convey sensation from periphery to CNS in the body.

Sensory Related to sensation in our body.

Sentiment Emotional attitude towards others or even towards nonliving things.

Sepsis Infection by bacteria which leads to the formation of pus.

Septic tank Latrine is connected to septic tank when there is no sewerage system, sanitary method of disposal of night soil.

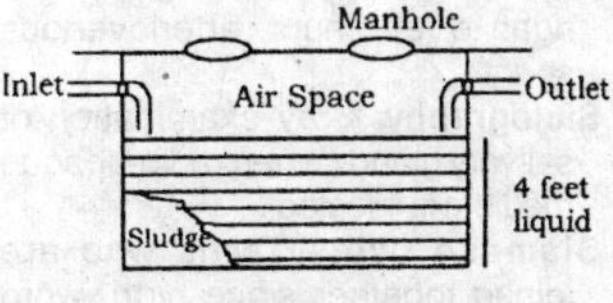

Septic tank

Septicaemia Bacteria and toxins are loaded in the blood which cause acute and emergency clinical condition.

Septum Septum of the nose, septum of the heart, partition wall between left and right side of heart or between two nostrils.

Sequela Clinical condition which occurs as a consequence of another illness lesion produced after the attack of a disease, after-effect of a disease.

Sequestrum Necrosed bony part called *dead bone* in a living bone.

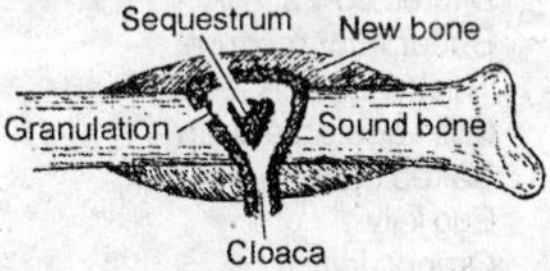

Sequestrum

Serological Anything which are related to serum, serological tests.

Serology Scientific study of serum of the body study of antigen antibody reaction for diagnosis of a disease.

Serosa Serous membrane which has two adjacent layers, visceral and parietal layers of serous membrane, lining of a cavity.

Serotonin It is a vasoconstrictor, produced from tryptophan, inactivated by monoamine oxidase,which is a platelet amine.

Serous Exudates of serum, serous exudates.

Serum Fluid residue of the blood which is devoid of cells and fibrin yellowish fluid of the blood which is left after the clot process; done in a test tube.

SET centre Survey Education Treatment unit under National Leprosy Elimination Campaign.

Sewage Liquid waste containing both liquid waste and human excreta.

Sex education The love of a husband and wife for each other and for their children is the very essence of good sex education, theme of sex education shall be sexual development, marriage, pregnancy love and affection in the community

Sex Gender of organism like male and female, reproductive act in nature, connected with sex organs of male and female.

Sexual dysfunction Sexual dissatisfaction by organic causes like no erection, no orgasm, painful intercourse.

Sexual Related to sex of both male and female.

Sexuality Male and female reproductive element which allow sexual attitude.

SGOT Serum **G**lutamic **O**xalacetic Transaminase, raised in M.I.

SGPT **S**erum **G**lutamic **P**yruvic **T**ransaminase, raised in I.H.

Shakes Refers to cold and fever, violent chills.

Shampoo Substance used in hair treatment, to reduce oily films, to treat dandruff.

Sheath Membranous covering of a muscle, of a structure, of an organ.

Sheepskin Sheepskin pad is used on the bed to help protect the patient's skin.

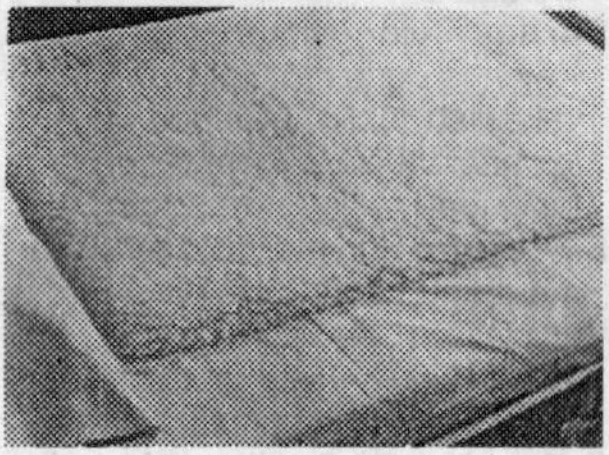

Sheep skin pad

Shegella Gram-negative bacteria which cause dysentery.

Shin Shin bone area, tibia bone area of lower leg.

Shingles Referred to herpes zoster infection.

Shirodkar's suture Surgical treatment for habitual abortion, purse string suture around cervix in incompetent cervix till 38 weeks of pregnancy.

Shock treatment Treatment of psychiatric patients by passing low voltage current, ECT or electro-convulsive therapy.

Shock Illness, trauma, bleeding, and extreme fear causes shock:

- Shell shock (warfare).
- Hypovolaemic shock.
- Allergic or anaphylactic shock.
- Cardiogenic shock.
- Neurogenic shock.

Shot One shot refers to one injection; also denote a dose of narcotic.

Shoulder Joining site of arm to the body, shoulder joint, junction of clavicle scapula and humerus.

Shunt Any diversion done to divert flow of liquid, common word in Cardiology like left to right shunt, right to left shunt, arteriovenous shunt.

Sialography X-ray examination of salivary glands when radio-opaque medium is injected .

Siamese twins Twins who are joined together since birth, word derived from Twins from Siam named Chang and Eng.

Sibling Born to same parents in a family, brothers, sisters.

Siccus Word meaning dry.

Sickle cell anaemia An inherited blood disease with anaemia.

Sickness Deviation from normal physiological state, an attack of illness an episode of sickness.

Sickroom cookery Food for invalids made best by quality, cooked in simple and digestible way.

Common sickroom cookery
Barley water
Diluted cow's milk
Butter flour mixture
Thickened milk feed
Milk vegetable soup
Baked custard
Egg jelly
Orange jelly
Bread and butter pudding
Scrambled eggs
High protein drinks

Side splint method Treatment of fracture of femur with well padded splint between the limbs extending from groin to the feet.

Siderosis Chronic inflammation of tissue by the deposit and reaction by iron dust particles or iron vapour.

SADS **S**easonal **A**ffective **D**isorder **S**yndrome, change in mood and feelings.

SIFT **S**emen **I**ntra **F**allopian **T**ube Transfer, a treatment for infertility.

Sigh maneuver It has value in managing routine tracheostomy care patients, in suctioning, the patient with a tracheostomy, using sign maneuver lung is inflated, when highinflating of patient is needed this maneuver is used.

Sigma Greek letter commonly used in scientific field (18th Greek alphabet).

Sigmoid Shaped like Greek letter S or S, sigmoid colon S-shaped anatomical structure, bent like letter S, sigmoid colon.

Sign Objective manifestation of illness, signs that a doctor observe during his clinical examination elicited clinical evidence for the diagnosis of disease by the Clinician, as observed by doctor on examination.

Signal Direction or signal sent by the brain to lower nervous system to act for a given situation.

Silicosis One of the common pneumoconiosis caused by inhalation of silica dust, miners silicosis, quarry workers silicosis.

Sim's position Common gynaecological position which is semi-prone in nature for gynaecological examinations.

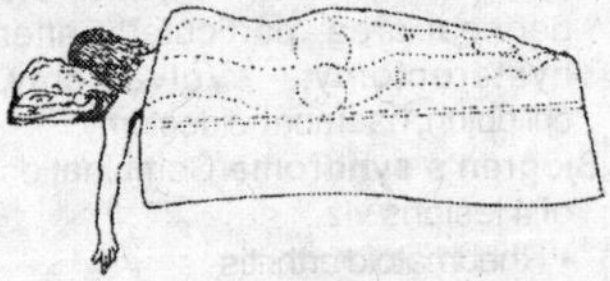

Sim's position

Simulium Black fly which transmits river blindness.

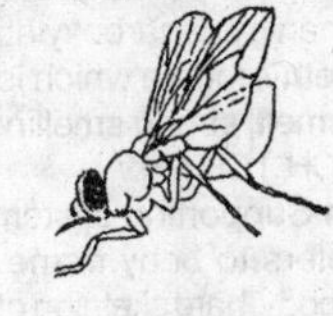

Black fly

Sinoatrial Refers to sinoatrial node the pace-maker of heart, anatomically in between sinus venosus and the atrium of the heart.

Sinus arrhythmia Condition in which the pulse quickens on inspiration and slows on expiration. It may be noticed in children and young people and is of no significance.

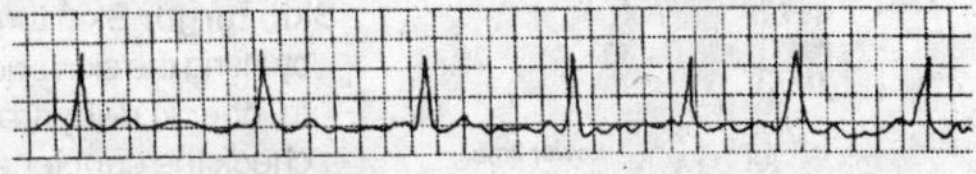

Sinus arrhythmia

Sinus Hollow space in the bone, cavity in bone, frontal sinus, maxillary Sinus, etc.

Sinusitis Infection and inflammation of sinus, frontal sinusitis.

Siphon Bent tube used to siphon liquid, tubes used in wound drainage.

Sitz bath It is prepared for patients who have vulvar pain and swelling and who require warmth to heal the perineal area; particularly after hysterectomy, vulvectomy, childbirth, haemorrhoidectomy.

Sjogren's syndrome Combination of 4 lesions viz.,
- Rheumatoid arthritis
- Xerostomia
- Keratoconjunctivitis sicca
- Parotid gland enlargement.

Skatole Decomposed protein from tryptophan by decarboxylation, it is Beta methyl indole which is strong faecal smell, strong smelling dung, $C_6H_4C(CH_3):CH.NH$.

Skeleton Supporting system of the body refers to bony framework of human body, hard skeleton of animal or human body, bony framework of higher animal.

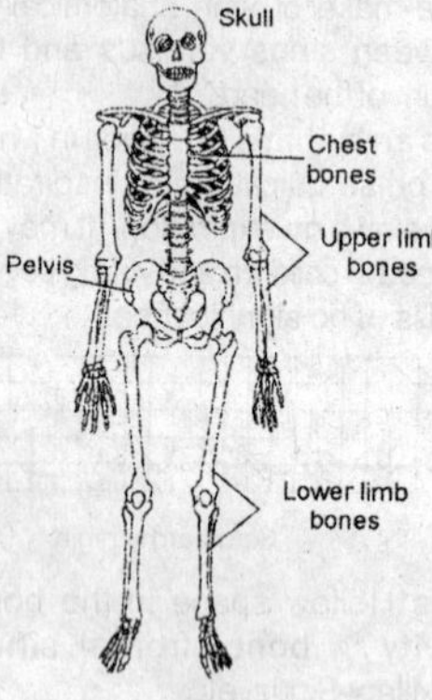

Skeleton

Skew One which is slant or asymmetrical, statistical word like skew to the right and skew to the left.

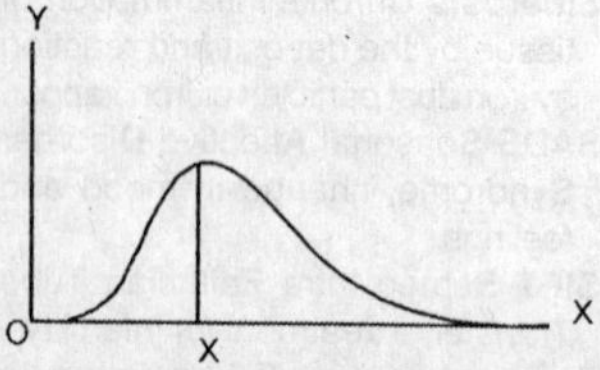

Positive skewness

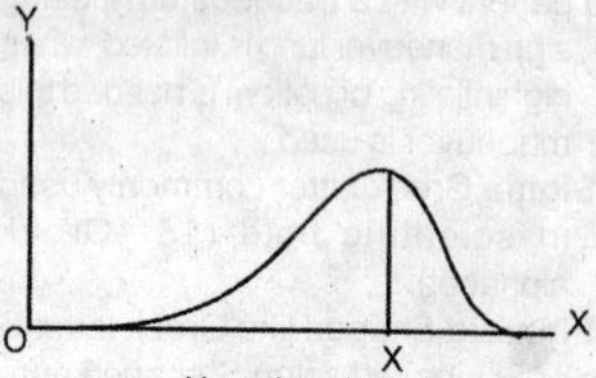

Nagative skewness

Skew to right and left

Skiametry Evaluation of refractory error of the eye by projecting beam of light into eye and observing illuminated reflection on retina, retinoscopy, shadow test.

Skin turgor Skin turgor is assessed by lifting the skin and leaving it back, to check dehydration states, to check the suppleness of the skin.

Skin Outer protecting cover of our body, true skin consists of epidermis inner dermis.

Skull Bony framework of head made of facial bones and cranium.

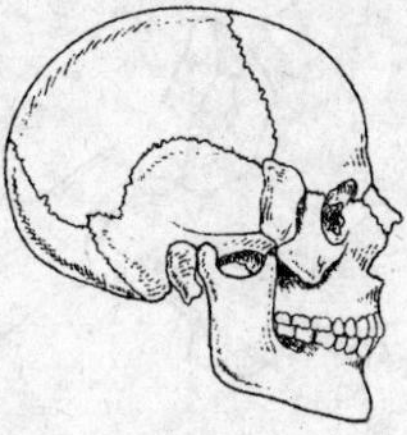

Skull

Sleep Mind and body taking rest constitute sleep, Types are:

NREM = Non Rapid Eye Movement sleep.
REM = Rapid Eye Movement sleep.

Sleeping sickness Trypanosoma infection transmitted by tsetse fly, a protozoal infection.

Slide projector One of the audio-visual aid in nursing teaching.

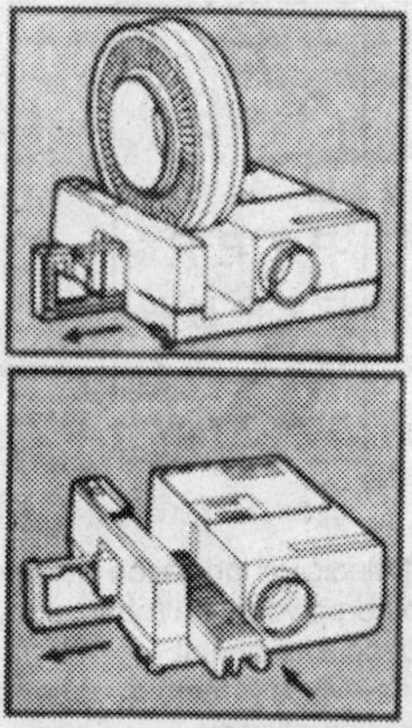

Slide projector

Slings They are triangular bandages used to support the forearm:

A = Clove hitch.
B = Narrow arm.
C = St.John.
D = Large arm.

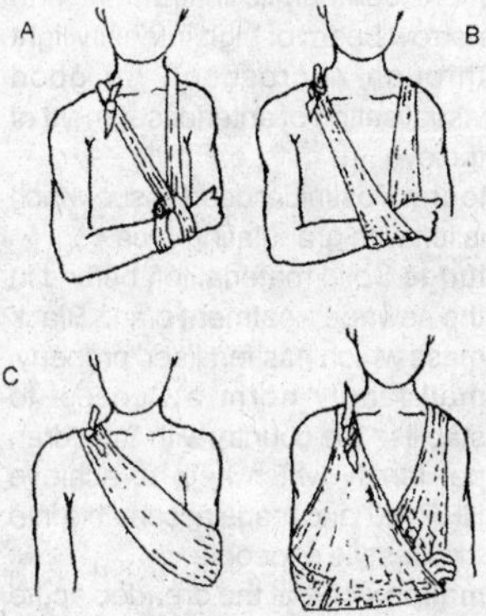

Arm slings

Sling psychrometer Mainly used to determine humidity of atmosphere, experiments from this also can give a) air temperature b)wind speed and c) absolute humidity.

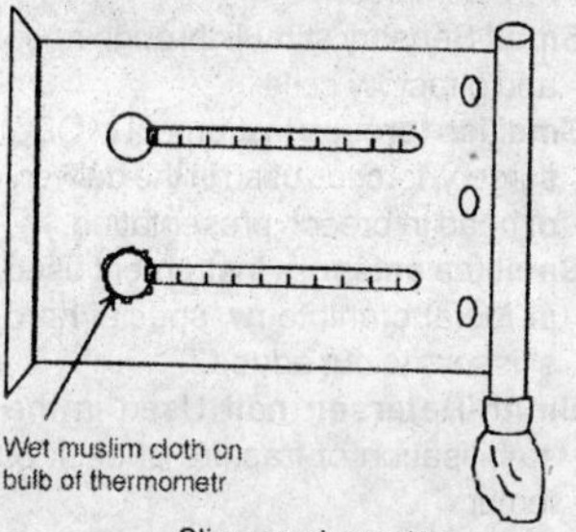

Sling psychrometer

Slipped disc prolapse of interverte-bral disc, spinal cord pressure by disc prolapse.

Slit lamp Microscopic examination of eye for in depth study of each layer by a special light source arrange-ment ophthalmic instrument with narrow beam of high intensity light through microscope for good visualisation of anterior segment of the eye.

Slough Postinjury dead tissue which is left with granulating area.

Sludge Solid material left behind in the sewage treatment plant, Black mass which has'fertiliser' property.

Small family norm a Concept to stabilise the country with 2 children per family which help to achieve NRR 1.0 and made acceptable into the lifestyle of people.

Smallpox one of the dreaded acute infectious disease of virus which is Totally Eradicated in the world.

Smear Thin film of smear on glass slide kept ready for microscopic examination.

Smegma Sebaceous glands secre-tion of prepuce in male and of clito-ris in females.

Smell Sensory stimuli through nose and olfactory cells.

Smellies forceps Instrument in OBG surgery, forceps used in the delivery of head in breech presentation.

Smellies scissors Instrument used in foetal craniotomy, special hard scissors to cut edges.

Smith-Patersen nail Used in the stabilisation of fracture of neck of femur.

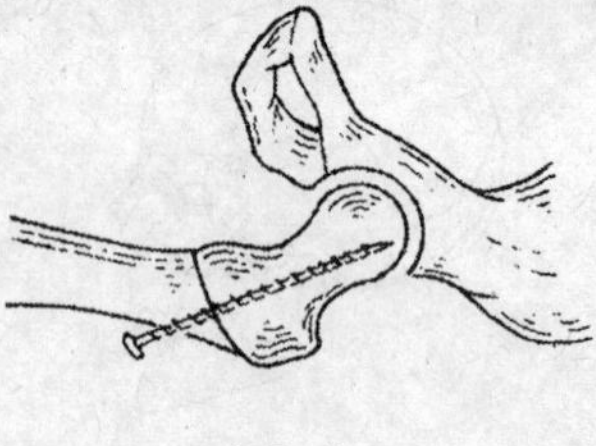

S. P.nail

Smoking Puffing out smoke of tobacco leaves powder in different forms beedi, cigarette, cigar.

Snake Reptile the serpents, types are poisonous and non-poisonous.

Snare A wire loop used to remove polyp or a tumour.

Sneeze Forcible expulsion of air from mouth and nose, involuntary audible expulsion of air from nose and mouth.

Snellen's chart Sight testing chart

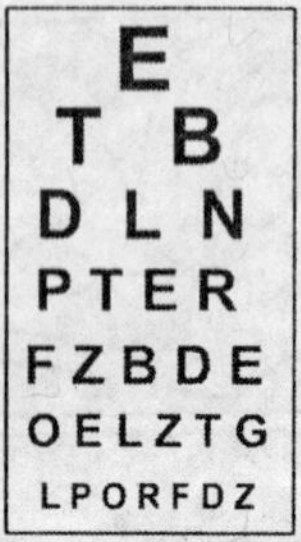

Snellen's chart

Snuff Medicinal inhalation into nose, errhine powder like tobacco snuff by people as a habit.

Snuffles Mucous membrane of nose becoming inflamed.

Soap It is a compound of fatty acids with alkali, a detergent.

Social action Direct or indirect interaction.

Social assistance Assistance to old age pension, widow pension, assistance to leprosy patients, old age homes, stipend for unemployed graduates, maternity assistance to the poor and senior citizen facility

Social benefit Financial benefit through states.

Social change Aspects of society move from one state to another.

Social class Hierarchical divisions of society by wealth, income and occupation.

Social closure monopoly of privileges and rewards for themselves.

Social construction Built up phenomenon by social process.

Social consumption Use of goods and services.

Social contract Utilitarian agreement in society.

Social control Social conformity to the dominant values and norms.

Social defence Like punishment of criminals, a ry Act, eradication of beggary, welfare of prisoner, alcohol prohibition, gambling control prostitution control and suicide counselling.

Social engineering Social change by social policy.

Social insurance Like ESI, crop insurance, accident insurance, insurance for health.

Social medicine It is the study of man as a social being in his total environment.

Social mobility Movement up and down the class structure.

Social order Regularities in social life.

Social policy Actions of government for the people.

Social problem Which produce negative effect on man.

Social problems No compliance to the given social norms like alcoholism, drug abuse, STD, Juvenile delinquency, prostitution, violent criminals, unmarried mothers, and physically challenged.

Social science Sociology, psychology economics and politics.

Social security System of welfare support.

Social status Honour or prestige given by members of society.

Social survey Systematic collection of information on population

Social system Patterned regularities and relationships in society.

Social trend Data by national statistics for sociologists.

Social worker One who identifies social aspect of disease, helps in social therapy and counselling.

Socialisation learning values, ideas, practices and roles of society adaptation of person with other members of the society, getting along with other is learnt by man.

Society The social totality of all the relationships in a given space.

Sociobiology Approach to human conduct by biological imperatives.

Sociometry technique of determining and identifying good respondents.

Sociology Study of human social relationships and organisation.

Sociogram Moreno method for information on how the members feel about each other, mapping of cooperation or non-cooperation of group.

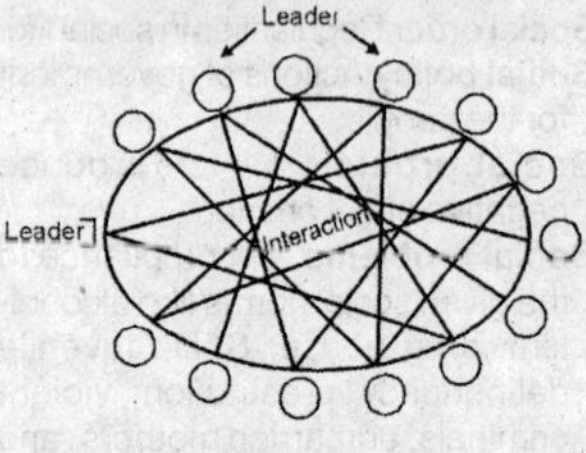

Sociogram

Sociopath Antisocial character of a person, similar to psychopath.

Socket Anatomically a socket into which a correspondence part fits.

Soda Baking soda, sodium bicarbonate.

Other terms of soda include:

Caustic soda = sodium hydroxide

Washing soda = sodium carbonate

Chlorinated soda = sodium chloride + sodium hypochlorite.

Sodium bicarbonate It is baking soda.

Sodium chloride Ordinary table salt, cooking salt, sea water salt commercially available

Sodomy A sexual perversion, sexual contact between animals and humans.

Soft palate Posterior portion of roof of mouth.

Soft sore One of the sexually transmitted disease by Ducrey bacteria.

Solar energy Heat from sun which is used in the production of fuel like electricity.

Solar plexus Nerve supply of abdominal organs below diaphragm, it is celiac plexus.

Solarisation Exposure to sun light and thereby its effect.

Sole Bottom of the foot.

Solid Substance which is not liquid or gaseous.

Saline rectal infusion Rectal administration of normal saline or water is a method of supplementing the fluid intake when the patient is unable to drink by mouth, 5% glucose can be added.

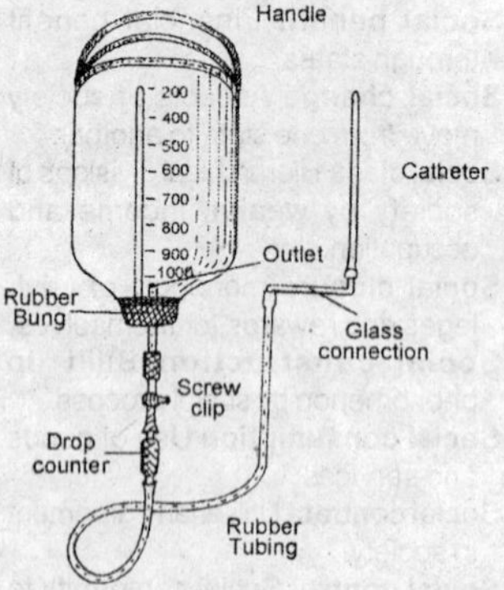

Apparatus for rectal infusion (enema)

Soluble If one can dissolve a substance in liquid, water soluble, fat soluble.

Solution Is a liquid in which given substance gets dissolved.

Solvent Power of dissolve of a liquid.

Solvent Water, alcohol and oil which are capable of dissolving other substances.

Somatic death A state where the body no longer can function for the living being, has irreversible unconsciousness.

Somatic Related with human body.

Somnambulism Carrying out activities during sleep habitual walk in the sleep, hypnotic state with full control but no recollection of any happening.

Somogyi effect Over treatment of diabetic patients with insulin induces hypoglycaemia which in turn result in rebound hyperglycaemia and ketosis.

Sone Unit of expression of loudness.

Sorbitol It is an alcohol, it is a type of sugar solution used in the treatment of patients who sweat a lot.

Sore throat Infection and inflammation of larynx, pharynx and tonsil.

Sore An open skin lesion like ulcer infection or inflammatory lesion of skin or mucous membrane, bed sore, oriental sore.

Soufflé Auscultatory finding where a blowing sound is heard, uterine soufflé.

Sound Probe like instrument to explore cavity, to dilate the stricture, sensory perception by the ear when a sound wave is or certain vibration have occurred, vibration in sound heard by ears.

Soya Chinese bean, high protein legume with little starch

Space medicine Branch of medicine which deals with pathology of aeronautics, Body changes of man in the space both physiological and pathological.

Spanish windlass In case of use of Thomas splint for fracture of any bone of lower limb, additional extension to the limb is obtained by means of Spanish windlass which is simply a skewer or piece of wood passed down between the extension bands of the clove hitch and twisted

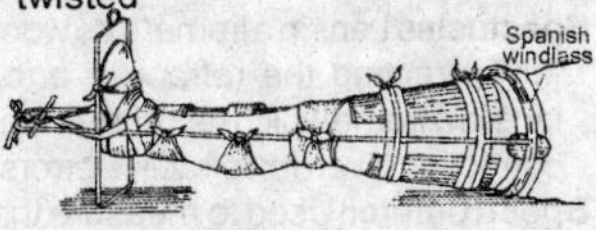

Spanish windlass

Spasm Sudden involuntary muscular contraction, types are:
- Tonic spasm.
- Carpopedal spasm.
- Clonic spasm.
- Nictitating spasm.
- Titanic spasm.

Spastic Cerebral lesion causing spasm or spasticity

Spatula Blunt blade used to spread ointment while preparing instrument used in the preparation of ointment and in spreading plasters, *flat bluht and knife like instrument*

Specific gravity The weight of a substance compared with that of an equal volume of another substance taken as a standard

Specific Meaning very relevant, specific gravity, specific drug in treatment

Specificity Quality of being specific, used term in screening test

Test	Disease +	Disease −	
+	a	b	= a + b
−	c	**d**	= c + d
	a + c	**b + d**	= a + b+ c+ d

specificity = d/bd x 100 = True negative

Diag: Formula for specificity

Specimen Collection of sample for chemical or pathological examination.

Spectacles Lens in a frame to be worn for correcting the refractive error lens in a frame which help the vision, correction given for refractive errors.

Spectrometer Used to measure the strength and wavelength of electromagnetic radiations.

Spectrum Component of white light VIBGYOR, range of drug action on Pathogens.

Speculum Instruments for examination of a canal like vaginal canal or ear canal.

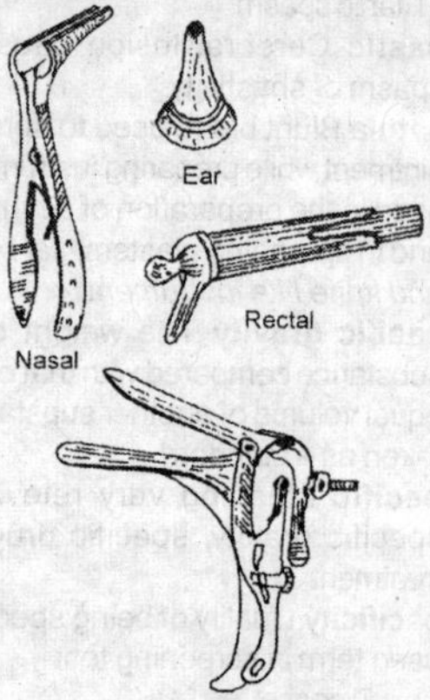

specula

Speech Use of linguistic code for communication by making sound of various pitch and loudness, types are:

- Explosive speech.
- Deaf speech.
- Clipped speech.
- Incoherent speech.
- Oesophageal speech.
- Staccato speech.

Spermatocele Swollen epididymis.

Sperm Meaning spermatozoon.

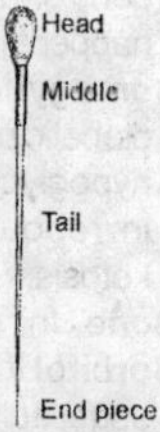

Sperm

Spermatocyte Mother cell of spermatid.

Spermatozoon Mature male germ cell, normal ejaculate contains 500 billion sperms.

Spermicide Agent used to kill sperms, contraceptives.

Spermine A chemical base from semen.

Sphenoid Wedge-shaped anatomically sphenoid bone with sinus located behind the nose in the centre of the head, a skull bone.

Sphere A structure which likes a globe.

Spherocytosis RBC shape is round as seen in acholuric jaundice and hereditary blood disorders.

Sphincter Circular muscle which can tighten an orifice small muscles surrounding certain parts of lumen which allow narrowing or widening of lumen, anal sphincter, oesophageal sphincter.

Sphincterectomy Surgical excision of a sphincter.

Sphygmogram Pulse recording, it has a primary elevation followed by fall and later with secondary elevation.

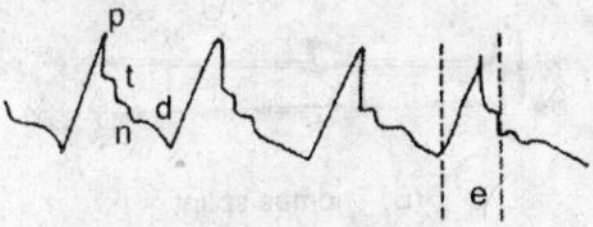

Sphygmogram

p = purcussion wave
t = tidal wave
n = aortic notch
d = dicrotic wave
e = period of semilunar valve opening.

Sphygmomanometer B.P. apparatus.

Spica bandage Used for joint where one part makes an angle with the other, bandage used in hip, shoulder and thumb.

Spica Figure of eight type bandage.

Spigot Small bung to close the opening of a tube.

Spina Thorn like projection of a bone.

Spinal cord Connecting big nerve of brain running downwards in the spinal column which contribute to the supply of peripheral nervous system.

Spinal Pertaining to spinal.

Spindle Fine threads radiating out from centrosomes, occurs in mitosis.

Spine Backbone vertebra.

Spinothalamic tract The spinothalamic tract transmits the sensations of pain, temperature, and crude touch, it can be assessed by checking sensory function using a dermatome chart.

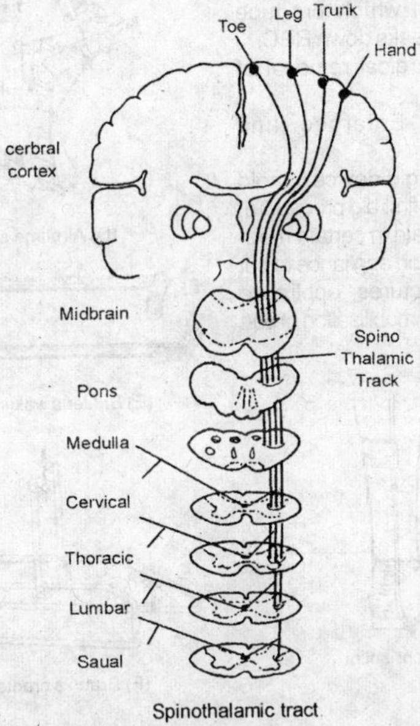

Spinothalamic tract

Spirillum Long motile spiral bacteria present in decaying organic matter.

Spirochete Coarse spiral micro-organism.

Spirochetes Spiral-shaped micro-organism, leptospira, treponema, borrelia.

Spirograph Graph representing respiratoy movements.

Spiro-meter Meter to measure air capacity of the lungs.

Spironolactone Drug used for promoting the excretion of sodium and water but not potassium.

Spleen rate Used in malaria measurement in the community, It is the percentage of children 2 to 10 years who show splenomegaly.

Spleen Large ductless organ in left hypochondrium which produce lymphocytes, breaks down RBC.

Splenectomy Surgical removal of spleen.

Splenomegaly Enlarged and palpable spleen.

Splint Hard and rigid device to hold broken bones as first aid procedure, Useful to ease pain in certain rheumatic diseases rigid appliance to put a safeguard fractures, appliance used in first aid, immobilisation of part of the body.

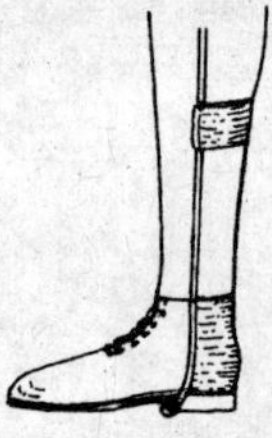

(A) Drop foot splint

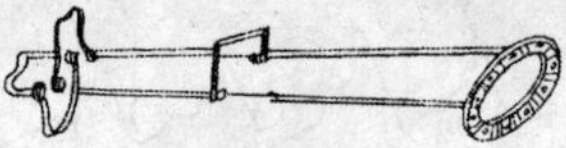

(B) Thomas splint

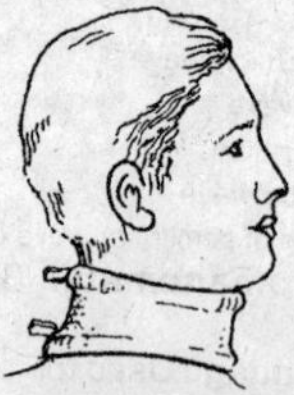

(C) Collar splint

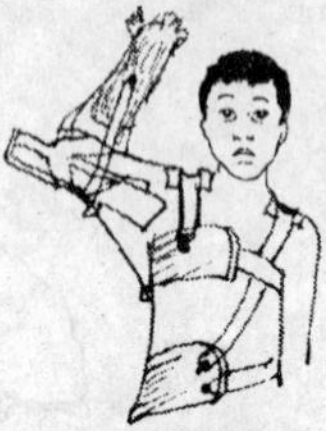

(D) Airplane splint

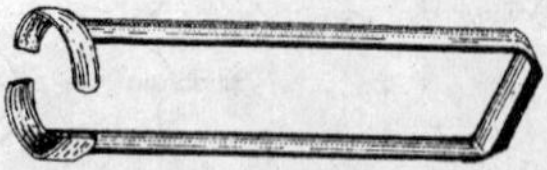

(E) Bohler's walking splint

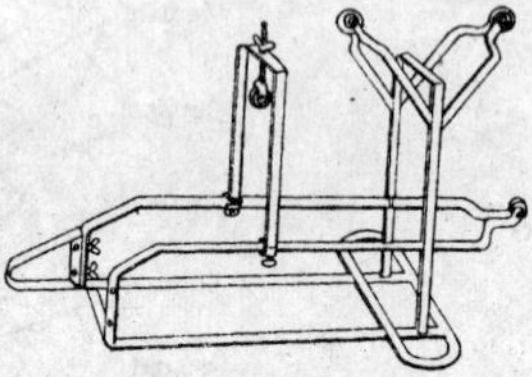

(F) Braun's cradle splint

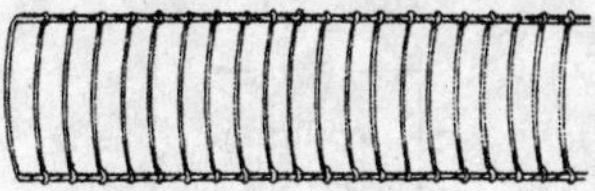

(G) Cramer's wire splint

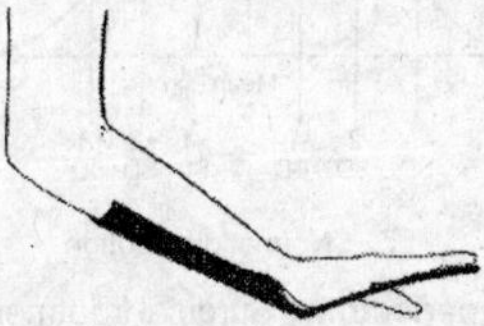

(H) Metal Cock up splint

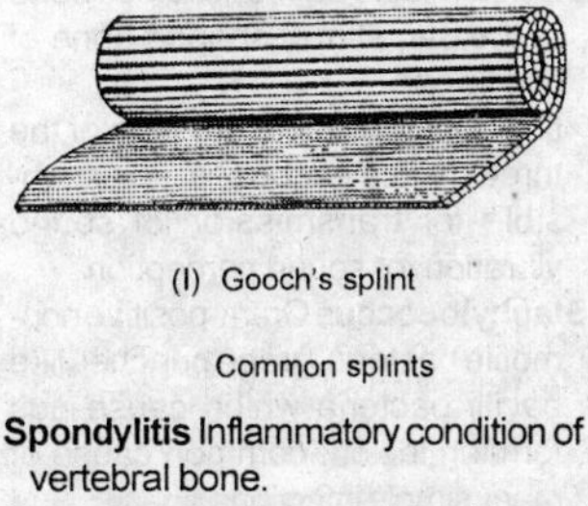

(I) Gooch's splint

Common splints

Spondylitis Inflammatory condition of vertebral bone.

Spondylosis Abnormal rigidity and ossification of vertebra, ankylosing spondylitis.

Sponge A cotton pad and gauze used for wound dressing which can absorb fluid and blood.

Sporadic Disease occurring in isolated places, cases here and there.

Spore Moulds, protective state of bacteria.

Spores Precursor or seed bodies of fungi, common cause of allergy.

Sporozoa One of the protozoal group which include plasmodia, toxoplasma and isospora organisms.

Sporozoite Infective form of malaria parasite.

Sports medicine Science that deals with sports injury treatment and improvements of sports training.

Spotted fever Fever with skin eruption, Rocky Mountain spotted fever, Tick borne rickettsial disease.

Spotting Blood discharge during no menstrual period or at the beginning of labour.

Sprain Tease of a ligament or an injury of a ligament around a joint, Sprain of ligament is associated with hair line fractures.

Sprengel's deformity it is a deformity where scapulae are usually small and located in the lower cervical and upper thoracic area causing the shoulders to be elevated.

Sprue Disease characterised by malabsorption, common features are Fatty loose motion, glossitis and anaemia.

Spore The reproductive element of lower animals.

SPS enema **S**odium **P**olystyrene **B**ulphonate enema is given to patients suffering from hyperkalaemia, Kayexalate enema.

Spur Projecting piece of a bone.

Sputum Phlegm liberated in lung and bronchi due to infection and inflammation.

Squamous Hard and scaly, Squamous cell.

Squeeze bottle Used in perineal care, use of squeeze bottle filled with tap water, Warm water at 100^0F for cleansing of perineum by postnatal mother.

Squint Deviated eye which looks abnormal, turned inwards or outwards are common which are called convergent squint and concomitant squint.

St.John method First aid method in the treatment of fracture of clavicle.

Staff of Aesculapius A rod or staff with a snake entwined around it which is a Representation of God of Medicine, It is the symbol of medicine and medical associations.

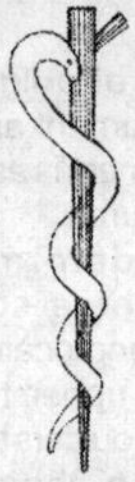

Staff of Aesculapius

Staging Refers to stages of a disease, cancer staging.

Stain Chemical, dye or reagent which is used to stain tissue for microscopic examination.

Stammering Speech disorder where words are uttered for a long duration.

Standard deviation (S D) It is a measure of dispersion.

$$S.D. = \sqrt{\frac{\sum (X - \bar{X})^2}{n-1}}$$

or

$$= \sqrt{\frac{\sum (X - \bar{X})^2}{n}}$$

Formula of S D

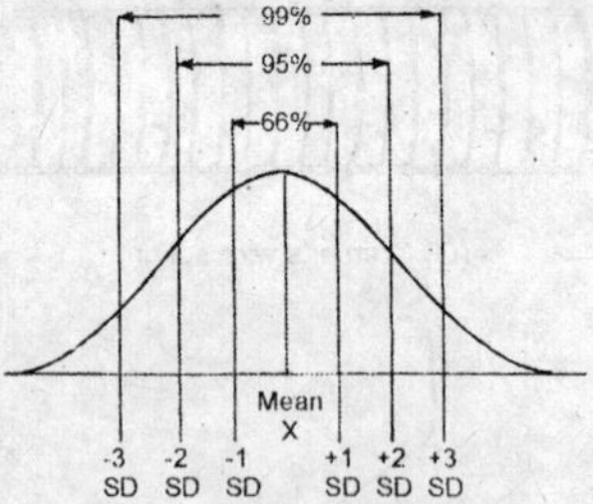

Normal distribution

Stapedectomy Surgical treatment of otosclerosis, removal of stapes and insertion of a graft.

Stapes Middle ear bone, small bone of the ear, stirrup-shaped bone of middle ear

tiny bone of middle ear, one of the three middle ear bones, is responsible for transmission of sound vibration for sound perception.

Staphylococcus Gram-positive nonmotile bacteria, grape bunches like bacilli bacteria which cause pus forming lesion, common cause of many simple infections.

Staphyloma Corneal protrusion due to injury of the eye.

Starch bath This is ordered as a soothing bath in eczematous skin conditions. It has 2 lb. of starch in 30 gallons of water.

Startle reflex Newborn will abduct and extend his arms when a loud noise is made, absence is indicative of a hearing loss or brain damage.

Stasis Stagnated movement of an item, stasis of vein and intestine are known.

Statistical significance Statistical test application to express that occurrence of a thing is by chance or not by chance, usually level of probability of 1 in 20, 1 in 100 and 1 in 1000 are considered which give P=0.05, P=0.01, P=0.001 ..and are expressed as Significant, highly significant and very highly significant respectively.

Statistics Science of collection, tabulation and analysis of numeral facts.

Status epilepticus In extreme cases of epilepsy there may be a sequence of convulsions without regaining consciousness, disease of CNS.

Status A described clinical condition, status asthmaticus, status epilepticus.

Statutory body Indian Nursing Council, Affiliated university, Board of studies which regulate the nursing education in India

STD **S**exually **T**ransmitted **D**iseases.

Steatoma Sebaceous cyst, a lipoma.

Steatorrhoea Malabsorption leading to fatty stool.

Stein Leventhal syndrome Polycystic ovaries with menstrual irregularities are associated with obesity, hirsutism and sterility.

Stellate Star-shaped item, expression given for fractures.

Stenosis Pathological narrowing of an orifice, mitral stenosis.

Stenson duct Parotid duct, duct from parotid gland to mouth opposite the second upper molar tooth.

Stent A device to be kept in a duct, tube or a canal to keep it patent, A surgical procedure of keeping steel or a plastic stent kept in an artery to keep it patent.

Stercobilin Bile derived pigment excreted in stool.

Sterile attire When a nurse is required to wear sterile attire for procedures in which surgical asepsis is necessary, wash hands, put on a hair cover, a facemask and then open the sterile gown to put on.

Sterile Free from pathogen, aseptic, also it means *no issues* any substance including live tissue when free from pathogens, not capable of procreating, infertile, free from contamination.

Sterilisation To render surgical dressings aseptic, family planning methods.

Steriliser An autoclave, instrument to sterilise linen and instruments.

Sterility Autoclaved material, woman without ovulation, man with azospermia infertility condition, incapable of procreating, condition of issueless.

Sterilisation Destruction of germs by heat, castration, vasectomy, tubectomy.

Sternum Breastbone, front bone of anterior wall of thorax.

Steroid Similar to cholesterol in their chemical nature, common steroids:

- Corticosteroids.
- Progesterone.
- Oestrogen.
- Androgen.

Sterol Steroid alcohol like ergosterol, cholesterol.

Stertorous Snoring in coma or in sleep.

Stethophone Instrument which transmits the sound of stethoscope which can be heard by many.

Stethoscope Instruments used by medical and nursing profession to hear or make audible of sounds with in the chest or abdomen.

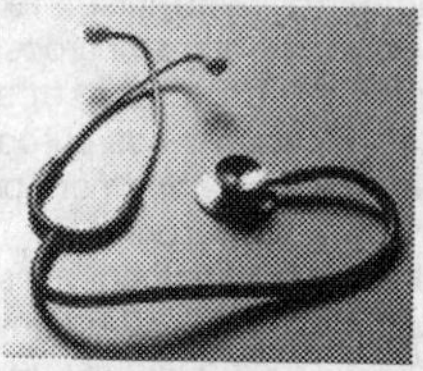

Stethoscope

Stevens-Johnson syndrome Erythema multiforme of oral and anogenital mucosa, eyes and viscera which produce constitutional symptoms.

STI Sexually **T**ransmitted **I**nfections.

Stigma spot or a dot on the skin.

Stilboestrol synthetic oestrogen used in cancer of prostate.

Still's disease Rheumatoid arthritis with lymphadenopathy.

Stillbirth Delivery of dead baby after its gestational age of 24 weeks.

Stimulant Any substance which influence the level of body activity, usually refers to a drug when it stimulates.

Stimuli It is a response of an organism to external stimuli, it is a goad to incite action, one which exert action of the other.

Stimulus Agent that influence functional change in a receptor.

Stitch Surgical suture, severe spasm of diaphragm.

Stoma care Care given in patients who have undergone colostomies and iliostomies.

Stoker's cramp In heat exhaustion if there is salt depletion there will be muscle cramps which is called stoker's cramp.

Stokes-Adams syndrome Syncopal attack by cerebral ischemia, effect of heart block.

Stoma Artificial opening made in surgical treatment with a tube of opening, colostomy, iliostomies.

Stomach Gaster, a dilated portion of intestine which accommodates food.

Stomatitis Inflammation of oral cavity, Types are:

- Angular stomatitis.
- Ulcerative stomatitis.
- Aphthous stomatitis.

infection and inflammation of the mouth or oral cavity.

Stomoxys Calcitrans Stable fly, leg sticker stable fly, annoying and disease transmitting.

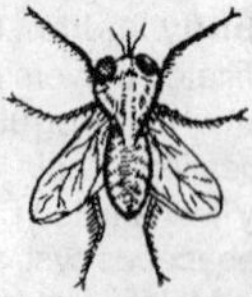

Stomoxys (stable fly)

Stone Name for a calculus.

Stool Digestive discharge from rectum in the form of faeces.

Strabismus Squint, heterotropia.

Strabismus Colloquially it is termed *crossed eye, wall eyes*, refers to squint inevitable deviation of eye which is a clinical condition, squint.

Strangulated Compressed and constricted hernia.

Strangulation Choking by air pipe compression, usually medicolegal.

Strapping Application of strips of adhesive plaster, one overlapping the other so as to cover a part and make pressure upon it.

Stratified When a thing is arranged in a layer, stratified epithelium.

Stratum lucidum epidermal layer which is translucent.

Stratum Layer covering the skin or mucous membrane.

Strep throat Sore throat caused by the infection of streptococci.

Streptococcus Gram-positive spherical bacilli which arrange in chain form.

Streptokinase Enzyme from streptococcus which is used to liquefy clotted blood.

Streptomycin Antibiotic drug used in the treatment of tuberculosis and other infections.

Stress Certain circumstances when a person is put under pressure which lead to his mental instability or mental illness, influences on emotion of an individual.

Stria Produced stripes, usually refers to strae gravidarum, singular , streak of a line

Striae Streaks or lines, bands of longitudinal fibres.

Striated muscle Voluntary muscles which are subject to control by human will.

Striated Striated, voluntary muscles.

Stricture narrowing of a canal, a duct or a passage.

Stridor Harsh vibrating sound due to laryngeal obstruction.

Strip Bressing the content of a canal by running finger along it, like as in urethra

Stroke Brain paralysis due to embolism which is sudden in onset, Cerebral haemorrhage.

Stroke Block, rupture or spasm of a brain artery which cause brain injury, Similar occurrence in the heart for heart stroke.

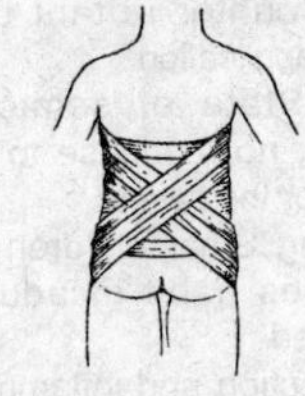

(A) Strapping dislocated disk

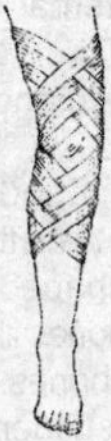

(B) Knee strapping

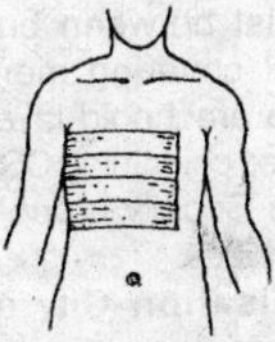

(C) Rib strapping

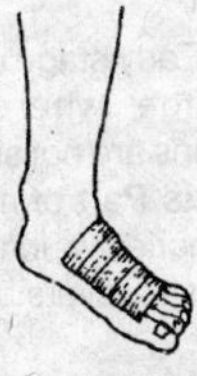

(D) Metatarsal strapping

Strapping

Stroma Ground substance of connective tissue, opposite of parenchyma.

Strongyloides Nematode worm which cause intestinal ulcer and diarrhoea.

Strontium Isotope used in bone scanning, used in radiotherapy for eye cancer and skin cancer.

Strophulus Infantile rashes like tooth rash and gum rash.

Strychnine Poisonous alkaloid, derived from nux vomica seed.

$$C_{21}H_{22}N_2O_2$$

Stryker wedge turning frame This frame in the patient's cot helps the nurse to change patients position from either prone to supine without disrupting alignment.

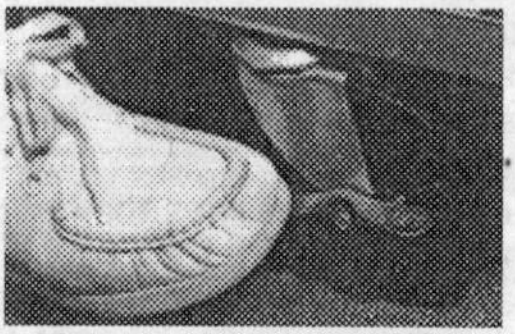

Stryker wedge turning frame

STS **S**erological **T**est for **S**yphilis.

Stump Distal part after amputation.

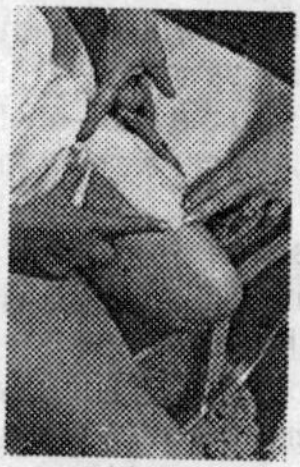

stump

Stupe Counter irritant used for topical application.

Stupor State of semiconsciousness, no response to external stimuli by the patient.

Stuttering Small children speech, becomes habit in adult if not corrected.

Stye Infection and inflammation of eyelash in eye eyelid, hardiolum, external or internal infection of hair follicle of eyelid.

Sty Sebaceous glands of eyelid are inflamed.

Styles of life Goods that people consume and taste that they exhibit.

Styloid Pen-shaped long pointed projection of bones like ulna, radium and temporal bones.

Subacute Not sudden and acute but slow in progression.

Subarachnoid Subarachnoid space which exist between brain and innermost covering membrane; Below the arachnoid layer of the brain, space containing CSF.

Subculture Society group sharing common values.

Suburbanisation City develop outlying districts.

Subclavian Structure below the clavicle.

Sub clinical Early stage of disease, illness stage where clinical manifestations are not seen.

Subconscious Part of mind which retains memories which cannot be taken out easily, reversible unconsciousness.

Subdural Below the dura mater of the brain, subdural haematoma.

Sub A suffix denoting below or moderate.

Subjective poverty Feels poor by comparisons.

Subjective Patient is aware of his symptoms, items related to individual.

Sublingual Below the tongue, floor of the mouth.

Subluxation Partial dislocation of a joint.

Submaxillary Below the lower jaw, submaxillary glands.

Sublimation Solid mass getting evaporated, an aspect of maturity by sublimation.

Sublimate Substance which is obtained by sublimation.

Submucous Below the mucous membrane, as in submucosal resection.

Subnormal Below normal, not average.

Subphrenic Below the diaphragm, subphrenic abscess.

Subscription It is the part of prescription which gives detail of directions for compounding medicine or chemicals.

Substance Substance is material out of which any body is made of.

Substitution To put one thing in place of the other, wet nursing replacement of one to the other, chemical replacement.

Substrate Enzyme acting upon a substance.

Suburbia City area where majority live.

Succussion Shaking patient to find out liquid in a cavity of his body.

Sucking reflex It is tested by keeping a finger in the neonatal mouth, one of care of the newborn.

Sucrose Table sugar, common sugar, a complex sugar it is a disaccharide, cane sugar, beet sugar,

$$C_{12}H_{22}O_{11}.$$

Suction Act of aspiration, act of sucking.

Suctioning airways Done in the care of the newborn, done in patients with tracheostomy.

Sudan A diazo compound, pigment brown, used to stain the fat.

Suet Internal fat of abdomen of sheep used in ointments.

Suffocation Cessation of breathing, asphyxia.

Sugar Saccharides under carbohydrate.

Suicide Committing ones own death by some means or the other, not homicide.

Suit Outer garment covering whole body.

Sulcus Fissures found on the brain which look like grooves.

Sulpha drug Originally derived from dye stuff, common chemotherapeutic agent in the use of infection by bacteria.

Sullage Liquid waste without human excreta.

Sulphone Drug used in the treatment of chronic disease leprosy, dapsone.

Sulphonylurea Oral hypoglycaemic agent for diabetes treatment.

Sum To be taken as a whole, to sum up.

Sump tubes Double lumen tubes used in lavage, gavage and decompression.

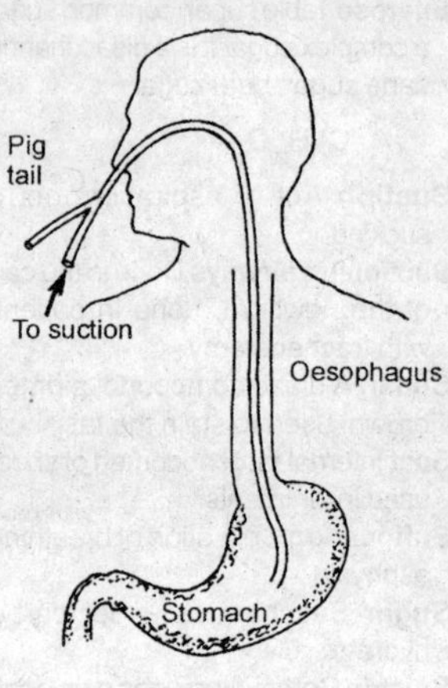

Sump tube

Sunburn Sun ray burn causing dermatitis.

Sunstroke Disturbance of body heat mechanism, fatality rate 40%.

Sunstroke High temperature of atmosphere causing brain injury and effect on cardiorespiratory centres.

Super class Fat cats like director of firm, lawyer, investment manager.

Superego It is developed from primary and secondary socialisation by a person, mental make up of acting on any impulses of ego.

Super fecundation More than one ova is fertilised , fertilisation of ova of same menstruation cycle but sperms are from different coitus

Superfetation After fertilisation of one ovum again second ovum is fertilised, both fertilised ova are of different state of maturity.

Superficial Situated near the surface, easily accessible

Super impregnation Fertilisation of second ovum after the first ovum is fertilised.

Superior Higher, upper portion in anatomical structure.

Supinator reflex It is to test the brachioradialis reflex which has C_5 and C_6 innervations, a deep tendon reflex.

Supine Person lying on the back, prone position.

Suppository It is for the use of medication by inserting into the rectum or into the vagina it is for giving rectal medications, in side lying position with upper leg flexed (Sims' position).

Suppuration It is the infection and inflammatory reaction by forming pus.

Supracondylar To mention the position as above the condyle, supracondylar fracture.

Supraorbital The position above the orbit of the eye.

Suprapubic Position above the pubic bone, suprapubic cystostomy.

Suprarenal Position above the kidney, suprarenal.

Surfactant It produceselastic property of pulmonary tissue, a mixture of phospholipids, that chemical which reduces the surface tension of pulmonary fluids, used in the treatment of respiratory distress syndrome.

Surgeon Person who is specialised in surgery or surgery and allied subjects.

Surgery Treatment modalities by operations or by surgical intervention.

Surgi-gator By using a Surgi-gator we can provide perineal care similar to Perineal care by squeeze bottle, useful for cleansing and providing warmth to the perineum.

Surrogate Substituted item, substance used as a substitute for another substitute for a person or for an object, surrogate mother is one who rents her womb for giving birth to a child for somebody.

Surrogate mother Rent a womb to infertile couple constitutes surrogate motherhood.

Survey Systematic data collection for obtaining base line information or for mapping out prevailing status on a clinical condition or of a public health aspect.

Susceptibility No immunity, absence of immunity, one who is susceptible for illness.

Suspension Temporary cessation, refers to vital function of the body.

Suture Surgical closure of a wound or incision it is a line of joining or closure of bones, material used in closeing the wound, commonly refers to catgut suture, types are:

- Continuous suture.
- Coronal suture.
- Facial suture.
- Interrupted suture.
- Lambdoid suture.
- Purse string suture.
- Tension suture.
- Sub cuticular suture.
- Everting suture.
- Atraumatic suture.

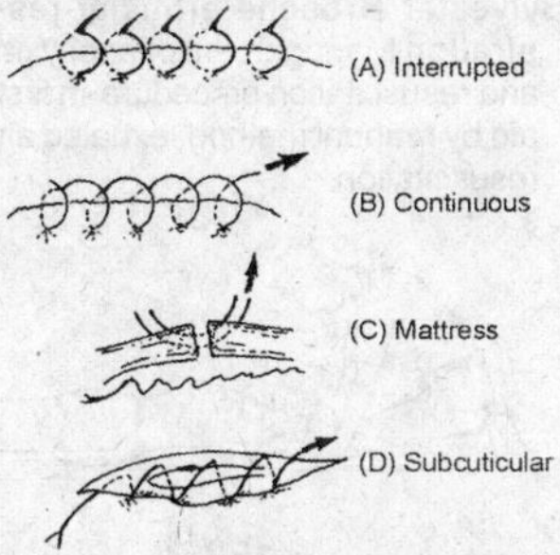

Suture

Swab Sterile stick of cotton used to collect specimen for pathological or bacteriological examination, cotton in spirit is used to cleansing the area or site of injection or operation.

Swallowing Voluntary and reflex action called deglutition, substance taken into mouth is swallowed by voluntary and reflex action through food pipe into stomach.

Swayback Exaggerated inward curve of the lumbar area which is called Swayback or lordosis, used in the assessment of musculoskeletal system.

Sweat Fluid secreted by sweat glands, physiologically it is referred to as perspiration.

Swimmer's itch Schistosomiasis among swimmers which cause itchy eruptions.

Sycosis Hair follicle infection with inflammation, pustular inflammation, Common in beard area.

Sydenham's chorea Saint Vitus' dance, CNS lesion with rheumatic fever, Irregular purposeless movement of involuntary muscles.

Sylvester Brosche artificial respiration Management of asphyxia and resuscitation procedure in first aid by manual method, exhaled air resuscitation.

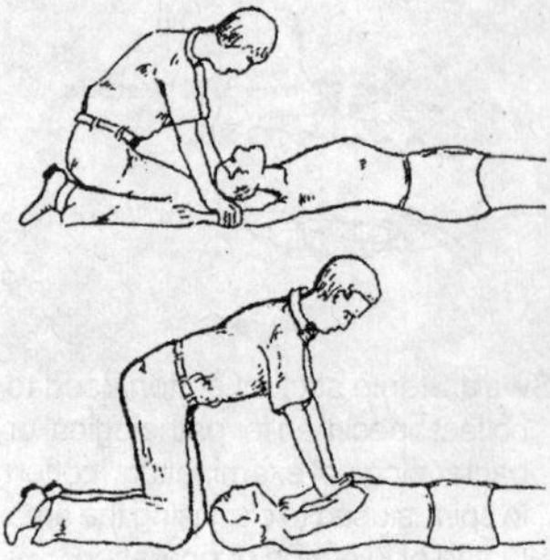

Sylvester Brosche method of artificial respiration

Symbiosis Good purposive association of two organisms.

Symblepharon eyelid is adhered to eyeball.

Sympathectomy Surgical treatment for Raynaud's disease, disconnecting autonomous nerve fibres which control involuntary muscles.

Sympathetic nerve It is a part of autonomic nervous system, this stimulates the smooth muscles of the body which are involuntary muscles help in involuntary activity which are required for normal and healthy living of organs or organisms.

Sympathetic It is an autonomic function by showing sympathy towards vital functions like respiration, circulation and ductless glands, sympathetic nervous system, sympathetic opthalmitis.

Sympathomimetic Drugs that act similar to sympathetic nervous system.

Symphysis Cartilaginous junction of two joints, symphysis pubis.

Symptom Subjective manifestation of illness manifestations, as perceived by the patient types are:

- Objective symptoms.
- Presenting symptoms.
- Signal symptoms.
- Withdrawal symptoms.
- Dissociation symptoms.
- Cardinal symptoms.

abnormality or manifestations that are unusual are felt by the Patients, subjective manifestations, patient's feelings.

Symptomatology Study of symptoms of illnesses.

Synapse Space where nerve impulse pass through, axon one nerve cell joins the dendrite of another nerve cell junction for nerve impulses, intervening of terminal branches of neurones so that nerve impulses may pass from one to the other, Anatomical relation of one nerve cell with another.

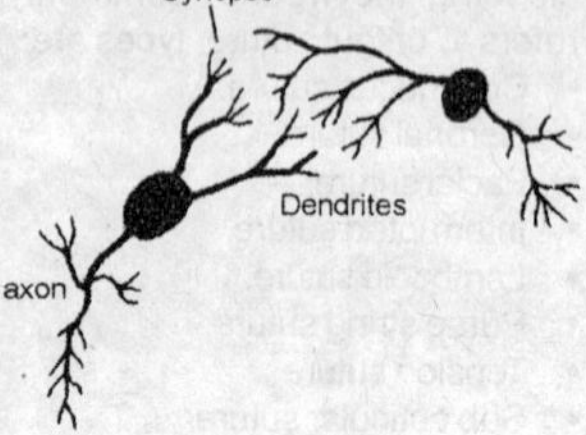

Synopse

Synchondrosis Connective tissue becoming cartilage.

Syncope Temporary loss of conscio-usness, cerebral ischemia, fall of B.P.

Syndactylism Having webbed toes, having webbed fingers.

Syndrome Combinations of symp-toms that are grouped under a condition called syndrome, obse-rved combination of symptoms.

Synechia Adhesion of iris to the lens, Types are anterior, circular and annular.

Synergist One muscle works with another muscle for an effective functioning, combination of two drugs for better effect.

Synopsis Preliminary briefing, a summary of study, summary of project, summary of dissertation.

Synovia Secreted fluid from synovial membrane in a joint, it contains synovin, mucin and mineral salts.

Synovial fluid Lubricating substance secreted by the synovial membrane for locomotor function.

Synovial membrane It is the lining of articular surface of joint which secrete synovial fluid for lubrication.

Synovitis Inflammation of synovial membrane.

Synthesis Organisms and plant do build up complex substances from simpler natural substances.

Syphilis STD caused by Treponema pallida a spirochete a spirochetal infection caused by Spirocheta pallida and transmitted through sexual contact, one of the STD or STI.

Syringe Mortin's Used in removal of collected fluid from the pleural cavity, Aspiration of chest instrument.

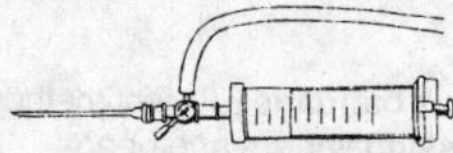

Martin's syringe

Syringe Medical instrument for aspiration of fluid, for injecting the medicine, specialised Syring like BCG syringe is known.

Syringomyelia Cavities with fluid in spinal cord, one of the progressive neurological diseases known, cause paralysis below the lesion.

Syringomyelitis Spinal cord infec-tion and inflammation which cause cavities with fluid.

Syringomyelocele Spina bifida in which central canal of the spinal cord is connected with protruded sac of fluid.

Syrup Water containing high quantity of sugar, concentrated sugary water.

Systemat-ic When everything is according to a system.

System Parts of an organ which perform common function:

- Nervous system.
- G I system.
- Cardiovascular system.
- Genitourinary system.
- Reproductive system.
- Excretory system.
- Respiratory system.

Systemic Clinical condition dema-rking whole body, affecting whole body, systemic circulation when whole body is influenced by an action, systemic effect of a drug or of a disease equivalent to systematic.

Systole In the cardiac cycle when heart contracts to squeeze out the blood. The phase is called systolic phase.

T

Tubegauz bandage Efficient method of dressing fingers and head.

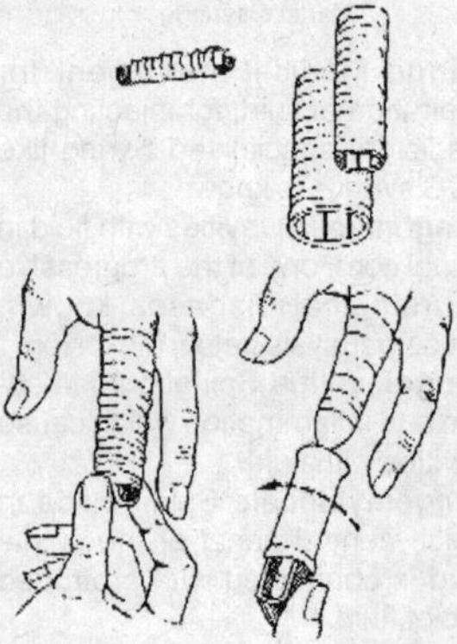

Tubegauz applicators and bandage

Triangular bandages Very useful bandage for all purpose, arm slings, clove hitch, scalp bandage, chest bandage, shoulder bandage and hip bandages are widely known.

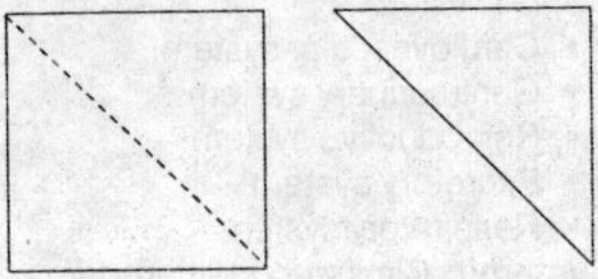

Square from a triangular bandage is made of

T cell Lymphocyte derived from thymus, responsible for cell mediated immunity.

T piece Similar to tracheostomy collar in use, it can be connected with an endotracheal tube.

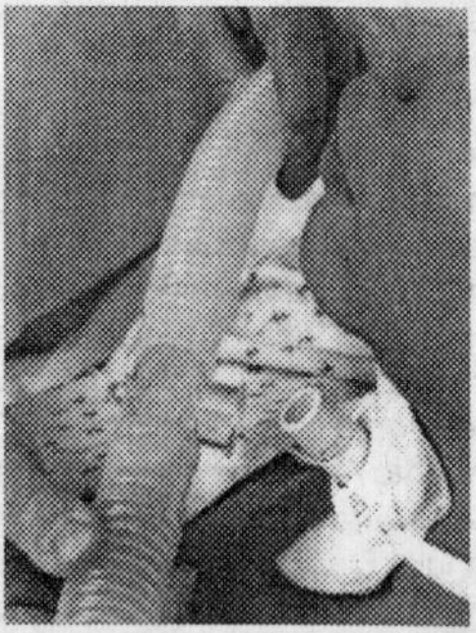

T piece for managing respiratory therapy

TAB vaccine Killed Salmonella vaccine to protect against typhoid infection,
Active immunising agent against typhoid.

Tabes Mean wasting, manifestation of syphilis leading to motor ataxia.

Table spoon Measure equivalent to 15 ml.

Tablet Moulded compressed solid round dosage containing medicinal substance for treatment , taken by oral route.

Taboo That which is forbidden by religious law or by custom, ritual prohibition of certain activities.

Tache Meaning spot, vascular skin lesion.

Tacho Denotes the relation of speed

Tachycardia In the assessment of CVS, greater than 100 beats per minute of heart, considered abnormal clinically, increased pulse rate.

Tachy Swift and rapidness in action.

Tactile Related to sense of touch.

Taenia Tapeworm group, helminthic infection.

TAF Toxoid Antitoxin Floccules, diphtheria vaccine.

Tagging Tagging isotope to chemical to trace its metabolism.

TAI Tuberculosis Association of India.

Taka diastase Digestive substance 3 formed by the action of spores of Aspergillus on the bran of wheat.

Talc A dusting powder used, hydrous magnesium silicate.

Talipes Clubfoot, congenital deformities of foot, types are Valgus, Varus, Calcaneus and Equines.

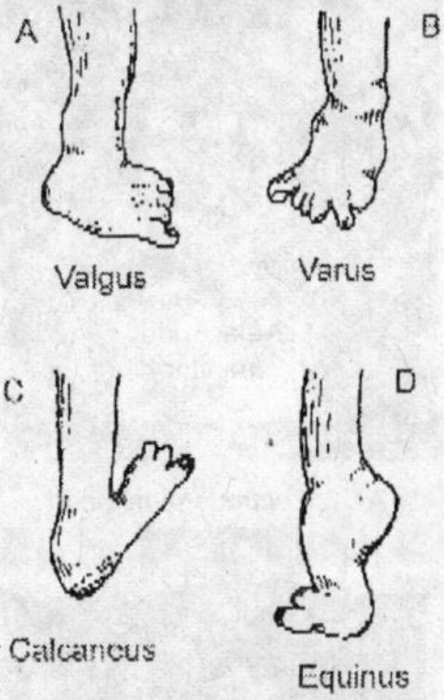

Talipes A, B, C, D

Talus Ankle bone.

Tampon Plug made of absorbent material for the use to plug to vagina, nose.

Tamponade Tampon used in surgical practice.

Tanning Skin changes produced by exposure to sunlight, varying grades like reddening, erythema, blistering, peeling of outer layer.

Tannin Acid substance of tea which is an astringent.

Tantalum Wire material used for suture or prostheses.

Tantrum Out bursting for every thing, behaviour disorder of child.

Tapeworm Cestode worms, intestinal parasite, most of them are Taenia group of helminths.

Taping IV needle Use of 3" strips of tape for fixing the IV needle introduced in IV therapy,
One strip over the wing of the needle
Second over the distal edge of the first strip
Third over the looped tubing.

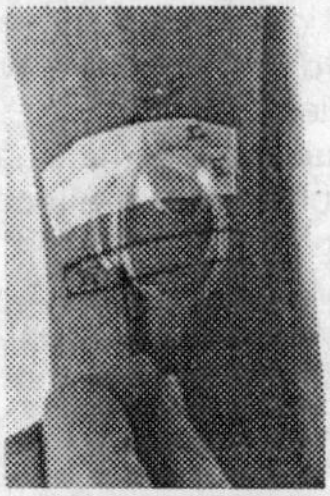
Taping (to tape the needle) the needle in I.V. therapy

Tapping Paracentesis, tapping of ascetic fluid, tapping of cystic fluid.

Tardieu' spots Sign of death by strangulation, subpleural spots of ecchymosis.

Target couple Age group of men and women in 15 to 45 years of age who are:
- Targeted for under NFPP.

Tarnish Used for discolouration.

Tarsal gland Meiobomian glands of eyelid.

Tarsal tunnel syndrome Weakness by the compression of tibial nerve, common cause of Numbness of sole of foot.

Tarsal Related to tarsus.

Tartar Deposits on the teeth, incrustation of teeth and dentures.

Taste bud Nerve organs on the tongue which enable the person to distinguish taste.

Taste Taste sense which detects the material eaten or drunk.

Tattoo Natural or chemical used in skin tattooing to produce permanent discolouration or a shaped picture.

Taxonomy The way of classification or grouping of animals and plants.

Tay-Sachs disease Amaurotic familial idiocy.

Teaspoon A measure which is equivalent to 5 ml.

Team nursing Shift nursing care in a hospital, group allocated for nursing care.

Tears Lacrymal gland secretion, conjunctival wetting agent.

Teat Bottle nipple used in artificial feeding of infants, breast nipple.

Technetium 99 mTc used in radiological diagnosis as tracer element.

Technician A person skilled in procedures requiring special knowledge and training which are applied under medical supervision, X-ray technician, laboratory technician.

Technology Scientific knowledge used for human activity in the world.

Teeth Refers to dentition temporary or permanent.

Teflon Used in surgical material and equipment since it is not made wet with water, plastic material which is inert.

Tegmentum Area of the brain containing red nucleus and oculomotor nuclei.

Tegument Refers to the skin of human beings.

Telangiectasis Wart like spot by dilatation of blood vessels.

Telangioma Tumour of the blood capillaries.

Telemetry monitoring Used in CVS monitoring, it will employ either 2 electrode or a 3 electrode monitor, ECG monitoring.

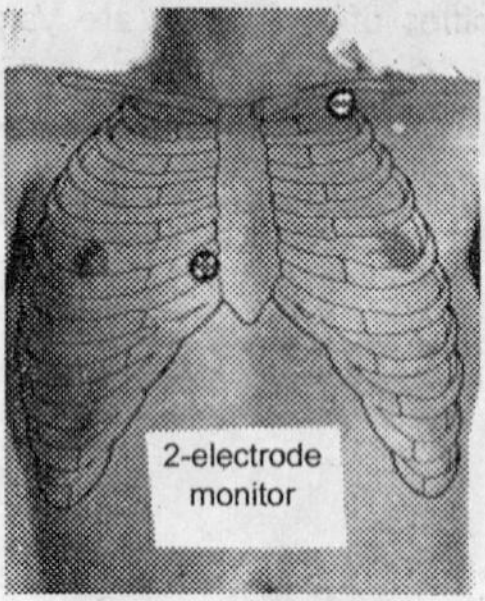

A 2 electrode monitoring

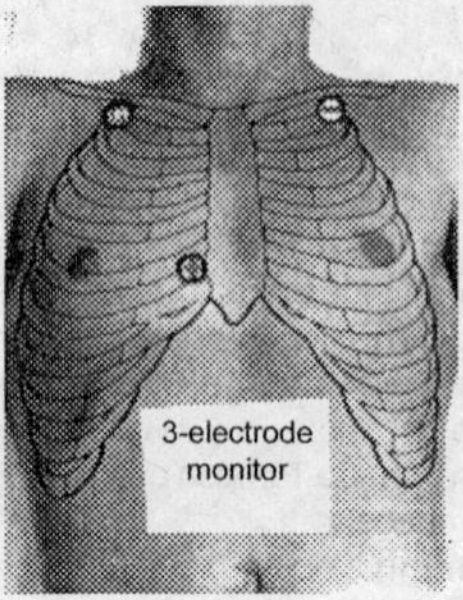

B 3 electrode monitoring

Electrode monitoring A and B

Telepathy Thought transmission from person to person by wireless means.

Telescopic stretcher A stretcher where the handles can be slid under the poles thus reducing its length to 6 feet.

Telophase Final stage of cell division.

Temperature It is a measure of body temperature which is 37^0 C normally.

Template Pattern prepared in diagnostic work, like gonads are protected At X-ray taking.

Temporal Related to temporal bone, side of the head.

Tenacious Thick and viscid material like sputum.

Tenaculum Used in surgery to hold a part or to seize a part, a surgical Instrument.

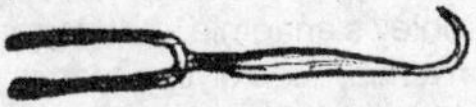

Tenaculum

Tendon Band of dense fibrous tissue forming the end of the muscle, It attaches the muscle to a bone.

Tendonitis Infection and inflammation of tendon.

Tenesmus Painful spasm of rectal spinter muscle, strain in defaecation.

Tennis elbow Occupation elbow where painful disorder develop in extensor muscle at elbow region.

Tenomyositis Inflammation of a muscle and tendon.

Tenon's capsule Eyeball situated in Tenon's capsule which is fibrinous in nature.

Tenositis Inflammation of tendon.

Tenosynovitis Infection and inflammation of tendon and synovial sheath tendon and its sheath gets inflamed.

TENS Care of patients with neurological disorders, it is battery operated device used to deliver electrical impulses to the body to relieve pain.

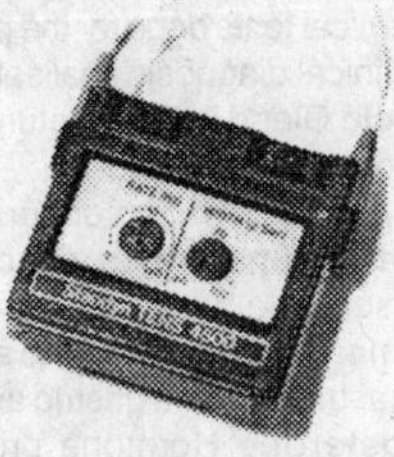

Transcutaneous electrical nerve stimulator device

Tension headache Sustained contraction of muscles of head and neck cause tension headache.

Tension Resistance or indirect pressure exerted to, types are ocular tension, arterial tension, premenstrual tension, surface tension.

Teratoblastoma Cancerous growth from embryonic tissue.

Teratocarcinoma Cancer of teratoma from epithelial element.

Teratogen Developmental defect causing agents.

Teratoma Most of the teratoma develop in ovaries and testes, similar to dermoid cyst.

Terminal care Care given to conditions which do not have reversal to normalcy at any professional cost like cancer.

Tertian Recurring once in 48 hours,or once in 2 days, Tertian malaria fever.

Tertiary Third level care in health care when defects and damage to tissues and organs have occurred, Institutional care or super speciality care in late phase of diseases.

Test A trial conducted, an examination done, an analysis done, usually refers to laboratory tests or chemical tests done for the purpose of clinical diagnosis finalisation.

Testicle Gland in the scrotum which produce spermatozoa.

Testimonial A written endorsement of a treatment by a nonmedical person who has suffered.

Test meal Meal given for the analysis of gastric content, gastric analysis.

Testosterone Hormone produced by the testes, an androgenic steroid, male testicular hormone, responsible for secondary sexual characters in male $C_{19}H_{28}O_2$ (3 keto 17 hydroxy Δ^4 androsterone)

Tetanus Acute infectious disease of nervous system caused by bacteria *Cl. tenani, lockjaw, hydrophobia.*

Tetany Hypocalcaemia causing excitability of nerves, produce carpopedal spasm.

Tetralogy Refers to Fallot's tetralogy with four characteristics:

a) pulmonary stenosis.

b) interventricular defect of the septum.

c) overriding of the aorta.

d) hypertrophy of the right ventricle.

Tetter Skin disease, denotes that it is from animals, intense itching.

Texas catheter For male patients when prolonged use of indwelling catheter is contraindicated, the external collection device like condom and Texas catheter is used.

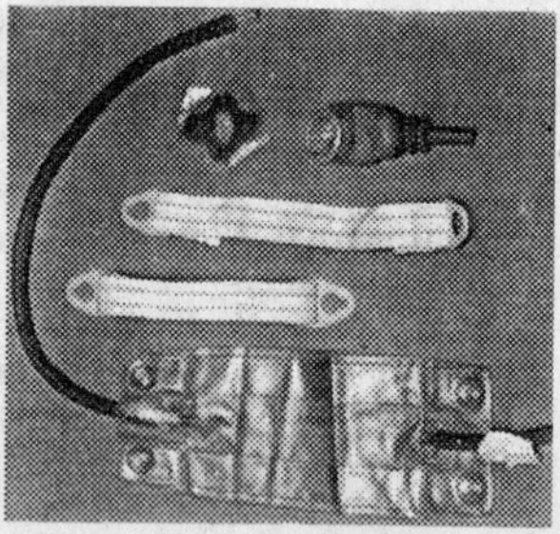

Texas catheter set

Thalamus Nerve cell mass at the base of the cerebrum.

Thalassaemia Inheritance of abnormal haemoglobin cause haemolysis,
Cooley's anaemia, mediterranean anaemia, haemolytic anaemia.

Thalidomide Teratogenic drug, has sedative effect, chemically it is alpha glutarimide.

Thanatology Forensic analysis of cause of death, study of cause of death.

Theca Covering of a tendon, thick sheath.

Thenar Base of the thumb where fleshy muscle mass is appreciated.

Theories of learning Theories of learning postulated for the man who has the great ability of learning, they are:

- Conditioning theory.
- Connectionism theory.
- Field theory.
- Learning model theory.

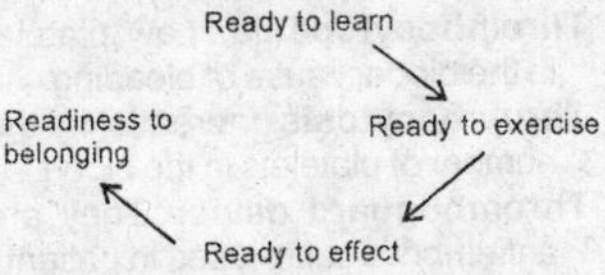

Connectionism theory of learning

Therapeutic diet Diet which is used as an adopted diet, therapeutic adaptation of normal diet, hospital diet like liquid diet, obesity diet, low calorie diet, peptic ulcer diet, diabetic diet, etc.

Therapeutic Related to the treatment of a disease or illness, therapeutic diet, therapeutic abortion,

Therapist occupational Rehabilitation by a trained person through constructive occupations which help overcome physical or mental disabilities.

Therapist speech One who deals with speech therapy for speech problems.

Therapist A person who is trained to give treatment by physical means, physiotherapy.

Therapy Mode of treatment of a disease.

Thermal Pertaining to heat.

Thermocautery Destruction of tissue by heat, warts treatment.

Thermometer Hospital instrument to measure patient's body temperature, Clinical thermometer.

Thermostat An automatic apparatus to maintain the temperature
an electronic device which controls temperature of air or water.

Thermotaxis Body balance for normal temperature through balanced heat production and heat loss.

Thiamine Vitamin B_1.

Thiazides Group of diuretics, inhibits reabsorption of sodium in proximal tubules and stimulates chloride excretion resulting in good urinary excretion of water.

Thiersch graft Partial thick skin graft developed by Thiersch.

Thiopentone Agent used in preoperative treatment, short-acting anaesthetic, short-acting barbiturate.

Thiouracil Drug used in thyrotoxicosis.

Thirty thirty forty society 30 : 30 : 40 society, advantage 40%, a newly insecure 30% and a disadvantaged 30% in a society.

Thomas splint Splint for the support of limb, weight bearing is shifted from knee to hip.

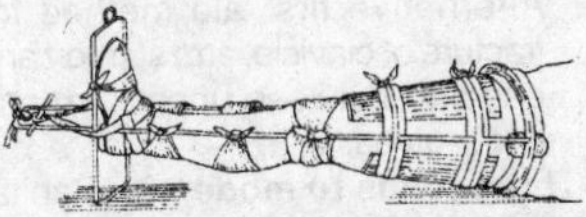

Thomas splint

Thomas test Positive Thomas test indicates flexion contracture of the hip,
Opposite hip also flexes when the patient pull bent knee inwards chest on one side.

Thoracic surgery Surgery on chest organs, heart surgery, lung surgery.

Thoracic Pertaining to thorax.

Thoracotomy Open surgery of the thorax.

Thorax Chest and chest cavity.

Three hand seat Used to carry a patient who is able to assist by using his arms.

A transport for the sick in first aid

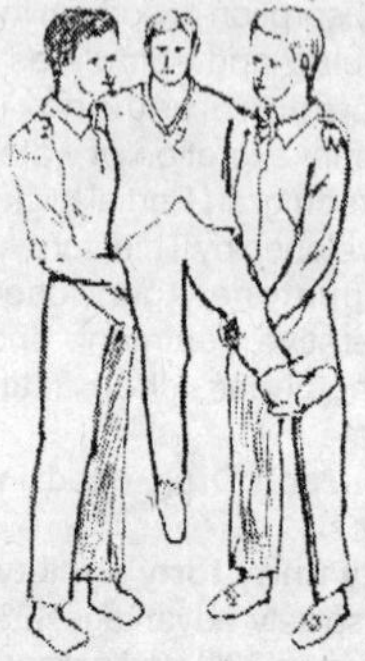

The three hand seat

Threadworm Nematode of children, helminthic infection of intestine.

Three handkerchief method Alternative first aid method for fracture of clavicle, arm support and padding between upper arm and chest given.

Three roads to modernity Capitalism, state socialism and state capitalism.

Thrill Vibration felt by applying our hand on the body, finger tips , Feeling of vibration on a particular region.

Throat Refers to pharynx which is anterior surface of neck.

Thyroglossal Related to thyroid gland and the tongue.

Thrombin Helps in clotting by converting fibrinogen to fibrin exists in the form of prothrombin in the circulating blood, in shed blood it gets converted to fibrinogen, fibrin ferment of the blood.

Thromboangitis Blood vessel inflammation which also has the clotting present.

Thrombocytopenia Low platelet in the blood, cause of bleeding.

Thrombocytosis Increase in the number of platelets in the blood.

Thromboguard device They are antiembolic cuffs, used in patients who are immobile over extended period of time.

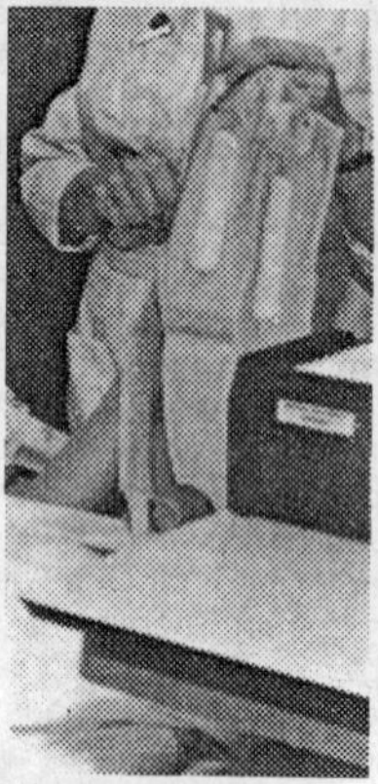

Thromboguard device

Thrombokinase Activates prothrombin to form thrombin, thromboplastin.

Thrombophelebitis Inflammation of lining of vein.

Thromboplastin Thrombokinase.

Thrombosis Formation of thrombus, complete or partial blocking of blood vessel by blood clot.

Thrombus Blood clot in vascular system including heart.

Thrush Vulvovaginal condition or Balanitis condition in fungal (candidiasis) infection contracted through sexual activity, fungal infection of mucous membrane.

Thumb sucking Normal in every infants, when older children do it could be by tiredness or unhappiness.

Thymine One of the pyramidine base of DNA.

Thymol Mouth wash antiseptic.

Thymus gland A structure lying beneath the breast bone which normally disappears at birth but continues functionally.

Thyroid Gland in front of neck, Adam's apple secretes thyroid hormone, situated in lower front region of neck.

Thyroiditis Inflammation of thyroid gland.

Thyrotoxicosis Hyperthyroidism.

Thyroxin Hormone secreted by thyroid gland.

TIA Transient Ischaemic Attack.

Tibia Shin bone, one of the long bone of the leg.

Tic Spasmodic involuntary twitching and certain muscles, tics, muscle twitch.

Tick Hard tick or soft tick, an insect that transmits disease in man.

Tidal volume Amount of air inspired and expired during respiration.

Tidal Refers to periodic rise and fall.

Tinea Fungal infection of skin, ringworm, named after infection region.

Tingling It is nervous disturbance, if associated with numbness it needs clinical examination.

Tinnitus Ringing in the ear, noise in the ear, a tinking, buzzing noise heard by patient.

Tissue Group of similar cells go to form a tissue to perform specific function.

Titration Qualitative analysis of liquid in the laboratory.

TNAI Trained Nurses Association of India.

TNM Classification Tumour, lymph node and metastasis method of classification of cancerous growth, local characteristics of tumours.

Toadstool They are known to produce food poisoning , mistaken for mushrooms.

Tobacco Dried leaves of a plant Nicotina, contain nicotine.

Tobacossis Nicotine in tobacco when inhaled constantly produce lung changes causing bronchitis, emphysema and bronchiectasis, it is associated with bronchogenic carcinoma.

Tocopherol Vitamin E, common source is wheat, milk and leafy vegetables.

Tolerance Ability to take high dose of drugs, diminished effect of medicine.

Tomography Radiological examination of a layer of tissue or organ of body.

Tone Normally required tone present in muscle.

Tongue Organ in the floor of the mouth responsible for taste, swallowing and speech.

Tonic Expression of tone of a muscle, vitamin supplemented to body.

Tonometer Instrument used to measure blood pressure, instrument used for measuring intraocular pressure.

Tonsil Lymphoid tissue mass in fauces.

Tonus Partial contraction of muscle which is normally noticed.

Tooth Dentine set used for mastication of food.

Topical Refers to skin part, for external application.

Topography Study of surface of body in relation to internal organs.

TORCH **To**xoplasmosis **R**ubella **C**ytomegalovirus and **H**erpes simplex.

Torsion Twisting of intestine or a cyst, torsion leads to gangrene.

Torso Body without the head and limbs.

Torticollis Twisted neck or wryneck, cervical muscle contraction leading to unnatural position of the neck

Total hip replacement Head of femur and acetabulum are replaced by silicone prosthesis surgical treatment for advanced hip disease.

Tourniquet Band applied to a limb to arrest haemorrhage.

Toxaemia Toxic condition due to toxins of bacteria in the body, toxaemia of pregnancy.

Toxic Related to toxin or poison of pathogen.

Toxicology Science that deals with poisons and its management.

Toxicosis Clinical condition due to toxin intoxication or due to poisoning.

Toxin Toxic substance liberated by bacteria, vegetable poison, animal poison, unstable antigenic material that can induce specific antitoxin.

Toxoid A toxin that has been deprived of power to injure but which still stimulates immunity formation bacterial endotoxin which has lost its toxicity but retains antitoxin property.

Toxoplasma Protozoal parasite is transmitted from birds and animals, sporozoan parasite found in endothelial cells of man, very common in birds and mammals, *Toxoplasma* gondii infection.

Toxoplasmosis Toxoplasma infection of man, congenital form is known to cause CNS lesion, acquired one cause pneumonia, nephritis and skin rashes.

TPA Tissue Plasminogen Activator.

Trabecula Connective tissue or connecting fibrous tissue between organ and its capsule refers to connective tissue, a connecting link between a capsule and the enclosed substance.

Trace elements They are chemical elements that are required by the body in small quantity.

Important trace elements
Iodine
Iron
Fluorine

Tracer It is a means to trace, to detect other item by following radioactive isotope tracer

Trachea The windpipe made of cartilage

Tracheostomy cuff Used to maintain patent airway in emergency case management

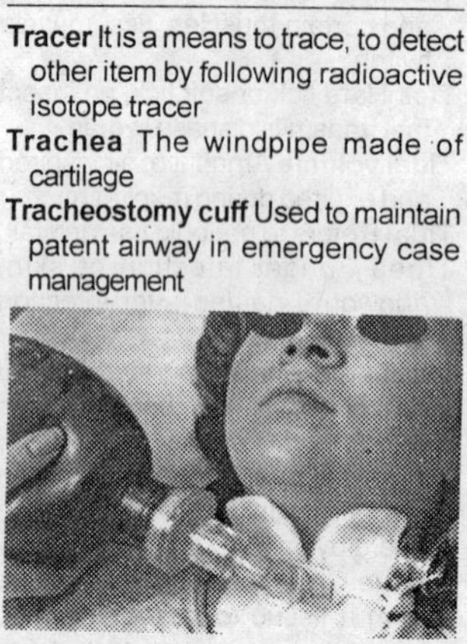

Managing tracheostomy cuffs

Tracheobronchitis Infection and inflammation of trachea and bronchi.

Tracheostomy Surgical opening in 4th cartilage for the purpose of artificial respiration, life saving procedure.

Trachoma Chronic viral infection of conjunctiva and cornea, a strain of *Chlamydia trachomatis* causing infection.

Traction Pulling force given to a limb with long bone fracture.

Tragus Goat-shaped, cartilaginous projection in front of the ear, Front cartilage of the pinna of the ear.

Training An organised instruction with specific purpose, systematic way of allowing development of skill in profession.

Trait Physical and mental characteristics those are due to inheritance or due to acquisition.

Trampline An apparatus for tumbling consisting of a frame on which a sheet or web of canvas is stretched by means of elastic ropes or springs.

Trance Semiconsciousness due to hypnosis or hysteria.

Tranquilliser Drug used to allay anxiety and tension; Drug which calms the disturbed nervous reaction, tranquillity producing drug.

Transaminase Which catalyse the transfer of amine group, like SGOT, SGPT.

Transcendental meditation Technique developed for mental relaxation as well as physical relaxation.

Transcription Synthesis of RNA with the help of DNA.

Transcutaneous blood gas monitor Applicator on the skin of baby to measure partial pressure of oxygen and carbon dioxide, a probe is used at 44^0 C to record pCO_2 and pO_2.

Transformation Change in the structure from one form to another.

Transfusion Blood or blood component given to a patient in blood loss, surgery, shock or septicaemia, types are exchange **T**, Direct **T**, replacement **T,** the transfusion of blood, plasma or packed cells with matching to a patient from a donor.

Transillumination Illumination of translucent body structure by strong light.

Translocation Chromosomal segment transfer which causes congenital anomaly.

Translucent Indistinct way of light passing through a structure.

Transmigration Moving from one place to the other, blood cells through capillary, ovum from ovary.

Transplacental mother to foetus transmission.

Transplant organ or tissue taken from one individual and grafted to another individual.

Transplantation Process of transplant, replacement of failed organ with a healthy organ donated by another healthy person.

Transposition Displacement of viscera from left to right or right to left.

Transsexualism gender identity is lost.

Transudate fluid that passes through membrane.

Transverse Horizontal or crosswise

Trauma indicate injury.

Traumatology Discipline that deals with care of injured patients by trauma.

Travel sickness Sea sickness, common complaint of travellers who experience vomiting and nausea.

Treatment Method of attending a clinical condition or a disease.

Treatment Care and management of patient for the cure from disease.

Trematoda Fluke worms, liver fluke, lung fluke.

Tremor Involuntary muscular movement due to fatigue, emotion or illness.

Tremor Trembling.

Trench foot Effect of cold on feet due to wet sacks or wet shoes over a longer period, exposure of foot to severe cold.

Trench mouth Vincent's infection due to unhygienic mouth conditions and lowered resistance of the mouth tissues.

Trendelenburg's position When patient's head is kept low as compared to lower extrimities.

Trendelenburg's sign It tests the stability of the hip, sign of dislocation of pelvis,
Standing on the affected leg and flexing other knee can show pelvis lower on the side of the flexed leg which is abnormal.

Trephine Circular hole on skull for haematoma.

Treponema Spirochete that causes syphilis.

Triad Refers to a group of three items, Charcot's triad, epidemiological triad, etc.

Triangle Any three cornered area in anatomical structure for the purpose of description,

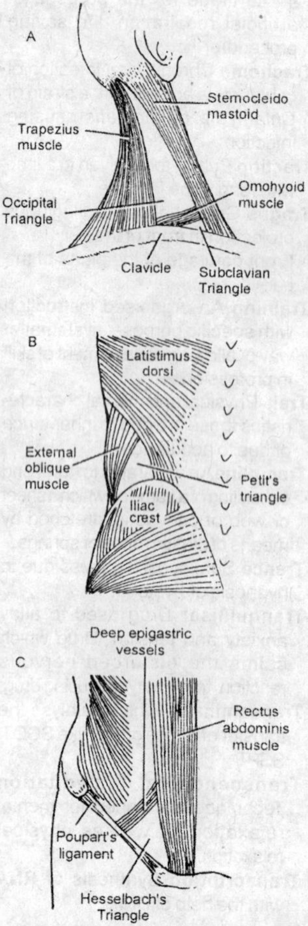

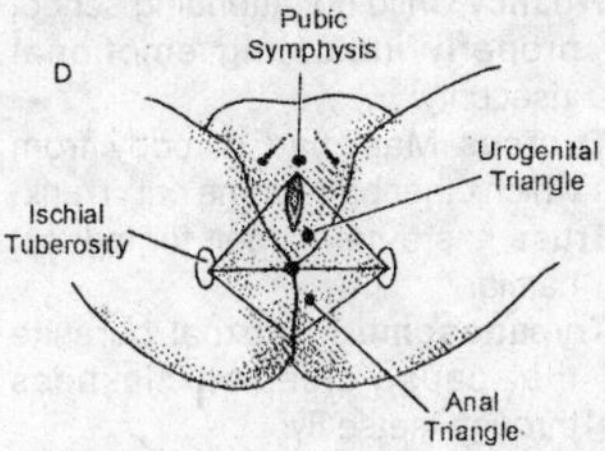

Common triangles A, B, C, D

T bandage It is used to fix dressings over the perineum.

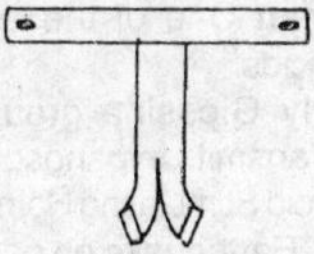

Pattern of T bandage

Tricarboxylic acid cycle Pyruvic acid metabolism, final path where proximate principles are utilised and energy is liberated.

Triceps Muscle of the arm which has three heads, back muscle of the arm.

Trichiasis In growing eyelashes , an ophthalmic clinical condition.

Trichinosis Infection of *Trichinella spiralis* through pork.

Trichobezoar Hair ball in the stomach, a surgical condition.

Trichophyton Fungal infection of nail, skin and hair.

Trichuriasis Whipworm infestation, nematode under helminths.

Tricuspid Valve having 3 cusps, valve between right atrium and right ventricle.

Trigeminal 5th cranial nerve which divides in to three parts to supply face.

Triglyceride Human glycerol and fatty acids.

Triiodothyronine Active form of thyroid hormone, represented as T_3.

Trimester Refers to the period of 3 months, used in pregnancy.

Trinitrophenol Used as dye, as reagent, as fixing agent, as an explosive,
Commonly known as picric acid, $C_6H_2(NO_2)_3OH$.

Triple response Redness, flare and wheal as responses to injury or inflammation.

Triplet Three foetal developments in single pregnancy giving rise to 3 births in a single delivery.

Tripod When there are 3 chromosomes at examination, a stand with 3 legs.

Trismus Lockjaw the symptom of tetanus spasm of masticating muscle because of motor disturbance of trigeminal nerve, early symptom of Tetanus.

Trisomy Presence of an extra chromosome, 3 homologous chromosomes
Instead of 2 chromosomes.

Trocar Instrument with cannula for paracentesis, sharp pointed instrument used with a cannula for tapping fluid from a cavity, used in paracentesis.

Trochanter Bony prominences by femur, greater one is on hip side and smaller one below the neck of femur.

Trochanter rolls To prevent abduction and external rotation of hip, a bath blanket which is folded and positioned from waist to midt-high for draping,
It is a positioning aid in such occasion.

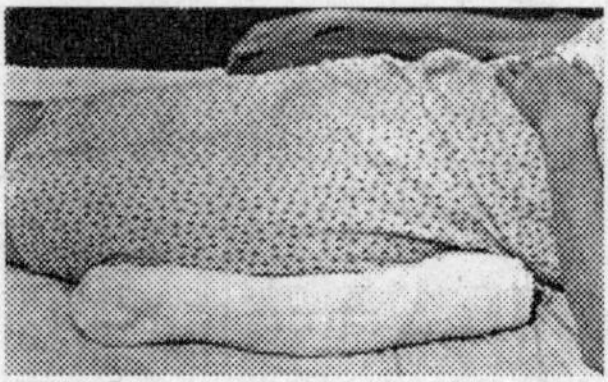

Positioning aid by trochanter roll

Trochlea Pulley-shaped, tendon of superior oblique muscle of the eye passes through angular process of frontal bone.

Trombicula Trombicular mite which transmits rickettsial infection.

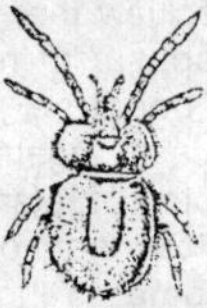

Trombicular mite

Trophoblast Cell layer around blastocyst responsible for implantation.

Tropia Squint manifested.

Tropical Related to tropics, hot climate countries.

Trousseau's sign Carpel spasm seen in Tetany, represents hypocalcaemia.

Truancy Child not attending school properly indicating emotional insecurity.

Truncus Main part of body from which other parts come out, Trunk.

Truss It is a hernia belt for indirect hernia.

Trypanosome Protozoal parasite that cause sleeping sickness through tsetse fly.

Trypsin Digestive enzyme which breaks protein in to amino acids.

Trypsinogen Precursor of trypsin it is secreted in pancreas, gets activated in intestine by enterokinase.

Tryptophan One of the essential amino acids.

Tsetse fly Glossina group of fly which transmits trypanosomiasis.

TSH Thyroid Stimulating Hormone.

Tsunami Earthquake on ocean bed gives rise to a dangerous, phenomenon called 'Tsunami' (Marcomoto) generating a several metres high sea wave which crashes down on the coasts and engulf people on the seashore or beach.

Tsutsugamushi disease Other name for scrub typhus, a mite borne disease.

Tubal One which is related to a tube like tubal pregnancy.

Tube feeding Feeding of a patient is done through any of the following tubes:

- Nasogastric tube.
- Gastrostomy tube.
- Enterostomy tube.

Indicated in patients who cannot take food by mouth.

Tubectomy Female sterilisation which provide permanent contraception for women.

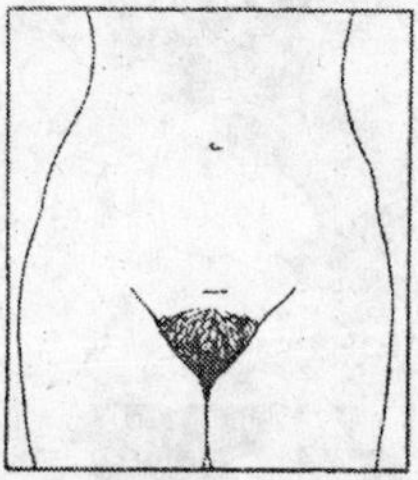

A: Minilaparotomy for tubectomy

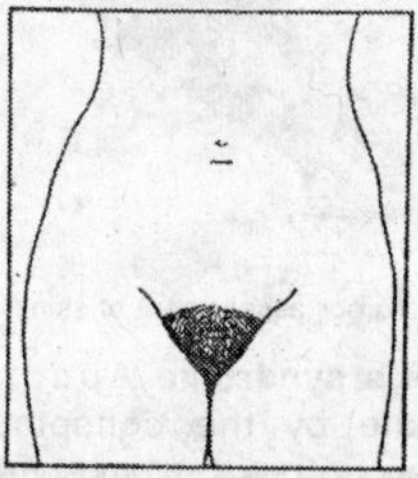

B: laparoscopy for tubectomy

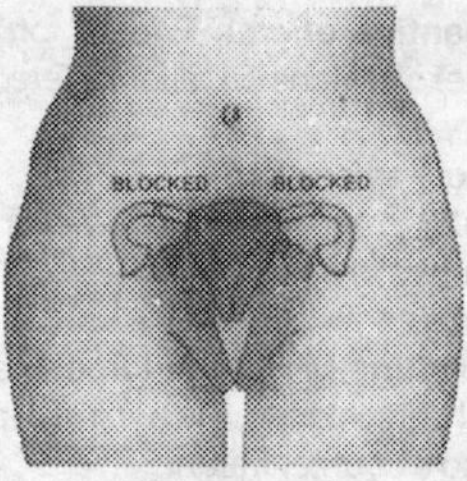

C: Tubes blocked in tubectomy

Tubectomy A, B, C

Tubule Refer to small tube like renal tubules.

Tubeless test for free gastric acid Done for free gastric acid in lab investigation, patient fasts overnight and breakfast is withheld

Procedure:

9AM empties bladder, takes diagnex capsule(caffeine sodium benzoate)

9.0 AM 0.8 mg histamine HCl is injected subcutaneously

10 AM control urine is collected for test, takes diagnex capsule (Quinine resin granules) in water

12 noon urine sample collected and sent for examination

Inference:

2 hour urine contains 25 mg or more of quinine, then free HCl is present in stomach.

Tubercle Lesion by tuberculosis, rounded bony prominence.

Tuberculin test A skin test which shows whether or not an individual has received tuberculus bacilli in his body.

Tuberculin Used in skin test for the diagnosis of tuberculosis, Mantoux test,

Heaf test, Old tuberculin test.

Tuberculosis Chronic bacterial infection caused by *Mycobacterium tuberculosis*

Types are Bovine **T.** Miliary **T.** Open T. Pulmonary **T.** Bone **T.**

Non-pulmonary T. infection with tuberculosis bacteria.

Tuberosity Protuberance of a bone where tendon attaches.

Tuberous Covered with tubers.

Tularaemia Diseases of rodents caused by pasteurella tularensis which is transmitted to man, plague like disease, a disease of wild animals which infects man through breaks in the skin.

Tulle Gras and Carbonet dressing A surgical dressing where an open mesh gauze dressing impregnated with water soluble non-adherent polyethylene glycol is used.

Tumbling A gymnastic exercise best described by its name.

Tumefaction Swollen wound, tumescence of a lesion.

Tumescence Swelling of a part, usually refers to penile erection.

Tumour Hugh growth of a tissue or an organ which may be benign or malignant.

Tunga penetrans Skin penetrating flea, chiggarosis.

Tunica Covering or a lining of a vessel,
Aponeurosis of abdominal muscles or big muscles.

Tuning fork A testing instrument in ENT to test for hard of hearing.

Tunnel Anatomical canal through which structure pass through like carpal tunnel.

Turbinates Baffles in the nose which increase its mucous surface.

Turgid Any distended organ, an organ swollen due to infection or inflammation.

Turgor skin assessment Lifted skin in forearm, lower abdomen or calf when left comes to original position which is called skin turgor, it is a test for testing suppleness of the skin in dehydration.

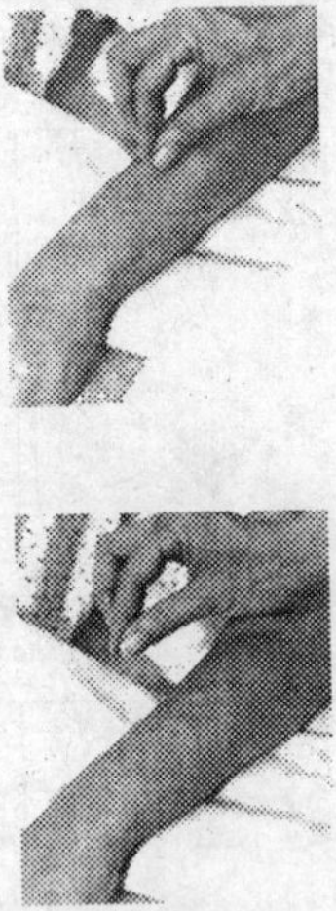

A

B

Turgor assessment of skin

Turner's syndrome Abnormal female by the conspicuous absence of one X chromosome, the syndrome has infertity, webbed neck, coarctation of aorta.

Turpentine enema Enema for the relief of distension, *enema Terebinthinae*.
Requirements are:
- 120 to 480 minims of turpentine.
- 1 pint of soap.
- Water.

Turpentine Mixture of turpene and its hydrochloride, it is a liniment and also a counter irritant.

TV infection Lower female genital tract infection by *Trichomonas vaginalis*,

Pathogenic protozoal infection of female genital tract.

Twin Two foetal growths in one pregnancy.

Two bin method Appropriate for ward management, Two portion one for immediate utility and the other for next requirement are kept.

Tylosis Callus formation on the skin

Tympanum The eardrum called tympanic membrane.

Type A behaviour Behaviour like aggression, progressive lifestyle and competitiveness are associated with development of coronary heart diseases, high-risk behaviour for CVS disorders.

Type I and II error When we make conclusion we are likely to make 2 types of error viz., Type I and Type II error (alpha and beta errors)

	Rejected	Not rejected
NH (True)	Type I (α)	No error
NH (False)	No error	Type II (β)

Type I and II errors

Typhoid fever Generalised infection with salmonella group of organisms

Typhoid Enteric fever caused by *salmonella typhosa*, water-borne disease.

Typhoral Oral vaccine to prevent typhoid, available in enteric coated form, one capsule on 1st, 3rd, and 5th day one hour before meal in tepid water gives protection from 15th day to 3 years.

Typhus Acute notifiable rickettsial infection, both louse-borne and flea-borne typhus are known.

Tyriasis Colloquial word for elephantiasis, common word for alopecia.

Tyrosine One of the essential amino acids which is a precursor of catecholamines, melanin and thyroid hormones.

U

U wave of ECG Low amplitude positive wave of ECG that appear after T wave,
Inversion of U wave indicates IHD.

Uraemia It indicates the presence of urinary constituents in the blood, types are retention **u**. prerenal **u**. eclamptic **u**. convulsive **u.**

Uberty Fruitfulness, indicates fertility in humans.

UIP Universal Immunisation Programme, most powerful and cost effective weapon of disease control, prevents 6 vaccine preventable diseases.

Pregnant	early pregnancy	TT I or booster dose
	4 weeks later	TT II*
Infants	at birth	BCG and OPV "0" dose
	6 weeks	$BCG@, DPT1, OPV 1
	10 weeks	DPT 2, OPV 2
	14 weeks	DPT 3, OPV 3
	9 months	measles
Children	16-24 months	DPT and OPV booster
	5-6 years	DT[m]
	10 years	TT
	16 years	TT

* last dose of TT should be given at least 1 month prior to expected date of delivery

@ in case of individual delivery/ if not given at birth

m 2 doses DT given at interval of 1 month

$ if there is no past history of immunisation

Table: U I P

Vaccine	*Syringe*	*Needle*
BCG	1 ml syringe	26 gauge (BCG syringe)
other vaccine	2 ml syringe	23 gauge
for reconstitution	5 ml syringe	20 gauge

Table: syringe and needle specifications

Ula From Greek *oulon* meaning gum, indicates gingiva.

Ulcer A sore, sore on mucous membrane, sore on the skin, peptic ulcer in stomach or intestine.

Ulcus Meaning ulcer.

Ultrafiltration Filter used to filter colloidal particles and suspending liquid.

Ultramicroscope Objects not visible under ordinary microscope are made visible by ultramicroscope, useful to visualise colloid particle, flagella of bacilli, spirochete, dancing granules of WBC.

Ultrasonic They refer to sound wave frequency which cannot be audible normally, beyond the audibility of human beings sound waves which have very high frequency range, inaudible, ultrasound rays are used as diagnostic agent.

Ultrasound Internal organs of the body can be examined by ultra sound waves, ultrasonic waves used in medical field.

Umbilical cord Connecting link between mother's uterus and foetus' naves, connects mother and foetus for the purpose of nutrition, immunity and hormonal action.

Umbilication Depression seen on a vesicle, any navel like depression.

Umbilicus Navel region, inward circular scar in adults, connected with umbilical cord.

Unconditioned reflex Reflex by nature, and not by any experience.

Unconscious Not capable to respond to external stimuli, not alert.

UNDA United Nations Development Programme to help poor nations to develop their own resources in social and economic areas.

Under five clinic Takes care of child care by integrating treatment prevention and surveillance activity in the community.

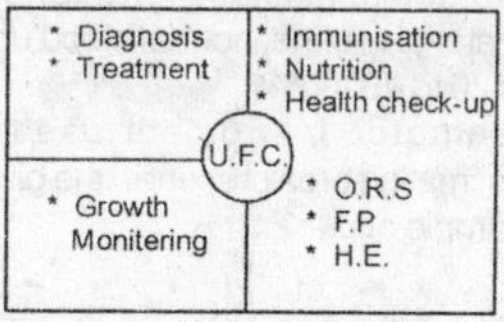

Functions of under five clinics

Under weight When the body weight is less than 10% of standard weight for the given age and sex.

Underclass People at bottom of class system.

Undeveloped society Original state of a society with no development.

Undine curse Apnoea seen during the sleep, a clinical condition.

Undulant fever Brucella infection, a bacterial infection.

Undulant Wavery, rise and fall are seen, refers to undulant fever caused by brucellosis.

Undulation Continuous wave-like motion, continuous wave-like pulsation.

Unemployment Working age people but without work.

UNFPA The United Nations Fund for Population Activities an international health organisation.

Unguentum It refers to the nature of ointment, ointment for external application.

Ungula Powerful claw of lower animals, an instrument to extract dead foetus.

UNICEF United Nations International Children Fund (E = emergency is Removed), an international health organisation.

Unicorn Single horn of a uterus.

Unilateral One sided, exist on one side only.

Union Tissue repair, joining together of two parts, join together of many items.

Unipara Woman who has one living child, one viable issue by a woman.

Unit It is an assumed quantity, a standard of measurement.

Universal antidote Oral remedy for unknown poisoning, it contains:

Tannic acid	....	1 part
MgO	....	1 part
Activated charcoal	.....	2 parts.

Universal donor 'O' Rh negative blood group is known as universal donor.

Universal precaution Procedure to protect oneself through precautions on universal blood and body fluid with all patients and at all time, measures to protect from HIV/AIDS.

Universal recipient 'AB' Rh positive blood group is known as universal Recipient.

Unmet need for FP It is 25% among eligible women, married women who prefer to avoid pregnancy are not attended to on priority basis, KAP gap correction is needed.

Unna's paste This application is a mixture of gelatine glycerine and Zinc powder, it is applied as a dressing and a support For varicose ulcers of the leg.

Unsaturated fats Fats which have a lower content of hydrogen than saturated fats, unsaturated fats are vegetable in their origin.

Unsaturated fatty acid Oleic acid, linoleic acid form unsaturated fatty acids, vegetable origin.

Unwed mother Unmarried expectant mother who need support for her life and the coming newborn in the society, has a fear of embarrassment.

Upward social mobility Movement from a subordinate social position to a higher one.

Urachal Refers to urachus.

Urachus A tubular connector of bladder and umbilicus in foetus.

Uraemia A disease state due to accumulation of wastes and in the blood and tissues consequent upon kidney failure.

Urate Salt of uric acid, sodium urate is present in goat.

Urban apartheid Segregate space in a class specific way like private space for rich, ghettos for the poor.

Urban areas High population density area.

Urban crisis Modern class struggle, unmet welfare.

Urban social movement Collective interest in community with concern.

Urban society Large dense and permanent settlement with civilised activities, it is 22% in India, 300 megacities in India 8637 towns and cities in India.

Urban villager Working class in city.

Urban zone Urban process in spread out zones.

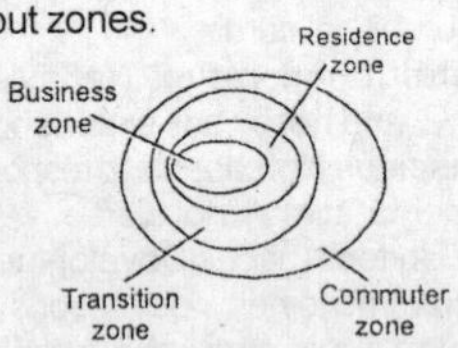

Urban zones

Urea cycle In nitrogen metabolism the process of urea formation is depicted in the cycle.

Urea It is an end product of protein metabolism, main nitrogenous material in urine, normal blood urea is 20 to 40 mg%.

Ureameter Instrument used in estimating urea present in the given sample of urine.

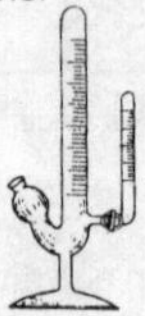

Ureameter

Ureter Conveying tube of urine from kidney to bladder.

Ureteric Related with ureters.

Ureterocele Bladder end of the ureter has cystic enlargement.

Ureterolith A stone in the ureter.

Urethra Urine discharging canal, canal from bladder to external opening of external genitalia, short urethra in female about 3.5 cm, longer in male about 18 cm.

Urethritis Infection and inflammation of the urethra.

Urethrocele Prolapse of female urethra, result of pelvic damage during delivery.

Uric acid End product of nucleic acid metabolism, normal constituent of urine, abnormal constituent of blood end result of body use of proteins rich in purine bodies, goat is the only form of arthritis which involves uric acid.

Urinary disinfectant A drug that tends to clear the urine of bacteria.

Urine analysis Physical chemical and bacteriological examination of urine.

Urine specimen collection Closed system collection of urine for lab examination in a patient who is catheterised, at port or at catheter urine is aspirated cleaned catheter just distal to the bifurcation by sterile procedure for urine sample.

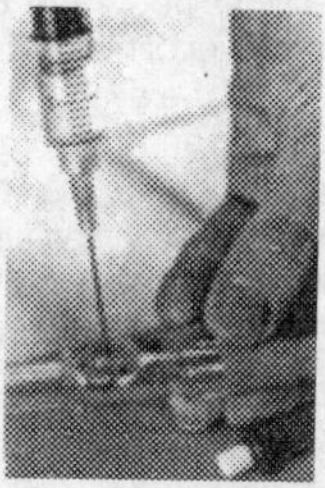

Urine aspiration through the port,

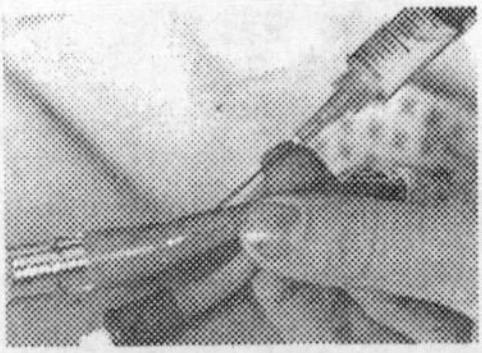

Urine aspiration through catheter from sterile syringe

Urine Main excretory product of human being, urea and uric acid are secreted , urine output renders fluid balance, sp.gr of normal urine is 1017 to 1020.

Urinaemia Refers to uraemia, urinary constituents in blood.

Urobilin Main urinary pigment from urobilinogen.

Urobilinogen It is a bilirubin pigment, its oxidation produces Urobilin.

Urochrome Colouring pigment present in urine which produces yellow urine.

Urogastrone Urinary polypeptide that inhibits gastric acid secretion.

Urogenital Pertaining to genital organs and urinary system.

Urogram Image produced by radiography examination, urography.

Urokinase Kidney enzyme secreted in the urine, does the lysis of fibrin.

Urolith Refers to urinary stone.

Urolithiasis Clinical manifestation due to stone in urinary tract.

Urology It is the study of the diseases of urinary system, medical specialty concerned with diseases of the urinary tract.

Urophobia Person has fear of passing urine.

Urosis Diseases of the urinary system.

Urostomy Artificial canal to abdomen for urine excretion.

Urticaria Hives, smooth elevated patches on the skin due to vascular reaction.

Use of life supporting system Comes under *death and dying* aspect of ethics, it achieves the maintenance of oxygenated circulation through the corpse, brainstem death is legal death and permission is granted to withdraw the life supporting system only with brainstem death.

Used blood Blood that has travelled through the body and exchanged its supply of oxygen for carbon dioxide.

USG Reflections of ultrasonic waves help in visualising deep organs of our body, Ultra Sono Graphy, US ray technique.

Usher's syndrome Complete blindness due to retinitis pigmentosa and associated with congenital deafness.

Uta Colloquial name for leishmaniasis.

Uterine soufflé Uterine vessel sound in a gravid uterus.

Uterine Related to the uterus.

Uterovesical Connected with uterus and urinary bladder.

Uterus Womb, main reproductive organ.

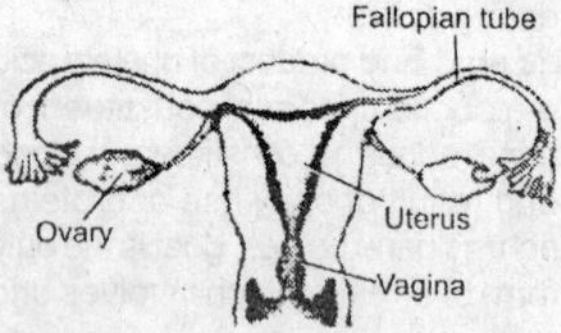

Uterus

Utricle Vestibular membranous labyrinth, refers to utriculus vestibuli.

UV light Skin exposure helps in the synthesis of vitamin D, used in physiotherapy.

UV rays Along with cosmic rays, this is present in sun light, high dose causes sun tanning.

Uvea Refers to uveal tract formed by iris, ciliary body and choroid pigmented layer of the eyeball, coloured layer of the eyeball.

Uveitis Infection and inflammation of uveal tract.

Uvula Free edge of soft palate which is found hanging from the Roof of the mouth.

V

Vaccination Introduction of vaccine into the body for producing immunity, vaccine administration under immunisation to protect the individual from infectious diseases, U I P, E P I, administration of active or passive immunising agents.

Vaccine preventable diseases Diphtheria, whooping cough, tetanus, polio, tuberculosis and measles are called VPD

Vaccine Suspension of organism, killed or attenuated, live attenuated for giving active immunity, common use in India are:

- DPT.
- BCG.
- OPV.
- Measles.
- TT.

a preparation of living or attenuated or killed micro-organisms used in the prevention of infectious diseases, tested agent for potency, clarity and safety and which can induce immunity

Vaccinia Name for cowpox virus

Vacuole Cavity formed in the protoplasm of the cell, clear space in cell.

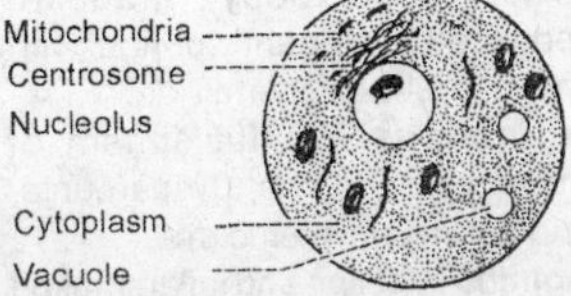

Cell showing vacuole

Vacutainer Collecting the blood sample with a vacuum container vacuum container is vacutainer.

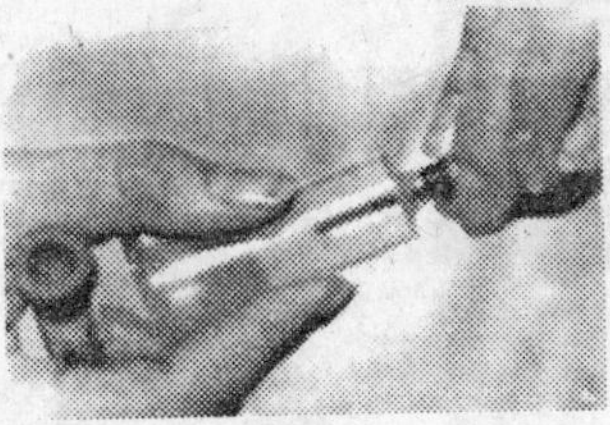

Vacutainer

Vagabonds disease Louse infestation and dermatitis among wandering people.

Vagal Related to 10th cranial nerve the vagal nerve.

Vaginal douching Done for cleansing purpose in cases of vaginal discharge, preoperative, when vaginal pessary is used, Hot pessary at 115^0 to 120^0 used in arresting uterine haemorrhage, Requirements are:

- A douche can
- Long piece of rubber tubing.
- Douche nozzle, rubber or glass, or a rubber catheter size 10.
- Clip.
- Douche lotion.
- libitane 1 percent (antiseptic).
- Sterile swab.
- Bowl.
- Douche pan.

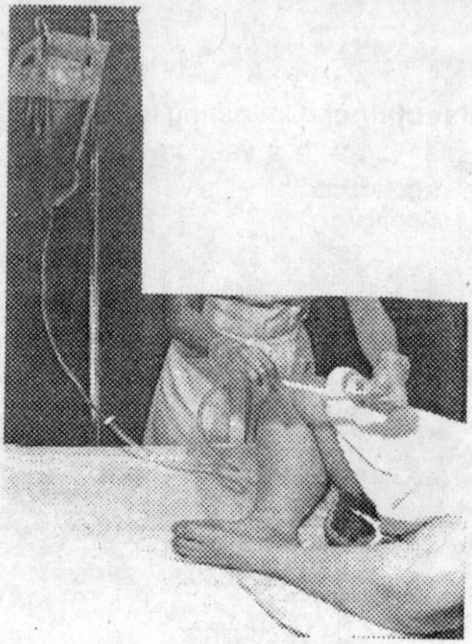

Vaginal douching

Vaginal examination Done for diagnosis, smear taking, preoperative, dorsal or lithotomy position are used, requirements for P V are:
- Right hand rubber gloves.
- Receptacle for soiled swab or instrument.
- Sterile glove if she is pregnant.
- A bowl with antiseptic lotion.
- Swabs.
- Swab holding forceps.
- Sims' specula or vaginal specula.

Requirement for smear in PV:
- Ferguson's speculum.
- Vulsellum forceps.
- Swabs and swab holder.
- Platinum wire loop or sterile throat wabs.
- Microscopic slides.
- Spirit lamp.
- Labels.

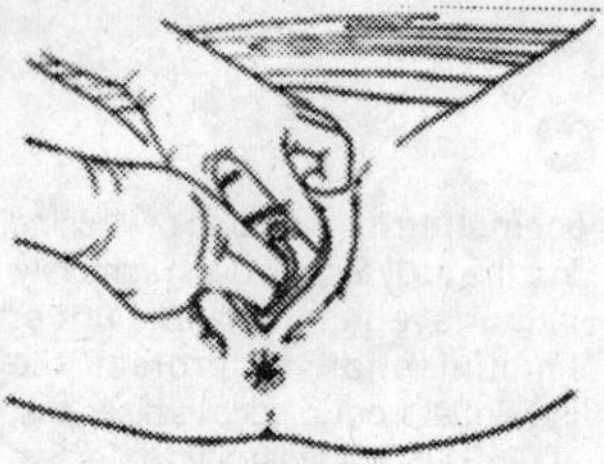

Positions for PV examination

Vaginal irrigation Douche, indicated in preoperative cleansing with providone-iodine solution.

Vaginal pessary It is introduced into the vagina to afford support in the case of a Prolapsed uterus, they are made of vulcanite, Perspex or coils of watch spring covered with rubber,

Requirements for insertion of pessary:
- Clip forceps.
- Sterilised pessary.
- Swabs in lotion of antiseptic.
- Sterile lubricant.
- Sterile gloves.
- Mackintosh.
- Receptacle for soiled swabs.
- Receiver for discarded gloves.
- Hand lamp.

Vaginal sponge It is available by trade mark 'today', made of polyurethane foam sponge with nonoxynol-9 as spermicide.

Vaginismus Painful spasm of muscles of vagina, dyspareunia, painful vagina intercourse

Vaginitis Infection and inflammation of vagina.

Vagina Female genital tract, passage from vulva to cervix which leads to uterus, a receptaculum for receiving semen during intercourse.

Vagotomy Surgical treatment for gastric ulcer, division of vagus nerves to minimise gastric secretion in duodenal ulcer cutting the vagus nerve, resection of vagus nerve, surgical treatment for gastric ulcer.

Vagotonia Clinical condition with hyperexcitability of the vagus nerve.

Vagus 10th cranial nerve which provide parasympathetic fibres to the organs of thorax and abdomen.

Valency Stability or strength, refers to chemical element.

Valgus Genu hallux, genu talipes, outward displacement of feet

Validity years Increase in lifespan with intervention, increased full health by intervention for prolongation of life, useful days of life.

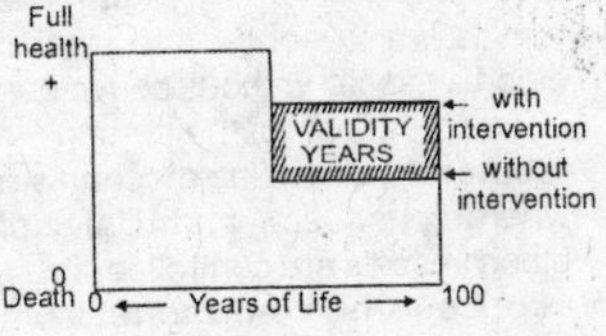

Validity years

Validity Quality of a measure or of an indicator is good and not biased, scientific judgement of a data found true.

Valine An amino acid, it is alpha amino iso valerianic acid,

Produced from digested protein $(CH_3)_2CH.CH(NH_2).COOH$

Valsalva maneuver It occurs in a person naturally when he strains for urination, defaecation, moving up in bed through arm and upper trunk, coughing, vomiting ,etc. It is a technique for increasing the intra-thoracic pressure by closing mouth and nose and blowing out the cheeks,Valsalva maneuver produces 3 consequential manifestation viz., increased intrathoracic pressure, tachycardia, and bradycardia,

This prevents air embolism in removal of a chest tube, this prevents air embolism during I V tubing on central lines.

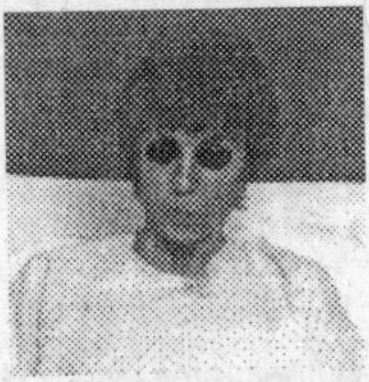

Valsalva maneuver

Value factor Fundamental value factor in nursing profession are treatment to cure, to relieve from pain, to relieve from suffering, to treat patient as an individual with human rights.

Value system It is one's personal life and one's professional life made dynamic influenced by civilisation. Value system of nurses' profession.

Value Desirability of a thing, often in respect of some property such as usefulness or exchangeability, Foundation of morality.

Values Ideas and beliefs which are thought to be valuable

Valve A device permitting control of an opening so as to allow free passage on one way but not in other way, structure that allow flow of liquid in one direction.

Valvotomy Surgical treatment for stenosed mitral valve.

Vampire A blood sucking bat, transmits rabies.

Van den Bergh test Blood examination in the laboratory for the detection of bilirubin.

Vanilla An aromatic substance, a flavouring agent.

Vaporiser Apparatus used to get fine spray of a medicine.

Variable Used in study or survey as a characteristic which is measurable.

Variance Statistical term denoting square value of S.D.

$$V = S^2 = \sum\frac{(X-\bar{X})^2}{n} or \sum\frac{(X-\bar{X})^2}{n-1}$$

Formula for variance

Varicella Other name for chickenpox.

Varicocele Varicose conditions of the veins, common sites are spermatic cord, ovarian, pelvic, uteroovarian veins.

Varicose Distended , dilated and tortuous vein which cause symptoms.

Variola Other name for smallpox, smallpox is not present in India, An eradicated viral infection.

Varix Enlarged and tortuous vein, artery or lymph vessel.

Varus Inward displacement of foot, genu talipes.

Vas Meaning a duct, vas deferens, vas efferens.

Vascular Pertaining to blood vessels

Vascularisation When new blood vessels are developed in the tissue.

Vasculitis Inflammation of blood vessel walls.

Vasectomy Permanent method of contraception in males.

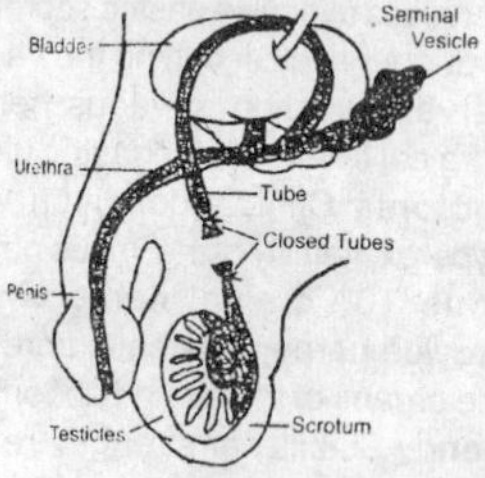

Vasectomy

Vasoconstrictor Drug that causes constriction of blood vessels.

Vasodilator Drug that causes dilatation of blood vessels, a drug that causes the smaller blood vessels to get enlarged.

Vasomotor nervous system The nerves which control the size of blood vessels without conscious effort on the part of the person.

Vasomotor Controlling mechanism where constructor and dilator of blood vessels are controlled.

Vasopressin A hormone from posterior lobe of the pituitary gland, an antidiuretic hormone.

Vasovagal Gower's syndrome, vagal and vascular, precardial and respiratory distress lasting for few minutes.

Vastus lateralis injection site Common site for neonatal vitamin K injection, middle third of vastus lateralis is selected because it is free of major nerves and major blood vessels at administering injectable medications.

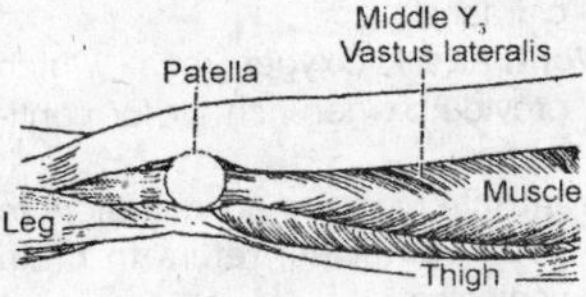

Anatomical site for vastus lateralis

Vector bionomics Breeding habit, biting habit, and life cycle of insects which are responsible for the transmission of human diseases.

Vector Lower species of animal including insects that carry pathogens or parasites that cause human disease.

VED method Best inventory control method at matron level in the hospital,
Categorisation of hospital requirement is done as essential, very essential at indent and supply.

Vegan Very strict and pure vegetarian who never takes even milk or milk products, person who never used animal or its product as food.

Vegetarian Person eating only plant origin foods.

Vegetation Pathological term denoting plant like growth of tissue.

Vehicle A medium for a drug in pharmacy, transport for movement, Media for transmitting diseases e.g., water is a vehicle of transmission of diseases.

Vein Vessel that carry blood from capillaries towards heart.

Veins Large vessels that carry blood to the heart bigger than venules or capillaries.

Venepuncture I.V. needle insertion to the vein with the intension of giving drugs or medication through parenteral route.

Venereal Diseases that spread through sexual intercourse, largely and not entirely through sexual intercourse, V.D. got a new nomenclature as STD, now again it is replaced by STI (sexually transmitted infections).

Venereology It is the study of sexually transmitted infections and their management (study of V.D.).

Venesection Surgical blood letting by opening a vein and introducing an I V needle, phlebotomy.

Venipuncture Performing a puncture of a vein is necessary for administering I V fluids and medications

Required materials for venipuncture
1. sterile gauze pad
2. tourniquet
3. air occlusive 7.5 cm tape (3" tape)
4. bed-saver pad
5. arm board , if necessary
6. antibiotic cream

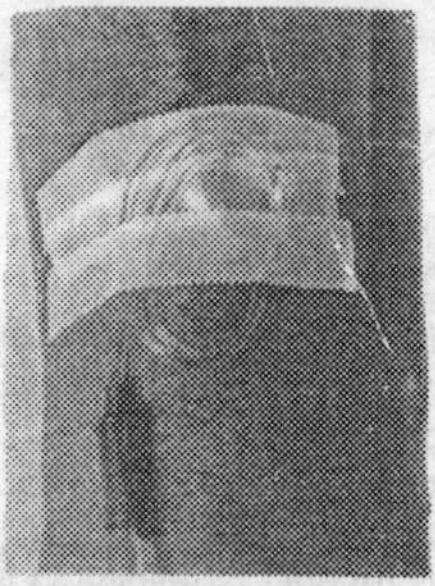

Venipuncture

Venogram Graphic recording of a vein pulsation.

Venography X-ray of the vein after introduction of contrast medium.

Venom The poisonous substance injected in bites by snakes, spiders, bees, wasps and hornets, snake poison.

Venous Related to veins.

Venous hums Common term in abdominal auscultation, venous hums are softer and more continuous than bruits and may be heard in the upper epigastric area and over the liver in advanced cirrhosis.

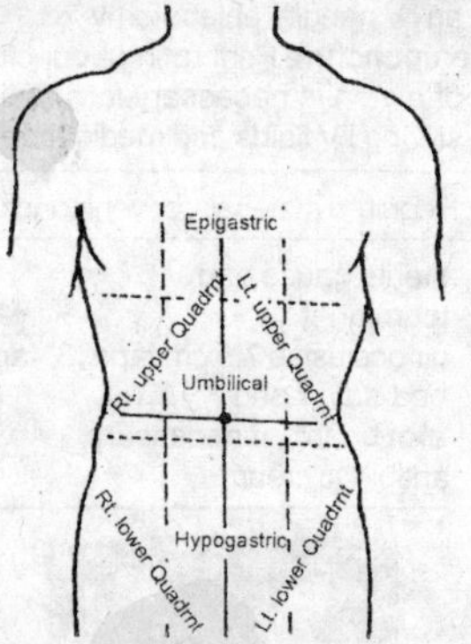

Dividing the abdominal area for the purpose of Palpation, percussion and auscultation

Ventilation Good air movement in the living space, refers to cross-ventilation,

Good respiratory function through exchange of airs,

Ventilator Artificial respirators which allow intermittent flow of air with oxygen under pressure to the patient connected to his mouth ,nose or trachea.

Ventimas k Oxygen mask which provide oxygen rich air for ventilation.

Ventricle Meaning pouch, refers to heart ventricles, refers to brain ventricles.

Ventricular gallop It is represented as S_3, it is a dull and low pitched sound, it is the first clinical signs of CCF.

Ventricular hypertrophy Strong and sustained heart beat is palpable in apical area of patients with ventricular hypertrophy.

Ventricular Referred to the ventricle.

Ventriculus Belly like, stomach, ventricle of the heart.

Ventrogluteal injection site site for I M injections

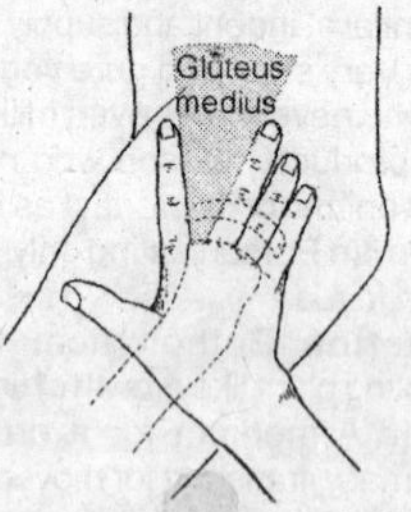

Ventrogluteal site for injection

Note that palm is over the greater trochanter, index finger is on the anterior superior iliac spine, with middle finger you can see a "V" shape for safety injection on ventrogluteal region (note these in above figure)

Venturi mask A disposable mask used to deliver a controlled oxygen, mask for 24 to 40 % delivery.

Venturi nebuliser Used in aerosol therapy, liquid enters the gas stream to break up into finer particles or spray.

Venule Smallest vein, small or minute vein.

Vermicide Chemotherapeutic agent against helminths or intestinal worms.

Verminous Louse infestation.

Vernix caseosa Lanugo and exfoliated skin with sebaceous deposit which cover the newborn.

Vernix Meaning varnish, fatty covering on the skin of the foetus.

Verruca Refers to wart, thickening of the horny layer wart, wart like elevation on the skin.

Version foetal turning to a given position, term used in delivery.

Vertebra One (single) bone from the spinal column which is made up of 33 vertebra, named after their regional positioning like Cervical, thoracic, lumbar, sacral and coccygeal.

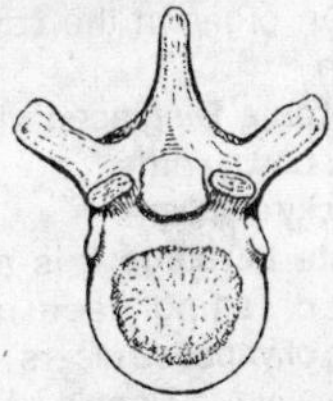

Thoracic vertebra

Vertex Vertex presentation of foetus in delivery, crown of the head.

Vertigo Feeling of rotation by self, feeling of rotation of surroundings, cerebellar lesions produce this symptom, vestibular nerve lesion can cause this symptom, other name for dizziness.

Vesicle Bladder which contain fluid, blister containing sebum, elevated skin lesion which contain serous fluid in it.

Vesicovaginal Related to the bladder and the vagina.

Vesicular That which contains vesicles.

Vessel Canal, duct or a tube that conducts fluid.

Vestibular Related to vestibule.

Vestibule Space at the entrance of a structure, vestibule of vagina, vestibule of the ear.

Vestibulocochlear Related to vestibule of ear and cochlea.

Vestigial Atrophied structure, rudimentary structure.

Vestigial Anything rudimentary, very old type, relic.

Viable One which can thrive independently.

Viagra Sildenafil citrate, oral drug for erectile dysfunction.

Vial A small glass container which contain drug for medication through parenteral route, sealed glass container with medication.

Vibration Motion of particles of a mass of air in a wave like manner and at different speed, usually with enough force to be packed up as 'sound' by receiving ear.

Vibrio Gram-negative bacteria which cause cholera or paracholera.

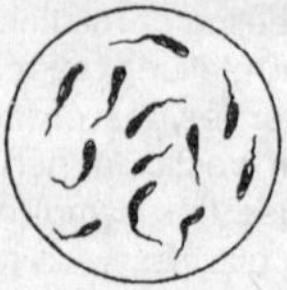

Vibrio cholerae

Vicarious Substituted organ for the purpose of performance of its function.

Village health guide A literate village volunteer who can secure people's participation in health care system, started in India in 1977.

Villi Vascular process or protrusion, chorionic villi.

Villus Finger like projections projecting from the surface of an organ,
small vascular process or protrusion.

Vinblastine Anticancer drug for Hodgkin's and cancer testes.

Vincent's angina Infection and ulceration of the tonsils by spirochete.

Vincent's infection Infection and inflammation by two infective agents of mouth.

Vincristine Anticancerous drug for lymphoma and leukaemia.

Vinegar Weak solution of acetic acid.

Vinyl Polyvinyl material for medical equipment, plastic used in the preparation of medical equipments.

Violent criminals Various causes including lack of social regulations in the family and mental illness due to organic lesions found to produce violent criminals.

Viraemia Appearance and manifestation of symptoms by virus in the blood.

Virchow angle Angle between nasosubnasal line and nasobasilar line.

Virchow node Supraclavicular lymph node.

Virgin Fresh, uncontaminated, woman not had sexual intercourse.

Virilism Ovarian tumour causing masculine traits on female, androgenic feature in a female, male secondary sexual characters in female.

Virility Masculine character, potent male.

Virion Complete infectious viral particle, virus with nucleic acid and capsid, extracellular virus.

Virology Study of viruses including their characteristics, multiplication, Site of harbour and disease manifestation.

Virulence Toxin producing pathogens.

Virulent Dangerous and acutely illness producing.

Virus Living entity which grows only in living tissues, ultramicroscopic in nature, viral infections are very common.

Viscera An organ in the cavity of abdomen.

Visceroptosis Displaced viscera towards downwards.

Viscid Sticky in nature.

Viscopaste bandage It is a supporting dressing used in the dressing of varicose ulcers,
An alternative to Unna's paste in varicose dressing.

Viscosity Physical property of a liquid which explains its sticky nature.

Viscus Organs in the cavity of abdomen.

Visible money It is called imprest amount, money provided to meet unforeseen emergency, a type of financial management.

Vision Sight sensation, faculty of seeing.

Visiting nurse Nursing care by the nurse in the community, nursing care at the doorstep , Public Health Nurse.

Visual Connected with sight.

Vital capacity Quantity of air expelled after forced inspiration.

Vital layer The biological layer which is made of algae, plankton, diatoms and bacteria help in removal of organic matter and oxidise. ammoniacal nitrogen, basic layer in slow sand filtration in water purification.

Vital statistics Statistics dealing with vital events of life like birth, death, and marriage.

Vital Life related item, vital statistics, vital capacity, vital sign.

Vitamin Accessory food factor in the diet, one which is essential for life, Micronutrient essential for metabolism, growth and development.

Vitiligo Leucoderma, absence of pigment in the skin.

Vitreous Jelly like substance between retina and lens, humour in the posterior chamber of the eye.

Viviparous Animals which give birth to fully developed offsprings.

Vocal cords Two transverse parallel folds of mucous membrane at the upper end of larynx which can either be relaxed towards the sides of the larynx during breathing, it is tightened and pulled toward each other to vibrate and produce or make sound.

Vocal Related to voice, vocal cord that produces voice.

Volatile Material which evaporates readily.

Volkmann contracture Contraction of fingers or toes resulting in loss of function of part, severe injury, improper tourniquet, improper cast culminates in Volkmann contracture.

Volume control IV set It is safe and effective procedure for administering precise dose of dilute medications to patients particularly to child patients, and for an extended period of IV drip.

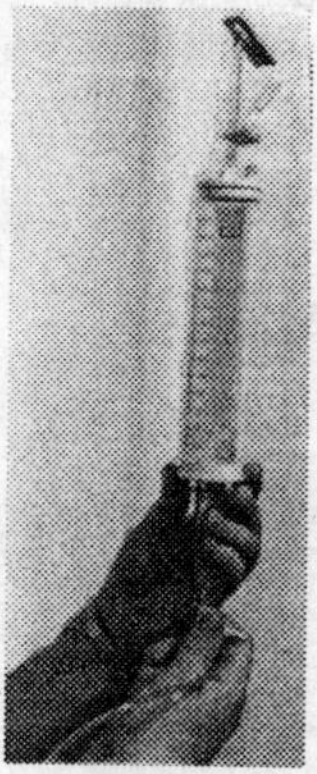

Volume control IV set

Volume Quantify the space occupied by a substance.

Voluntary The act that is done under the control of will of a person.

Voluntary muscle Striated muscle, since they attach skeleton they are skeletal muscle, voluntary muscle.

Volvulus Twisting of intestine causing intestinal obstruction.

Vomit To eject material from stomach.

Von Graefe's sign A sign of thyrotoxicosis, failure of lid to roll downward on looking down.

Von Recklinghausen's disease A clinical condition called neurofibromatosis.

Voyeurism A form of sexual offence, observing nude persons, observing sexual activity.

VSD Congenital heart defect, ventricular septal defect.

Vulgaris Expression for *ordinary.*

Vulva External genitalia of female.

Vulval toilet In obstetric cases where vulval or perineal area is sutured, careful vulval toilet is necessary for comfort and to prevent infection,

Types of vulval toilet are:

- Vulval swabbing which follow dressing of suture
- Jug douching.

Vulvovagititis Infection and inflammation of vulva and vagina.

VVM Vaccine vial monitor used in polio vaccine potency.

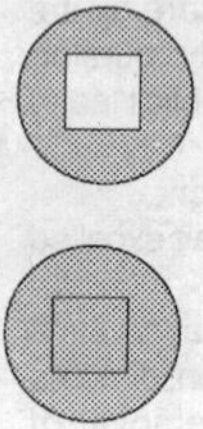

Inner square lighter than outer circle = Fit

Square and outer circle same = Un fit

VVM

VZIG Varicella zoster immunoglobulin against Varicella zoster virus.

W

Wafer A flat vaginal pessary.

Waist Part of the body between trunk and hip.

Waldeyers ring Lymphoid tissue in pharynx which is circular form, lingual faucial and pharyngeal tonsil area.

Walkers Patient who is to be assisted to walk is provided four pointed walker, patient moves the walker forward and walk into it and then repeats.

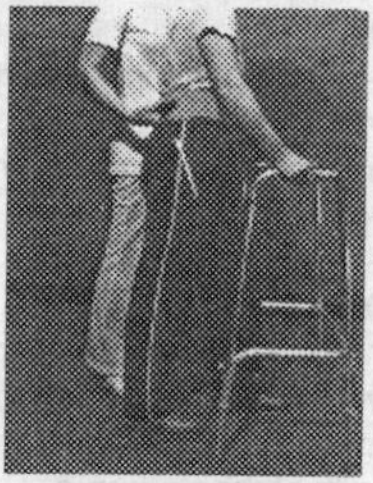

Walker

Wall plate Electrical apparatus for a current of low tension and low voltage.

Wallerian degeneration Nerve fibre degeneration along with myelin sheath, tubular structure instead of a nerve.

Walnut Juglans fruit, butternut, an astringent.

Wangensteen tube GI aspiration tube which has the tip which is radio-opaque.

Wantedness Making a person feel wanted in his group or in his family.

War wounds Wounds caused by bullets and the fragments of shells and bombs which are associated with complications.

Warburg apparatus Capillary monometer used in the study of oxygen consumption studies or carbon dioxide production studies.

Ward bathroom It is one of the domestic ward management.

Ward management Management of sick through medical and nursing care in the ward.

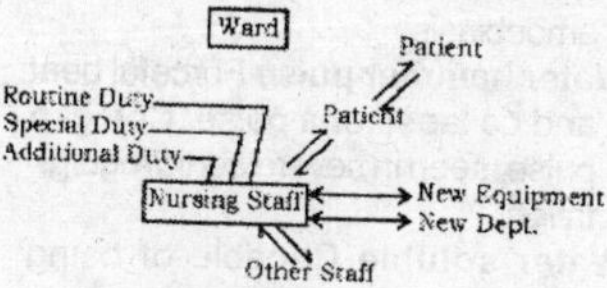

Ward management

Ward Hospital room to accommodate the sick for medical care and nursing care.

Warfarin Oral anticoagulant drug, used in coronary artery thrombosis, used in venous thrombosis.

Warm blooded Referred to animals which maintain a uniform temperature whatever the temperature changes of the surrounding.

Warmth In an illness due to injury body temperature is to be maintained by blanket and rug as a part of treatment.

Warts A virus infection of skin hypertrophy of papillae in the dermis upon viral infection.

Wash bottle Bottles with two tubes from the cork, used in washing the chemical material, blowing in one tube allow water to force in other tube for washing purpose.

Wasp Stinging bee, stinging insect, insect which injects wasp.

Wassermann reaction Laboratory test for syphilis, a complement fixation test.

Water balance Common term for fluid and electrolyte balance.

Water bed It is common apparatus used to prevent bedsore, rubber tube with water used for bedridden patients.

Waterborne disease Diseases that are transmitted through water, typhoid, diarrhoea, cholera, polio, amoebiasis.

Water hammer pulse Forceful beat and collapse of a pulse, Corrigan pulse, seen in severe aortic regurgitation.

Water soluble Capable of being dissolved in the water.

Waterhouse Friderichsen syndrome Meningococcal meningitis associated with fever, coma, cyanosis, haemorrhage from skin or mucous membrane and adrenal dysfunction due to bleeding.

Wax Hard brittle solid that become pliable on warming and melt on further heating, high molecular weight fatty acids, substance from animal source or plant source or mineral source.

Weal Whip injury markings, urticarial rash.

Weaning Discontinue breastfeeding at 4th month onwards to substitute cows milk and supplementary feeds like:

- Cow's milk.
- Fruit juice.
- Soft coked rice.
- Dhal soup.
- Vegetable soup.

Webbing Connecting by a fold of skin or a membrane, webbing of hand, foot and neck occur in congenital conditions.

Weber test Test with tuning fork for hard of hearing, activated tuning fork is placed on forehead which will be heard by both ears (normal).

Weber Classical sociologist who gave idea of social change.

Weight Heaviness expressed for compounding prescriptions, for ordinary commodities and for gold or precious stones

apothecaries – for compounding prescriptions

1. Grain
2. Scruples
3. Dram
4. Ounce
5. Pound

atomic – in comparison with oxygen which is 16

avoirdupois–for ordinary commodities

1. Grain
2. Dram
3. Ounce
4. Pound

combining–relative weight compared with hydrogen which is 1 of an element that enters into combination with other elements

equivalent – substance weight is equivalent in a chemical reaction to 1.008 G. of hydrogen

troy – by Jewellers

1. Grain
2. Penny weight
3. Ounce
4. Pound

Metric weight	*Metric measure*
microgram	microlitre
milligram	millilitre
centigram	centilitre
decigram	decilitre
gram	litre
decagram	dekalitre
hectogram	hectolitre
kilogram	kilolitre
metric ton	myrialitre

Measure capacity	*Measure length*
minim	micron
fluid dram	millimetre
fluid ounce	centimetre
gill	decimetre
pint	meter
quart	decametre
gallon	hectometre
	kilometre
	myriameter
	megameter

Weighing Weighment of food in diet survey, body weight recording in anthropometry, weighing of chemicals in pharmacy.

Weil Felix reaction Agglutination test for the diagnosis of rickettsial infection.

Weil's disease Jaundice caused by spirochete infection transmitted by rats leptospiral infection, leptospira ictero haemorrhagica.

Well baby clinic MCH service for the promotion of child health through growth monitoring immunisation health education on ORS and breast-feeding.

Well disinfection Water in the well is disinfected with bleaching powder to present water-borne diseases.

Wellbeing Feeling of good health from all angles.

Wenckebach phenomenon Incomplete heart block, detected by ECG changes of progressive lengthening of PR interval.

Wen A sebaceous cyst, plugged sebaceous glands in which the secretion hardens.

Wernicke's encephalopathy Thiamine deficiency manifestation, alcoholics suffers from this encephalopathy, delirium, eye paralysis and memory loss present.

Wertheim's operation A surgical procedure of hysterectomy.

Western blotting An immunological test done in case of HIV/AIDS.

Wet nurse Lactating mother breastfeeding other's babies.

Wet to dry dressing Refers to packing a wound either with medication or without medication.

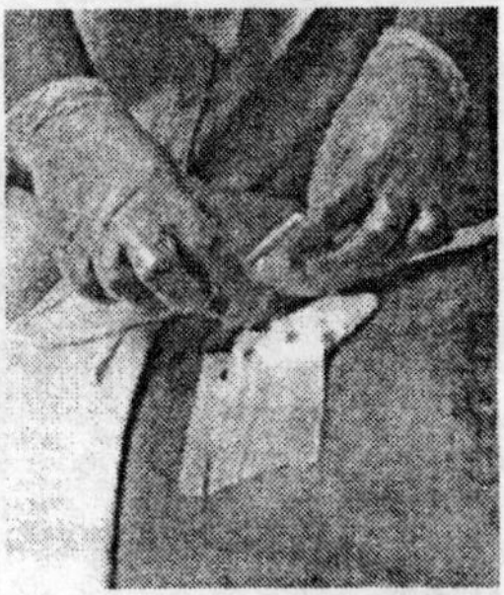

Wet to dry nursing

Wharton's jelly Name given to the connective tissue of the umbilical cord.

Wheelchair Chair with wheels are used to transfer cases, ambulatory for patients with lower limb paralysis or trauma or acutely ill.

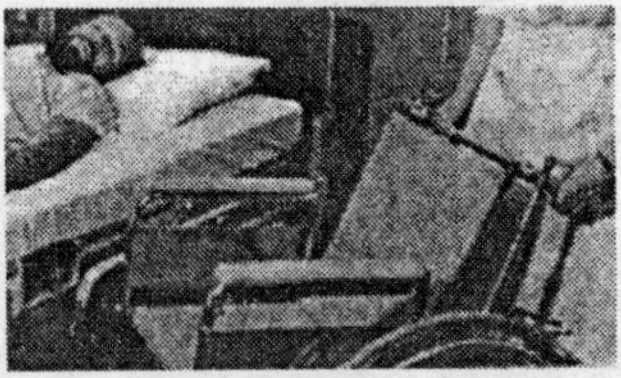

Wheelchair

Wheezing Spasm of smooth muscle of respiratory system giving rise to whistling sound during breathing, allergic bronchitis.

Whey Milk remaining after the curd and cream have been removed.

Whipples' disease Lipophagia granulomatosis, lipodystrophy.

Whipworm One of the nematode infection, trichuris infection.

Whisky Drinks containing 50% ethyl alcohol.

White cells Leucocytes, bodies in blood about 1/3rd larger than RBC, cells that war against infection, WBC.

White line Midline of, front of the body; linea alba, white tendinous attachment of external oblique and transverses muscle.

White matter myelinated nerve fibre of CNS.

White's disease Keratosis follicularis.

Whitefield's ointment Benzoic and salicylic acid ointment.

Whitlow The term applied to the formation of an abscess near the nailbed in a finger or toe, infection either superficial or deep.

WHO World Health Organisation, an international organisation.

Whooping cough Childhood preventable disease caused by B pertussis, a notifiable disease.

Whorl Whorl of finger print, circular arrangement of a part around a point, whorl of sun flower.

Widal reaction Blood test done for the diagnosis of typhoid and paratyphoid, an agglutination test.

Willett forceps A vulsellum forceps for applying scalp traction in the control of haemorrhage from placenta praevia.

Will Controlling one's own action and thoughts, firm decision.

Willi's circle Circle of arteries at the base of the brain, circle formed by internal carotid artery, anterior cerebral artery, posterior cerebral artery, and basilar artery.

Williams position For pelvic counter traction and for comfort this position is used in which patient's hips and knees are flexed to approximately 45^0 and the head of the bed is elevated to 20^0 to 30^0.

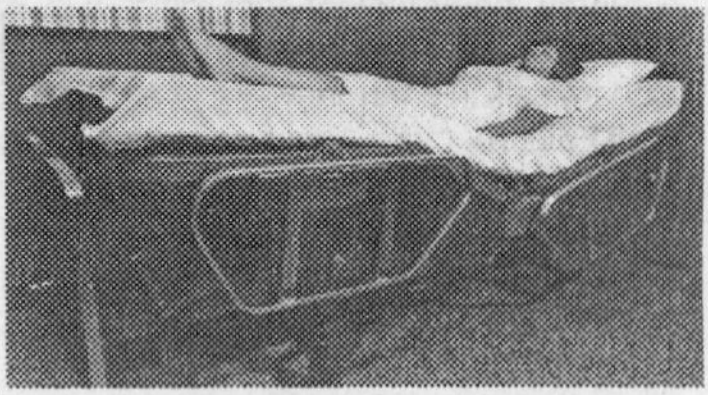

William's position

Wilms' tumour Cancer of kidney in young age, nephroblastoma.

Wilson's disease Deranged copper metabolism, hereditary in nature, neurological degeneration, and hepatolenticular degeneration.

Wine Fermented fruit juice with 5 percent alcohol.

Wing tipped needle Butterfly needle is called wing tipped needle used in the administration of IV fluid.

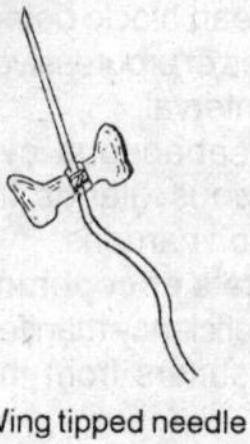

Wing tipped needle

Winging Displacement of the scapula seen in scoliosis.

Wintergreen oil A counter irritant, methyl salicylate.

Wire splints One of the types of splint for first aider, Kramer's wire splinting is common, framework of metal which is strengthened by struts placed across it.

Wiring Orthopaedic correction by fixing of fractured bones by using wire, repair of jaw, patella and sternum.

Wisdom tooth Third molar tooth which sprouts at puberty, back molar which erupt after maturity.

Withdrawal syndrome Seen in addicts of alcohol or drugs when they are withdrawn by force.

Withdrawl Abnormal shyness, unwilling to mingle, taking away of drug from an addict, taking away of male organ before ejaculation.

Wolffian body The mesonephros, , embryonic organ on either side of vertebral column.

Wolffian duct Duct running from mesonephros to cloaca in foetus.

Wolman's disease Inherited metabolic disease, infantile hepatosplenomegaly.

Womb Refers to uterus the main organ of reproduction.

Wonder drugs Public usage for sulphonamide in older times, later to penicillin group of drugs, now fourth generation of drugs.

Wood alcohol Methyl alcohol which causes blindness.

Wooden splints Varying lengths of wood is used for splints in first aid.

Wool fat Lanolin from sheep wool, a base used in ointment preparation.

Wool sorter's disease Clinical condition of anthrax involving lungs, a bacterial infection from animals.

Word blindness Clinical condition called dyslexia where difficulty in learning to read or learning to write.

Workmen' compensation Is an act which require employers to furnish medical care to employees whose injuries or occupational illness occur from an in the course of their employment.

World bank A specialised agency of United Nation to help countries to raise their living standards.

Worm Parasitic invertebrates which cause disease in man.

Wound drainage system post-surgical indwelling drain that connects to a portable vacuum container.

Wound Injury or surgery cause a break in tissue continuity types are contused **w**. incised **w**. lacerated **w**. open **w**. penetrating **w**. septic **w**.

Wright's syndrome A neurovascular syndrome caused by hyperabduction of the arm which occludes subclavian artery leading to gangrene.

Wrist bandage This is used to retain a dressing on the palm of the hand, useful for sprains of the wrist.

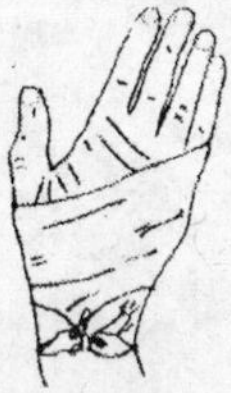

Wrist bandage

Wrist drop Radial nerve paralysis cusing wrist drop paralysis of the extensor muscles of the hand and fingers.

Wrist restraint Method of restrain the wrist in disoriented patient who may potentially dislodge the needle or catheter in the opposite arm.

Wrist Point of joining carpal bones and forearm bones.

Wry neck Torticollis, neck torsion of neck due to contraction of cervical muscles.

Wuchereria Filaria worm which causes elephantiasis.

Wylie's operation Surgery for prolapse of uterus, shortening of round ligament.

X

X chromosome Female chromosome denoted XX for female.

X-linked X-linked disorders are caused by genes of X chromosomes.

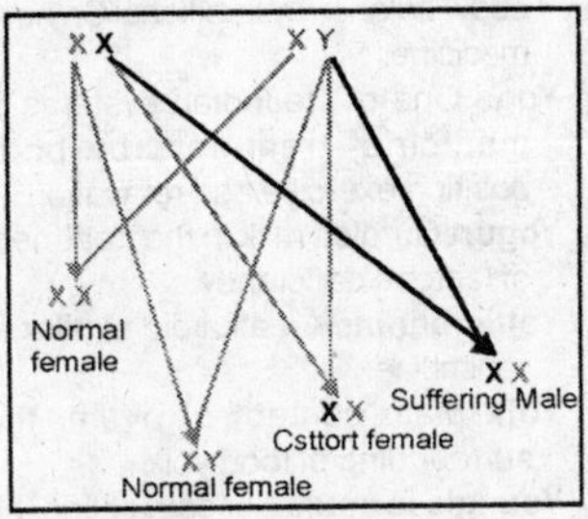

Sex-linked disorder

X ograph X-ray taken, Roentgenograph.

X-rays They are used for the diagnosis and for the treatment of diseases, electromagnetic waves of short length.

Xanthosis Yellow skin pigmentation on patients suffering from diabetes and poliomyelitis.

Xanthine Forerunner of uric acid in nucleoprotein metabolism.

Xanthochromia Skin changes and CSF changes to yellow is referred to as xanthochromia.

Xanthocyte Cell containing yellow pigment.

Xantho Meaning *yellow*.

Xanthoma Flat plaques of yellow colour in the skin, lipoids deposits foam cells or xanthoma cells.

Xanthophyll Yellow colour matter of plants, alpha carotene.

Xenology Science that deals with parasite and host relationship living parasites and man relationship study.

Xenopsylla Genus belonging to fleas responsible for disease spread rat flea Xenopsylla cheopis transmits plague.

Xeroderma Dryness of skin, hereditary dry skin.

Xerophthalmia Dryness of conjunctiva and cornea due to vitamin A deficiency.

Xerosis Dryness of an organ, of eye, of mouth, of vagina, of skin.

Xerostomia Dryness of the mouth, absence of saliva secretion.

Xiphoid process Lower portion of the sternum.

Xiphoid Sword-shaped, refers to xiphoid sternum.

Xylem Woody portion of plant.

Xylene Used for pathological laboratory microscopes cleaning, dimethyl benzene, a solvent.

Xylocaine Lignocaine used in anaesthesia.

Xylol Xylene.

Xylose A pentose sugar, connective tissue sugar.

Xyphisternum Lower end of the sternum which is pointed.

Xyrospasm Occupational disease among barbers, wrist and forearm muscle spasms.

Xysma Shaved material seen, stool containing thrown out mucous membrane.

Xyster File maintained by the surgeon.

Xystos Scraped lint.

XYYsyndrome Klinefelter's syndrome with 47 chromosomes, super male.

Y

Y chromosome Male sex chromosome, male has XY component, not present in females who has XX component.

Yard A unit of linear measure which is equivalent to 3 feet, 0.914399 meter.

Yawning Involuntary movement of mouth opening to breathe air in, which is associated with tiredness.

Yaws A tropical disease caused by Treponema pertenue.

Yeast Fungus belonging to group *Saccharomyces*, malt producer.

Yellow body It is corpus luteum

Yellow fever A viral infection transmitted by Aedes mosquito, present in South America and Africa.

Yellow marrow Found in the hollow center shaft of bones.

Yellow spot Central point of retina.

Yeo's treatment Treatment of obesity by giving large quantity of hot drinks and avoiding carbohydrates.

Yersinia One of the Gram-negative bacteria, include plague bacilli.

Yielding joint This is a term applied to a joint which permits slight movement intervertebral joints.

Yin and yang Principles of Chinese medicine, harmony of the body by dark and bright; positive and negative: feminine and masculine, body balance by traditional Chinese medicine.

Yoga One of the Indian systems of medicine, treatment by body position exercise and relaxation.

Yogurt Curdled milk in the treatment of lactose deficiency.

Yohimbenine An alkaloid similar to yohimbine.

Yolk Main content of ovum, the surrounding of food yolk.

Young's formula For calculating the proportion of the adult dose of a drug

To be given to a child =

$$\frac{\text{Age of the child}}{\text{age of child + 12}} \times \text{adult dose}$$

Young's rule Similar to Young's formula.

Youth culture Way of life and attitude same in youths.

Z axis Axis in the graphic representation, anteroposterior axis.

Z line Indicate the clear zone of a muscle fibre, indicate the position of sarcomere.

Z N stain Bacteriological staining method employed in staining *acid fast bacilli*, common stain for tuberculosis bacilli, Ziehl-Neelsen stain.

Z plasty A plastic surgery procedure, removal and repair of deformity, common surgical procedure to repair scar produced by contraction by injury or burns.

Z test Significant test done for a large sample, test of significance for large sample, normal deviate

$$Z = \frac{\overline{X}-\mu}{SD/\sqrt{n}} \quad \text{Where}$$

X = mean of sample (150 cm)

μ = Population mean (All India) (154 cm)

SD = 10 cm

n = 100 nurses

$$Z = \frac{150-154}{10/\sqrt{100}} = \frac{4}{1}$$

Infer :- Z calculated is more than 2.54 indicating that it is highly significant.

Z track injections When medication like iron injection may potentially seep into the injection tract and stain the skin and surrounding tissue, Z-track method into gluteal muscle is needed procedure:

1. Use 2 inch long needle.
2. Prepare the skin.
3. Displace tissue downwards, keep traction.
4. Continue displacement of tissue while injecting.
5. Aspirate to check.
6. Wait for 10 seconds after injection.
7. Remove the needle and traction given.
8. No massaging.

A

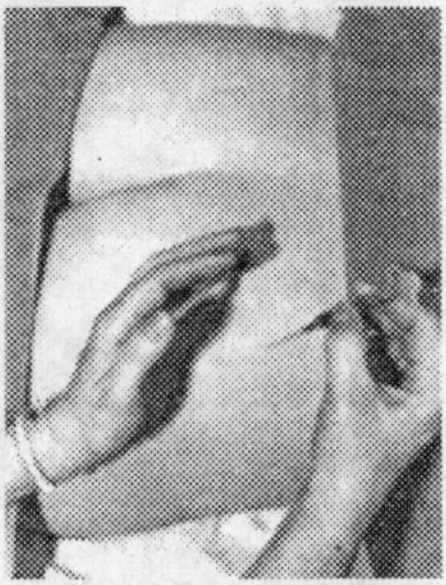

B

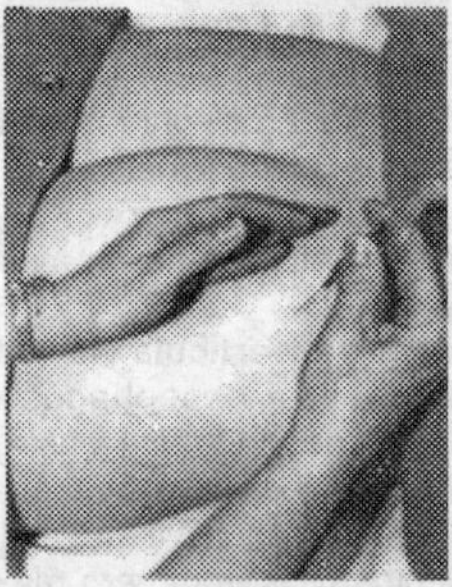

C

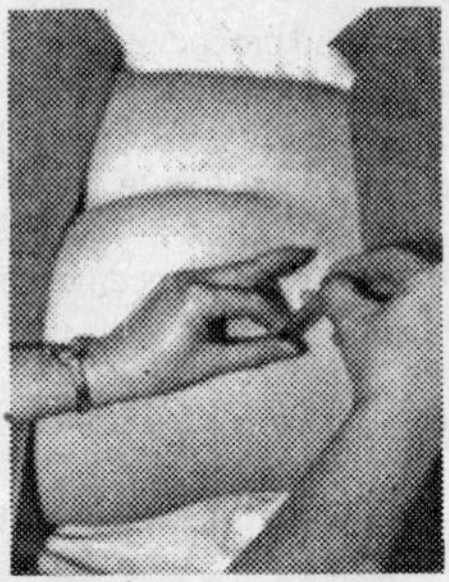

D

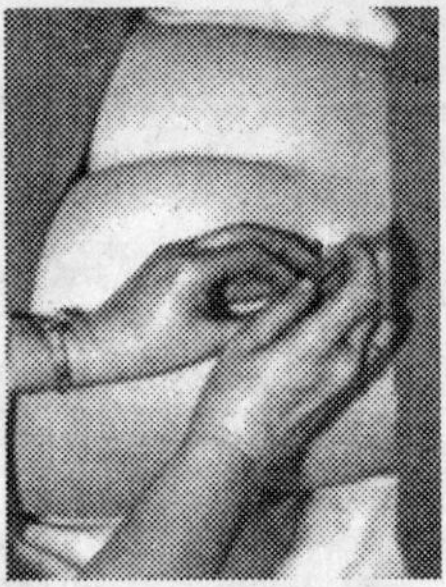

Steps in Z tract injection

Zappert's chamber A chamber for counting RBC with the help of microscope.

Zelotypia Zeal which is insane, jealous of insane nature.

Zenker degeneration Hyaline degeneration of skeletal muscles in typhoid.

Zenker's diverticula Herniation in the wall of oesophagus which cause oesophageal obstruction, defect in the wall of oesophagus.

Zero Any measure where graduation begins, it is *from zero* maximum possible lowest rate in any scale.

Zidovudine It is azidothymidine or AZT, an antiviral drug which retard the progress of AIDS.

ZIFT Zygote Intra Fallopian Tube Technique, a variant of I V F – E T i.e., In Vitro Fertilisation and Embryo Transfer, it is an ethics of human life, a procedure in fertility clinic.

Zimmer Zimmer metal is used in light weight walking aid , metal for elderly rehabilitations.

Zinc oxide Common smoothening agent, used for external application.

Zinc Astringent, antiseptic, 20% as ZnO used for external application.

Zipp Wound applicator for quick healing, a paste containing ZnO, iodoform and liquid paraffin (1: 2:2).

Zirconium A metallic element used in dentistry as a white pigment.

Zoetic When it is related with life or living material.

Zollinger-Ellison syndrome Resistant peptic ulcers present, 60% of ulcers are malignant gastrin producing tumour, causing ulcer.

Zonary placenta Placenta is shaped like a broad ring around the chorion.

Zona A belt, or a zone, zona pellucida, zona radiata, etc.

Zone A region, area with specific boundary.

Zonula Small circular area, a zonule.

Zonular cataract When opacity is limited to certain layers of lens.

Zonules of zin They are suspensory ligament of the lens.

Zonulysin An enzyme used in ophthalmic surgery.

Zoobiology It is the biology of animals.

Zoogeny Evolution and development of animals.

Zooglea Congregation of living material like algae, fungi, microbe zooglear layer in slow sand filtration has algae and planktons.

Zoology Biology of animals.

Zoonoses A disease transmitted from animals to man and sometimes back again.

Zoonosis Singular word for zoonoses.

Zoophilism Love for animals which is uncalled for, abnormality of human behaviour.

Zoophobia Fear for animals which is uncalled for, abnormality of human behaviour.

Zoopsia Hallucination of man where he sees that he is seeing animals though it is not real.

Zoster Herpes zoster a viral infection which attach cutaneous nerve path.

Zygocyte It is called zygote meaning yoked together, fusion of two gametes.

Zygoma It is a bony arch in front of ear formed by temporal bone and malar bone.

Zygomatic process Projection of the temporal bone.

Zygomatic reflex Lower jaw movement towards percussed side when zygoma is percussed.

Zygote Union of male and female gamete.

Zymase Yeast enzyme or bacterial enzymes which convert carbohydrate into water and carbon dioxide.

Zymogen Precursor of an enzyme which is not active.

Zymology Science of enzyme function, study of fermentation.

Zymosis A process of fermentation.

APPENDIX

1. COMPOSITION OF HUMAN BODY

Element	Percent	Element	Percent
Oxygen	65.00	Sulphur	00.15
Carbon	18.00	Chlorine	00.15
Hydrogen	10.00	Magnesium	00.05
Nitrogen	03.00	Fluorine	Traces
Calcium	01.50	Silicon	Traces
Phosphorus	01.00	Other elements	Traces
Potassium	00.35		

2. PHYSIOLOGY OF NORMAL LABOUR

Labour is a series of increasingly strong and painful rhythmical contraction of the uterine cavity, assisted in the later stages by the abdominal muscles, which expel the foetus. Uterine contraction in labour is painful and not painful in pregnancy (before labour).

Nursing care need the understanding of terms used for an act in an emergency. Foetus lies in uterus in an attitude of universal flexion with the head at the lower pole and the back lying against the anterior abdominal wall. Vertex presentation is normal and all other presentations like occipito-posterior, face, brow, breech, cord are abnormal presentations.

LOA (Left Occipito Anterior) where vertex position is the most common and the one is described in normal labour.

Stages of Labour

First Stage of Labour

It is from the onset of labour to full dilatation of cervix. Per vaginal examination is done to ascertain if the cervix has begun to dilate. There is little bleeding from torn capillaries, in the beginning then with mucous "The Show" starts with fore water in front of head (liquor amnii). When tension rises, membrane ruptures, fluid escapes by which time foetal head starts getting brunt of the pressure. This may produce "Caput succedaneum" which, however, is soon reabsorbed. The interval between the pains gives the mother rest and allows free flow of blood, through the uterine muscle to the placental site. The average duration of this stage is 10 to 12 hours in primi and lesser (4 to 6 hours) in multi.

Second Stage of Labour

It is from full dilatation of cervix to the birth of baby. This takes 2 hours in primi and lesser in multi. Retraction of uterine muscle presses down from above and advances with each pain. Head descends through vagina, perineum is stretched and head passes through vulva and is delivered between contractions. The shoulders rotate and are born with the next contraction and rest of the body is delivered at the same time.

Third Stage of Labour

It is from the birth to the delivery of placenta. The baby breathes and often cries lustily immediately after it is born and the cord may be cut as soon as convenient. There is no need to wait until it has ceased to pulsate.

3. OBSTETRIC DATE TABLE

Month in which menses occurred	*Day of the month to the day of the month noted*	*Number to be added to be noted*	*Month of expected confinement*
January	e.g., 01 (1.1.05)*	7	October
February		7	November
March		5	December
April		4	January
May		4	February
June		7	March
July	e.g., 08 ** (8.7.1979)	6	April
August	e.g., 25*** (25.8.2005)	7	May
September		7	June
October		7	July
November		7	August
December		6	September

*LMP = 1.1.2005, EDD = 8.10.2005
**LMP = 8.7.1979, EDD = 14.4.1980
***LMP = 25.8.2005, EDD = 1.6.2006
(EDD = LMP + 9 months + No. of days according to table)

Steps in finding out obstetric date from table

Step 1: The English calendar month in which menses occurred is noted e.g., **July**** (example illustrated is 8.7.1979).

Step 2: Date of **first day of menses** in taken e.g., **8th** [8th of July 1979 in illustration]

Step 3: To the numerical taken in Step 2, **table value for the given calendar month** is added.
[**8**th is the date of first day of menses, to this **6** is the value to be added (see table) which is **14** which could be the actual date of confinement.]

Step 4: Expected month is noted from the table. It is **April** for illustration.
[So, EDD is 14th April 1980]
Inference: **LMP = 8.7.1979, EDD = 14.4.1980.**

4. MIDWIFERY KIT CONTENT

Contents of maternity care kit

Sr.No	*Item*	*Nos.*
1.	Umbilical (cotton 0.3 cm x 25 cm)	2
2.	Blade with holder	1
3.	Cotton swab 7.5 cm x 7.5 cm (2.5 gm)	3 pieces
4.	Surgical gauze pieces 5 cm x 7.5 cm-12 ply	2 pieces
5.	Sanitary pad no. 4	1
6.	Drape - polyethylene sheet 75 cm x 100 cm	1
7.	Trolley cover	1

Contents of Dais Kit

Sr. No	*Item*	*Nos.*
1.	Aluminum kit box	1
2.	Stainless steel straight scissors (blunt - pointed)	1
3.	Stainles steel teaspoon	1
4.	Enamel irrigator with rubber tubing and ebonite nozzle	1
5.	Enamel bowl (large)	1
6.	Aluminum bowl	2
7.	Mackintosh sheeting (90 cm square)	1
8.	Hand towel	2
9.	Soap dish with soap	1
10.	Nail brush	1
11.	Absorbent cotton wool (sterilized)	1 packet
12.	Gauze (sterilized)	1 packet of 12 pieces
13.	Umbilical cord tape (sterilized)	6 pieces
14.	Dusting powder in a plastic container	1
15.	Antiseptic lotion	1 bottle

5. HEALTH WORKER FEMALE KIT CONTENT

List of Contents of Kit for Health Worker Female

A. General Kit

Sr.No.	*Item*	*Quantity*
1.	Kit bag (brown) with nylon tray, rectangular aluminum tray, side pocket, rear pocket, cover flap and shoulder strap.	1
Cover flap		
2.	Spring type dressing forceps—stainless steel (150 mm)	1
3.	Surgical straight scissors (blunt-stainless steel) (140 mm)	1
4.	Pencil with eraser	1
5.	Teaspoon – stainless steel	1
Side pocket		
6.	Nail brush	1
7.	Soap dish	1
8.	Soap	1
9.	Nail clipper	1
Rear pocket		
10.	Clear vinyl plastic sheeting (910 mm wide)	1 metre
11.	Huck towel (430 × 500 mm)	2
12.	Folding aluminum shield (BCG)	1
13.	Polythene self-sealing bag (125 × 200 mm)	12
14.	Sterile gauze pads (12 ply) (76 × 76 mm square)	6
15.	Arm circumference scale	1
16.	Nylon tray	1
17.	Absorbent non-sterile cotton wool (113 gm)	1roll
18.	Vinyl-coated fiberglass tape measure (1.5 metre/60")	1
19.	Safety pins (medium/40 mm)	1bag of 12
20.	Adhesive zinc oxide tape (25 mm × 0.9 metre)	1roll

(Contd.)

(Contd.)

Sr.No.	*Item*	*Quantity*
21.	Alcohol lamp with screw cap—metal (60 ml)	1
22.	Safety razor blades (double edge)	1 pkt of 5
23.	Clinical oral thermometer (35 to 42°C)	1
24.	Clinical rectal thermometer (35 to 42°C)	1
25.	Gauze bandage (non-sterile) (25 mm × 9 metres)	1 roll
26.	Triangular cloth bandage (910 mm slides)	1
27.	Microscope slide box	1
28.	Microscope slides (plain) (75 mm × 25 mm)	1 pkt of 10
29.	Cloth for cleaning micro-slides	1
30.	Stick swabs	1 bag
31.	Rubber solid stopper (bottom 16 mm top 20 mm)	1 for
32.	Specimen tube - glass (1900 × 75 mm)	1 hagedorm needle
33.	Keith abdominal suture needle (44 mm)	1
34.	Anaemia recognition card(English/Hindi)	1
35.	Nelaton solid-tip one eye urethral catheter (12 Fr)	1
36.	Urinalysis outfit (test tubes/bottle/clamp)	1 set
37.	Mayo Ochsner haemostat straight forceps-stainless steel (160 mm)	1
38.	Umbilical tape (non-sterile)	1
39.	DeLee tracheal catheter with glass mucus trap	1
40.	Rectangular aluminum tray	1
41.	Medicine cup – polypropylene (30 ml)	1
42.	Lubricant jar – plastic	14
43.	Amber dropping bottle – glass (10 ml)	3
44.	Wide—mouth screw cap square bottle – polyethylene (60 ml)	9
45.	Screw cap sputum container	4

B. Immunization Kit (one for each Subcentre)

Sr.No.	*Item*	*Quantity*
46.	Rubber ring	2
47.	File for BCG ampoules (6 mm × 50 mm)	1
48.	Wooden block for ampoules	1
49.	Sharpening stone (50 mm × 19 mm x 6.3 mm)	1
50.	Bifurcated needles— stainless steel (65 mm)	12
51.	Luer hypodermic needles (0.90 mm × 25 mm/20 G x 1")	1 box of 12
52.	Luer hypodermic needles (0.60 mm x 25 mm/23 G x 1")	2 boxes of 12 each
53.	Luer hypodermic needles (0.45 mm × 10 mm/26 G × 3/8")	1 box of 12
54.	Luer nylon hypodermic syringe (2 ml × 0.1ml)	2
55.	Luer glass hypodermic tuberculin syringe (1ml × 0.01ml)	2
56.	Test tube holder— two piece plastic	1
57.	Vacum insulated thermocontainer (300 ml)	1
58.	Aluminum box (180 mm × 100 mm × 40 mm)	1

6. FIRST AID BY DUTY NURSE

In case of accident or in case of emergency, nurse has to attend to the First Aid of the patient pending the arrival of the duty doctor or till the transport of the patient to the hospital.

Send the note to the duty doctor in writing. Without waiting the duty doctor, attend the emergency like cessation of breathing, profuse haemorrhage and shock.

In case of unconscious patient, put him on prone position, make sure that tongue is not obstructing his airway, do not give anything by mouth to a patient who is vomiting or who is unconscious.

Keep the body of patient warm by putting him on rugs. Assure and send the attendants to outside to avoid overcrowding round the patient.

Nursing Management of Shock

Check for pallor, cold skin, weak pulse and low BP. Observe for thirst, sweating, restlessness, dyspnea and vomiting in such admitted cases.

In case of blood loss, arrange for blood transfusion or to be sent by ambulance to the nearest hospital if the case seen in peripheral centres. Throughout rest, reassurance and conservation of body heat are to be taken care of. Withhold oral fluids till the case is transferred to a hospital and examined there, since, the case may need administering anaesthesia and surgery.

Nursing Management in Case Haemorrhage

If blood is red and escapes in spurts it is arterial haemorrhage. If blood is dark and pours out in steady stream it is venous haemorrhage. If it is capillary haemorrhage it is controllable by pressure.

Observe for pallor of skin and mucous membranes, lowered body temperature, deep and sighing respiration, restlessness, anxiety, rapid pulse, thirst, feeling of faintness, blurred vision and gradual loss of consciousness.

Arrange for blood grouping and cross-matching and wait for the duty doctor to come.

Let the patient lying flat with head in low position. Apply direct pressure at bleeding point. Apply a tourniquet in case of limb. Available pressure points are brachial artery, ulnar artery, radial artery, femoral artery, subclavian artery, carotid artery, temporal artery and popliteal artery.

Keep a watch on special types of haemorrhages like bleeding from varicose vein, GI tract, haemoptysis, epistaxis, cerebral haemorrhage and report to the duty doctor.

Nursing management in Fractures:

Ask and elicit pain, tenderness, swelling, bruising, loss of function, unnatural mobility, crepitus, grating of bone, shock, history of accident.

Let the patient be lying down, treat for shock, if there is an open wound do dressing, immobilise by splints, arrange safe transport.

Bring to the notice of duty doctor if special fractures are notice like rib fracture, spine fracture, pelvis fracture, femur fracture, skull fracture because they are dangerous and can be fatal if not noticed by the nurse.

Nursing Management in Dislocations

Observe for deformity, loss of movement, pain and swelling.

Put the patient in comfort position. Use bandage or splint when necessary. Call the duty doctor at the earliest.

Nursing Management in Sprains

Observe for pain, swelling and discolouration. Keep in mind the possibilities of dislocation and fracture and send words to the duty doctor to attend.

Immobilise, elevate the part and apply cold applications to prevent swelling. In case of swelling, application of hot application gives relief to the patient.

Nursing Management in Burns and Scalds

Early hospitalisation by emergency ambulance is requested. Morphine to relieve pain may be needed. Cover the burnt area with clean dressings.

Do not cover any, used or dirty clothing to cover the burns and scalds. In case of common accidental burns, water soluble cream containing penicillin or sulphonamide and 1 percent cetrimide with dressings is recommended.

In case of scalds of throat and mouth, patient may need tracheostomy and arrange for the same while sending call to duty doctor. Sips of olive oil given by mouth is recommended.

In case of chemical burns, washing with water is advocated. If nature of chemical is known a neutralising agent is to be used.

Chemical burns of the eye needs thorough wash with clean water, eye is covered with pad and bandage. Immediate call to the duty doctor is imminent.

Nursing Management of Poisons

Should have an idea about corrosives, irritants, narcotics, convulsants.

Any clue to the poison should be obtained for an effective treatment of the case.

To remove the poison, emetics and stomach wash are given. Common emetics like salt and water, mustard and water are usually tried.

To neutralise poison appropriate antidote are given.

To combat poisonous effect, respiratory stimulants and oxygen are given. Milk, white of egg, starch, corn flour mucilage or gruel are used in poisoning since they can buffer the effect of poison.

Nursing Management in a Patient with Loss of Consciousness

Nurse is expected to observe the signs of pallor, restlessness, perspiration round the mouth and on the forehead, nausea, faintness, feeble and slow pulse.

Patient is allowed to lie down flat, all tight clothing is loosened. A quick feeble pulse may indicate a concealed haemorrhage.

Nursing Management in Convulsions

If there is no danger of fall to injure him, nothing need be done in the tonic stage except to loosen any tight clothing. Mouth gag slipped to mouth prevents tongue biting.

Nurse should look for hysterical fit which is common in young women. High temperature and rickets in children are to be taken care of in case of convulsion among infants and children.

Nursing Management in Asphyxia

Clearing the air way, carrying out artificial respiration is undertaken along with sending for the duty doctor. Use of mechanical respirators is undertaken in hospital under the care of the duty doctor.

Nursing Management in CO Poisoning:

Patient is taken to area with fresh air to breath. Ammonia is tried as respiratory stimulant. Artificial respiration is needed in case of cessation of respiration.

Oxygen and carbon dioxide mixture is allowed for breathing which is followed by removal to hospital at the earliest.

Nursing Management in Electric Shock:

If patient is with live circuit, cut of the current, pull him away with the help of wooden stick.

After disconnecting, patient may need artificial respiration.

Electric burns sustained by the patient needs specific treatment.

Nursing Management in Snake bite:

History of snake bite followed by burning stinging pain and swelling of the part should allow the nurse to come to conclusion that common snake must have bitten and rush to the first aid of the case. The patient may tell about Cobra, Common Krait, Russel's viper or saw scaled viper.

Apply ligature to the limb some distance above the bite. It should be tight to stop circulation but should be slackened off once in 10 minutes.

Cross-incisions be made over snake bite area.

Suction of poison is done by some suction apparatus like breast pump or by mouth sucking if nothing is available.

As soon the duty doctor comes, administration of antisnake venom serum is done.

Associated treatment with analgesics, tranquilliser may be needed.
If the duty doctor orders for transfusion of blood or plasma nurse should arrange at once.

Nursing Management in Insect Bite, Bee Sting, Wasp Sting:

Mild local reaction is very easily attended with ice pack application. In hospital or health centre, diluted vinegar or antihistaminic ointment is applied. Severe cases need injection of adrenaline.

Sting should be carefully removed and remaining venom is expressed from the gland with the help of forceps.

7. WARD MANAGEMENT

Unit of a hospital which host the sick for medical care and nursing care form a ward in the hospital.

According to WHO the hospital is "an integral part of a social and medical organisation, the function of which is to provide for the population the complete health care, both curative and preventive and whose out-patient services reach out to the family and its home workers and for Bio-social research".

Expected functions of professional care are:

- Care of the sick.
- Care of the injured.
- Prevention of diseases.
- Promotion of health.
- Diagnosis.
- Treatment.
- Rehabilitation.
- Vocational training.
- Nursing education.
- Research.

Nursing Management include

- Division of work starting from nursing superintendent, Matron, Dept sister, charge nurse, staff nurse, ANM, clerk, Ward aides, cleaning staff.
- Division of work starting from principal senior sister tutor, junior sister tutor at nursing college level.
- Authority and responsibility in nursing duties.
- Discipline as per nursing code.
- Unity of command from one source.
- Unity of direction of work or activity.
- Subordinate coordination.
- Adequate remuneration.

Nursing Skills at Hospitals and Health Centres are

- Conceptual skills.
- Human relation skill.
- Technical skill.

Nursing Ward Management is summarized by following diagram

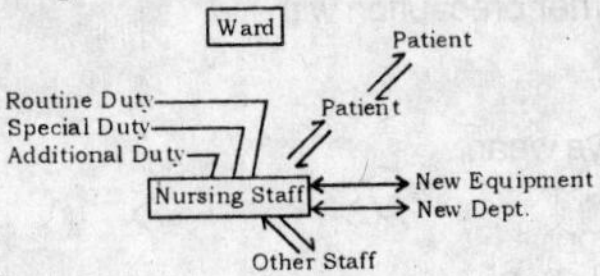

Ward Management

8. UNIVERSAL WORK PRECAUTION

For bio safety, a nurse is instructed to follow

- Persons who are trained in management of potential hazards only should handle infectious material.
- All laboratories must be biohazard free area.
- Working coat and working gown should be worn by all workers working in laboratory.
- Gloves should be worn when handling infectious material. Adequate supply of gloves of good quality should be made available.
- Disinfection of all working surface and working area should be done each time.
- Use of syringes, sharp instruments and needles should be avoided. When used utmost care must be used.
- Used needles should not be recapped and they should not be removed from syringes.
- Always use pipetting device and avoid mouth pipetting of substances
- Aerosols droplets, splashes and spills should be avoided by skill work.
- Frequent hand wash and not touching mouth, nose, eyes and organs are avoided.
- In working area eating, drinking smoking or storing food should be avoided.

Care by the nurse at samples collections

- Inspect your skin for any cut or abrasions.
- If gloves are contaminated or blood tinge discard them.
- Wash hands before and after sample collection.
- Always use working gown at work.
- Used needles and syringes should be put in a puncture resistant container.
- Seal all contaminated specimen and wipe the outer surface with a hypochlorite solution with a concentration of 0.1% available chlorine.
- Take suggested precaution in needle prink injury.
- Report to your senior for any doubt of contamination at work.

Professional precautions by the working nurse are:

- Always take barrier precaution with
  - i. Gloves.
  - ii. Masks.
  - iii. Protecting eye wear.
  - iv. Facial shields.
  - v. Gown or apron.
- Wash your hands before and after all nursing care activities. Even do this after removal of gloves after any nursing procedure.

- Take care to prevent injury by needle, scalpel and sharp instruments.
- In emergency nursing care use mouth pieces, resuscitation bags and other ventilation devices as precaution to HIV transmission.
- If you have skin lesions or weeping dermatitis, refrain from work.
- If you are pregnant , avoid attending HIV patients.
- Always prefer disposables in your nursing care services.

9. PRESCRIPTION AND PHARMACY TERMS IN NURSING PROFESSIONAL CARE

a.	ante, before
aa.	ana,of each
a.c.	ante cibum, before food
ad lib.	ad libitum, at pleasure
ae.p.	aequales partes, equal parts
aq	aqua, in water
b.i.d	bis in die, twice a day
c.sem.	cum semisse, and a half
coch.	cochleare, spoonful
div.	divide
fl.	fluid
gtt.	gutta, a drop
h.	hora, an hour
h.d.	at bed time
h.s.	at bed time
h.s.s.	hora somni sumendus, to be taken at bedtime
liq.	liquor
mist	mixture
m	mane, morning
m.d.	more dicto, as directed
m.p.	mane primo, early in the morning
n.	note, night
NP	nomen proprium, desired that drug name is written
om.	omni., every
o.h.	omni hora, every hour
o.n.	omni nocte, evry night
o.m.	omni mane, every morning
pil.	pill
pulv.	powder
p.c.	post cibum, after food
p.prandium,	post prandial, after dinner
p.r.n.	pro re nata, when necessary
q.i.	quantum libet, enough

q.s.	quantum sufficiat, sufficient
q.v.	quantum volueris, as much as you wish
rep.	repeat
sum.	take, sumatur
s.	solve or dissolve
st.	statim, immediately
s.o.s.	si opus sit, if necessary
t.d.s.	ter die sumendus, take thrice a day
tr.	tincture
u.d.	ut dictum, as directed
2 tis.	every 2 hours
3 tis.	every 3 hours
4 tis	every 4 hours
6 tis.	every 6 hours
i.m.	intra muscular
i.v.	intra venous
s.c	sub cutaneous
Proph	prophylactic
Thera	Therapeutic

10. FOOD SOURCE FOR NUTRIENTS

Source of food for nutrients

Nutrient	*Food*
Energy	Cereals, pulses, roots, tubers, fats, oils, sugar, jaggery
Protein	Milk, egg, fish, meat, liver, pulses, nuts, oilseeds.
Fat	Butter, ghee, vegetable oils, hydrogenated fats, nuts and oilseeds
Carbohydrate	Cereals, pulses, sugar, jaggery, roots, tubers.
Fiber	Green leafy vegetables, fruits, unrefined cereals, pulses, legumes
Calcium	Milk, milk products, ragi, green leafy vegetables
Iron	Liver, green leafy vegetables, rice flakes, wholewheat flour, ragi, pulses
Vitamin A	Fish, liver oil, butter, ghee, milk, carrot, green leafy vegetables, papaya, mango
B complex	Milk, egg, liver, home-pound rice, whole wheat, whole gram, pulses, green leafy vegetables, nuts, oil seeds.
Vitamin C	Gooseberry, lime, orange, guava, tomato, lettuce, sprouted gram
Vitamin D	Milk, sunlight

FOOD STUFF	PROTEIN	FAT	CARBOHYD.	CALORIES
Cereal	9.9	2.3	71.0	344
Bread	7.8	0.7	51.9	245
Salt biscuit	6.6	32.4	54.6	534
Sweet biscuit	6.4	15.2	71.9	450
Pulses	22.6	2.0	58.4	342
Green leafy vege.	3.8	0.6	6.0	45
Roots, tubers	1.2	0.2	16.0	70
Other vegetables	2.2	0.3	6.3	36
Nuts, oilseed	15.2	46.6	20.4	578
Condiment, spice	9.8	6.6	40.6	261
Fruit	1.1	0.4	7.6	79
Meat	21.0	4.9	0.8	131
Egg	13.3	13.3	0.0	173
Milk	3.6	5.8	4.7	85
Curd	3.1	4.0	3.0	60
Butter	0.0	81.0	0.0	729
Ghee	0.0	100.0	0.0	900
Oil	0.0	100.0	0.0	900
Sugar	0.1	0.0	99.4	398
Honey	0.3	0.0	79.5	319
Jaggery	0.4	0.1	95.0	383
Sago	0.2	0.2	87.1	351

Table: Nutritive value of common foods

11. PERIOD OF INFECTIVITY OF INFECTIOUS DISEASES

Chickenpox	6 days after the onset of rashes
Cholera	3 days after tetracycline started
German measles	cannot be ascertained
Hepatitis A	3 weeks from onset of illness
Herpes zoster	6 days after herpes rash
Influenza	3 days after clinical manifestations
Measles	upto 3rd day of the rash
Mumps	until parotid swelling subsides
Meningococcal meningitis	upto 6 hours of starting antibiotics
Polio	6 weeks in children
Pertussis	till paroxysms ceses about 1 month
Shigellosis	till 3 stool culture negative (3 successive)
Salmonellosis	till 3 stool culture negative (3 successive)
Streptococcal pharyngitis	upto 6 hours of starting antibiotics
Tuberculosis	Till sputum is negative

12. TRANSPORTATION OF THE SICK AND INJURED

Sick and injured may require life saving attention before being transported to hospital .

Injured person may be trapped in debris and may need removal and some first aid treatment.

Nurse should wait for rescue service to arrive and for equipment arrive. After the accident, patient need removed to hospital for emergency treatment.

Manual and by stretcher the sick and injured are transported which are learnt by the first aider in their training.

During transport some of the rules to be followed are:

- safety.
- steadiness.
- speed.
- observation of sick or injured.

Manual method of transport of the sick and injured

(a) The cradle carry method help in carrying children and light persons.

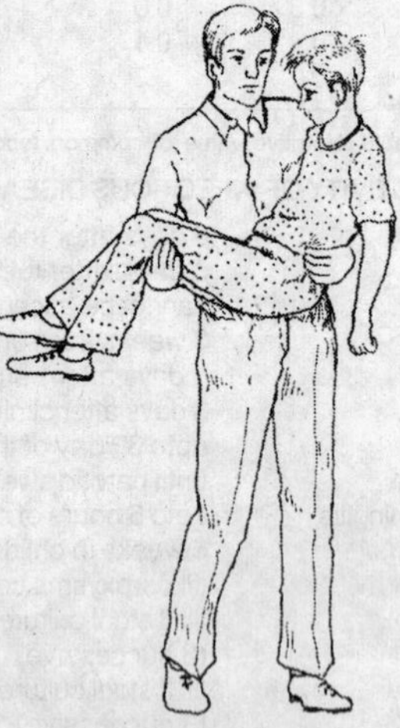

The cradle carry

(b) The Human crutch method help in carrying one leg injured person who can be helped to move to required place.

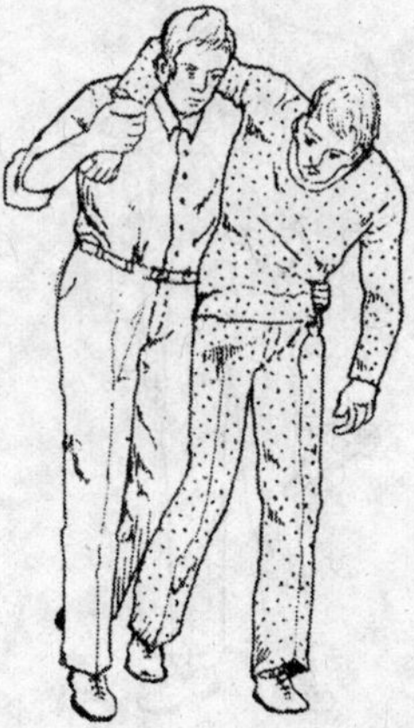

The human crutch

(c) The pick a back to carry conscious person who can be carried on the back of first aider.

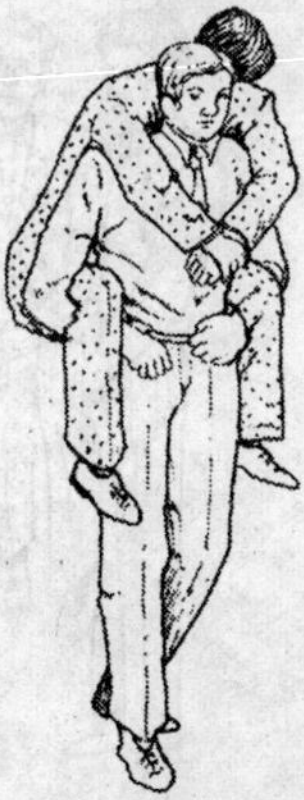

The pick a back

(d) The Fireman's lift and carry to carry a patient who is unable to walk but is lighter in weight.

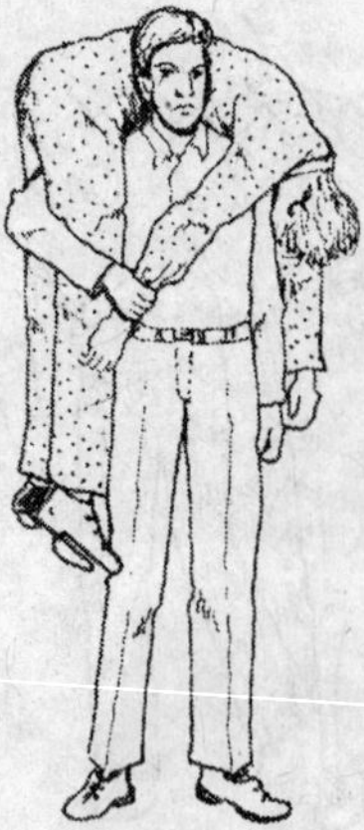

The Fireman's lift and carry

(e) The two hand seat to carry conscious patient who is unable to use his arms.

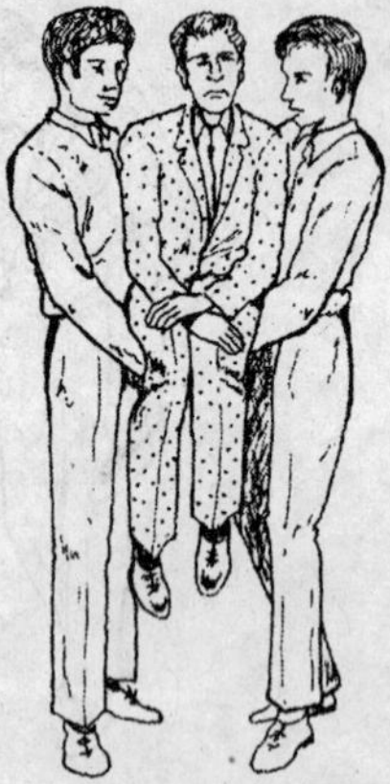

The two hand seat

(f) The human stretcher to carry a patient in the lying down position who is nconscious.

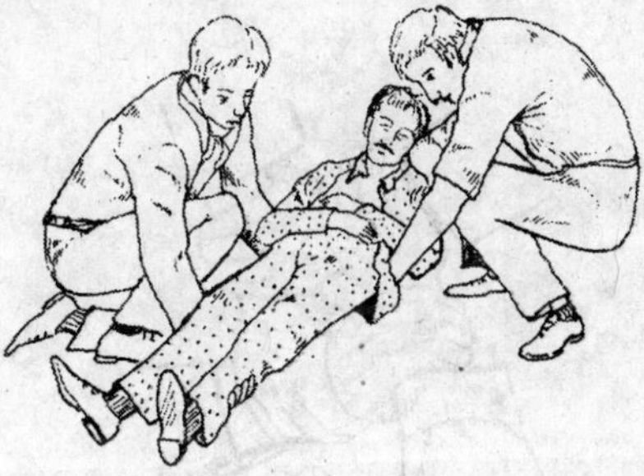

The human stretcher

(g) The three hand seat to carry patient who uses his arms and who is conscious.

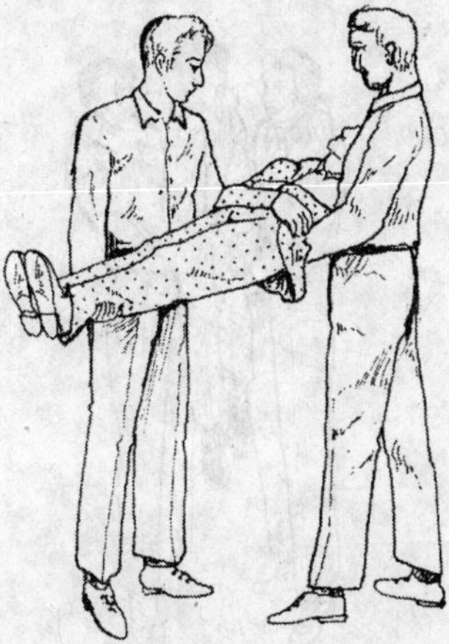

The three hand seat

(h) The four hand seat to carry conscious patient who can help first aiders with his arms and who does not require support for lower limbs.

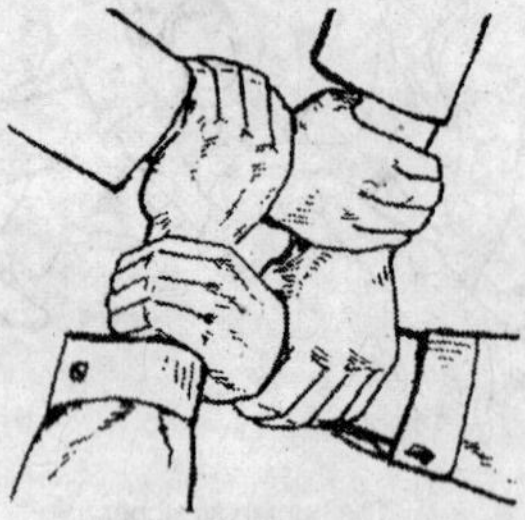

Hand position (for four hand seat)

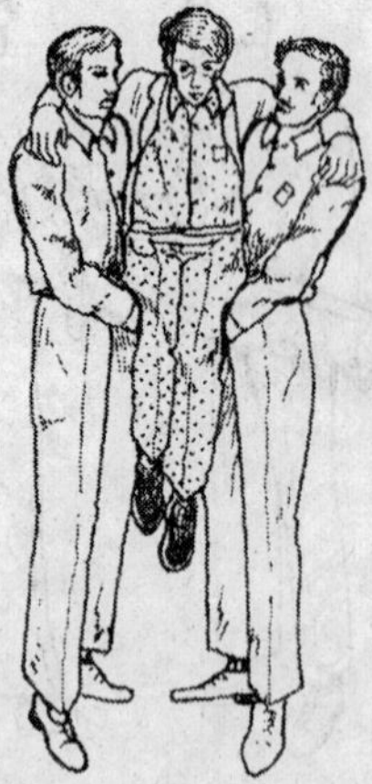

The four hand seat (Read to carry)

(i) Transport by stretcher of severely injured and severe sick careful loading the patient, after preparation, by following steps.

Preparing the patient to lift
Lifting the patient to place onto stretcher
Placing the stretcher under patient
Lowering the patient to stretcher
Moving or advancing the patient

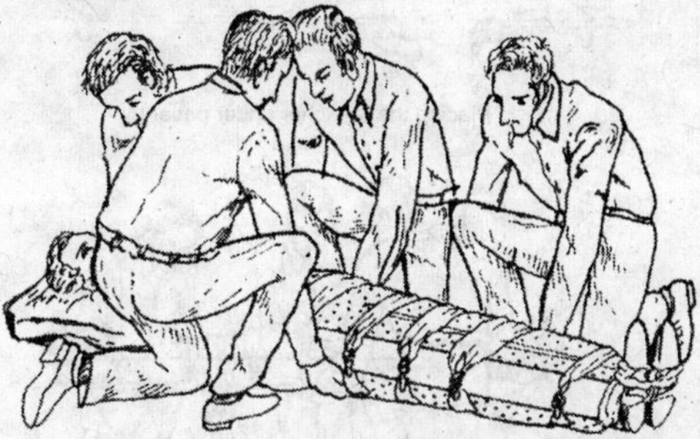

Preparing the patient to lift

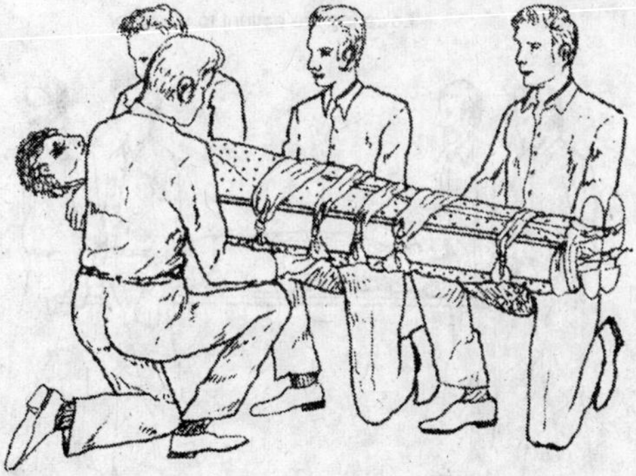

Lifting the patient to place onto stretcher

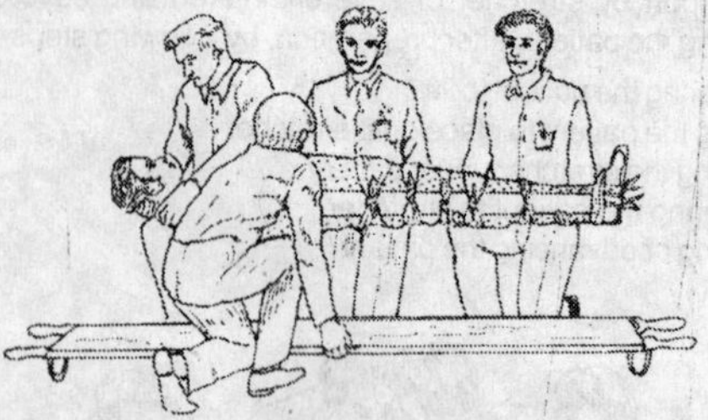

Placing the stretcher under patient

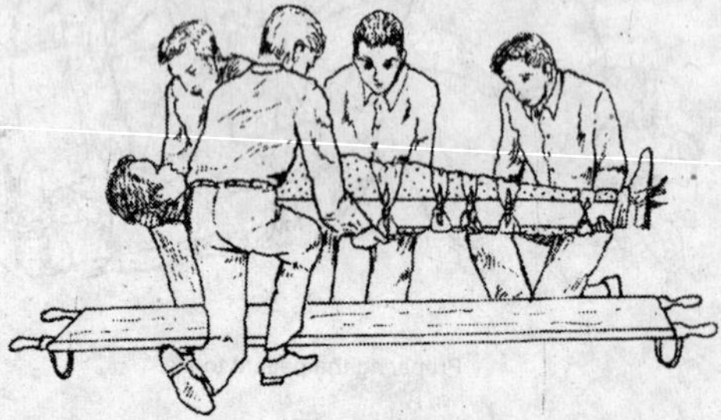

Lowering the patient to stretcher

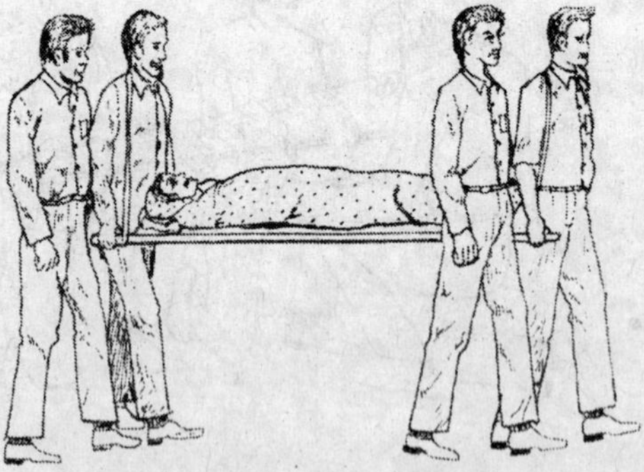

Moving or advancing the patient

13. SYNDROME APPROACH FOR STD

(i) Lower Abdominal Pain in the Female (PID)

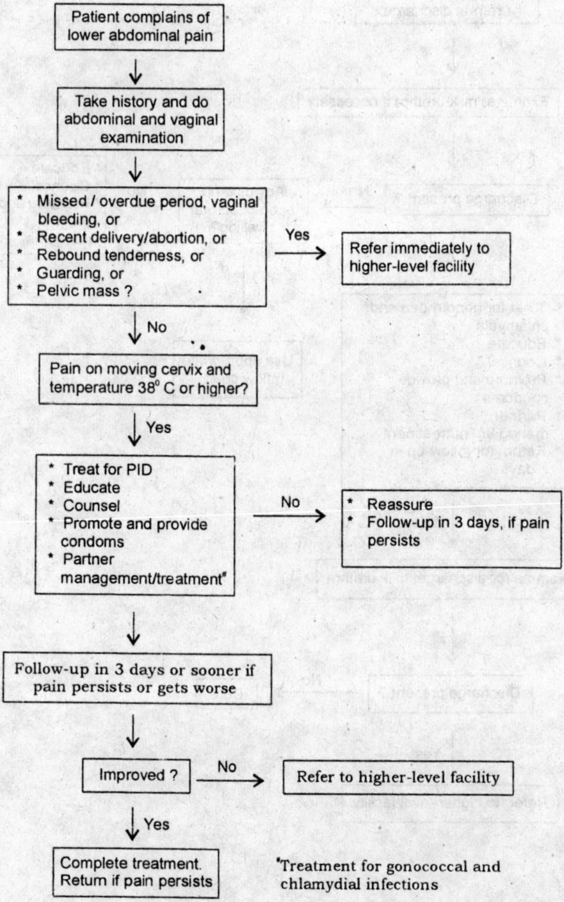

#Treatment for gonococcal and chlamydial infections

(ii) Urethral discharge

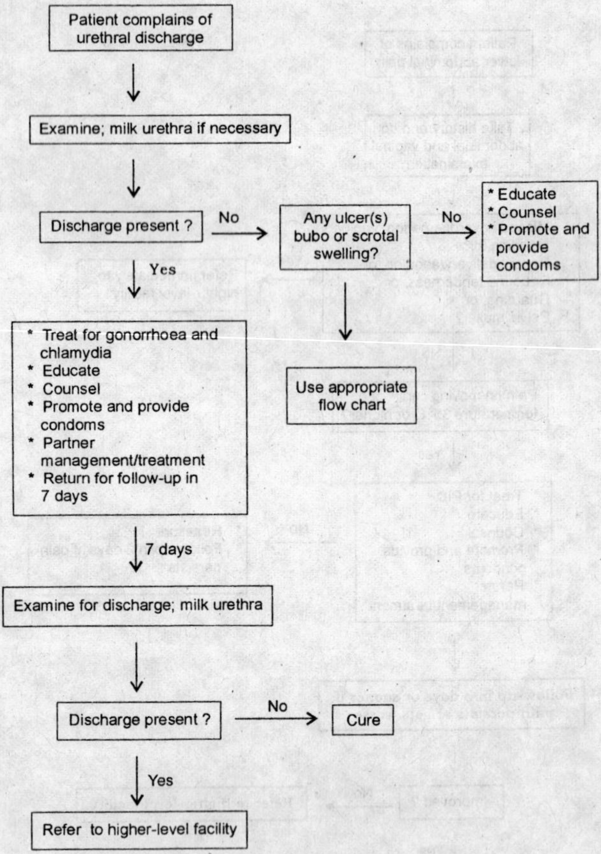

(iii) Vaginal Discharge
(With speculum Examination)

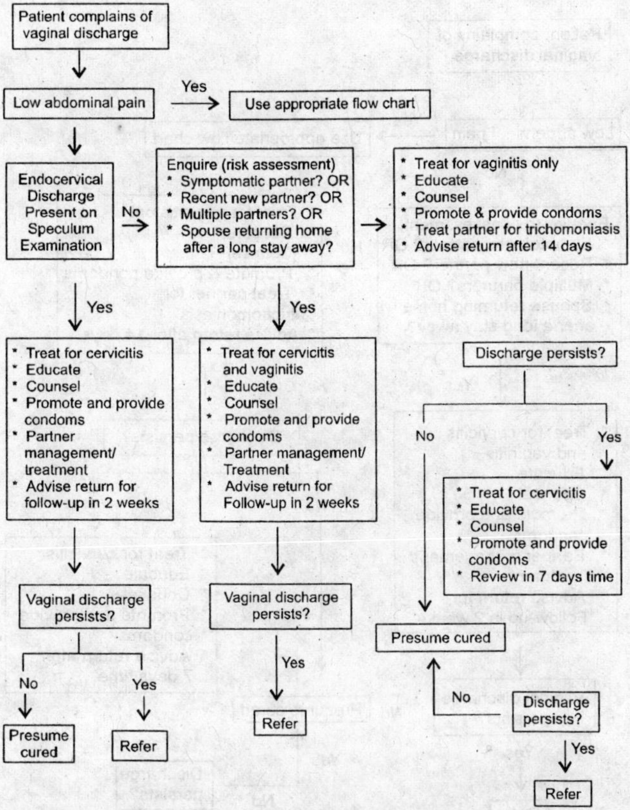

(iv) Vaginal Discharge

(No speculum Examination)

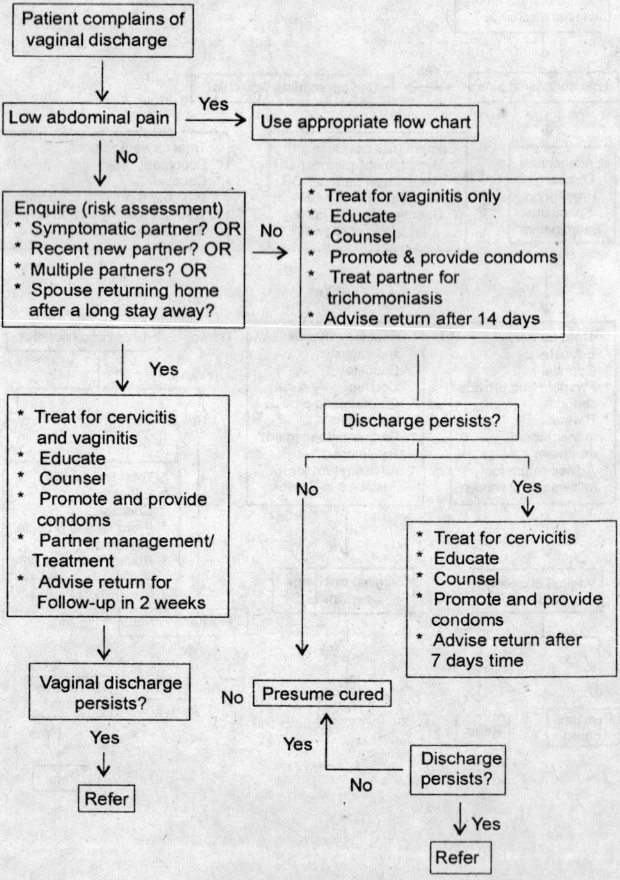

(v) Genital Ulcers

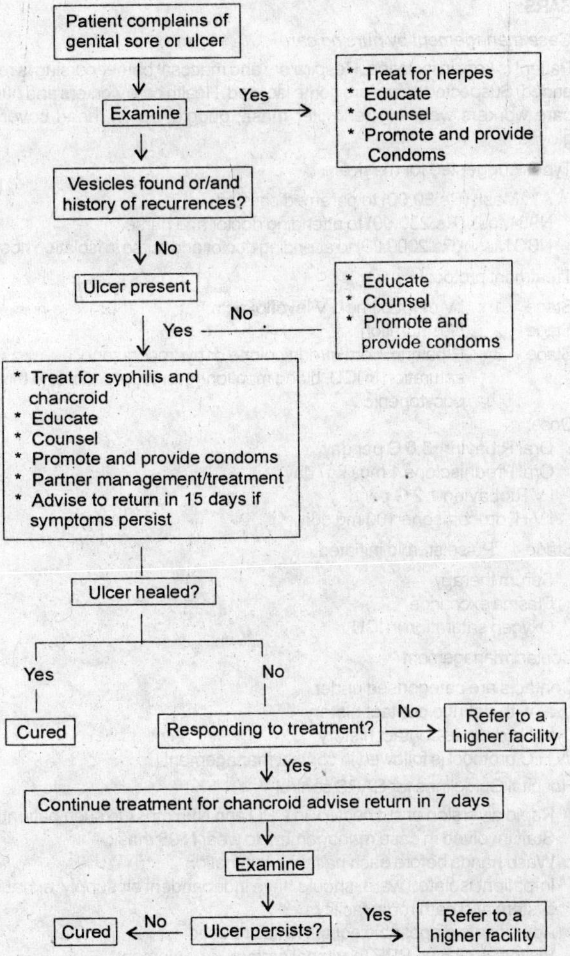

14. NURSING CARE IN COMMUNICABLE DISEASES

SARS:

Case management by nursing care

Patient is kept in isolation. Respiratory and mucosal barrier nursing is recom ended. Suspected cases are home isolated. Health care workers and nursing care workers wear efficient filter mask, goggle, apron, head cover and gloves.

Types suggested for mask are

A71Mask (Rs.80.00) to paramedical staff.
N95 Mask (Rs.230.00) to attending doctor and nurse.
NBC Mask (Rs.2000.00) to attending doctor and nurse in isolation hospital.

Treatment protocol

Stage 1 : I V cefotaxime/ I V levofloxacin
Stage 2 : Desaturation
Stage 3 : Ribavirin + oral prednisolone or hydrocortisone, oxygen saturation in ICU, blood monitoring for leucopenia and throm bocytopenic

Dose:

Oral Ribavirin 3.6 G per day
Oral Prednisolone 1 mg / kg / day
I V Riobavirin 1.2 G per day
I V Hydrocortisone 100 mg q6h

Stage 4 : Pulse steroid initiated

Serum therapy
Plasma exchange
Oxygen saturation in ICU

Contact management

Contacts are categorised under

a) with definite contact history.
b) No definite contact history.

W.H.O protocol is followed in contact management.

Hospital Guidelines for SARS control

Rapid diversion of suspected, in OPD and N95 mask to such patients.
Staff involved in case management to wear N 95 mask.
Wash hands before each patient examination.
In-patient isolated ward, should have independent air supply, exhaust. system and bath room facility.
Appropriate disposable equipments are used.
Visitors are given PPE (personal protective equipment).

Restriction to non-essential staff to SAS ward is followed.
Alcohol based skin disinfectants are used.
Special care is given in interventions like nebuliser, chest physiotherapy, bronchoscopy and gastroscopy.

ANTHRAX

Case management with nursing care

Skin lesion is readily curable with early diagnosis and prompt treatment. Treatment is started with ciprofloxacin 500 mg daily until penicillin sensitivity result comes. Then change of treatment is 6 lakh unit penicillin-G intravenously 6 hourly (or penicillin V 500 mg 6 hourly). Aggressive fluid resuscitation and addition of aminoglycoside improve the condition. In pneumonia (of inhalation type), ventilatory assistance is needed.

Nursing staff and medical staff attending the case need prophylaxis with ciprofloxacin 500 mg 12 hourly.

DENGUE

Case management and nursing care:

There is no specific drug. Paracetamol is given for pains. Sometimes opiates are given; aspirin should be avoided. Capillary leak syndrome causing shock requires volume replacement, blood transfusion and management of shock; corticosteroids are not useful.

Incubation period is usually 5 to 6 days. Patients are infective for mosquito from the day before onset to 5th day of disease. The mosquito becomes infective 10 days after blood meal and remains for life.

AIDS

Nursing Management of Needle Stick Injury:

Being risk group, nursing professionals have to deal with anticipated accidental exposures to HIV. Average risk is 1 in 300 (0.3%) and prevention is the main strategy to avoid occupational exposure to HIV.

Use of protective barrier:

- Latex or vinyl gloves.
- Heavy duty rubber glove at cleaning.
- Gloves and apron at surgery.
- Protective eye wear.
- Safe handling of sharps.

In case of injury (after exposure):

- Wash injury with soap and water.
- Splash to the nose, mouth, skin should be flushed with water.
- Eyes are irrigated with clean water.

- Don't put prinked finger into mouth.
- Report to authorities.
- Postexposure prophylaxis (PEP) may be recommended.

When source material are blood, bloody fluid or other potentially infectious material, determination of the exposure code (EC) and determination of HIV status code (HIVSC) as EC_1, EC_2, EC_3, EC_4 and $HIVSC_1$, $HIVSC_2$ and HIVSC unknown will help in case management with recommended prophylaxis.

INFLUENZA

Case management with nursing care

Bed rest is advocated until fever subsides. Paracetamol 0.5 to 1.0 gram 6 hourly can relieve headache and generalised pains. Amantadine and Rimantidine 100 mg BD for 3 days is found effective. Pholcodine 10 mg every 6 hours may be given to suppress cough. Specific treatment for pneumonia may be necessary.

DIPHTHERIA

Case management with nursing care

Clinical diagnosis of diphtheria should be notified to local authorities. Swab is taken for confirmation and treatment is started at once. Regimen is:

- Antitoxin.
- Antibiotic.
- Isolation.

For mild case antidiphtheria serum (ADS) 4000 to 8000 units, moderately severe cases 16000 to 40000 units and severely ill 100,000 units are given I M route. Care is taken to see adrenaline is kept available for immediate type-reaction along (0.5 ml 1 in 1000 I M) with an antihistaminic.

Penicillin 1200 mg 6 hourly I V or amoxicillin 500 mg 8 hourly should be administered for 2 weeks to eliminate bacteria. Erythromycin is a choice in penicillin sensitive cases. Patient is managed in strict isolation. Nursing management should adhere to strict nursing barrier. Patient is clear only when 3 swab 24 hour apart are culture negative.

TETANUS

Case management in nursing care

Neutralise toxin by I V injection of 3000 IU human tetanus antitoxin

Prevent further toxin by debridement of wound.

Benzyl penicillin 600 mg IV 6 hourly (alternative is metronidazole).

Control the spasm by nursing in a quiet room; avoid noise, light and other stimuli,

IV diazepam for spasms

General nursing by hydration, nutrition (tube feeding) and treating secondary infections

Wound treatment strategy in hospital:

Action is taken on the nature and type of injury or would as under:

	Less than 6 hours	*Other wounds*
TT taken before 5 years	No treatment	No treatment
TT taken between 5-10 years	TT(1) dose	TT (1) dose
TT taken above 10 years Immunisation	TT(1) dose	Active + passive
TT history not known	TT course given	Immunoglobulin TT course given

MEASLES

Management with nursing care

Only symptomatic treatment. Antibiotic should be given only if the child has clinical signs of pneumonia or other evidence of sepsis.
Isolation of cases for 7 days from rash.
Immunisation of contacts within 2 days of exposure.
Routine immunisation to be done.
Community measures against malnutrition.

MALARIA

Case management and nursing care

P.vivax, P.ovale, P.malariae infections should be treated with chloroquine 600 mg base followed by 300 mg base in 6 hours, later 150 mg base 12 hourly for 2 more days. Relapse is overcome by antimalarial drugs in suppressive doses. Primaquin 15 mg daily for 14 days will destroy hypnozoits phase in liver. Haemolysis and cyanosis are common but not dangerous.

P.falciparum is best treated with quinine 10 mg/kg body weight 8 hourly by mouth till clinical improvement and till M.P. smear is –ve. This is followed by single dose of sulfadoxine 1.5 G combined with pyrimethamine 75 mg. In pregnancy 7 days Quinine is given. Alternatively Atovaquone 250 mg + Proguanil 100 mg 4 tablets once daily for 3 days is given.

Nursing Care

Good nursing care of the patient with severe malaria is of vital importance.

i) Ensure meticulous nursing care. This can be life saving for unconscious patient. Maintain clear air way. Nurse the patient in the lateral or semiprone position to avoid aspiration of fluid. Insert a nasogastric tube and suck out the stomach contents to minimize the risk of aspiration pneumonia. Since aspiration pneumonia is fatal, it is dealt with by attending nursing staff by giving :

a) Parenteral antimicrobials.
b) Change position of patient.
c) Give physiotherapy and.
d) Give oxygen.Turn the patient every 2 hours. Do not allow him to lie in a wet bed. Pay attention to pressure points.

ii) Keep a careful record of fluid intake and output. If this is not possible, weigh the patient daily in order to calculate the approximate fluid balance.
iii) Note any appearance of black urine (Haemoglobinuria).
iv) Check the speed of infusion of fluids frequently. Too fast or too slow infusion can be dangerous.
v) Monitor temperature, pulse, respiration and blood pressure every 4 hours.
vi) Monitor level of consciousness.

a) Glasgow coma scale for adults :

Eyes open	Spontaneously	4
	To speech	3
	To pain	2
	Never	1
Best verbal response	Oriented	5
	confused	4
	In appropriate word	3
	In comprehensible sound	2
	None	1
Best motor response	Obeys commands	5
	Localises pain	4
	Flexion to pain	3
	Extension to pain	2
	None	1
	Total	3 to 14

If score is 10 it is unrousable coma.
It has to be done repeatedly to assess improvement or deterioration.

b) Paediatric coma scale for child Blantyre coma scale)

Best motor response	Localises pain stimuli (Rub knuckle onchild sternum)	2
	Withdraw limb from pain (Firm pressure on thumb-nailbed with pencil)	1
	No response	0

(contd.)

(contd.)

Verbal response	Appropriate cry	2
	Moaning	1
	None	0
Eye movement	Directed	
	(Follow mother face)	1
	Not directed	0
	Total	0-5

If score of 3 is unarousable coma.
It has to be repeated to assess either improvement or deterioration.

vii) Report level of consciousness, convulsions or change in behaviour to duty doctor. All such changes need additional treatment.

viii) Rectal temperature if above 39°C, rectal paracetamol is given, tepid sponging is done. Fanning continued.

As duty nurse, never allow duty doctor to give chloroquine to treat severe falciparum malaria, in view of chloroquine resistance in severe malaria.

Special Nursing Care in Severe Malaria of a Child

Nursing care should include all well established principles of the care of unconscious child. Every 2 hours frequent turning of the child, careful attention to airways, eyes, mucosae, skin and fluid requirements. The child should be nursed in the lateral or semiprone position.
Special paediatric nursing care should include:

- Insert nasogastric tube to minimise risk of aspiration pneumonia.
- Correct hypoglycaemia.
- Restore circulating volume.
- Treat anaemia.

Special Immediate Nursing Care of Complications of Malaria

All cases are attended with suggested chemotherapy for severe malaria. Apart from that, immediate nursing management of complications include the following :

1. Hyperpyrexia
   - Paracetamol 15 mg /kg.
   - Tepid sponging.
   - Fanning.
2. Spontaneous bleeding, coagulopathy
   - Transfuse fresh whole blood.
   - Transfuse clotting factor.
   - I.V. Vit-K 10 mg.
3. Shock due to algid malaria
   - Suspect gram negative septicaemia.

- Take blood sample for culture.
- Give parenteral antimicrobial.
- Correct hemodynamic disturbances.

4. Acute pulmonary oedema
   - Avoid excess rehydration.
   - Prop up the patient.
   - Give oxygen.
   - Give frusemide 15 mg I.V.
   - Withdraw 3 ml/kg by venesection into donor bag.
5. Metabolic acidosis
   - Treat hypoglycaemia.
   - Treat hypovolaemia.
   - Treat septicaemia.
   - Give isotonic saline 20 ml/kg rapidly.
   - Give whole blood 10 ml/kg over 30 min.
   - Do not allow Hb% fall below 5 G%.
6. Hypoglycaemia
   - R.B.S. take blood and check.
   - 50% dextrose 50 ml followed by 5 or 10% dextrose infusion.
7. Acute renal failure
   - Exclude dehydration.
   - Maintain fluid balance.
   - If indicated dialysis.
8. Severe anaemia
   - Whole blood transfusion.
   - Packed cell transfusion.
9. Hyper parasitaemia
   - Parenteral antimalaria therapy.
   - Exchange transfusion.
10. Malaria haemoglobinuria
    - Continue antimalaria treatment.
    - Fresh blood transfusion.
11. Convulsion
    - Maintain airway.
    - I.V. diazepam (0.15 mg/kg).
    - Intrarectal (0.5mg/kg).
    - I.M. paraldehyde (0.1mg/kg).
12. Coma
    - Maintain airway.
    - Exclude hypoglycaemia, exclude bacterial meningoencephalitis.
    - Avoid corticosteroids.
    - Avoid heparin.
    - Avoid adrenaline.

YELLOW FEVER: (not present in India)

Nursing management:

Whole treatment is supportive, with meticulous attention to fluid and electrolyte balance. Blood pressure and urine output need to be recorded. There may be requirement of blood transfusion, plasma expanders and peritoneal dialysis. Patient is infectious and must be isolated during illness.

STD :

Nursing management

Nurse has to manage a case of STD by syndrome approach which is a method of management of cases based on a group of symptoms and signs. Treatment is targeted towards all diseases that could cause that syndrome. It allows diagnosis without extensive laboratory tests and treatment within a single visit. This approach is relevant in the context of Indian condition where laboratory facilities for diagnosis are limited. Syndrome approaches for "Five Field Approach" are given in appendix under the following heads:

- Genital discharge.
- Vaginal discharge (no speculum examination).
- Vaginal discharge (with speculum examination).
- Urethral discharge.
- Lower abdominal pain in the female (PID).

CHOLERA

Making oral fluid in nursing care:

One litre glucose salt solution should contain

- Sodium chloride 3.5 G
- Sodium bicarbonate 2.5G
- Potassium chloride 1.5 G
- Glucose 20.0 G

They are measured, prepacked in aluminium foil and sealed by drug companies. They are distributed through health service network. The above packet is dissolved in 1 litre of drinking water which is suitable size for use in home visiting.

For clinics, hospitals, bags or bottles containing 10 times this amount for dissolving in 10 litres of water is more practical.

Standard measure is used at dispensing. Once prepared, the ORS should be used within 24 hours. Every 24 hours, fresh solution is prepared. It should not be boiled.

TYPHOID

Case management and nursing care:

- Ciprofloxacin 500 mg 112 hourly.
- Cotrimoxazole 2 tablet 12 hourly.

- Amoxicillin 750 mg 6 hourly.
- Chloramphenicol 500 mg 6 hourly.
- In resistant case, third generation antibiotics like cephalosporins, ceftriaxone and cefotaxime are used with caution.
- The treatment is continued for 14 days. Pyrexia exists for 5 days with treatment. Chronic carriers are treated with ciprofloxacin for 4 weeks. In some cases of carriers' stage, cholecystectomy may be needed.

MENINGOCOCCAL MENINGITIS

Case management with nursing care:

Benzyl penicillin 2.4 G. IV 6 hourly even before hospitalisation is advocated. Hospitalisations, regular nursing care, CSF analysis for any treatment regimen change, are advocated. Steroid therapy is useful in paediatric patients. Contact management by Rifampicin 600 mg BD for 2 days for adults is given.

PLAGUE

Case management and nursing care:

- Streptomycin 1 G 12 hourly.
- Gentamicin 1 mg per Kg 8 hourly.
- Tetracycline 500 mg 6th hourly.
- Chloramphenicol 12.5 mg per kg 6 hourly.
- Management of acute circulatory failure.
- Management of disseminated intravascular coagulation.
- Management of hypoxia.

ARI

Nursing management:

Infant below 2 months

Very severe disease	–	refer urgently to hospital, keep infant warm, give first dose of antibiotic
Severe pneumonia	–	Refer urgently to hospital, keep infant warm, give first dose of antibiotic
No pneumonia only cough or cold	–	Advise mother to give home care like keep young infant ward breastfeed frequently clear nose if it interferes with feeding to return if infant has difficulty breathing fast breathing problem to feed increased sickness

Child 2 months to 5 years

Very severe disease — Refer urgently to hospital
Give first dose of antibiotic.
Treat fever if present.
Treat wheezing if present.

If cerebral malaria is possible give antimalarial.

Severe pneumonia — Refer urgently to hospital

Give first dose of antibiotic

Treat fever if present

Treat wheezing if present

Pneumonia — advice home care

Give antibiotic treat fever, wheezing if present advise mother to return in 2 days for reassessment cough and cold - Attend symptomatic treatment

Advice home care

Feed the child * feed during illness
* increase feed after illness

Clear nose if interferes with feeding

Increase fluids * Offer extramilk
* increase breastfeeding

Soothe throat and relieve cough with safe remedy

Watch the signs to ask to return quickly such as
* breathing become difficult
* breathing becomes fast
* child is not able to drink
* child becomes sicker
* think the child may have pneumonia

HEPATITIS A

Case management and nursing care:

Acute cases need hospitalisation for required nursing care to allow early detection of acute hepatic failure. Reassurance is needed for posthepatitis syndrome. Balanced diet should provide 2000 to 3000 calories per day which should have light diet supplemented by fruit drunks and glucose. The diet should be as per wish of patient for taste. This should take care of high protein intake. IV fluid and glucose may be needed in some of the patients. Drugs like sedatives and hypnotics should be avoided. Oral contraceptives are avoided during illness. Except for life saving surgery no surgery is allowed in hepatitis patients. Mortality of acute viral hepatitis is about 0.5%.

HEPATITIS B

Nursing management

Nursing care should focus attention on monitoring acute liver failure. There is no specific treatment. Interferon 5 micrograms daily for patients with high serum transminase are advocated.

HEPATITIS C

Nursing management

Case management and nursing care include use of Interferon and Ribavirin.

RABIES

Nursing management:

As soon as a case of a dog bite by an infected dog is received, steps are taken to assure patient and his family to overcome unnecessary anxiety state. At the earliest, postexposure prophylaxis with ARV is the need of the hour. In all cases, postexposure prophylaxis must be started before 5 days from the day of bite to save the life of patient.

When once symptoms are started, only palliative treatment is ascertained. The patient is sedated with diazepam 10 mg 6 hourly. This is supplemented by chlorpromazine 100 mg. Nutrition and fluids are given IV route or through gastrostomy. The patient is kept in dark room and silent zone to avoid external stimulus. The patient may need intensive care with facilities to control cardiac failure and respiratory failure.

Nursing personnel attending patient should use protective devices like face-mask, glove, goggle and working white coat to protect them. Because patient secretes virus in saliva, tears, vomits and in other body fluids nursing staff with cuts, wounds, aberrations are not allowed to nurse the patient. In case of encounter with Rabies case, the attending nursing staff should get a course of pre-exposure prophylaxis with 3 doses of HDC vaccine.

RELAPSING FEVER

Nursing care in management:

Procaine benzyl penicillin 300 mg IM followed by next day 500 mg tetracycline. Doxycycline 200 mg orally is alternative to tetracycline.

Since it produces Jarish Herxheimer reaction, the case is best managed in a high dependency unit with expert nursing care.

SCABIES

Case management and nursing care:

All the members of the family of case are given simultaneous treatment. 20% emulsion of benzyl benzoate is applied from neck down after a bath and allowed to dry and clothing is put. The next day second bath and clothing wash are a must. The treatment is repeated on 6th day.

Secondary infection is treated by penicillin one course for 5 days.

Alternative drugs are:

— NBIN emulsion (1 : 15 water before us)

• Benzyl benzoate	68%
• DDT	6%
• Benzocaine	12%
• Polysorbate	14%

— BHC malathion lotion

• Malathion	0.5%
• BHC	1.0%

— Crotamiton daily application for 5 days. It is suitable for infants since it is an antipruritic

—Tetmasol 5% solution.

15. UNIVERSAL IMMUNISATION PROGRAMME

WHEN	*WHAT*	*WHY*
As early as pregnancy is detected	2 doses of TT at 4 weeks apart At least four weeks before expected date of delivery	Given to mother to protect both mother and the new Second dose should be given born from tetanus
At birth or till 12 months	One injection of BCG vaccine	To protect the child from tuberculosis
6 weeks to 9 months	3 doses each of DPT and OPV at minimum 4 weeks interval: I dose at 6 weeks II dose at 10 weeks III dose at 14 weeks In case of institutional deliver a dose of OV at birth is given which is called 'O'dose	To protect the child from Diphtheria, Pertussis (Whooping cough) Tetanus and Poliomyelitis
9 to 12 months	One injection of measles vaccine	To protect the child from measles
16 to 24 months	Booster doses of OPV and DPT	To protect the child from Diphtheria, Pertussis (Whooping cough) Tetanus and Poliomyelitis
5 to 6 years	Two doses of DT*	To protect the child from Diphtheria and Tetanus
10 years	Two doses of TT*	To protect from Tetanus
16 years	Two doses of TT*	To protect from Tetanus

* One dose of DT / TT if vaccinated earlier

16. PHYSIOLOGICAL RANGES

A. Temperature, Pulse, Respiration, Dentition

(i) Comparison of Fahrenheit and Centigrade Thermometers

Degree centigrade	*Degree fahrenheit*
35	95
35.5	95.9
36	6.8
36.5	97.7
37	98.6
37.5	99.5
38	100.4
38.5	101.3
39	102.2
39.5	103.1
40	104
40.5	104.9
41	105.8
41.5	106.7
42	107.6

(ii) and (iii) Pulse and respiration at different ages:

	Pulse per min.	*Resp. per min*
In utero	150 to 140	
In new born	140 to 130	
During 1st year	130 to 115	35 = 1st year
During 2nd year	115 to 100	25 = 2nd year
During 3rd year	100 to 95	20 = Puberty
8th to 14th year	average 84	18 = adult
Adult	average 72	
Old age	average 76	

(iv) Dentition Table:

Milk Teeth – The first dentition begins at the sixth or seventh month and is completed by about the second year.

Central incisors	(1) lower, 6th month
	(2) upper 7th month
Lateral incisors	(1) upper 9th month
	(2) lower 10th month

First molar	12th month
Canines	18th month
Second molars	2nd year (often later)

The full primary dentition is 20 tooth: 10 in each jaw.

Permanent Teeth

First molars	6.5 years
Lower central incisors	7 years
Upper central incisors	8 years
Lateral incisors	9 years
First bicuspid	10 years
Second bicuspid	11 years
Canines	12 years
Second molars	13 years
Third molars (wisdom)	17 to 25 years or at any later period
The full permanent dentition is 32 tooth,	16 in each jaw.

B. Standard weight for height:

Height in feet and inch	*Men in kg.*	*Women in kg*
5' 0"	-	50.8 to 54.4
5' 1"	-	51.7 to 55.3
5' 2"	6.3 to 60.3	53.1 to 56.7
5' 3"	57.6 to 61.7	54.4 to 58.1
5' 4"	58.9 to 63.5	56.3 to 59.9
5' 5"	60.7 to 62.2	57.6 to 61.2
5' 6"	60.8 to 65.3	58/9 to 63.5
5' 7"	64 to 68.5	60.8 to 65.4
5' 8"	65.8 to 70.8	62.2 to 66.7
5' 9"	67.6 to 72.6	64 to 68.5
5' 10"	69.4 to 74.4	65.8 to 70.3
5' 11"	71.2 to 76.2	67.1 to 71.1
6' 0"	73 to 78.5	68.5 to 73.9
6' 1"	75.3 to 80.7	-
6' 2"	77.6 to 83.5	-
6' 3"	79.8 to 85.9	-

C. BMI chart (Body Mass Index)

4' 10" Height	*41 – 54 kg. wt.*	*56 – 65 kg wt.*	*67 – 76 kg wt.*	*78 – 87 kg. wt.*
4' 11"	43 - 56	58 - 67	70 - 79	81 - 90
5'	44 - 58	60 - 70	72 - 81	84 - 93
5' 1"	45 - 60	62 - 72	75 - 84	86 - 96
5' 2"	47 - 62	65 - 75	77 - 87	89 - 99
5' 3"	49 - 64	66 to 77	80 - 90	92 - 102
5' 4"	50 - 66	69 - 79	82 - 93	95 - 105
5' 5"	52 - 68	71 - 82	85 - 95	98 - 109
5' 6"	54 - 70	73 - 85	87 - 98	101 - 112
5' 7"	55 - 72	75 - 87	90 - 101	105 - 116
5 ' 8"	57 - 75	78 - 90	92 - 105	107 - 119
5 ' 9"	58 - 77	80 - 92	95 - 107	110 - 123
5' 10"	60 - 79	82 - 95	98 - 110	114 - 126
5' 11"	62 - 81	85 - 98	101 - 114	117 - 130
6'	64 - 84	87 - 100	104 - 117	120 - 134
6' 1"	65 - 86	90 - 103	107 - 120	124 - 137
6' 2"	67 - 88	92 – 106	109 - 124	127 - 141
6' 3"	69 - 91	95 - 109	113 - 127	130 - 145
6' 4"	71 - 93	97 - 112	115 - 130	134 - 149
	normal	**overweight**	**Obesity grade**	**Obesity grade**
			1	**2**
	BMI=19 to 25	**BMI=26 to 30**	**BMI=31 to 35**	**BMI=36 to 40**

D. Laboratory Values:

Of serum:	Albumin	3.6 to 5.0 g/dl
	Total bilirubin	0.3 – 1.1 mg/dl
	Direct bilirubin	0 – 0.03 mg/dl
	Arterial pH	7.35 – 7.45
	Calcium	8.6 – 10./3 mg/dl
	Cholesterol	
	desirable	below 200 mg/dl
	borderline high	200 – 239
	High	above 240 mg/dl
	HDL cholesterol	below 35 mg/dl

Creatinine	
adult male	0.7 – 1.5 mg/dl
adult female	0.6 – 1.4 mg/dl
FBS	65 – 109 mg/dl
Total protein	6.5 – 8.5 g/dl
Urea nitrogen	8 – 25 mg/dl
Uric acid	3 – 8 mg/dl
Of serum enzyme	
SGOT	11 – 47 IU/L
SGPT	7 – 53 IU/L
Of serum hormone	
Aldosterone	10 – 160 ng/l
Parathyroid	12 – 72 pg/ml
Total thyroxine	4.5 – 12.0 ìg/dl
Of urine	
Calcium	50 – 250 mg/d
Creatinine	0.6 to 1.8 g/d
Protein	0 – 150 mg/d
Of blood	
Bleeding time	2.5 – 9.5 min
Prothrombin time	10.5 – 14.5 sec
Hb%	12.1 – 17.2 g/dl (14.5%)
RBC count	5 million/cub mm
Haematocrit value	45%
MCH	27 – 32 picogram
MCV	80 – 93 cubic microns
MCHC	32 – 38%
WBC count	5 – 8 thousand / cub mm
Polymorphs	65 – 70%
Eosinophils	2 – 5 %
Basophils	0.5 – 1.0%
Lymphocytes	20 – 25%
Monocytes	3 – 8%
Reticulocyte count	0.15%

17. COMMON INSTRUMENTS A NURSE SHOULD KNOW

A. Allis Forceps

It is called Allis tissue forceps used in OBG surgery such as

- Episiotomy.
- Repair of perineal tear.
- D & C.
- LSCS.

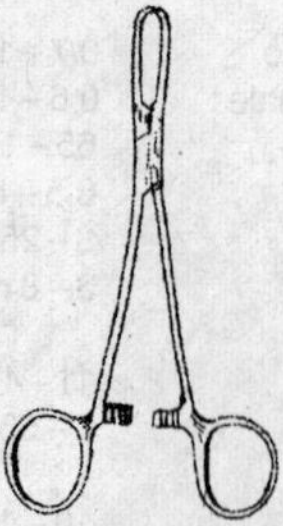

Allis forceps

B. Cervical Dilator

Used in dilatation of cervix prior to D & C. Required in the following:

- In complete abortion.
- In suction evacuation.
- In MTP by D & C.

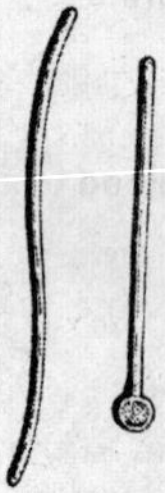

Cervical dilators

C. Disposable Cord Clamp

- It is disposable clamp supplied in a sterile pack.
- Used in clamping detached stump of umbilical cord.

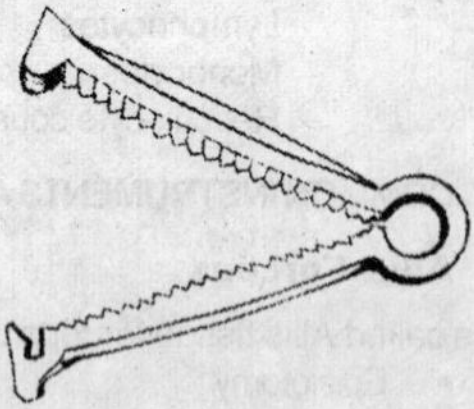

Disposable cord clamp

D. Doppler (USG)

Use in U.S. examination of abdomen in pregnancy.

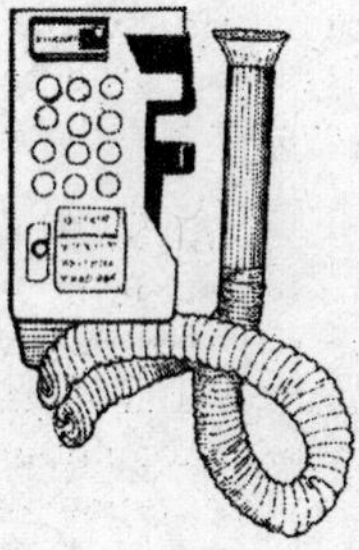

Doppler (ultrasonic)

E. Pelvimeter (External)

Use in external pelvic measurement.

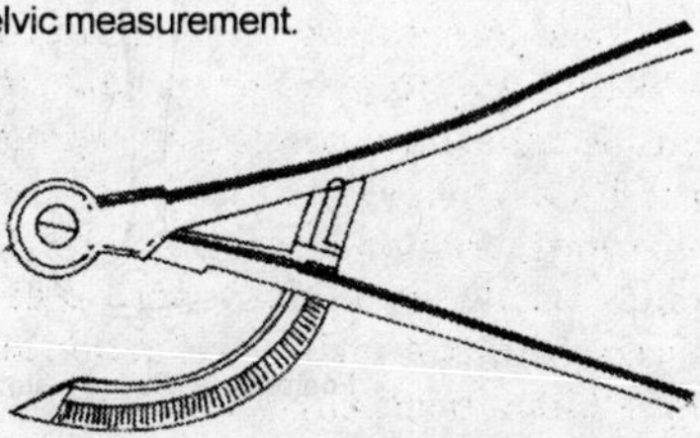

External pelvimeter

F. Female Rubber Catheter

Indicated in the following:

- Urinary retension in prgnancy.
- Urinary retension in delivery.
- Urinary retension in puerperium.
- Before conducting delivery.

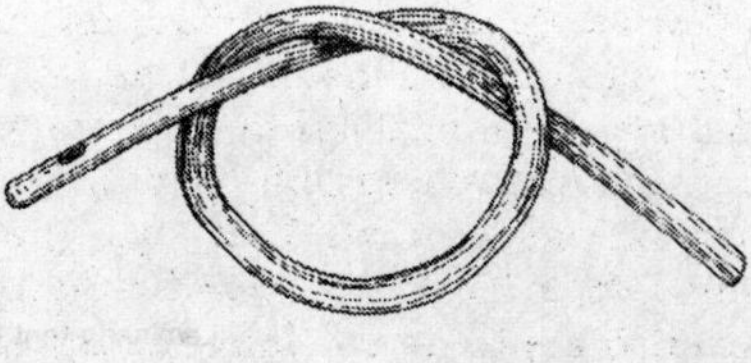

Female rubber catheter

G. Curette (Flushing)

Used in D & C.

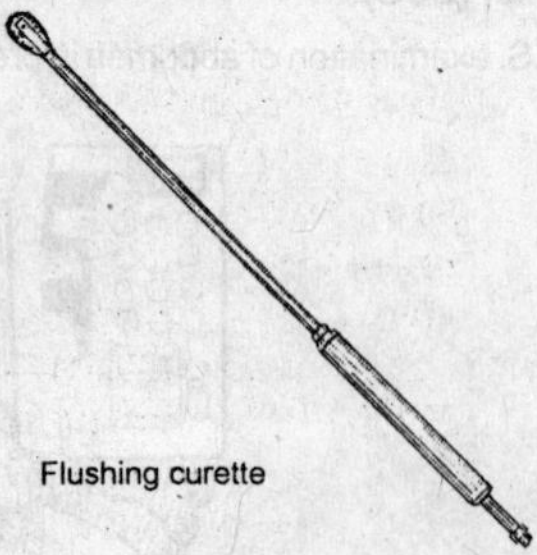

Flushing curette

H. Foetoscope

Used to ausultate foetal heard sound.

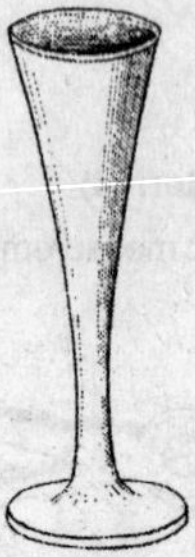

Foetoscope (Pinard's stethoscope)

I. Lamanaria Tent Forceps

Used to introduce Lamanaria Tent which has hygroscopic action and swels to dilate cervical canal.

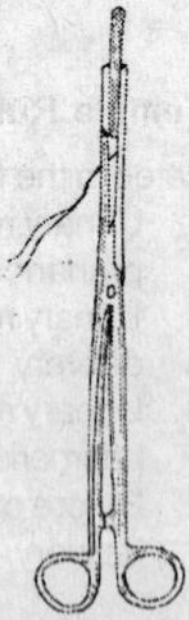

Laminaria tent forceps

J. Multiple Toother Vulsellum

Used in D & C.

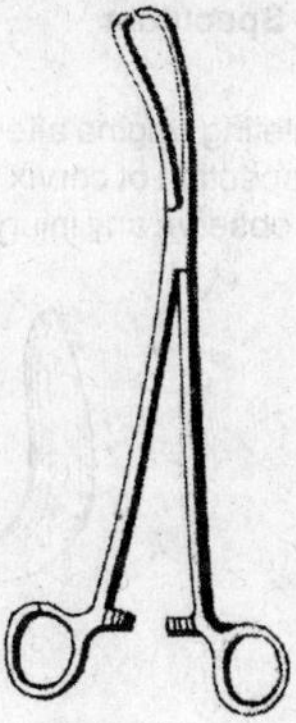

Multiple toother vulsellum

K. Obstetric Forceps

Used in low forceps operation.

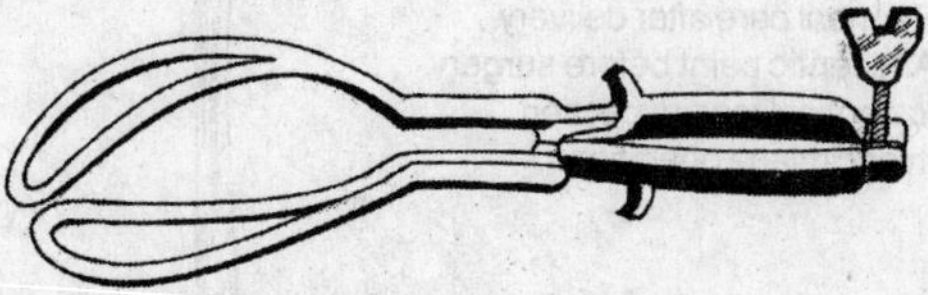

Obstetric forceps

L. Ovum Forceps

- Introduced with uades closed.
- Opened inside uterine cavity to grasp the product to take out with slight rotatory movement.

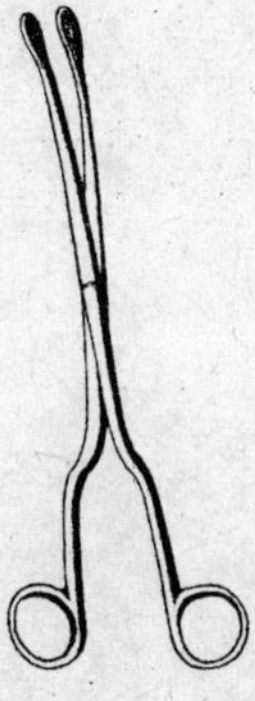

Ovum forceps

M. Sim's Speculum

Used in

- Toileting vagina after delivery.
- In spection of cervix.
- To observe any injury.

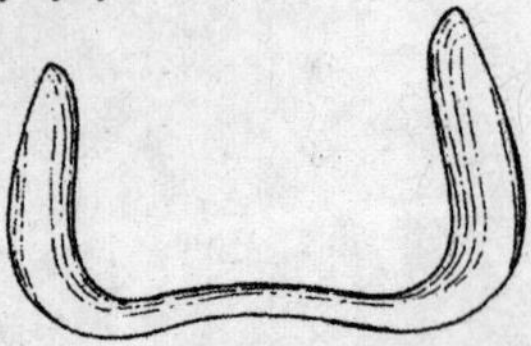

Sim's speculum

N. Sponge Holding Forceps

This is curved forceps used to hold sponge.
used in

- Perineal care after delivery.
- Antiseptic paint before surgery.
- In cervical tear inspection.
- In encirclage operation.

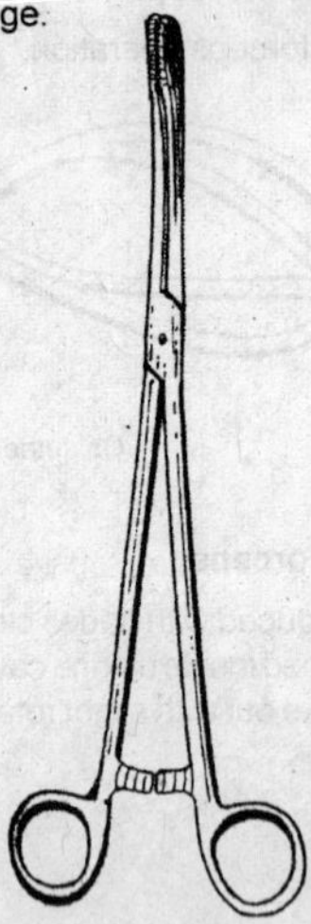

Sponge holding forceps

O. Straight Scissor

Used in

- Episiotomy.
- Cutting umbilical cord.
- Caesarean section.

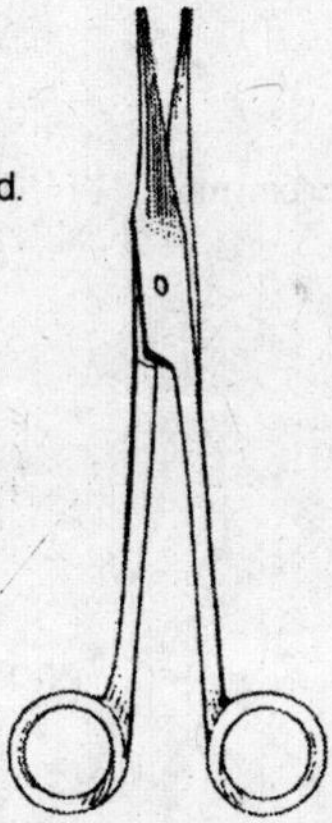

Straight scissor

P. Uterine Sound

Used in measuring length of uterine cavity before D & C.

Uterine sound

Q. Uterine Curette

Used in

- D & C.
- Evacuation & hydatidiform mole.

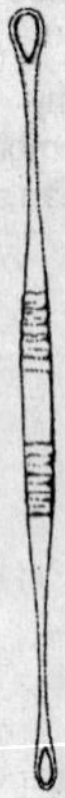

Uterine curette

R. Uterine Dressing Forceps

- Used in dressing uterus following D & C.
- Sometimes to dilate cervix in pyometra.

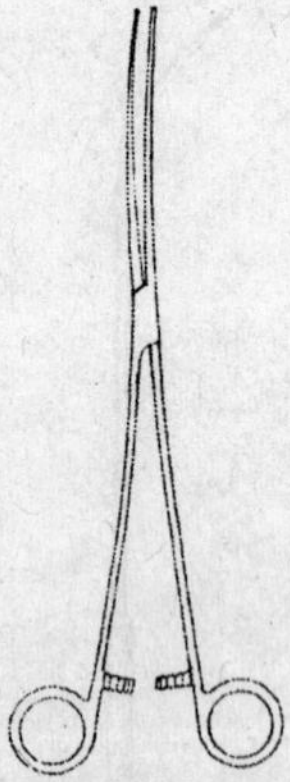

Uterine dressing forceps

18. NATIONAL NURSING PROGRAMME

In this focus of attention I for updating the knowledge and skills of nursing personnel to provide qualitative nursing care to the patients. Rs. 100 lakhs is allocated for 2000-01 to conduct 200 courses at various centres in the country and to train about 6000 in-service nurses.

Under these new nursing colleges are encouraged.

Under the scheme 3 lakh per institution is provided towards AV aids, library books, equipments and transport.

This scheme allows attending the housing problems faced by the nurses in the capital

Nursing courses come under Para medical Courses. Degree courses come under the affiliated universities.

Speciality nursing training is encouraged.